PHENOTHIAZINES

AND

STRUCTURALLY RELATED DRUGS

Advances in Biochemical Psychopharmacology

Series Editors

Erminio Costa, M.D.

Chief, Laboratory of Preclinical Pharmacology
National Institute of Mental Health
Washington, D.C., U.S.A.

Paul Greengard, Ph.D.

Professor of Pharmacology
Yale University School of Medicine
New Haven, Connecticut, U.S.A.

International Symposium on Phenothiazines and Structurally Related Drugs, 3d, National Institute of Mental Health, 1973

Phenothiazines and Structurally Related Drugs

Advances in Biochemical Psychopharmacology

Volume 9

Editors:

Irene S. Forrest, Ph.D.
Biochemical Research Laboratory
Veterans Administration Hospital
Palo Alto, California

C. Jelleff Carr, Ph.D.
Life Sciences Research Office
Federation of American Societies for Experimental Biology
Bethesda, Maryland

Earl Usdin, Ph.D.
Psychopharmacology Research Branch
National Institute of Mental Health
Rockville, Maryland

Raven Press, Publishers ▪ New York

Proceedings of the Third International Symposium on Phenothiazines and Structurally Related Drugs

Held at the National Institute of Mental Health, Rockville, Maryland, June 25–28, 1973

Welcoming Address

Bertram S. Brown

I welcome you to the Third International Symposium on Phenothiazines in several capacities: as Director of the National Institute of Mental Health, as representative of the Department of Health, Education and Welfare's Parklawn building, and, last but not least, as a psychiatrist.

As Director of the Institute, I am proud of the support which NIMH has given to the development of phenothiazine chemotherapy. It is hardly necessary to point out how the advent of chlorpromazine and other phenothiazines not only has halted the rapidly rising rate of hospital beds required for the mentally ill, but also has actually resulted in a sharp decrease in the number of psychiatric beds required. Not only have billions of dollars been saved for the nation but, more significantly, many patients have been enabled to lead useful, productive lives instead of wasting their lives behind the bars or quasi bars of an institution.

However, we at the NIMH recognize that not all of the problems are solved, that not all schizophrenics respond to existing chemotherapy, that some patients do develop undesirable side effects, that it would be desirable to develop drugs which need to be administered less frequently for long-term patient maintenance, etc. It is for these reasons that we continue to support research on phenothiazines in both our intramural and our extramural programs.

I take note of the fact that the official title of this conference is the Third International Symposium on Phenothiazines and Structurally Related Drugs. This latter rubric has been included, I am sure, to cover such drugs as the imipramines and thioxanthenes. The decision seems justified to me since the imipramines and thioxanthenes have become so important to practicing psychiatrists.

I look forward to finding out about the current state-of-the-art ranging from the physical chemical aspects and methodology to the applied clinical aspects. I hope essential unsolved problems will be identified and profitable collaborative arrangements will be initiated between investigators from the diverse laboratories and the different countries represented here.

Foreword

With a delay of a year, missing chlorpromazine's 20th anniversary and commemorating instead its coming of age, the Organizing Committee was finally able to convene the Third International Symposium in this series of conferences.

The untimely death of Dr. Daniel H. Efron was a personal sorrow for his many friends and a serious setback to the Committee's plans. The generosity of the National Institute of Mental Health and the friendly cooperation of the staff of its Psychopharmacology Research Branch facilitated the translocation from the originally planned site of the meeting in Sarajevo, Yugoslavia, to Rockville, Maryland. The invited participants proved to be as flexible as the Organizers: there were no drop-outs.

The interdisciplinary nature of the Symposium is reflected in the broad scope of the papers presented. Basic scientists and clinicians are equally interested in developing new insights linking basic biochemical and pharmacological mechanisms to clinical findings. Admittedly it is difficult to sustain the rapprochement generated at interdisciplinary conferences held at 5 or 6 year intervals between such disparate disciplines as physical chemistry, neurochemistry, toxicology, and clinical psychiatry. This difficulty in fact remains one of the reasons for holding the present Symposium.

In the meantime, it is encouraging to note that increasing numbers of psychiatrists profess a need for pharmacokinetic studies to help them understand, provide, and hopefully predict adequate patient response, while avoiding drug toxicity.

The reader should recognize that the research reports in this volume reflect ongoing studies rather than completed work permitting general conclusions. Also, the published version of the reports cannot adequately reflect the true degree of interaction between the scientists of the various disciplines represented, since many of the discussions following the presentation of papers may have been initiated in the conference room, but were concluded without the benefits of microphones. Discussion remarks and the speakers' responses that were recorded are included in the proceedings in form of a reporter's summary for each session.

The Organizing Committee wishes to acknowledge the very generous financial support provided by the Roerig Division of Pfizer, Inc., as well as the contributions of Dow Pharmaceuticals, Schering Corporation, Smith Kline and French Laboratories, and Wyeth Laboratories. These funds made it possible for many of the foreign participants to travel to the meeting site. In addition, we should like to thank the National Institute of Mental Health for providing a meeting site.

Irene S. Forrest
C. Jelleff Carr
Herman C. B. Denber
Earl Usdin

Contents

Session VI. Thioxanthenes
Chairmen: Nathan Kline and Herman C. B. Denber

Session VII. Specific Chlorpromazine Metabolites
Chairmen: Irene S. Forrest and George J. Cosmides

Session VIII. Clinical Session:
Pharmacological Effects of Phenothiazines and Related Drugs
Chairmen: Samuel C. Kaim and Pavel Stern

List of Participants

Dr. M. Ackenheil
Nervenklinik der Universität München
8 München 2, Germany

Dr. H. Richard Adams
Department of Pharmacology
Southwestern Medical School at Dallas
The University of Texas
Dallas, Texas 75235 USA

Dr. Liisa Ahtee
Department of Pharmacology
University of Helsinki
SF-00170 Helsinki 17, Finland

Dr. Tai Akera
Department of Pharmacology
Michigan State University
East Lansing, Michigan 48823 USA

Dr. Frank J. Ayd, Jr.
912 West Lake Avenue
Baltimore, Maryland 21210 USA

Dr. Thomas A. Ban
Department of Psychiatry
Division of Psychopharmacology
McGill University
Montreal, Canada

Dr. Allen Barnett
Department of Pharmacology
Schering Corporation
Bloomfield, New Jersey 07003 USA

Dr. H. Beckmann
Nervenklinik der Universität München
8 München 2, Germany

Dr. Marcel H. Bickel
Universität Bern
Medizinisch-Chemisches Institut
3000 Bern, Switzerland

Dr. Ursula Breyer
Institut für Toxikologie der Universität
*   Tübingen*
74 Tübingen, West Germany

Dr. Joseph P. Buckley
Department of Pharmacology
School of Pharmacy
University of Pittsburgh
Pittsburgh, Pennsylvania 15213 USA

Dr. Benjamin S. Bunney
Department of Pharmacology
Yale University School of Medicine
New Haven, Connecticut 06519 USA

Dr. L. Rivera-Calimlim
Department of Pharmacology
University of Rochester
*   School of Medicine and Dentistry*
Rochester, New York 14620 USA

Dr. C. Jelleff Carr
Director, Life Sciences Research Office
Federation of American Societies for
*   Experimental Biology*
9650 Rockville Pike
Bethesda, Maryland 20014 USA

Dr. Lim Castaneda
Department of Psychiatry
University of Rochester
*   School of Medicine and Dentistry*
Rochester, New York 14620 USA

Dr. Tin Lok Chan
Department of Psychiatry
New York University Medical Center
550 First Avenue
New York, New York 10016 USA

Dr. Mervin L. Clark
Central State Griffin Memorial Hospital
Norman, Oklahoma 73069 USA

Mr. Michael Conway
Department of Pharmacology
University of Oklahoma
Norman, Oklahoma 73069 USA

Mr. Thomas Cooper
Research Laboratories
Rockland State Hospital
Orangeburg, New York 10962 USA

Dr. George J. Cosmides
Pharmacology and Toxicology Programs
National Institute of General Medical
*   Sciences*
National Institutes of Health
Bethesda, Maryland 20014 USA

Dr. John C. Craig
Department of Pharmaceutical Chemistry
School of Pharmacy
University of California
San Francisco Medical Center
San Francisco, California 94122 USA

Dr. George E. Crane
Director of Research
Spring Grove State Hospital
Baltimore, Maryland 21228 USA

Dr. Stephen H. Curry
Department of Pharmacology
  and Therapeutics
The London Hospital Medical College
Turner Street
London El, England

Dr. John M. Davis
Department of Psychiatry
School of Medicine
Vanderbilt University
Nashville, Tennessee 37203 USA

Dr. Herman C. B. Denber
Department of Psychiatry
College of Medicine
University of Florida
J. Hillis Miller Health Center
Gainesville, Florida 32601 USA

Dr. R. L. Dillenkoffer
Veterans Administration Hospital
New Orleans, Louisiana 70140 USA

Dr. Alan M. Duffield
Department of Genetics
Stanford University School of Medicine
Stanford Medical Center
Stanford, California 94305 USA

Dr. Alina Efron
5419 Burling Road
Bethesda, Maryland 20014 USA

Ms. Dorothy M. Eisel
Pharmacology Section
Psychopharmacology Research Branch
National Institute of Mental Health
Rockville, Maryland 20852 USA

Dr. Helmut Fenner
Freie Universität Berlin
Fachbereich Pharmazie
D—1000 Berlin 33, Germany

Dr. Fred M. Forrest
Biochem. Research Lab. (151F)
Veterans Administration Hospital
Palo Alto, California 94304 USA

Dr. Irene S. Forrest
Biochem. Research Lab. (151F)
Veterans Administration Hospital
Palo Alto, California 94304 USA

Dr. Charles A. Free
Department of Biochemical Pharmacology
The Squibb Institute for Medical Research
Princeton, New Jersey 08540 USA

Dr. Sabit Gabay
Biochem. Research Lab.
Veterans Administration Hospital
Brockton, Massachusetts 02401 USA

Dr. George Gardos
Boston State Hospital
Boston, Massachusetts 02124 USA

Dr. Samuel Gershon
Neuropsychopharmacology Research Unit
New York University School of Medicine
550 First Avenue
New York, New York 10016 USA

Dr. Alexander H. Glassman
Department of Biological Psychiatry
New York State Psychiatric Institute
722 W. 168th Street
New York, New York 10032 USA

Dr. Vera Glocklin
Food and Drug Administration
5600 Fishers Lane
Rockville, Maryland 20852 USA

Dr. Fred Goodwin
NIMH Intramural Program
National Institutes of Health
Bethesda, Maryland 20014 USA

Dr. John W. Gorrod
Department of Pharmacy
University of London
Chelsea College of Science
  and Technology
271, Kings Street
London W6, England

Dr. Frederick W. Grant
Research Laboratory
Marcy State Hospital
Marcy, New York 13403 USA

Dr. Donald E. Green
Biochem. Research Lab. (151F)
Veterans Administration Hospital
Palo Alto, California 94304 USA

Dr. T. A. Grover
Department of Biochemistry and Biophysics
University of Hawaii
Biomedical Sciences Building
1960 East-West Road
Honolulu, Hawaii 96822 USA

Dr. Felix Gutmann
Department of Physical Chemistry
The University of Sydney
Sydney, NSW 2006
Australia

Dr. I. Hanin
NIMH, St. Elizabeth's Hospital
Washington, D.C. 20032 USA

Dr. Sidney M. Hess
Department of Biochemical Pharmacology
The Squibb Institute for Medical Research
Princeton, New Jersey 08540 USA

Dr. Leo E. Hollister
Medical Investigator (151H)
Veterans Administration Hospital
Palo Alto, California 94304 USA

Dr. P. C. Huang
Biochem. Research Lab.
Veterans Administration Hospital
Brockton, Massachusetts 02401 USA

Dr. Turan M. Itil
Missouri Institute of Psychiatry
5400 Arsenal Street
St. Louis, Missouri 63139 USA

Dr. Donald J. Jenden
Department of Pharmacology
University of California (UCLA)
Los Angeles, California 90024 USA

Dr. Samuel C. Kaim
VA-SAODAP Cooperative Studies
Department of Medicine and Surgery
Veterans Administration
Washington, D.C. 20420 USA

Dr. Joyce J. Kaufman
Department of Chemistry
Johns Hopkins University
Charles and 34th Streets
Baltimore, Maryland 21218 USA

Dr. Pushkar N. Kaul
College of Pharmacy
The University of Oklahoma
625 Elm
Norman, Oklahoma 73069 USA

Dr. Ari Kiev
Department of Psychiatry
Cornell University
525 East 68th Street
New York, New York 10021 USA

Dr. Nathan S. Kline
Director of Research
Rockland State Hospital
Orangeburg, New York 10962 USA

Dr. Anant S. Kulkarni
Medical Department
Dow Pharmaceuticals
The Dow Chemical Company
P. O. Box 10
Zionsville, Indiana 46077 USA

Dr. William C. Landgraf
Manager, Applications Research
Syntex Laboratories
3401 Hillview Avenue
Palo Alto, California 94304 USA

Dr. Alice Leeds
Psychopharmacology Research Branch
National Institute of Mental Health
5600 Fishers Lane
Rockville, Maryland 20852 USA

Dr. Heinz E. Lehmann
Department of Psychiatry
McGill University
Montreal, Canada

Dr. François Leterrier
Division de Biophysique du Centre de
*   Recherches du Service de Santé*
*   des Armées*
1 bis rue du Lt. Raoul Batany
92140 Clamart, France

Dr. Jerome Levine
Chief, Psychopharmacology Research
*   Branch*
National Institute of Mental Health
5600 Fishers Lane
Rockville, Maryland 20852 USA

Dr. Nils-Gunnar Lindquist
Uppsala University
Biomedical Center

Department of Toxicology
S-751 23 Uppsala, Sweden

Dr. Peter Lomax
Department of Pharmacology
University of California (UCLA)
Los Angeles, California 90024 USA

Dr. Roger P. Maickel
Department of Pharmacology
Indiana University
Medical Sciences Program
Myers Hall
Bloomington, Indiana 47401 USA

Dr. Albert A. Manian
Assistant Chief, Pharmacology Section
Psychopharmacology Research Branch
National Institute of Mental Health
5600 Fishers Lane
Rockville, Maryland 20852 USA

Dr. E. Markianos
Nervenklinik der Universität München
8 München 2, Germany

Dr. J. J. H. McDowell
Physics Department
University of Cape Town
Cape Town, South Africa

Dr. J. Neye
Freie Universität Berlin
Fachbereich Pharmazie
D−1000 Berlin 33, Germany

Dr. Eugene C. Palmer
Department of Pharmacology
School of Medicine
The University of New Mexico
915 Stanford Drive, N.E.
Albuquerque, New Mexico 87106 USA

Dr. James M. Perel
Department of Biological Psychiatry
New York State Psychiatric Institute
722 W. 168th Street
New York, New York 10032 USA

Dr. Lawrence H. Piette
Department of Biochemistry and
* Biophysics*
University of Hawaii
Biomedical Sciences Building
1960 East-West Road
Honolulu, Hawaii 96822 USA

Dr. William Z. Potter
National Institutes of Health
Building 10, Room 8-N-113
Bethesda, Maryland 20014 USA

Dr. Krishnaswamy S. Rajan
Physical Chemistry Research
IIT Research Institute
10 West 35th Street
Chicago, Illinois 60616 USA

Dr. H. Roebke
Schering Corporation
Bloomfield, New Jersey 07003 USA

Dr. H. Rössler
Freie Universität Berlin
Fachbereich Pharmazie
D−1000 Berlin 33, Germany

Dr. W. S. Ryback
Dixon State School
Dixon, Illinois 61021 USA

Dr. George Sakalis
Department of Psychiatry
New York University Medical Center
550 First Avenue
New York, New York 10016 USA

Dr. Nina Schooler
Psychopharmacology Research Branch
National Institute of Mental Health
5600 Fishers Lane
Rockville, Maryland 20852 USA

Mr. Robert Schultz
Food and Drug Administration
5600 Fishers Lane
Rockville, Maryland 20852 USA

Dr. J. Schwarz
Sandoz Inc.
Route 10
East Hanover, New Jersey 07936 USA

Dr. Philip Seeman
Department of Pharmacology
University of Toronto
Toronto 181, Canada

Dr. Michael Shostak
Department of Experimental Psychiatry
New York State Psychiatric Institute
722 W. 168th Street
New York, New York 10032 USA

Dr. George M. Simpson
Rockland State Hospital
Orangeburg, New York 10962 USA

Dr. Sydney Spector
Roche Institute of Molecular Biology
Nutley, New Jersey 07110 USA

Dr. Morris A. Spirtes
Veterans Administration Hospital
1601 Perdido Street
New Orleans, Louisiana 70140 USA

Dr. Pavel Stern
Chief, Department of Pharmacology
Medical Faculty
71001 Sarajevo, Yugoslavia

Dr. B. Suplich
Smith Kline and French Laboratories
Philadelphia, Pennsylvania 19101 USA

Dr. Richard Templeton
Biochemistry Division
May & Baker Ltd.
Dagenham
Essex RM10 7XS
England

Dr. Sarah Tjioe
Department of Pharmacology
The Ohio State University
5086 Medical Basic Science
333 West Tenth Avenue
Columbus, Ohio 43210 USA

Ms. Patricia Turano
Research Division
Central Islip State Hospital
Central Islip, New York 11722 USA

Dr. William J. Turner
Research Division
Central Islip State Hospital
Central Islip, New York 11722 USA

Dr. Earl Usdin
Chief, Pharmacology Section
Psychopharmacology Research Branch
National Institute of Mental Health
5600 Fishers Lane
Rockville, Maryland 20852 USA

Dr. Melvin H. Van Woert
Department of Internal Medicine
School of Medicine

Yale University
333 Cedar Street
New Haven, Connecticut 06510 USA

Dr. Oldrich Vinar
Psychiatric Research Institute
Prague 8 – Bohnice
Czechoslovakia

Mrs. Evelyn Volkman
Life Sciences Research Office
Federation of American Societies of
  Experimental Biology
9650 Rockville Pike
Bethesda, Maryland 20014 USA

Dr. Sidney S. Walkenstein
Associate Director, Biochemistry
Smith Kline and French Laboratories
Philadelphia, Pennsylvania 19101 USA

Dr. Lee W. Wattenberg
Department of Pathology
Health Sciences
  Medical School
University of Minnesota
198 Jackson Hall
Minneapolis, Minnesota 55455 USA

Dr. Albert Weissman
Pfizer Inc.
Groton, Connecticut 06340 USA

Mr. Gerald K. Wilburn
Roerig Pfizer
235 East 42nd Street
New York, New York 10017 USA

Dr. David H. Wiles
Littlemore Hospital
Oxford, England

Dr. B. G. Winsberg
Child Psychiatric Evaluation Research
  Unit
524 Clarkson Avenue
Brooklyn, New York 11203 USA

Dr. Richard J. Wittenborn
The Interdisciplinary Research Center
Rutgers University
The State University of New Jersey
New Brunswick, New Jersey 08903 USA

Dr. Maria Wollemann
Institute of Biochemistry

Biological Research Center
Hungarian Academy of Sciences
Szeged POB 521
Hungary

Dr. George J. Wright
Drug Metabolism Unit
Merrell-National Laboratories
Cincinnati, Ohio 45215 USA

Dr. Rita Wroblewski
Roerig Pfizer
235 East 42nd Street
New York, New York 10017 USA

Dr. N. Zampaglione
Schering Corporation
Bloomfield, New Jersey 07003 USA

Dr. Virginia L. Zaratzian
Pharmacology Section
Psychopharmacology Research Branch
National Institute of Mental Health
5600 Fishers Lane
Rockville, Maryland 20852 USA

Dr. Charles Zirkle
Associate Director, Chemistry
Smith Kline and French Laboratories
Philadelphia, Pennsylvania 19101 USA

The Phenothiazines and Structurally Related Drugs, edited by I. S. Forrest, C. J. Carr, and E. Usdin. Raven Press, New York © 1974.

The Search for a Relationship Between Phenothiazine Drug Metabolism and Clinical Effectiveness

C. Jelleff Carr

Life Sciences Research Office, Federation of American Societies for Experimental Biology, Bethesda, Maryland 20014

In 1962, approximately 10 years after the discovery of chlorpromazine, a meeting was convened in Paris to review the studies under way in a number of laboratories in many countries on the absorption, distribution, and excretion of this remarkable drug. At that time, there was the exciting possibility that a clear relationship might be shown between the metabolic characteristics of chlorpromazine and its effectiveness in individual patients. Were those patients who did not respond favorably to drug therapy simply not taking their medication, did they not absorb the drug, or was there some bizarre metabolic or excretion pattern at work in these individuals?

At that time, the Forrests introduced their urine tests for phenothiazine drugs, and it was possible to document what was suspected: many non-responders were simply not taking their drug dosage—a fact that even today seems to be curiously overlooked. However, analytical methodology was just beginning to be employed in a search for key metabolic fragments of the chlorpromazine molecule thought to be responsible for the pharmacologic effects.

The difficulties of obtaining repeated blood samples, or even 24-hr urine samples from psychiatric patients, were formidable. Quantitative measures of clinical changes under drug therapy or placebo were only in a primitive evolutionary state at the time. Although it is difficult to recall, the clinical efficacy of the then relatively new psychotropic drugs was not universally accepted. The biochemical pharmacologist had little opportunity to team up with the psychiatrist in a research setting that included a climate for controlled studies.

The Psychopharmacology Service Center of the National Institute of Mental Health sponsored the first International Conference on Phenothiazine Metabolism through a grant to the organization of Friends for Psychiatric Research under the able leadership of Dr. Albert Kurland of Baltimore,

1

Maryland. Dr. Irene S. Forrest and I were cochairmen in bringing together all the workers interested in the field at that time. They numbered less than 50.

Five years later (1967) we organized with Dr. Laborit the second International Conference on Phenothiazine Metabolism. This meeting was also held in Paris and was successful with over 150 participants meeting in the Hôpital Militaire D'Instruction du Val-De-Grace. By this date, there was no longer any debate about the clinical efficacy of the phenothiazine drugs. Analytical methods had evolved to a considerable degree and the major excretory products had been identified: the sulfoxide, the mono- and didemethylated forms of chlorpromazine, the glucuronides, and sulfoxides. By this time also, it was recognized that drug dosage, blood, tissue, and urine levels were going to be difficult to correlate with clinical effectiveness or pharmacologic effects in animals or man. The prolonged excretion of the phenothiazine drugs in the urine after discontinuing medication was discovered, and it was suspected but not yet proved that relapse was related to the rate of tissue "wash-out" or the excretion kinetics. It is remarkable that only traces of unchanged chlorpromazine are detected in the urine of patients receiving daily medication, and this still remains a pharmacologic puzzle.

By the time of the 2nd Phenothiazine meeting, it was recognized that the pharmacokinetics of these drugs were not the same as that of many other drugs acting on the central nervous system. The models of the barbiturates or similar CNS depressants did not seem to apply to chlorpromazine, the single phenothiazine that continues to be studied in greatest detail. Absorption, liver metabolism, blood and tissue levels, and excretion patterns for the barbiturates that correlate so well with their sedative properties do not hold for the phenothiazines – at least as far as we know at the present time. The mechanisms of the antipsychotic properties of the phenothiazines may indeed pose a new pharmacologic phenomenon as yet to be discovered and explained. By 1967 the first suggestions of such a possibility were made. There remained the nagging idea that if only the analytical methodology could be made more precise, i.e., able to detect smaller and smaller amounts of significant drug fragments, then the puzzle could be unraveled. This has been the thrust of much research in the past 5 years.

In 1970, plans were made to hold a third phenothiazine meeting in 1972 on the occasion of the 20th anniversary of the discovery of chlorpromazine. Elegant new analytical tools had appeared on the scene and were being employed in the search for new metabolites. The analysis of nanogram amounts of drugs or drug metabolites in untreated body fluid specimens was being correlated with clinical rating scales of patients' behavioral changes that had proved their value. The excellent response to the letters of invitation is demonstrated by the crowded program for this meeting.

One of the most intriguing concepts of pharmacologic actions relates to molecular electron exchange and charge-transfer complex as influencing cell membranes. Is it possible that these drugs exert their effects on brain function via a charge phenomenon of this character? Can loci of sites be identified by some analytical device now available? Mass spectrometric methods combined with mass fragmentography and with computerization of the readout data do indeed permit the detection of exquisitely small amounts of these drugs. Is the radioimmune assay to be the most precise and the most finite? When we approach fractions of a nanogram amount, we must be getting very close to the limits of chemical and physical analytical tools.

The extrapolation of animal test data to man, always hazardous, is especially difficult for behavior-modifying drugs. The similar metabolic pathway approach in both species is well known and useful. However, a way must be found to assay the specific amounts of the phenothiazine drugs or their active metabolites, in discreet neuroanatomic sites in man during the time sequence of drug effect and recovery. We have autoradiographic methods in animals and a few studies suggesting similar metabolic pathways in rhesus monkeys and man; we know that the hydroxy derivatives are active and can enter the brain; and we have excellent methods to assess enzymic changes. Some workers feel that techniques must be discovered that are capable of simultaneously measuring many chlorpromazine metabolites before we can explain the total metabolic picture as reflecting clinical effectiveness. In an exhaustive review of this subject in 1971, Dr. Usdin concluded that, indeed, the fate of chlorpromazine in the human body remains an open question.

I fear that the total metabolic fate of the phenothiazines, as reflected in urine excretion values for metabolites or blood plasma levels, will not yield the data we must eventually have to understand the site and mechanisms of action. Overall pharmacokinetic data are useful and necessary as first steps. Certainly, drug-protein binding values permit a better understanding of the distribution of the drug to central nervous system tissues. However, the binding capacity of tissue proteins can be influenced and the half-life of the drug controlled in this manner. I suggest that selective binding on receptor sites related to the geometry of the molecule as demonstrated for other CNS drugs might be applied to the phenothiazines. However, where is one to look? Where are the receptor sites? Is the issue simply one of controlling the so-called blood-brain barrier for these drugs? Do they exert their effects by modifying brain blood circulation, electrical functions, or neurotransmitter formation, storage, or release?

It is apparent that since the biochemical lesions responsible for mental disturbance have not been delineated, it is unlikely we will find the locus of action of the phenothiazine drugs. The chapters in this volume will show how we can measure the factors such as dosage, distribution, and excretion patterns that appear to correlate with patient responses. We now have the tools to give us excellent answers to some analytical questions, even if a full understanding of all the facts is not yet available.

Session I

Physical Chemical Aspects and Methodology

Chairmen: Earl Usdin and Felix Gutmann

The Phenothiazines and Structurally Related Drugs, edited by I. S.
Forrest, C. J. Carr, and E. Usdin. Raven Press, New York © 1974.

EPR Studies on the Mechanism of Biotransformation of Tricyclic Neuroleptics and Antidepressants

Helmut Fenner

Fachbereich Pharmazie, Freie Universität Berlin, D-1000, Berlin 33, Germany

Within the series of drugs affecting the central nervous system (CNS), it is more difficult to ascertain all parameters which influence the behavior of these drugs during absorption, distribution, biotransformation, and elimination than in most other classes of drugs. It is not enough to describe their general behavior in the biological system with well-known methods of pharmacokinetics. It is necessary to know more about their plasma concentration in relation to their availability in the CNS (especially in particular brain areas) and to define the amount of the drug really responsible for pharmacodynamic effects. These difficulties are of extraordinary importance in the phenothiazine series because of their striking "bioreactivity." The tricyclic antidepressants related to diphenylamine show a similar reactivity in the biological system. All the problems concerning the uncertainty in characterizing the availability of these drugs within the CNS cannot be settled by *in vivo* studies only. As much as possible, *in vitro* methods, which have been applied successfully in molecular biology, must be used—especially NMR and EPR spectroscopy.

The redox activity of phenothiazine derivatives was already known before their use as antipsychotic drugs. In my opinion, however, pharmacologists did not really recognize the unusual "bioreactivity" of these agents until 1958 (1) when I. S. Forrest discovered free radicals as metabolites of chlorpromazine-like drugs in the urine of patients after ingestion of these compounds. These studies focussed attention on several questions concerning the mechanism of action of these drugs and the possible significance of free radicals as reactive intermediates in their biotransformation. In the meantime, several authors described the use of EPR techniques in this field but the importance of EPR studies in biochemical pharmacology is not yet established (2–19).

From the results of our studies in this field during the last 5 years, high-resolution EPR spectroscopy, in my opinion, is applicable to several problems concerning the bioavailability of these drugs, and the structure-activity relationship in the tricyclic series.

In the phenothiazine series, the effects of substituents can be ascertained. The relationship between electronic effects of substituents and bioavailability (16, 17) will be discussed first. The effects of electron-donating and electron-attracting groups can be correlated qualitatively and quantitatively with the course of oxidative reactions involving biotransformation. In connection with other molecular properties of these drugs, which are important for their behavior in absorption, distribution, and elimination processes, these effects of substituents elucidate the different "bioreactivity" of phenothiazines. Electron-attracting groups, such as the CF_3-substituent in fluphenazine or the CN- and CO—C_2H_5 group in periciazine and butyrylperazine render the radical formation more difficult and are responsible for the differences in the delocalization of the unpaired electron in the tricyclic system (Fig. 1).

There is just the opposite influence on the formation and electronic structure of the radicals from phenothiazine derivatives with electron-donating properties of their substituents; O—CH_3 and S—CH_3-groups lower the stability of the radicals and activate the sulfur in the thiazine system and the 3-position in electrophilic reactions (Fig. 2).

In the phenothiazine series, EPR techniques can also be applied in studies on steric effects of the side chain. It was surprising to us that there was a difference in the formation of cation radicals between promazine and alimemazine, a drug with a branched side chain and different pharmacodynamic properties. Alimemazine forms cation radicals only during photolysis.

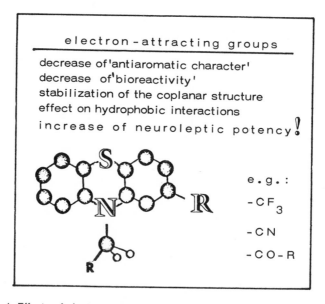

FIG. 1. Effects of electron-attracting groups on the phenothiazine system.

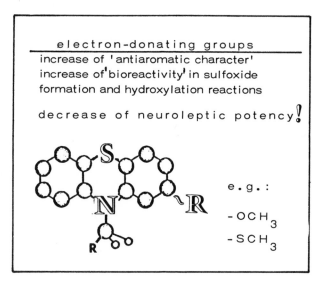

FIG. 2. Effects of electron-donating groups on the phenothiazine system.

The influence of the side chain on the formation of radicals demonstrates the correlation between the redox activity of the phenothiazine nucleus and some dynamic aspects of stereochemistry. Three types of concurrent processes must be considered regarding the possible mechanism of an interaction of the tricyclic system and the side chain (Fig. 3).

The "butterfly wing conformation" of the tricyclic nucleus does not change when ring inversion occurs. The two isomeric "boat conformations"

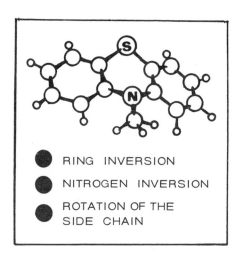

FIG. 3. Dynamic aspects of stereochemistry in the phenothiazine series.

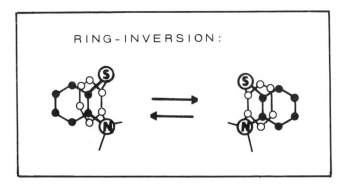

FIG. 4. Structure of the two isomeric "boat conformations" interconverted by ring inversion.

are interconverted without changing the steric shape of the molecule. The energy barrier mainly due to the stretching of bond lengths and the widening of bond angles is very low in this process (Fig. 4).

In contrast to this, another process changes the steric shape of the molecule: the pyramidal nitrogen inversion. The two isomeric pyramidal forms (invertomers) have a different configuration at the nitrogen center passing an energy barrier which is influenced by steric effects, especially the interaction with the side chain, and also by electronic effects of substituents which influence the stabilization of the coplanar transition state (Fig. 5).

The transition state is of interest regarding the redox activity of the phenothiazine nucleus: when the substituent at the nitrogen center changes its position from "quasiequatorial" to "quasiaxial," the free electron pair at the nitrogen pyramide is interconverted from "quasiaxial" to "quasiequatorial." Only in the "nontetraedric" transition state, when the electrons

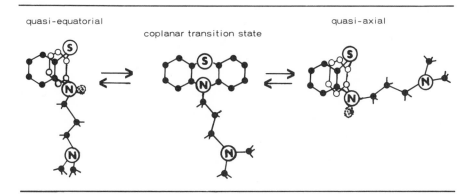

FIG. 5. Change of the steric shape of promazine during pyramidal nitrogen inversion.

at the nitrogen center are localized in a *p*-orbital, is a maximal mesomeric interaction with the aromatic π-electron system possible. This "antiaromaticity" of the thiazine system is the determinant factor regarding the electron-donating properties of these drugs.

Together with these processes, the rotation of the side chain must be discussed. Nitrogen inversion means a change of ligand position at the ring nitrogen from axial to equatorial, and both structures involve different energy barriers for the rotation of the methylene group of the side chain. The hindrance of the free rotation is minimized in the "quasiaxial" structure, increases when the coplanar transition state is formed, and in the "quasiequatorial" structure the free rotation is hindered maximally by interaction of the side chain and the peri H-atoms of the tricyclic system. It is obvious that there is a difference in these concurring processes between alimemazine and drugs with an unbranched side chain due to the space-filling side chain of alimemazine (Fig. 6).

Considering these stereochemical properties of the tricyclic system and the side chain, the importance of the interaction of both components for the steric shape of the whole molecule is evident. The energy barriers of all concurrent processes cannot be regarded as isolated from one another. This interaction is important for our understanding of molecular aspects of phenothiazine action. Earlier discussions in this field had the tendency to separate the two structural components (20, 21). From our studies, it is obvious that dynamic aspects of stereochemistry can be correlated to structure-activity relationships, and it should be understood that the differences in these molecular properties might be the reason for their different pharmacodynamics regarding high stereospecifity of the active site.

These studies in the phenothiazine series suggested that in the case of similar tricyclic systems with an antidepressant activity, biotransformation reactions could also be explained by substituent effects.

Some structural characteristics of antidepressants are represented by the

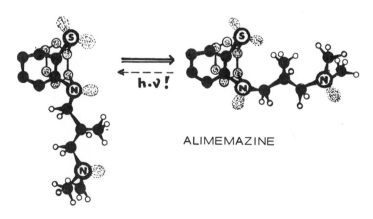

ALIMEMAZINE

FIG. 6. Structure of the two invertomeres of alimemazine.

general structure (Fig. 7), and the most important drugs of this series can be correlated to these structural essentials (22).

Since the discovery of a large number of new structures with an established antidepressant activity, it is no longer possible to maintain that the

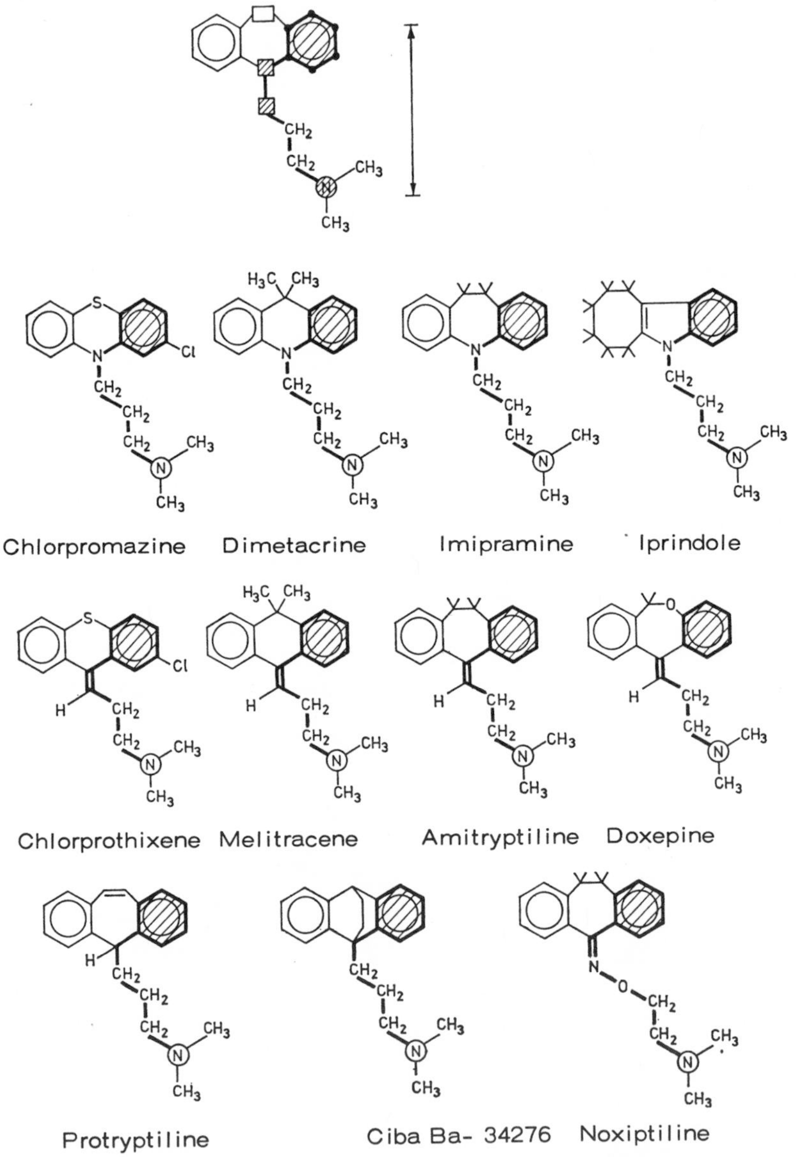

FIG. 7. General structure of tricyclic antidepressants and structural correlation to some types of drugs.

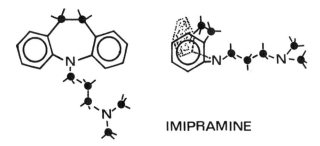

IMIPRAMINE

FIG. 8. Structure of imipramine.

relation between the steric shape of the tricyclic system and its antide-pressant activity establishes a correlation between the structure and the pharmacodynamics in this class of drugs.

A comparison of stereochemical properties of imipramine and dimetacrine in relation to their redox activity demonstrates the importance of dynamic aspects of their stereochemistry. These antidepressants with the closest structural relationship show striking differences in their LD_{50} and their anti-depressant potency which can be explained only by their different molecular properties in relation to stereochemical effects (Figs. 8 and 9).

The differences in the bridged diphenylamine systems can be studied by EPR spectroscopy. The formation and the stability of the free radicals from imipramine and other dihydrodibenzoazepines differs very much from those of their analogs in the acridane series. Some data are given in Fig. 10 (23).

The coplanar cation radicals obtained from acridanes can be stabilized by delocalization of the unpaired electron involving high electron density in the *para* position, the preferred position of electrophilic attack in redox re-actions. The dihydrodibenzoazepines are hindered from forming a coplanar

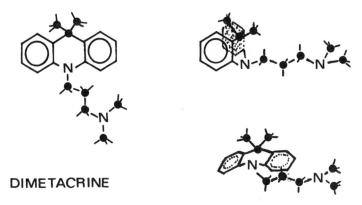

DIMETACRINE

FIG. 9. Structure of dimetacrine.

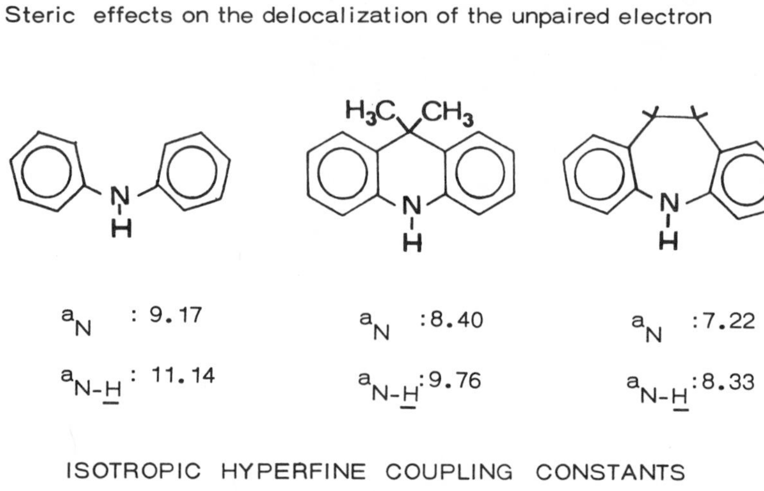

Steric effects on the delocalization of the unpaired electron

a_N : 9.17

a_{N-H} : 11.14

a_N : 8.40

a_{N-H} : 9.76

a_N : 7.22

a_{N-H} : 8.33

ISOTROPIC HYPERFINE COUPLING CONSTANTS

FIG. 10. Isotropic hyperfine coupling constants of diphenylamine-related cation radicals.

system because of the distortion of the two aromatic nuclei. Their radicals are more unstable (Fig. 11).

These differences in the molecular properties of imipramine and dimetacrine can explain the fact that the behavior of these two compounds in the biological system differs so much. In spite of their structural similarity, their different lipoid affinities, pK values, and redox activity, the determinant properties regarding their bioavailability, indicated a different dosage in clinical use of both drugs. The elimination of dimetacrine after the ingestion of the threefold amount of this drug in comparison to imipramine was studied. A clinical administration of 400 to 600 mg of dimetacrine daily is required to produce an equivalent effect to imipramine, which leads to a correspondingly higher rate of elimination.

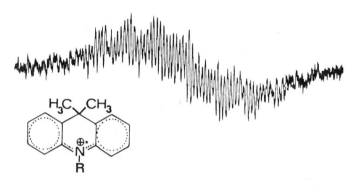

DIMETACRINE CATION RADICAL

FIG. 11. EPR-spectrum of dimetacrine cation radical [$CF_3COOH/Pb(OAc)_4$] AEG × 12, 25'.

These studies in the field of tricyclic antidepressants show the application of EPR spectroscopy in clinical pharmacology. They indicate the importance of *in vitro* studies for the determination of all extrabiological parameters of drugs whereby predictions and clarifications of effects in the biological system can be made. If we know more details concerning the availability of tricyclic systems in the CNS, we have a better basis for discussing the mode of action of these drugs.

SUMMARY

Substituent effects observed in high-resolution EPR spectroscopy of phenothiazines can be correlated qualitatively and quantitatively with the course of biotransformation reactions. Studies on the influence of the side chain on the formation of cation radicals indicate the importance of dynamic aspects of stereochemistry regarding structure-activity relationships. In the field of tricyclic antidepressants related to diphenylamine, EPR spectroscopy elucidates the correlation between steric parameters and redox activity of these drugs whereby the differences in biotransformation can be determined.

ACKNOWLEDGMENTS

EPR spectra were recorded in cooperation with S. Bamberger at the Max-Planck-Institut für Medizinische Forschung, Heidelberg. Thanks are due to Dr. F. Neugebauer for his interest in this work.

REFERENCES

1. Forrest, I. S., Forrest, F. M., and Berger, M., *Biochim. Biophys. Acta*, **29**, 441 (1958).
2. Billon, J. P., *Ann. Chimie*, **7**, 183 (1962).
3. Piette, L. H., and Forrest, I. S., *Biochim. Biophys. Acta*, **57**, 419 (1962).
4. Lagercrantz, C., *Acta Chem. Scand.*, **15**, 1545 (1961).
5. Borg, D. C., and Cotzias, G. C., *Proc. Natl. Acad. Sci. U.S.A.*, **48**, 623 (1962).
6. Schiesser, D. W., and Tuck, L. D., *J. Pharmac. Sci.*, **51**, 694 (1962).
7. Billon, J. P., Cauquis, G., and Combrisson, J., *J. Chim. Phys.*, **61**, 374 (1964).
8. Piette, L. H., Bulow, G., and Yamazaki, I., *Biochim. Biophys. Acta*, **88**, 120 (1964).
9. Lhoste, J. M., and Tonnard, F., *J. Chim. Phys.*, **63**, 678 (1966).
10. Machmer, P., *Z. Naturforsch.*, **21b**, 934 (1966).
11. Meunier, J., et al., *Ann. Pharmac, Franc.*, **25**, 683 (1967).
12. Meunier, J., et al., *Agressologie*, **9**, 37 (1968).
13. Thiery, C., Capette, J., Meunier, J., and Leterrier, F., *J. Chim. Phys.*, 134 (1969).
14. Fenner, H., and Möckel, H., *Tetrahedron Letters*, 2815 (1969).
15. Fenner, H., *Arch. Pharmaz.*, **303**, 919 (1970).
16. Fenner, H., *Arch. Pharmaz.*, **304**, 36 (1971).
17. Fenner, H., *Arch. Pharmaz.*, **304**, 47 (1971).
18. Fenner, H., *Pharmakopsychiatrie*, **3**, 332 (1970).
19. Fenner, H., *Arzneimittel-Forsch.*, **20**, 1815 (1970).
20. Bente, D., Hippius, H., Pöldinger, W., and Stach, K., *Arzneimittel-Forsch.*, **14**, 486 (1964).
21. Stach, K., and Pöldinger, W., *Fortschr. Arzneimittelforsch.*, **IX**, 129 (1966).
22. Fenner, H., *Dtsch. Apoth. Ztg.*, **111**, 1495 (1971).
23. Part of a dissertation Renner, I., Freie Universität Berlin, *in preparation*, 1973.

The Phenothiazines and Structurally Related Drugs, edited by I. S.
Forrest, C. J. Carr, and E. Usdin. Raven Press, New York © 1974.

Charge Transfer Interactions of Chlorpromazine with Neural Transmitters

F. Gutmann, Lynne C. Smith, and *M. A. Slifkin

*Department of Physical Chemistry, The University of Sydney, Sydney, Australia, and
Department of Physics, University of Salford, Salford, England*

INTRODUCTION

The electrical properties of chlorpromazine (CPZ) and related psychotropic compounds have been studied (1) by one of us and his associates as
well as by others (2). It has been shown that these substances can act, in
the formation of charge transfer complexes, as electron donors although
CPZ itself is also capable of acting as an electron acceptor (3). These preceding studies were concerned with the interaction of CPZ and its relations
with well-known acceptors such as iodine, tetracyanoquinodimethane
(TCNQ), tetracyanoethylene (TCNE), and others. In this chapter, we wish
to report results on the complexation of CPZ with neural transmitters *viz.*
acetylcholine, serotonin, and 6-hydroxydopamine. In these interactions,
CPZ is still expected to act as the donor although acetylcholine in its interactions with thiamine (4), chloranil (4, 5), hexanitrodiphenylamine, and
picric acid (6) behaves as a donor. Serotonin (5-hydroxytryptamine) also
has been reported (7) to be an electron donor. A molecule, however, may
be capable (8) of donating and accepting electrons depending on its partner
and other conditions such as the solvent, if any. CPZ itself has been shown
(3) to exist in two valency states so that it can act both as a donor and as an
acceptor, and a similar amphoteric function has been reported (9) for hema-
toporphyrin.

Several complexes between CPZ and biomolecules are known (10), as
well as complexes between acetylcholine and catecholamines (12), hista-
mines (13), and thiamine (4).

At least in molluscs, acetylcholine, serotonin, and adrenaline act as
competitive antagonists on apparently the same receptor site (14) and
complexes have been reported between serotonin and pteridines (15),
nicotinamide adenine dinucleotide (16), and flavins (17). There appear to
be no studies of complexes involving 6-hydroxydopamine although CPZ is
known, e.g., to raise the dopamine concentration in the brain (18) as well

as its release rate from and concentration in the adrenal glands (19). Interactions between the parent compound, *viz.* dopamine, and serotonin and acetylcholine have been reported (20) on the basis of nonadditive conductivity and molar refraction.

The interactions of phenothiazine itself as well as methylphenothiazine with acetylcholine have also been studied.

METHODOLOGY AND EXPERIMENTAL

The complexes were formed *in vitro* and their formation followed conductometrically (11) as well as spectrophotometrically. The solvents were A.R. grade or better. CPZ · HCl, recrystallized, was obtained from Messrs. May and Baker Ltd. Melbourne. Acetylcholine · Cl, serotonin creatinine sulfate and 6-hydroxydopamine · Br were A.R. grade.

Acetylcholine was used as the chloride and serotonin as the creatinine sulfate. 6-Hydroxydopamine chloride was prepared from the bromide by Dr. K. Calderbank of the Department of Organic Chemistry, who also prepared the 10-methylphenothiazine; the former was purified chromatographically whereas the latter was recrystallized. 6-Hydroxydopamine was obtained from Fluka A. G. Buchs, Switzerland. CPZ · HCl was partially converted to the free-radical form by prolonged exposure of an acidulated aqueous solution to direct sunlight until it became deep pinkish red in color, and exhibited a strong ESR signal.

The CPZ free base was obtained from the hydrochloride as described by Keyzer (22) and recrystallized. The water was triply distilled and demineralized conductivity water.

The other solvents were A.R. grade. Conductance measurements were carried out by means of a Wayne-Kerr Admittance Bridge Model B–221A and at 37°C unless stated otherwise. The electrodes were plane parallel, either bright or platinized platinum as reported later, and had a geometric capacitance of a few pF. They were standardized against 0.01 N KCl solutions.

The solution was thermostated to ± 0.5°C and after every addition of titrant, sufficient time was permitted to elapse for the attainment of thermal equilibrium before taking readings. The solutions were stirred either by the bubbling through of dry N_2 or else manually. The stirring was discontinued while taking readings.

Spectra were taken with a Unicam SP-700 spectrophotometer.

ACETYLCHOLINE INTERACTIONS

With CPZ · HCl

A plot of the conductivity titration of CPZ · HCl versus acetylcholine · Cl, each 10^{-3}M, in water is shown in Fig. 1. The electrodes were bright

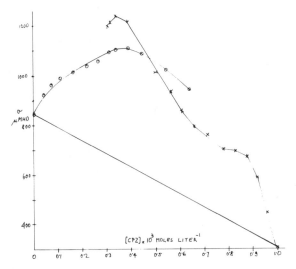

FIG. 1. Conductivity titration curves of chlorpromazine-hydrochloride versus acetyl-choline-chloride, both 10^{-3} M in water, at 37°C, using bright platinum electrodes.

platinum. Although the two branches of the titration curve do not coincide, it is seen that both peak at about 0.33 CPZ · HCl:0.67 acetylcholine, indicating the formation of a 1:2 complex. A shoulder at about 0.75 CPZ · HCl: 0.25 acetylcholine suggests a contribution from a 3 CPZ · HCl:1 acetylcholine adduct.

Plotting the conductance differences above a baseline connecting the conductances of the pure donor and acceptor solutions, shown in Fig. 2, confirms the 1:2 stoichiometry and also suggests a contribution from a 1:1 adduct. The failure of the converse titration curve to match indicates that one component is being preferentially adsorbed on the electrode surfaces. In the present case, this is the CPZ · HCl which is well known to be highly surface active and to be readily adsorbed from aqueous solutions (24). Moreover, the capacitance values encountered during the titration suggest that the failure of the titration curves to coincide is due to differences in the adsorption regime: the measured capacitance for the pure CPZ · HCl stock solution was 2.96×10^{-4} μF whereas that for the acetylcholine-Cl stock solution it was 7.13×10^{-4} μF. It is clear that these are double layer capacitances because the geometric capacitance was only a few pF, such as were indeed measured in the case of DMSO (dimetylsulfoxide) as the solvent. Thus, it is reasonable to assume that the lowering of the capacitance in the case of the CPZ · HCl solution is due to preferential adsorption of the CPZ. Acetylcholine adsorbs on the electrode to a lesser degree than the more surface-active CPZ and thus fails to displace the CPZ from the double layer in proportion to its bulk concentration. During the titrations, the capacitance values exhibit considerable changes, peaking in both directions at the stoichiometry indicated by the conductance values, *viz.* at 1:2 CPZ · HCl:

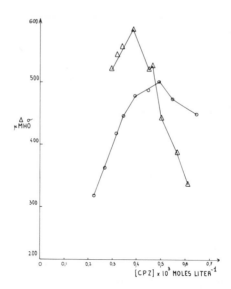

FIG. 2. Δ-plot of the data of Fig. 1. The ordinates are the differences between the titration curves and the base line which linearly connects the conductivities of the two stock solutions, *viz.* CPZ and acetylcholine; the base line is also indicated in Fig. 1.

acetylcholine. The peak capacitance values were 12.8×10^{-4} μF when adding CPZ and 34.6×10^{-4} μF for the converse, i.e., when adding acetylcholine. Thus, complex formation by addition of CPZ · HCl to acetylcholine causes an about twofold rise in capacitance while the converse, i.e., complex formation by adding acetylcholine to the CPZ · HCl solution, causes an about 10-fold rise. Such large capacitance changes cannot be associated with a bulk effect, seeing that the concentrations were only 10^{-3} M, but must be due to processes occurring within the double layer.

In DMSO as the solvent, there is little evidence for such preferential adsorption and both branches of the titration curve coincide quite well, see Fig. 3. The peak is seen to be flat and compatible with stoichiometries ranging from 1:2 to 1:1 CPZ · HCl:acetylcholine-Cl. The Δ plot suggests a 1:1 ratio. From other experience (25) it seems probable that the flatness of the peak is due to the presence of adducts of both stoichiometries in different concentrations.

At 25°C, also in DMSO, there was evidence for only the merest trace of an interaction.

The capacitances measured were about two orders of magnitude below those observed in aqueous solution: the CPZ · HCl solution yielded 27×10^{-6} μF and acetylcholine-Cl solution 50×10^{-6} μF. Thus, while CPZ is still more readily adsorbed than acetylcholine, the effect is smaller in DMSO than in water. The capacitances also exhibited a flat peak indicating a 1:2 CPZ · HCl:ACHOL · Cl interaction.

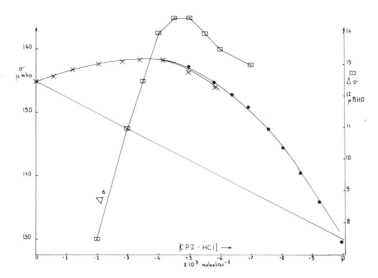

FIG. 3. Conductivity titrations of chlorpromazine-hydrochloride versus acetylcholine-chloride, both 10^{-3} M in DMSO at 37°C, using bright platinum electrodes. The points marked ⊡ are a Δ plot of the same data; the base line is also shown. Ordinate values on the right refer to the Δ-plot.

With CPZ · HCl Free Radical

Conductivity titrations of a CPZ · HCl aqueous solution containing the CPZ mainly in the form of its free radical, against acetylcholine-Cl in water with bright platinum electrodes gave results which were very poorly reproducible and varied with time. The two titration branches do not even meet. However, there is a pronounced break in the slope of the curve resulting from the addition of the free radical solution to acetylcholine solution, at the 1:2 CPZ:acetylcholine ratio although there is no evidence for any such discontinuity in the converse titration, i.e., when adding acetylcholine-Cl.

With CPZ Free Base

These titrations were carried out in DMSO (dimethylsulfoxide), the free base being insoluble in water. The Δ plots are shown in Fig. 4 and indicate a 1:1 stoichiometry. The behavior of the system in the case of bright platinum electrodes is rather similar to that exhibited on platinized platinum electrodes, although in the latter case the two branches of the titration curve, which match well on platinized platinum, fail to coincide. This again is probably due to adsorption effects. The capacitance values changed nearly linearly during the course of the titration, without showing any evidence of a peak.

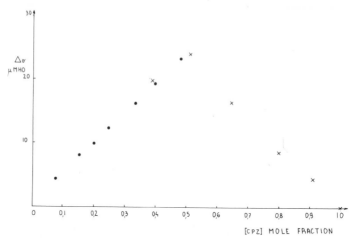

FIG. 4. Δ-plot of conductivity titrations of chlorpromazine free base 5 × 10⁻³ M versus acetylcholine-chloride, both in DMSO at 37°C, using platinized platinum electrodes.

There is no spectroscopic evidence for any charge transfer interaction in DMSO between acetylcholine-Cl and CPZ, either as the free base or the hydrochloride; also infrared spectra of these adducts in KBr discs show no evidence of an interaction in the solid state.

This may be due at least in part to a high degree of complex dissociation (40): "strong charge transfer complexes, with predominantly dative character in the ground state can dissociate into the component ions in solvents of high dielectric constant" so that the charge transfer band is replaced by the spectra of the individual ions. Such has been observed (25), e.g., in the phenothiazine-iodine complexes. Moreover, if the reaction is indeed an electrode reaction as proposed in this chapter, then the mere addition of donor and acceptor in the absence of an electrocatalytic surface should not suffice for a charge-transfer interaction. It is likely that both these causes contribute to the absence of a charge-transfer band in cases where a conductivity titration shows a definite ionic interaction. Moreover, complexes involving donors of relatively high ionization potential and acceptors of relatively low electron affinity would cause the charge-transfer band to appear in the far ultraviolet where it would be very hard to detect. The two techniques — conductometry and spectroscopy — are complimentary.

The Concentration versus Conductivity Relations for the Chlorpromazine-Acetylcholine Adducts

The CPZ · HCl-acetylcholine 1:2 adduct was preprepared in conductivity water at 10^{-2} M concentration and then diluted with conductivity water. The resulting equivalent conductivities Λ are proportional to (concentration)$^{1/2}$ and extrapolate to a conductivity at infinite dilution, Λ_∞, of 470 mho equ^{-1}cm^2; with bright platinum electrodes.

The above dilution experiment shows that the Debye-Hückel-Onsager equation (26) for the equivalent conductivity Λ_{eq}

$$\Lambda_{eq} = \Lambda_\infty - (A + B \Lambda_\infty) \, C^{1/2},$$
$$= \Lambda_\infty - \text{Const.} \; C^{1/2}, \tag{1}$$

is obeyed. The value of $\Lambda_\infty = 470$ (ohm-cm)$^{-1}$ equ^{-1}cm^2 is of the same order as that of known "strong" or "true" electrolytes (27) such as HCl.

The conductivity Λ is given by

$$\Lambda = (\mu_+ \, n_+ + \mu_- n_-) \, ez, \tag{2}$$

where the μ's refer to the ionic mobilities, the n's to the ionic concentrations and ez to the number of electronic charges e carried by an ion. It is assumed that cations and anions have the same valency. Since the solution must be electrically neutral, $n_+ = n_- = n$, so that

$$\Lambda = 2 \, \bar{\mu} n \, ez, \tag{3}$$

where $\bar{\mu}$ stands for the mean ionic mobility, $(\mu_+ + \mu_-)/2$. The carrier concentration n can be estimated by assuming that the conductance ratio $\Lambda_{e_2}/\Lambda_\infty$ can be equated to the coefficient of dissociation α. Thus, for 0.01 M, $\alpha = 0.61$ to 0.66, the latter value referring to platinized platinum electrodes while the former refers to bright platinum electrodes. The degree of dissociation changes relatively little with concentration up to 10^{-2} M. An extreme case of this behavior has been reported for the phenothiazine-iodine complex (25) where Λ_{eq} remains independent of concentration below 3×10^{-3} M. For that complex the majority carriers have been shown to be I_3^- ions and it has been suggested (25) that charge transfer occurs via a Grotthus-like handing on of charge.

For $z = 1$, $\bar{\mu} = 0.86 \times 10^{-3}$cm^2/V-sec at infinite dilution as the mean of four determinations on platinized and bright platinum electrodes, the values ranging from 0.62 to 1.15×10^{-3}cm^2/V-sec. The majority carrier mobility $\mu' = 2 \, \bar{\mu}$, on a single carrier model, then has a mean value of 1.7×10^{-3}cm^2/V-sec at infinite dilution.

Calculating μ' from the slope of the dilution curve under the assumption that the coefficient of dissociation, α, remains constant, yields a value of 4.3×10^{-3}cm^2/V-sec. Since α does alter somewhat with dilution, the agreement is not unsatisfactory.

This relatively high mobility is comparable (29) with that of the (hydrated) proton $\mu_H^+ = 3.6 \times 10^{-3}$ and it appears that the step which determines the rate of charge transfer in aqueous solution of the CPZ · HCl acetylcholine · Cl complexes is proton transfer. The assumption of a univalent majority carrier is thereby confirmed.

This behavior contrasted with that of both the hydrochloride and the free base as donors in DMSO instead of water as the solvent. While the acetylcholine CPZ · HCl complex dissolved in water behaves like a classical "strong," or better "true" electrolyte (26), the complex dissolved in DMSO shows the behavior typical of a "weak" or better "potential" (29) electrolyte; no linear extrapolation to yield a conductivity at infinite dilution is possible.

The CPZ free base acetylcholine 1:1 preprepared complex, dissolved in DMSO, behaves like a typical liquid organic semiconductor (30): its conductivity rises linearly with concentration over a concentration range from 10^{-2} to 10^{-5} molar. The hydrochloride as donor yields a plot which exhibits a definite curvature over the same concentration range. The conductivity of the 10^{-2} M preprepared acetylcholine-Cl complex solution in DMSO at 38°C was 3.33×10^{-4} (ohm-cm)$^{-1}$ for the free base as the donor, and 6.98×10^{-4} (ohm-cm)$^{-1}$ for CPZ · HCl as the donor. For comparison, the CPZ · HCl acetylcholine-Cl complex 10^{-2} M in water has a conductivity of 29.2×10^{-4} (ohm-cm)$^{-1}$.

Since for CPZ free base acetylcholine-Cl in DMSO, a plot of conductivity versus concentration is linear and very nearly passes through the origin, one may assume that the mobility as well as the coefficient of dissociation remain independent of concentration. On a one-carrier model, the (majority) carrier mobility may then be calculated from the slope of the dilution curve and results as $\mu' = 3.36 \times 10^{-4}$ cm^2/V-sec, thus about one order of magnitude below the value reported above for the CPZ · HCl/acetylcholine in water system. It is a mobility of the order to be expected if the carrier is a relatively large molecular ion (31).

The CPZ · HCl/acetylcholine complex in DMSO and diluted with DMSO yields a nonlinear relation between conductivity and concentration. Therefore, α and/or μ depend on concentration. If one neglects this dependence and assumes $\alpha = 1$, a mobility value of 6.9×10^{-4} cm^2/V-sec results, which is quite compatible with the other mobility values here reported.

Acetylcholine acts as an electron acceptor, at least against CPZ. The CPZ · HCl interaction is considerably stronger than that of the free base; the peak obtained in the conductometric titration of the hydrochloride is higher than that resulting from the free base as the donor. The role which the free radical plays in the interaction is still undetermined; the present results give no indications of any definite trend.

Interactions of Acetylcholine with Phenothiazine and with 10-Methylphenothiazine

A conductivity titration curve of the parent compound of CPZ, *viz.* phenothiazine, against acetylcholine-Cl in acetonitrile shows no evidence for any charge transfer interaction. Phenothiazine appears to be adsorbed at the electrode surfaces because the capacitance of its pure stock solution was about 1 pF while that of the pure acetylcholine-Cl stock solution was 60 pF. The capacitance values changed very nearly linearly during the course of titration without any evidence of a maximum.

The titration was repeated with DMSO as the solvent. The low conductivity of the phenothiazine stock solution causes the base line to rise steeply, rendering the location of any conductance peaks somewhat imprecise, although the phenothiazine stock solution was 10^{-2} M while that of the acetylcholine-Cl was 10^{-3} M. A definite ionic interaction is indicated and the two branches of the titration curve match well. A Δ plot indicates a stoichiometry of about 3 phenothiazine:1 acetylcholine which is the same ratio at which a shoulder has been observed in the CPZ · HCl versus acetylcholine-Cl in water titration, see Fig. 1.

Conductivity titrations of 10-methylphenothiazine against acetylcholine-Cl in DMSO as the common solvent showed no trace of any ionic interaction. Both branches of the titration curve are linear and match well, exhibiting only small and insignificant deviations.

The conductance peak produced in the phenothiazine interaction is of a height comparable to that obtained with CPZ · HCl or with CPZ itself as the donor, also in DMSO. In an aprotic solvent such as DMSO, the proton conductance mechanism suggested for charge transport in aqueous media cannot apply. Conduction must again be due to molecular ions.

It appears that phenothiazine itself is at least as good an electron donor as CPZ although it has no psychotropic activity, while it is physiologically not inactive (41). This agrees with previous studies (1) based upon iodine as the acceptor. Thus, the main locus of electron donation is the ring system as has already been suggested (1): the phenothiazines are $n-\pi$ donors. Introduction of a methyl group blocks the electron-donating ability by reducing the delocalization of the electron derived from the N atom.

THE CHLORPROMAZINE-SEROTONIN INTERACTION

Serotonin (usually as the creatinine sulfate) in most cases acts as an electron donor (7); its ionization potential is about 8.1 eV compared (42) to that of CPZ · HCl of 7.4 eV. CPZ can act not only as a donor but also as an acceptor. However, the terms "donor" and "acceptor" are only relative (8) and a weak donor may act as an acceptor versus another donor of significantly lower ionization potential and relatively high electron affinity.

CPZ · HCl forms a number of adducts if combined with serotonin in water; conductometrically stoichiometries of 1:3, 1:2, 1:1, and 2:1 are evidenced. The behavior of this system, in a general way, parallels that of the CPZ · HCl-acetylcholine system although preferential adsorption of CPZ is even more evident than in the case of acetylcholine; serotonin is far less surface active than acetylcholine (32). The interaction leading to complex formation is much weaker than that between CPZ and acetylcholine though this may at least partially be due to the serotonin being kept away from the electrode surface by adsorbed CPZ.

The capacitance values remained essentially constant at about 1.7×10^{-3} μF, after a slight initial rise, using platinized platinum electrodes. The two branches of the titration curve fail to match. With bright platinum electrodes, however, a definite capacitance peak at 1 CPZ · HCl:3 serotonin is observed, the values rising from 5 to 12×10^{-3} μF at the peak.

In view of the several stoichiometries observed, it is likely that the CPZ-serotonin interaction is quite complex, both components acting as donors as well as acceptors.

Spectroscopically no charge transfer bands could be observed for serotonin and either CPZ free base or CPZ · HCl, whether in water or in DMSO.

6-HYDROXYDOPAMINE INTERACTIONS

With Chlorpromazine Free Base

6-Hydroxydropamine was first used as the hydrochloride and titrated against CPZ · HCl in order to maintain the anion invariant and its concentration constant. However, this titration proved to be difficult due to the rapid oxidation of the rather unstable hydrochloride. The solutions, including the stock solution, rapidly tended to become discolored during the course of the experiment. 6-Hydroxydopamine itself was then titrated against CPZ free base, in DMSO. While the departures from the base line were only small they did suggest a 2 CPZ:1 6-hydroxydopamine interaction. The complex solution also exhibited a distinct purplish discoloration. The interaction was confirmed spectroscopically by the appearance of a new band centered at 19.2 kK and about 6 kK wide. It was verified that this band was indeed a charge transfer band, by observing the reversible[1] decrease of the peak with increasing temperature. It was concluded that the complex fails to dissociate appreciably in DMSO, its ground state being predominantly nondative. A further conductivity titration was therefore carried out at 40°C in a medium of permittivity higher than that of DMSO, *viz.* in dimethylformamide (DMF). A definite ionic interaction was obtained, indicating again a 2:1 CPZ:6-hydroxydopamine stoichiometry. The titration curve is shown in Fig. 5. The 6-hydroxydopamine stock solution became immediately discolored, acquiring a

---

[1] A charge-transfer band should diminish reversibly upon heating (23) because the equilibrium between the complex and its constituent ions then shifts toward dissociation so that the band tends to be replaced by the spectra of the constituent ions. A chemical reaction, conversely, will cause the peak amplitude to rise with increasing temperature because the equilibrium then shifts towards a higher concentration of the reaction product. Only ions contribute to the peak obtained in conductivity titrations; thus the conductivity peak due to a charge transfer complex increases upon heating.

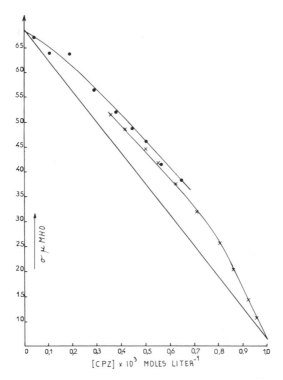

FIG. 5. Conductivity titrations of 6-hydroxydopamine versus chlorpromazine free base, each 10^{-3} M in dimethylformamide, at 40°C, using bright platinum electrodes.

pinkish hue and was used as such. Most of this discoloration tends to disappear within about 4 days. 6-Hydroxydopamine in DMF by itself yields[2] a new absorption band at 20 kK, about 6 kK wide. The peak amplitude drops reversibly[1] increasing temperature, thus indicating that it is due to a charge-transfer complex. A day later, however, the peak has disappeared; only a shoulder is left. The interaction apparently commences as a charge transfer complex which slowly gives place to chemical bonding.

The interaction of 6-hydroxydopamine with CPZ free base in DMF indicates a definite charge-transfer interaction between the 6-hydroxy-

---

[2] This is an extreme case of the solvent interactions which occur so frequently (34). A basic assumption in the conductivity titration of charge-transfer complexes is that the solvent is inert. It has always been recognized that no such solvent exists; in particular DMSO as well as DMF are known (35) to be electron donors. CPZ, as the free base and as the hydrochloride, however, is a much stronger electron donor than either DMSO or DMF so that their interaction with the acceptor should predominate. This has indeed been observed, as evident from the present report.

dopamine acceptor and both donors then present, *viz.* the DMF solvent as well as the CPZ: the band shifts to 19.7 kK and becomes somewhat wider; its temperature reversibility indicates that it is a charge-transfer band. If a solution of 6-hydroxydopamine in DMF, aged for 24 hr, is used as the acceptor solution, the shoulder is increased and addition of fresh 6-hydroxydopamine causes the original 19.7 kK peak to reappear. With effluxion of time, however, the initial charge transfer complex again goes over into a new chemical compound by means of a chemical reaction subsequent to the charge transfer (49). This is similar to what has been observed for the phenothiazine-chloranil reaction (33).

In acetonitrile, a definite charge-transfer band was observed centered at 20.4 kK and about 5.8 kK wide.

With Chlorpromazine-HCl

There is no evidence from either spectroscopy or conductivity for any interaction between 6-hydroxydopamine and CPZ · HCl or with the pre-prepared CPZ · HCl free radical; neither in the ultraviolet nor in the visible spectra, neither in water nor in DMSO.

OTHER CHARGE-TRANSFER INTERACTIONS OF 6-HYDROXYDOPAMINE

6-Hydroxydopamine in the above interactions behaved as an acceptor. This was verified by forming complexes with the known donor anthracene; in acetonitrile a charge-transfer reaction was observed resulting in a new band at 20.8 kK, about 5.8 kK wide. At higher concentrations, the band shifted to 20.6 kK. No interaction could be observed with pyrene in DMSO.

6-Hydroxydopamine also complexes with noradrenaline in water, giving rise to a new and very wide band centered at 20.4 kK.

The interaction with acetylcholine-chloride in water yields a narrow and structured peak at 25 kK which is ascribed to a chemical rather than a charge-transfer interaction.

Likewise, a new, skewed peak results from the reaction of 6-hydroxy-dopamine with serotonin in water, situated at 24.1 kK. The height of this peak increases with rising temperature, thus again indicating a chemical rather than a charge-transfer interaction. The color of the solution changes to beige.

No trace of any interaction, chemical or charge transfer in nature, was observed between 6-hydroxydopamine and phenothiazine.

FURTHER DISCUSSION

CPZ-hydrochloride has been shown in this chapter to complex with acetylcholine in the ratios of 1:2, 1:1, and 3:1, with 1:2 predominant.

The free base, however, only yields a 1:1 stoichiometry. The 1:1 adduct thus seems to be associated with the CPZ molecule while the other stoichiometries involve the hydrochloride group: the hydrochloride behaves differently from the free base. This might be associated with the different mode of charge transfer: the protonic transfer, which has been shown to be the main contribution to the current, cannot occur in the case of the free base in an aprotic solvent such as DMSO.

CPZ · HCl does not complex with 6-hydroxydopamine which interacts strongly with the free base although both are comparably good donors — if anything, the hydrochloride is the stronger donor. Thus it may well be that this is yet another case of charge transfer involving localized (donor) sites as suggested (35) by Pullman and Pullman, and indeed observed (36) for the guanidine-chloranil complex; again the hydrochloride fails to react.

Adsorption processes, especially preferential adsorption of CPZ, are seen to play a major role in the electrochemical behavior of these interactions, particularly in aqueous solution. The interaction appears to take place at the electrode surface within an "active space" (39) which includes, but needs not be confined to, the double layer facing the electrode. In other words, the CPZ-acetylcholine interaction is an electrode reaction.

That a biological membrane is capable of acting as an electrode has been demonstrated (37) by Pant and Rosenberg; it also has been shown by Hameister (38) that CPZ attaches itself to biological membranes. Since the free base is water-insoluble, Hameister's experiments (38) must refer to the hydrochloride although the author does not explicitly say so.

The capacitance changes observed during the titrations also support the hypothesis that the interaction is an electrode reaction: (1) the capacitance peaks at the stoichiometry which yields a conductivity maximum, (2) the two- to 10-fold rise in the capacitance values measured cannot possibly be caused by any reasonable increase in the permittivity of the bulk of the solutions, which were only about 10^{-3} molar. The bulk permittivity thus is mainly determined by that of the solvent. The capacitance changes observed must therefore be due to changes within an "active space" (39) or reaction zone, which comprises the double layer. During the titration, the reaction proceeds within that reaction zone and concentrations therein may differ significantly from the bulk concentrations.

There exists a great deal of direct experimental evidence for the *in vivo* interactions between chlorpromazine and acetylcholine (43), serotonin (44), and dopamine (45). On the basis of the experimental results here reported it is suggested that these *in vivo* processes involve the formation of charge-transfer complexes on the surface of a biological membrane which acts as an electrode.

CPZ is still the drug of choice (46) in the treatment of schizophrenia. Biochemical evidence (47) suggests that the causative agent of the disease is 6-hydroxydopamine and a recent theory (47) of schizophrenia presents a coherent picture for this aberration which also, in a general way, explains why CPZ should be active: the drug is assumed to "protect the reward system of the schizophrenic by blocking the uptake of endogeneously formed 6-hydroxydopamine into the noradrenalergic nerve endings."

This hypothesis is supported by the results presented here on the 6-hydroxydopamine–CPZ interaction. 6-Hydroxydopamine fails to displace adsorbed CPZ from an electrode surface. If, as has been suggested, the synaptic membrane acts as an electrode, then it is reasonable to assume that likewise access of the 6-hydroxydopamine to the nerve endings will be prevented by the presence of the CPZ: the drug is firmly adsorbed and immediately complexes with any 6-hydroxydopamine present. This charge-transfer reaction then goes over into a true chemical reaction involving the formation of a new chemical compound which is then decomposed by a series of enzymatic reactions; at no time, however, is free 6-hydroxy-dopamine available to attack the nerve endings.

However, if adsorption followed by charge-transfer complex formation followed by chemical interaction protects the nerve endings against 6-hy-droxydopamine — would not the very same effect also prevent neural transmitters such as acetylcholine from acting on the postsynaptic membrane? It has been pointed out, e.g., by Karlin (48) that all activators act in the same way, i.e., by providing a bridge between a negative subsite and a second region of positive interaction, the receptor activation being characterized by a decrease of a few Å in the distance between the two sites. However, it is known that CPZ does not block cholinergic synapses.

This is explained by the formation of charge-transfer complexes between CPZ and acetylcholine which are largely, to 61 to 66%, dissociated into free ions, as shown in this chapter. Moreover, acetylcholine is sufficiently surface active to compete with CPZ on the membrane surface. The extent of the involvement of the CPZ free radicals is just one of many questions which remain to be answered.

SUMMARY

Chlorpromazine (CPZ) acts as the donor in forming charge transfer complexes with acetylcholine (as the chloride), serotonin (as the creatinine sulfate) and with 6-hydroxydopamine evidenced from conductometric titrations and from spectroscopy. CPZ · HCl forms 1:2 complexes with acetylcholine as acceptor; with a contribution from a 1:1 ratio in water and in dimethylsulfoxide (DMSO) as solvents. In water, the complex behaves like a typical "strong" or "true" electrolyte obeying the Debye-Hückel-Onsager equation in its concentration dependence; the equivalent conductivity at infinite dilution is 470 mho equ^{-1} cm^2 and thus comparable to, say HCl. The degree of dissociation $\alpha = 0.61$ to 0.66 at 0.01 M changes but little to 0.1 M. In a single carrier model, the majority carrier mobility $\mu = 1.7 \times 10^{-3}$ cm^2/V-sec as the mean of four determinations, is comparable to the mobility of the (hydrated) proton or OH ion. It is concluded that in this system conduction is due to proton transfer. The very large — two- to 10-fold — capacitance changes as well as the high-capacitance values — of the order of 0.001 μF cm^{-2} — observed during the titrations suggest that the complex formation is an electrode reaction at the electrode surface. This is further supported by the changing adsorption effects. The *in vivo* interaction likewise might involve a sort of electrode reaction with the synaptic membrane acting as an electrode.

In DMSO, CPZ · HCl acts as a more powerful electron donor against acetylcholine than CPZ free base: the conductometric peak obtained from the former is much higher. The free base complexes with acetylcholine in DMSO in a 1:1 ratio plus a contribution from 3:1. The conductivity of the CPZ acetylcholine in DMSO system changes linearly with concentration over a 1,000-fold range. The dissociation and the mobility thus do not change with concentration; $\mu = 3.36 \times 10^{-4}$ cm^2/V-sec comparable to other molecular ions. In contradistinction, CPZ · HCl acetylcholine in DMSO neither obeys the Onsager relation nor is the concentration dependence linear. The mobility of the majority carrier may be estimated as about 7×10^{-4} cm^2/V-sec.

There is no spectroscopic evidence for these complexes; it appears that they are formed at the electrode surfaces and that their ground state is mainly ionic; in high permittivity solvents they are largely dissociated. The parent compound of CPZ, phenothiazine, complexes with acetylcholine in a 3:1 stoichiometry which also contributed to the CPZ complex. Methylphenothiazine, however, fails to complex with acetylcholine in any way.

Serotonin, although generally considered as a donor, also forms complexes with CPZ · HCl. Several ratios are evident, mainly CPZ · HCl: serotonin, 1:3. Spectroscopy reveals no charge transfer band.

6-Hydroxydopamine appears to be a good electron acceptor: a charge transfer band about 5.8 kK wide was found at 20.8 kK with the well-known donor anthracene, in acetonitrile as well as in DMSO. No interaction could be ascertained with the donors pyrene or phenothiazine. New bands, probably due to chemical rather than charge transfer reactions, were obtained from the 6-hydroxydopamine versus acetylcholine and serotonin adducts. A charge transfer complex is formed between 6-hydroxydopamine and noradrenaline in water, yielding a typical charge transfer band at 20.4 kK.

6-Hydroxydopamine forms a charge transfer complex with CPZ free base in DMSO and in dimethylformamide, as is seen from the appearance of a new, wide, temperature-reversible band at 19.2 kK in DMSO and at 19.7 kK in dimethylformamide. Conductometric titrations indicate a CPZ:6-hydroxydopamine stoichiometry of 2:1 for the adduct. Within a day or so, however, the charge transfer interaction gives place to mainly chemical bonding as evidenced from spectroscopy. In CH$_3$CN, likewise, there occurs a definite charge transfer interaction.

There is no evidence from either spectroscopy or conductometry for any interaction between 6-hydroxydopamine and CPZ · HCl, in neither ultraviolet, visible, nor infrared spectra, in neither water nor DMSO.

It is suggested that the *in vivo* interaction of 6-hydroxydopamine with CPZ involves the formation of an initial charge transfer complex on the surface of a biological membrane which acts as an electrode, more specifically at the postsynaptic membrane where CPZ is preferentially adsorbed. The therapeutic activity of CPZ may thus involve a fast charge transfer interaction between 6-hydroxydopamine and adsorbed CPZ in the form of the free base; this complexation prevents the accumulation of free 6-hydroxydopamine and consequent attack of the nerve endings. CPZ does not block cholinergic synapses because the CPZ-acetylcholine complex dissociates into free ions in an aqueous medium. Moreover, acetylcholine is far more surface active than 6-hydroxydopamine, sufficiently so to compete with CPZ for adsorption sites.

REFERENCES

1. Gutmann, F., and Keyzer, H., *J. Chem. Phys.,* **50,** 550 (1969); *Electrochim. Acta,* **13,** 693 (1968); **12,** 1255 (1967); *Nature,* **205,** 1102 (1965); *Rev. Aggressol. (Paris),* **7,** 27 (1968); Gutmann, F., and Netschey, A., *Nature,* **191,** 1390 (1961); *J. Chem. Phys.,* **36,** 2355 (1962); Gooley, C. M., Keyzer, H., and Setchell, F., *Nature,* **223,** 80 (1969); Brau, A., Farges, J. P., and Gutmann, F., *Electrochim. Acta,* **17,** 1803 (1972).
2. Cann, J. R., *Biochem.,* **6,** 3435 (1967). Foster, R., and Hanson, P., *Biochim. Biophys. Acta,* **112,** 482 (1966); Fulton, A., and Lyons, L. E., *Aust. J. Chem.,* **21,** 873 (1968); Labos, E., *Nature,* **209,** 201 (1966); Seghatchian, M. J., et al., *Chem. Biol. Interact.,* **3,** 413 (1971); Bloor, J. E., et al., *J. Med. Chem.,* **13,** 922 (1970); Foster, R., and Fyfe, C. A., *Biochim. Biophys. Acta,* **112,** 490 (1966); Foster, R., *Organic Charge Transfer Complexes,* Academic Press, New York, 1969.
3. Gutmann, F., and Keyzer, H., *Nature,* **205,** 1102 (1965).
4. Galzigna, L., *Biochem. Pharmacol.,* **18,** 2485 (1969); *Int. J. Vitamin Res.,* **40,** 38 (1970).
5. Saucin, M., et al., *Bull. Cl. Sci. Acad. Roy. Belge,* **54,** 1006 (1968).
6. Eksberg, S., et al., *private communication,* 1972.
7. Szent-Györgyi, A., *An Introduction to Submolecular Biology,* Academic Press, New York, 1960. Allison, A. C., et al., *Life Sci.,* **12,** 729 (1962).
8. Slifkin, M. A., *Charge Transfer Interactions of Biomolecules,* Academic Press, New York, 1971. Woronkow, M. G., and Deitsch, A. J., *Öst. Chemiker Ztg.,* **67,** 1 (1966); Allison, A. C., et al., ref. 7.
9. Heathcote, J. G., et al., *Biochem. Biophys. Acta,* **153,** 13 (1968); Kearns, D. R., et al., *J. Chem. Phys.,* **32,** 1020 (1960); and Gouterman, M., and Stevenson, P. E., ibid., **37,** 2266 (1962).
10. Saucin, M., and Van de Verst, A., *J. Chim. Phys.,* **67,** 507 (1970); Cann, J. R., *Biochemistry,* **6,** 3427 (1967). Foster, R., and Hanson, P., *Biochim. Biophys. Acta,* **112,** 482 (1966); Slifkin, M. A., *Charge Transfer Interactions of Biomolecules,* Academic Press, New York, 1971, pp. 123, 169, 182, 200, 208, 213, 217; Seghatchian, M. J., and Winder, A. F., *Chem. Biol. Interact.,* **3,** 413 (1971); Guth, P. S., and Spirtes, M. A., *Internatl. Rev. Neurobiol.,* **7,** 231 (1964); Yagi, R., et al., *Nature,* **184,** 982 (1959).
11. Gutmann, F., and Keyzer, H., *Electrochim. Acta,* **11,** 555, 1163 (1966); Gutmann, F., *J. Sci. Ind. Res.,* **26,** 19 (1967); Job, P., *C.R. Acad. Sci. (Paris),* **180,** 928 (1925).
12. Galzigna, L., *Nature,* **225,** 1085 (1970).
13. Saucin, M., et al., *Bull. Cl. Sci. Acad. Roy. Belge,* **54,** 1006 (1968).
14. Manukhin, B. N., and Turpaev, T. M., *Zh. Evol. Biokhim. Fiziol.,* **7,** 229 (1971).
15. Slifkin, M. A., ref. 8, p. 101.
16. Slifkin, M. A., ref. 8, pp. 112, 182, 235.

17. Isenberg, I., and Szent-Györgyi, A., *Proc. Natl. Acad. Sci.*, **44**, 857 (1958); Slifkin, M. A., ref, 8. pp. 136, 148, 241, 242.
18. Cegrell, L., et al., *Res. Commun. Chem. Pathol. Pharmacol.*, **1**, 479 (1970).
19. Vapaatalo, H., *Ann. Med. Exp. Biol. Fenn.*, **49**, 89 (1971).
20. Galzigna, L., and Naurel, P., *J. Theoret. Biol.*, **31**, 553 (1971).
21. Slifkin, M. A., ref. 8, pp. 200 ff; Gutmann, F., and Keyzer, H., *J. Chem. Phys.*, **46**, 1969 (1967).
22. Keyzer, H., Ph.D. Thesis, University of New South Wales, Sydney, Australia (1967).
23. Slifkin, M. A., ref. 8, p. 23. Rao, C. N. R., and Bhat, S. N., *Appl. Spectrosc. Rev.*, **5**, 1 (1971).
24. e.g. Seeman, P. M., and Bialy, H. S., *Biochem. Pharmacol.*, **12**, 1181 (1963); Kitler, M. E., and Lamy, P., *Pharm. Acta Helv.*, **46**, 1483 (1971).
25. Brau, A., Farges, J. P., and Gutmann, F., *Electrochim. Acta*, **17**, 1803 (1972).
26. Bockris, J. O'M., and Reddy, A. K. N., *Modern Electrochemistry*, Plenum Press, New York, 1970, p. 434.
27. ref. 26, p. 179.
28. Gutmann, V., and Mayer, U., *Monatshefte f. Chem.*, **100**, 2048 (1969); see also ref. 25.
29. ref. 26, p. 472.
30. Gutmann, F., and Lyons, L. E., *Organic Semiconductors*, Wiley, New York, 1967.
31. De Groot, K., et al., *J. Chem. Phys.*, **47**, 3084 (1967); see also ref. 30, p. 767.
32. Kurk, J., *Zesz. Nauk Uniw. Jagiellon. Ph. Chem.*, **16**, 101 (1971).
33. Barigand, M., et al., *Bull. Soc. Chim. Belges*, **79**, 177 (1970); ibid., *in press*. Tondeur, J. J., et al., *Bull. Soc. Chim. Belges*, **79**, 401 (1970).
34. e.g. Slifkin, M. A., ref. 8; Kosower, E. M., and Tanizawa, K., *Chem. Phys. Lett.*, **16**, 419 (1972); Taniguchi, Y., and Mataga, N., ibid., **13**, 6 (1972); Kosower, E. M., *J. Amer. Chem. Soc.*, **80**, 3253, 3261 (1958), **78**, 3497 (1956).
35. Slifkin, M. A., *Spectrochim. Acta*, **25 A**, 1037 (1969); see also ref. 49; Pullman, B., and Pullman, A., *Quantum Biochemistry*, Interscience, New York, 1963.
36. Slifkin, M. A., and Kushelevsky, A. P., *Spectrochim. Acta*, **27 A**, 1999 (1971); Moxon, G. H., and Slifkin, M. A., *Biochim. Biophys. Acta*, **286**, 98 (1972).
37. Pant, H. C., and Rosenberg, B., *Chem. Phys. Lipids*, **6**, 39 (1971).
38. Hameister, W., *Arzneimittel Forschg. (Drug Res.)*, **20**, 1818 (1970).
39. Breyer, B., and Bauer, H. H., *AC Polarography and Tensammetry*, Interscience, New York, 1963; Breyer, B., and Gutmann, F., *Aust. J. Sci.*, **8**, 163 (1946); Smith, D., *Crit. Revs. Anal. Chem.*, **2**, 247 (1971); Breyer, B., and Hacobian, S., *Aust. J. Chem.*, **7**, 225 (1954).
40. ref. 8, p. 24.
41. Pamukcu, A. M., et al., *J. Natl. Cancer Inst.*, **47**, 155 (1971).
42. Fulton, A., and Lyons, L. E., *Aust. J. Chem.*, **21**, 873 (1968).
43. e.g. Machotra, C. L., *Indian J. Physiol. Pharmacol.*, **11**, 69 (1967); Liang, C. L., and Quastel, J. H., *Biochem. Pharmacol.*, **18**, 1187 (1969).
44. Massini, P., and Lüscher, E. E., *Thromb. Diath. Haem.*, **25**, 13 (1971); Jansson, S. E., *Acta Physiol. Scand.*, **78**, 420 (1970); Akira, I., et al., *Eur. J. Pharmacol.*, **8**, 200 (1969); Chase, T. N., et al., *J. Neurochem.*, **16**, 607 (1969).
45. Vapaatalo, H., *Ann. Med. Exp. Biol. Fenn.*, **49**, 89 (1971); Cegrell, L., et al., *Res. Commun. Chem. Pathol. Pharmacol.*, **1**, 479 (1970).
46. e.g. Cole, J. O., and Davis, J. M., in *Psychopharmacology*, Effron, D. H., ed., U.S. Govt. Printing Office, Washington, D.C., 1968; Forrest, I. S., *Proc. West Pharm. Soc.*, **12**, 36 (1969).
47. Stein, L., and Wise, C. D., *Science*, **171**, 1036 (1971) and references cited therein.
48. Karlin, A., *J. General Physiol.*, **54**, 245 (1969) p. 261 ff.
49. Slifkin, M. A., *The Purines—Theory and Experiment; The Jerusalem Symposia on Quantum Chemistry and Biochemistry*, **IV**, Jerusalem, 1972; p. 392 ff.

The Phenothiazines and Structurally Related Drugs, edited by I. S.
Forrest, C. J. Carr, and E. Usdin. Raven Press, New York © 1974.

The Molecular Structures of Phenothiazine Derivatives

J. J. H. McDowell

Department of Physics, University of Cape Town, Cape Town, Republic of South Africa

INTRODUCTION

The crystallographic study of a series of derivatives of phenothiazines
has been undertaken in the laboratory of the University of Cape Town with
the eventual hope of correlating molecular structure with psychopharmacological properties.

The phenothiazines are divided into three groups according to the chemical nature of the side chain attached to the nitrogen atom: (a) dimethylaminopropyl, (b) piperazine, and (c) piperidine radical. Chlorpromazine, pyscho-
tropically potent, belonging to the first group, and thiethylperazine, with
relatively little tranquilizing or sedative action, belonging to the second,
were chosen for complete structural analyses and are here described. For
control purposes, the structural parameters of a potent drug as compared
with a less potent one could be of great significance. The structure of
thioridazine, a potent representative of the third group, has been determined
and will shortly be reported.

The crystal data on the three compounds and also on phenothiazine and
chlorpromazine hydrochloride are given in Table 1. Owing to the problems
experienced in obtaining high-quality crystals of chlorpromazine hydrochloride which disintegrated even when sealed in nitrogen-filled capillaries,
it was decided not to proceed with the structure determination. Work is,
however, continuing on the orthorhombic form of phenothiazine, as it will
be of interest to compare the results obtained with those of Bell et al. (1)
for monoclinic phenothiazine.

CHLORPROMAZINE

Chlorpromazine is 3-chloro-10 (3′ dimethylamino–*n*–propyl) phenothiazine, which since its first introduction into clinical psychiatry by Delay
and Deniker in 1952 (2) has been one of the best known derivatives of
phenothiazine (3).

TABLE 1. Crystal data of phenothiazine and four derivatives

	Phenothiazine	Chlorpromazine hydrochloride	Chlorpromazine base	Thiethylperazine	Thioridazine
R_1	H	Cl	Cl	SC_2H_3	SCH_3
R_2	H	$(CH_2)_3N(CH_3)CH_3$ +HCl	$(CH_2)_3N(CH_3)CH_3$	$(CH_2)_3N \bigcirc NCH_3$	$(CH_2)_2-C \bigcirc$ (CH₃, N-piperidine)
Formula	$C_{12}H_9NS$	$C_{17}H_{20}N_2SCl_2$	$C_{17}H_{19}N_2SCl$	$C_{22}H_{29}N_3S_2$	$C_{21}H_{26}N_2S_2$
Molecular weight	199.266	355.326	318.861	399.602	370.566
Density Flotation liquids	Water+mercury potassium iodide	Benzene+carbon tetrachloride	Water+mercury potassium iodide	Water+mercury potassium iodide	Water+mercury potassium iodide
g/c.c. meas.	1.355	1.31	1.289	1.187	1.19
g/c.c. calc.	1.342	1.28	1.285	1.198	1.24
No. of mols.	4	8	8	4	8
Crystal system	Orthorhombic	Monoclinic	Orthorhombic	Orthorhombic	Orthorhombic
Space group	$Pnma$	$P2_1/c$	$Pbca$	$P2_12_12_1$	$Pna2_1$
$a(Å)$	7.94±0.01	11.96±0.02	23.50±0.04	12.057±0.01	18.3369±0.002
$b(Å)$	21.02±0.01	31.77±0.06	15.20±0.02	19.953±0.01	12.4353±0.002
$c(Å)$	5.91±0.01	9.84±0.01	9.23±0.01	9.215±0.01	17.3764±0.004
β	–	98.9°±1°	–	–	–
Volume ($Å^3$)	986.4	3,694	3,297	2,217	3,962
Solvent	Carbon tetrachloride or methyl alcohol	Benzene+ethanol under nitrogen	Low b.p. petrol ether under nitrogen	Petrol ether	Low b.p. petrol ether

Solution and Refinement of the Structure

Needle-shaped crystals were formed from a solution of powdered chlor-promazine dissolved in low-boiling-point petrol ether. Because of the deleterious effects of light, air, and X-rays and the consequent difficulties, the following procedure was finally adopted, with successful results: the crystals were grown in darkness under an atmosphere of nitrogen; single crystals were sealed in nitrogen-filled, Lindemann glass capillaries; and exposure to light rays was avoided as much as possible throughout the photographic process. X-ray rotation and equi-inclination Weissenberg photographs, using Cu Kα radiation, Ni-filtered, taken about the y and z axes gave an orthorhombic system with $a = 23.50 \pm 0.04$ Å, $b = 15.20 \pm 0.02$ Å, and $c = 9.23 \pm 0.01$ Å. The conditions for nonextinction are: hko, $h = 2n$; okl, $k = 2n$; hol, $l = 2n$; hoo, $h = 2n$; oko, $k = 2n$; ool, $l = 2n$; which lead uniquely to the space group $Pbca$. $D_m = 1.289$ g/cc, $D_c = 1.285$ g/cc for 8 molecules per unit cell (4, 5).

Eight layer-lines (hko to $hk7$) were photographed using the standard multiple-film technique. On each film $I_{(hkl)}$, $I_{(h\bar{k}l)}$, plus either $I_{(\bar{h}kl)}$ or $I_{(\bar{h}\bar{k}l)}$ were measured; for $Pbca$ these are all equal. Thus, by collating their symmetry relationships, about 6,000 measured intensities were reduced, by averaging, to 1,895 independent reflections. Scale factors for the individual layer-lines were obtained by the following two methods: (a) the crystal was rotated about the y-axis and a five-film Weissenberg gave 120 independent $h1l$ intensities with which to set the z-axis photographs on to the same scale; and (b) Wilson's method (6) of obtaining absolute K's for each layer-line was used. The second method was found to give results more closely consistent with the refined scale factors obtained by the least-squares method. All the usual correction factors were applied, but absorption was neglected since the value of μR < 0.5.

A three-dimensional Patterson function, sharpened in accordance with the formula

$$|F|^2 = \frac{(\sin^2 \theta / \lambda^2 + 0.16) F_0^2 e^{B \sin^2 \theta / \lambda^2}}{(\Sigma f_i)^2},$$

was calculated. The S—S and the Cl—Cl inversion peaks and the eight corresponding S—Cl peaks were correctly located, and a three-dimensional Fourier synthesis phased on S and Cl gave initial values of the coordinates of the C and N atoms. Structure factors were calculated using the analytical f values of Berghuis et al. (7).

The structure was refined by further Fourier and difference Fourier syntheses and five least-squares cycles using the Busing et al. program *ORFLS* (8). Initially, an overall temperature factor of 3.8 obtained by Wilson's method (6) was applied; subsequently individual isotropic temperature factors for each atom were used. The value of R for observed reflections

TABLE 2. Chlorpromazine: Final atomic fractional coordinates (× 10⁴) and thermal
parameters (× 10⁴) with estimated standard deviations

Temperature factor $= \exp\{-(h^2\beta_{11} + k^2\beta_{22} + \ell^2\beta_{33} + 2hk\beta_{12} + 2h\ell\beta_{13} + 2k\ell\beta_{23})\}$ with $\beta_{11} = 2\pi^2 a^{*2} U_{11}$,
$$\beta_{12} = 2\pi^2 a^* b^* U_{12}, \text{ etc.}$$
The least-squares standard errors are given in parentheses.

	x	y	z	β_{11}	β_{22}	β_{33}	β_{12}	β_{13}	β_{23}
Cℓ	4520 (1)	0199₅(2)	3710 (3)	23 (0₄)	102 (2)	176 (4)	20 (1)	4 (1)	11 (2)
S	2164 (1)	0515 (1)	0643 (2)	28 (0₄)	41 (1)	107 (3)	-6 (0₅)	-16 (1)	-13 (1)
N(1)	2687 (2)	1874 (3)	2481 (6)	17 (1)	29 (2)	107 (9)	-1 (1)	-0 (2)	-9 (3)
N(2)	4192 (2)	3325 (4)	3565 (7)	19 (1)	58 (3)	122 (10)	-5 (1)	10 (3)	-5 (4)
C(1)	3855 (3)	0261 (5)	2893 (8)	23 (2)	58 (4)	88 (12)	7 (2)	10 (3)	14 (5)
C(2)	1344 (4)	4537 (5)	2131 (9)	27 (2)	55 (4)	92 (13)	-5 (2)	-17 (4)	11 (5)
C(3)	1870 (4)	4617 (5)	1478 (9)	34 (2)	36 (3)	138 (14)	-1 (2)	-21 (4)	1 (5)
C(4)	2802 (3)	0398 (4)	1597 (8)	24 (2)	32 (3)	88 (11)	-1 (2)	5 (3)	-5 (4)
C(5)	3020 (3)	1111 (4)	2379 (7)	20 (1)	42 (3)	50 (10)	3 (2)	6 (3)	-5 (4)
C(6)	3548 (3)	1045 (5)	3073 (7)	21 (1)	52 (4)	58 (11)	5 (2)	11 (3)	-11 (4)
C(7)	1807 (3)	1156 (5)	1926 (8)	21 (2)	45 (3)	102 (12)	-2 (2)	-15 (3)	15 (5)
C(8)	1206 (3)	1052 (5)	2119 (11)	23 (2)	48 (4)	232 (17)	-3 (2)	-19 (4)	27 (6)
C(9)	0921 (4)	1579 (6)	3109 (13)	22 (2)	53 (5)	281 (20)	5 (2)	4 (5)	27 (8)
C(10)	1214 (4)	2194 (6)	3942 (11)	24 (2)	53 (4)	233 (18)	9 (2)	15 (5)	20 (7)
C(11)	1807 (3)	2288 (5)	3780 (9)	22 (2)	39 (3)	145 (13)	6 (2)	8 (3)	17 (5)
C(12)	2097 (3)	1782 (4)	2747 (8)	18 (1)	36 (3)	104 (12)	-0₄(2)	-7 (3)	21 (4)
C(13)	2973 (3)	2709 (4)	2992 (8)	20 (1)	34 (3)	91 (11)	-4 (2)	2 (3)	-17 (4)
C(14)	3394 (3)	3028 (4)	1840 (8)	26 (2)	42 (3)	80 (11)	-10 (2)	1 (3)	-6 (4)
C(15)	3802 (3)	3713 (5)	2522 (9)	27 (2)	43 (3)	112 (13)	-8 (2)	-3 (4)	2 (5)
C(16)	4662 (4)	2836 (7)	2845 (15)	24 (2)	83 (6)	395 (26)	5 (3)	28 (6)	-62 (11)
C(17)	4426 (4)	4024 (7)	4476 (11)	35 (2)	89 (6)	161 (16)	-17 (3)	-15 (5)	-28 (8)

dropped to 18.9%. At this stage, 675 unobserved reflections, estimated as $\frac{1}{3} |F_{min}|$ of the appropriate layer line, were included, and a further six cycles with anisotropic temperature factors for all atoms (excluding hydrogen atoms) were computed. In the last cycle the average parameter shifts expressed as fractions of the e.s.d.'s were about 0.3 for x-coordinates, 0.5 for y- and z-coordinates. The final R-index for 2,560 reflections is 11.4%. The f-values used in the least-squares calculations are those given by Hanson et al. (9). Final atomic parameters and their standard deviations are given in Table 2.

Discussion

Figure 1 shows the structure of the molecule and bond lengths and angles. Table 3 gives interatomic distances, angles, and thermal-motion parameters with associated standard deviations which were calculated from the results of the last refinement cycle by the Busing-Levy program ORFFE (10). The quoted errors include allowance for errors in cell dimensions.

The C—C bond lengths within the benzene rings are all between 1.38 and 1.43 Å; the average value for each benzene ring is 1.40 Å which is in good

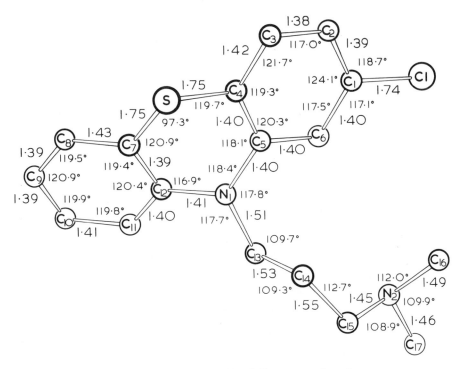

FIG. 1. Chlorpromazine: Bond distances and angles.

TABLE 3. *Bond lengths and angles of chlorpromazine*

Bond		ℓ	Angle			θ
C(1)	– C(2)	1.39 Å	C(6)	– C(1)	– C(2)	124.1(7)°
C(2)	– C(3)	1.38	C(1)	– C(2)	– C(3)	117.0(7)
C(3)	– C(4)	1.42	C(2)	– C(3)	– C(4)	121.7(7)
C(4)	– C(5)	1.40	C(3)	– C(4)	– C(5)	119.3(7)
C(5)	– C(6)	1.40	C(4)	– C(5)	– C(6)	120.3(6)
C(6)	– C(1)	1.40	C(5)	– C(6)	– C(1)	117.5(7)
C(7)	– C(8)	1.43	C(12)	– C(7)	– C(8)	119.4(7)
C(8)	– C(9)	1.39	C(7)	– C(8)	– C(9)	119.5(8)
C(9)	– C(10)	1.39	C(8)	– C(9)	– C(10)	120.9(8)
C(10)	– C(11)	1.41	C(9)	– C(10)	– C(11)	119.9(8)
C(11)	– C(12)	1.40	C(10)	– C(11)	– C(12)	119.8(8)
C(12)	– C(7)	1.39	C(11)	– C(12)	– C(7)	120.4(7)
C(7)	– S	1.75	C(4)	– S	– C(7)	97.3(3)
C(4)	– S	1.75	S	– C(7)	– C(12)	120.9(6)
C(12)	– N(1)	1.41	C(7)	– C(12)	– N(1)	116.9(6)
C(5)	– N(1)	1.40	C(12)	– N(1)	– C(5)	118.4(5)
			N(1)	– C(5)	– C(4)	118.1(6)
N(1)	– C(13)	1.51	C(5)	– C(4)	– S	119.7(5)
C(13)	– C(14)	1.53				
C(14)	– C(15)	1.55	C(12)	– N(1)	– C(13)	117.7(5)
C(15)	– N(2)	1.45	C(5)	– N(1)	– C(13)	117.8(5)
N(2)	– C(16)	1.49	C(1)	– C(13)	– C(14)	109.7(5)
N(2)	– C(17)	1.46	C(13)	– C(14)	– C(15)	109.3(6)
			C(14)	– C(15)	– N(2)	112.7(6)
Cl	– C(1)	1.74	C(15)	– N(2)	– C(16)	112.0(8)
Cl	– C(16)	4.10	C(15)	– N(2)	– C(17)	108.9(7)
Cl	– S	6.24	C(16)	– N(2)	– C(17)	109.9(7)
Cl	– C (T)	3.34	Cl	– C(1)	– C(2)	118.7(6)
Cl	– S(4)	4.47	Cl	– C(1)	– C(6)	117.1(6)
Cl	– S(4)	6.26				
N(2)	– S(3)	5.37				
N(2)	– S(2)	5.45				
N(2)	– Cl(3)	4.71				
N(2)	– Cl(3)	5.28				

The estimated standard deviations in the bond lengths are all 0.01Å.
Deviations in the bond angles ($\times$ 10) are given in parentheses.

agreement with the values reported for benzene: 1.397 Å (11), 1.392 Å (12), 1.394 Å (13).

The C—Cl bond length is 1.74 ± 0.01 Å; this is a typical C (aromatic)—Cl bond distance, although the value given by Sutton (13) is 1.70 ± 0.01 Å. Palenik et al. (14) tabulated 26 C—Cl bond distances reported between the years 1959 and 1968 in various aromatic molecules. Each distance involves a chlorine atom bonded to only one other atom. Of the bond lengths tabulated, four are equal to or greater than 1.76 Å, six have values between 1.71 and 1.72 Å, and 16 have values between 1.73 and 1.75 Å. The average value of the 26 bonds reported is 1.737 ± 0.016 Å, which is in excellent agreement with the result reported above.

The S—C bonds are 1.75 ± 0.01 Å, which implies double-bond character of about 13%. This is close to other values in similar aromatic substances: e.g., thianthrene, 1.76 Å (15); phenoxthionine, 1.75 Å (16); phenothiazine, 1.77 Å (1). The C—S—C angle (97.3°) is much less than the C—N—C angle (118.4°). The implication of the difference in angles and the contraction of the S—C bond will be discussed in the next section.

The best planes for the two benzene rings were obtained by the method of Schomaker et al. (17) with the program *LSPLANE,* and are given by

$$-0.4353x - 0.3576y + 0.8262z = -1.8684 \text{ for C(1)—C(6),}$$
$$0.1603x - 0.6920y + 0.7039z = 0.7144 \text{ for C(7)—C(12).}$$

The maximum displacement of any carbon atom from these planes is 0.01 Å, which is not significant. The Cl atom is 0.035 Å from the plane of the attached benzene ring; S and N however are not at the intersection of the two planes; i.e., the tricyclic group does not have a plane of symmetry through the S—N axis.

The dihedral angle between the two planes of the benzene rings is 139.4°, and is very close to that found by Hosoya (16) for phenoxthionine. The folding of the molecule, the difference in the angles of the type C—N—C and C—S—C, and the shortening of the C—S bond are characteristic of a number of heterocyclic compounds derived by replacing anthracene *meso*–CH groups by atoms A and B. It has been found that molecules are planar if both A and B are any of C, N, or O, but folded if at least one of A and B is S, Se or Te. The X—S(Se,Te)−X angles that have been determined are in the range 93 to 100° e.g., thianthrene (15), phenothiazine (1, 18, 19), phenoxthionine (16, 18). According to Lynton and Cox (15) and Hosoya (20), this is explained by assuming the participation of *d* orbitals in the bonding of S and S-like atoms. The valence orbitals in atoms of the second period such as C, N, and O are limited to 2*s* and 2*p* or hybrids of the two, but sulfur can be converted to the excited configuration $(3s)^2 (3p)^3 (3d)$. The folding of the molecule enables the sulfur atom to retain its "natural" valency angle. The quantum mechanical treatment of Craig and Magnusson (21) lends support to the above theory.

The molecular packing in the unit cell is given in Figs. 2 and 3. Four of the molecules are "left-handed," and the other four are "right-handed" enantiomorphs. Figure 3, which represents half the contents of the unit cell from 0 to *b*/2, shows clearly that the molecules are arranged in layers of width *a*/2, with the axis of the fold alternately left and right in the *z*-direction.

THIETHYLPERAZINE

Thiethylperazine (trade name Torecan®) is 2-ethylthio-10-|3-(4-methyl-piperazine-1-yl)propyl|phenothiazine. It is valued mainly for its antiemetic properties and is used for the control of postoperative vomiting, vomiting associated with malignant disease, radiation therapy, etc.

Although the phenothiazines have been subjected to extensive clinical tests, their chemical structural features have not so far been found to have a sufficiently constant association with pharmacological, psychological,

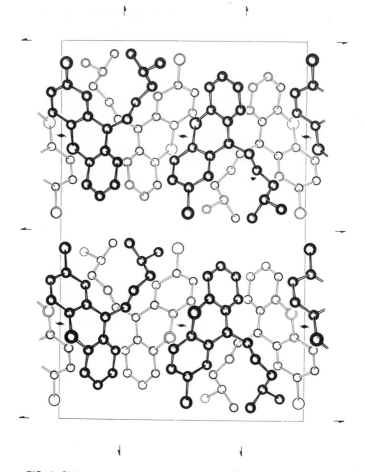

FIG. 2. Chlorpromazine. The structure viewed down the c axis.

and clinical effects to develop a theory of their mode of action. It seems likely that in seeking the precise mechanism of action of the drugs, the problems must be "viewed through the glasses of the submolecular" (22).

Solution and Refinement of the Structure

Colorless transparent prismatic crystals were prepared by evaporation from a warmed solution of thiethylperazine in petroleum spirit. X-ray oscillation and Weissenberg photographs, with the use of Ni-filtered $CuK\alpha$ radiation, taken about the x and y axes, gave an orthorhombic system with $a = 12.056 \pm 0.02$, $b = 19.952 \pm 0.03$, and $c = 9.204 \pm 0.01$ Å, in close agreement with the diffractometer values obtained subsequently: $a = 12.057 \pm 0.01$, $b = 19.953 \pm 0.01$, and $c = 9.215 \pm 0.01$ Å. The latter

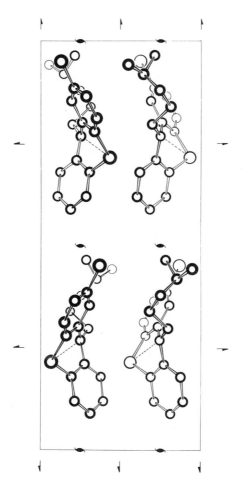

FIG. 3. Perspective drawing of half the contents of the unit cell (from 0 to $b/2$) viewed down the b axis. All molecules from 0 to $a/2$ are folded downward about the S–N axis (dashed lines); all molecules from $a/2$ to a are folded upward.

values were considered more accurate and were used in all calculations. The conditions for nonextinction were found to be hoo, $h = 2n$; oko, $k = 2n$; ool, $l = 2n$, which uniquely determined the space group as $P2_12_12_1$. $D_m = 1.187$ g/cc, $D_c = 1.198$ g/cc for four molecules per unit cell.

Using specially devised apparatus, cubic-cut crystals were ground into near-perfect spheres of 0.04 cm diameter and mounted on glass rods along one of their axes, the directions of which were located as the directions of extinction under a polarizing microscope. Because crystals exposed to air turned yellow within a few hours, it was found necessary to coat selected crystals immediately with a thin layer of low-absorbent polyvinylacetate.

The most suitable crystal was mounted on a Hilger and Watts automatic diffractometer and exposed to Zr-filtered MoKα radiation. The measured data extended to h, k, l(max) = 14, 23, 10, respectively; subsequently it was found that more than 98% of the reflections with h, k, $l >$ 12, 17, 8, respectively, were not measurable; therefore, the 2,200 reflections originally recorded were reduced to about 1,400 in the refinement (i.e., about 56% of the CuKα sphere was utilized).

The standard deviation was calculated and I_{min} was estimated to be approximately $3 \times \dfrac{\Sigma\sigma^2}{n(n-1)}^{1/2}$. Peak intensities which were less than I_{min} were recorded as $\frac{1}{2} I_{min}$ and the corresponding F values are treated as F_{unobs}.

Preliminary scale and temperature factors were estimated by Wilson's method. Absorption corrections were not applied since the value of μR for MoKα = 0.05.

A three-dimensional, unsharpened Patterson function was computed and gave 30 possible Harker vectors in $\frac{1}{8}$th unit-cell. A more useful, sharpened Patterson function, $P'(uvw)$, was also calculated which, by a considerably improved resolution of closely neighboring peaks, provided 63 vectors. The sharpened Patterson function was developed by Jacobson et al. (23) and Spencer and Lipscomb (24) and may be expressed as

$$P'(uvw) = Q(uvw) + KP(uvw), \tag{1}$$

where P is the usual sharpened Patterson function and Q is a "gradient" sharpened Patterson function, given by

$$Q(uvw) = V \int_0^1 \int_0^1 \int_0^1 \nabla\rho(xyz) \cdot \nabla\rho(x+u,y+v,z+w)$$

$$\times \, \mathrm{dx} \, \mathrm{dy} \, \mathrm{dz} \, \alpha \frac{1}{V} \sum_h \sum_k \sum_l \frac{\sin^2 \theta}{\lambda^2} \tag{2}$$

$$\times |F_{hkl}|^2 \cos 2\pi(hu + kv + lw).$$

The value empirically chosen for K was $\frac{1}{6}$, as it was found that a small contribution of the function P added to the gradient function decreased the negative regions around the sharpened peaks. In both functions Q and P, the $|F_{hkl}|^2$ were the usual sharpened coefficients,

$$|F_{hkl}|^2 = F_0^2 \exp (B \sin^2 \theta/\lambda^2)/(\Sigma_i f_i)^2. \tag{3}$$

Equations 1, 2, and 3, together with the value of $\frac{1}{6}$ for K, lead to the relation

$$|F|^2 = \left(\sin^2 \theta/\lambda^2 + \frac{1}{6}\right)F_0^2 \exp (B \sin^2 \theta/\lambda^2)/(\Sigma_i f_i)^2,$$

for the sharpened Patterson coefficients, which was the formula used for thiethylperazine.

TABLE 4. *Thiethylperazine: Final atomic fractional coordinates* $(\times 10^4)$ *and thermal parameters* $(\times 10^4)$ *with estimated standard deviations*

Anisotropic temperature factor = exp $\{-(h^2\beta_{11} + k^2\beta_{22} + l^2\beta_{33} + 2hk\beta_{12} + 2hl\beta_{13} + 2kl\beta_{23})\}$ with

$$\beta_{11} = 2\pi^2 a^{*2} U_{11}, \quad \beta_{12} = 2\pi^2 a^* b^* U_{12}, \text{ etc.}$$

The least-squares standard errors are given in parentheses.
Isotropic temperature factors are given in the last column.

	x	y	z	β_{11}	β_{22}	β_{33}	β_{12}	β_{13}	β_{23}	B
S(1)	1729 (4)	3003 (2)	0905 (6)	91 (4)	28 (1)	264 (10)	-9 (2)	30 (6)	8 (3)	5.83
S(2)	0079 (3)	5809 (2)	3137 (5)	73 (3)	41 (2)	138 (6)	-3 (2)	16 (4)	-24 (3)	4.93
N(1)	2181 (8)	5584 (5)	1552 (13)	45 (8)	22 (4)	145 (18)	-10 (5)	36 (10)	4 (7)	3.50
N(2)	5626 (8)	5272 (6)	2031 (13)	38 (7)	36 (5)	112 (18)	-9 (5)	-5 (9)	4 (7)	3.66
N(3)	6933 (9)	4193 (7)	3230 (15)	68 (9)	44 (5)	165 (22)	1 (6)	16 (13)	15 (9)	4.80
C(1)	1302 (12)	3823 (8)	1455 (16)	64 (11)	30 (5)	130 (24)	4 (7)	-38 (15)	-19 (9)	4.24
C(2)	1941 (10)	4380 (7)	1168 (16)	44 (9)	13 (4)	188 (25)	-14 (6)	-23 (15)	-1 (8)	2.98
C(3)	1567 (10)	4998 (7)	1689 (15)	39 (9)	26 (5)	106 (20)	-11 (6)	10 (12)	26 (8)	3.13
C(4)	0525 (12)	5030 (7)	2401 (16)	90 (13)	23 (5)	121 (23)	-11 (7)	15 (15)	10 (8)	3.79
C(5)	-0127 (14)	4449 (9)	2565 (16)	84 (14)	45 (7)	88 (20)	-5 (8)	-5 (14)	9 (9)	4.20
C(6)	0252 (13)	3837 (8)	2125 (18)	75 (14)	33 (6)	154 (26)	-6 (7)	12 (16)	-2 (10)	4.52
C(7)	0604 (11)	6354 (8)	1770 (15)	69 (11)	29 (5)	75 (18)	-1 (6)	-7 (13)	-15 (8)	3.69
C(8)	1602 (12)	6194 (7)	1106 (16)	80 (12)	25 (5)	107 (21)	-9 (7)	18 (14)	3 (8)	4.13
C(9)	2024 (13)	6608 (7)	0010 (17)	91 (14)	17 (4)	163 (26)	-8 (7)	10 (16)	-9 (8)	4.10
C(10)	1440 (16)	7188 (9)	-0348 (22)	100 (17)	43 (7)	217 (34)	-8 (9)	-39 (22)	-9 (13)	6.18
C(11)	0449 (17)	7340 (9)	0313 (23)	121 (19)	36 (7)	230 (37)	-18 (10)	-17 (23)	-15 (14)	5.77
C(12)	0003 (14)	6930 (9)	1390 (21)	81 (13)	33 (6)	256 (35)	-4 (8)	-65 (21)	-41 (12)	5.40
C(13)	3374 (12)	5534 (7)	1176 (19)	61 (11)	22 (5)	213 (29)	1 (6)	4 (16)	-4 (9)	3.67
C(14)	4044 (11)	6067 (7)	2007 (18)	57 (10)	29 (5)	147 (24)	-7 (6)	4 (14)	-3 (9)	4.12
C(15)	5288 (10)	5957 (7)	1690 (16)	61 (10)	23 (5)	136 (23)	-2 (6)	-11 (14)	24 (9)	3.98
C(16)	5698 (13)	5151 (8)	3652 (15)	81 (13)	36 (5)	87 (20)	8 (7)	4 (14)	9 (8)	4.84
C(17)	5934 (12)	4408 (9)	3925 (21)	65 (12)	47 (7)	223 (33)	6 (8)	46 (17)	8 (13)	5.29
C(18)	7176 (15)	3469 (9)	3484 (26)	118 (17)	38 (6)	349 (48)	25 (9)	16 (26)	77 (15)	7.66
C(19)	6923 (12)	4325 (8)	1645 (17)	79 (12)	37 (6)	130 (25)	1 (7)	-4 (15)	1 (10)	4.93
C(20)	6688 (11)	5081 (8)	1389 (15)	66 (11)	44 (6)	77 (20)	9 (7)	-1 (13)	20 (9)	3.95
C(21)	3192 (18)	3104 (9)	0453 (27)	136 (21)	33 (7)	380 (52)	9 (10)	97 (30)	21 (16)	7.71
C(22)	3673 (24)	2454. (14)	0180 (39)	207 (33)	69 (10)	559 (75)	26 (16)	210 (45)	-11 (24)	12.43

The combination of the Harker vectors of the sharpened function led to 34 possible sets of coordinates, of which two were eventually correctly assigned to the two sulfur atoms. Six successive three-dimensional Fourier and difference Fourier syntheses gave the locations of the three nitrogen and 22 carbon atoms. The Fourier synthesis gave evidence of considerable thermal motion among some of the atoms, notably $C(22)$, $C(21)$, $C(18)$, $C(10)$, and $C(11)$, as well as of the anisotropic character of the S atoms. At this stage the value of R for observed reflexions was 18.7%.

The structure was refined by four least-squares cycles with the use of the Busing et al. program $ORFLS(8)$. The function minimized was $R_1 = \Sigma W(hkl)\{|F_0(hkl)| - |F_c(hkl)|\}^2$ with equal weight given to each term. Individual isotropic temperature factors were assigned and F_{unobs} were included. The number of F_{obs} was only 892, which was unfortunately insufficient to carry out a meaningful anisotropic cycle in which there were 244 parameters to be varied. From this point, therefore, the refinement was continued along two separate lines: six cycles were carried out using 1,418 F values (including about 500 F_{unobs}) and anisotropic temperature factors, resulting in a final R index for all reflections of 0.113; six cycles were carried out using 892 F_{obs} and isotropic temperature factors, resulting in a final R index of 0.105. The refinement was terminated when the average parameter shifts were approximately 10% of the estimated standard deviations. The analytical f values used in all calculations are those given by Hanson et al. (9). Table 4 gives the final atomic positional parameters and anisotropic thermal-motion parameters with their standard deviations which were obtained in the final cycle. The last column of Table 4 lists the isotropic temperature factors obtained at the end of the 13th cycle.

Patterson and Fourier syntheses were carried out on an ICT 1301 computer. An IBM 360/65 computer was used for the correction calculations and the least-squares refinements.

Discussion

The structure of the molecule and bond lengths and angles are shown in Fig. 4. Table 5 lists the interatomic distances and angles with associated e.s.d.'s, which were calculated from the results of the last refinement cycle using the Busing et al. program $ORFEE(10)$.

The Tricyclic Group

All C—C distances are between 1.37 and 1.42 Å, and the mean length of the C—C bonds within the first benzene ring, $C(1)$—$C(6)$, which is 1.396 Å, and that of the second ring, $C(7)$—$C(12)$, 1.393 Å, compare favorably with accepted values for benzene: 1.397 Å (25) 1.394 Å (13).

Applying Cruickshank's (26) criterion to the two C—N(1) bonds of 1.39,

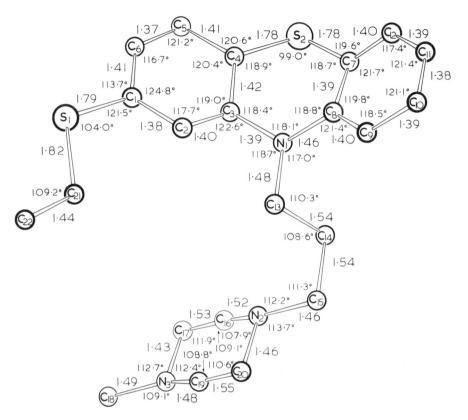

FIG. 4. Thiethylperazine: Bond distances and angles.

1.46 ± 0.015 Å, which should be expected to be chemically equivalent, the value obtained for $(l_1 - l_2)/(\sigma_1^2 + \sigma_2^2)^{1/2}$ is 3.5, which is in the zone of probable significance. However, no explanation for a significant difference in the two bonds can be suggested, as the N(1) atom is in a symmetrical environment and secluded from short intermolecular contacts. It appears more likely that the discrepancy would be reduced if the following factors, *inter alia,* were taken into consideration: (a) the bonds are not independent since a change in the position of N(1) would affect both lengths; (b) corrections for temperature librations, which could amount to as much as 0.02Å (27), have not been applied; and (c) as discussed above, the number of measurable reflections was unfortunately limited by the nature of the compound.

Abrahams (28) has calculated a value of 1.82 Å for a C—S single-bond distance, which is close to the sum of the covalent radii for sulfur and carbon given by Pauling (25). Using Pauling's relation $R = R_s - (R_s - R_D)3x/(2x + 1)$ for the resonance-interatomic distance curve, the value of x obtained for the C—S(2) bond lengths (which are both 1.78 ± 0.015 Å) is

TABLE 5. *Bond lengths and angles of thiethylperazine*

Bond		ℓ	Angle			θ
C(1)	– C(2)	1.38(2) Å	C(6)	– C(1)	– C(2)	124.8°(1.4°)
C(2)	– C(3)	1.40(2)	C(1)	– C(2)	– C(3)	117.7 (1.2)
C(3)	– C(4)	1.42(2)	C(2)	– C(3)	– C(4)	119.0 (1.2)
C(4)	– C(5)	1.41(2)	C(3)	– C(4)	– C(5)	120.4 (1.4)
C(5)	– C(6)	1.37(2)	C(4)	– C(5)	– C(6)	121.2 (1.4)
C(6)	– C(1)	1.41(2)	C(5)	– C(6)	– C(1)	116.7 (1.4)
C(7)	– C(8)	1.39(2)	C(12)	– C(7)	– C(8)	121.7 (1.5)
C(8)	– C(9)	1.40(2)	C(7)	– C(8)	– C(9)	119.8 (1.4)
C(9)	– C(10)	1.39(2_5)	C(8)	– C(9)	– C(10)	118.5 (1.6)
C(10)	– C(11)	1.38(2_5)	C(9)	– C(10)	– C(11)	121.1 (1.9)
C(11)	– C(12)	1.39(2_5)	C(10)	– C(11)	– C(12)	121.4 (1.9)
C(12)	– C(7)	1.40(2)	C(11)	– C(12)	– C(7)	117.4 (1.6)
C(4)	– S(2)	1.78(1_5)	S(2)	– C(4)	– C(3)	118.9 (1.1)
C(7)	– S(2)	1.78(1_5)	C(4)	– C(3)	– N(1)	118.4 (1.3)
C(3)	– N(1)	1.39(1_5)	C(3)	– N(1)	– C(8)	118.1 (1.0)
C(8)	– N(1)	1.46(1_5)	N(1)	– C(8)	– C(7)	118.8 (1.3)
S(1)	– C(1)	1.79(1_5)	C(8)	– C(7)	– S(2)	118.7 (1.2)
S(1)	– C(21)	1.82(2)	C(7)	– S(2)	– C(4)	99.0 (0.7)
C(21)	– C(22)	1.44(3)	C(6)	– C(1)	– S(1)	113.7 (1.2)
N(1)	– C(13)	1.48(1_5)	C(2)	– C(1)	– S(1)	121.5 (1.1)
C(13)	– C(14)	1.54(2)	C(1)	– S(1)	– C(21)	104.0 (0.8)
C(14)	– C(15)	1.54(2)	S(1)	– C(21)	– C(22)	109.2 (1.6)
C(15)	– N(2)	1.46(1_5)	C(3)	– N(1)	– C(13)	118.7 (1.1)
N(2)	– C(16)	1.52(2)	C(8)	– N(1)	– C(13)	117.0 (1.1)
C(16)	– C(17)	1.53(2)	N(1)	– C(13)	– C(14)	110.3 (1.2)
C(17)	– N(3)	1.43(2)	C(13)	– C(14)	– C(15)	108.6 (1.2)
N(3)	– C(19)	1.48(2)	C(14)	– C(15)	– N(2)	111.3 (1.1)
C(19)	– C(20)	1.55(2)	C(15)	– N(2)	– C(16)	112.2 (1.2)
C(20)	– N(2)	1.46(1_5)	C(15)	– N(2)	– C(20)	113.7 (1.1)
N(3)	– C(18)	1.49(2)	C(20)	– N(2)	– C(16)	107.9 (1.1)
			N(2)	– C(16)	– C(17)	109.1 (1.3)
			C(16)	– C(17)	– N(3)	111.9 (1.4)
			C(17)	– N(3)	– C(19)	112.4 (1.3)
			N(3)	– C(19)	– C(20)	108.8 (1.3)
			C(19)	– C(20)	– N(2)	110.6 (1.2)
			C(17)	– N(3)	– C(18)	112.7 (1.5)
			C(19)	– N(3)	– C(18)	109.1 (1.5)
			C(2)	– C(3)	– N(1)	122.6 (1.2)
			N(1)	– C(8)	– C(9)	121.4 (1.4)
			C(5)	– C(4)	– S(2)	120.6 (1.2)
			S(2)	– C(7)	– C(12)	119.6 (1.3)

The estimated standard deviations in the bond lengths ($\times 10^2$) and deviations in the bond angles are given in parentheses.

0.07; i.e., they have 7% double-bond character. (Abrahams' bond-order, bond-length curve gives a value of 25%.)

The angles of the heterocyclic ring are all approximately 118° except for the C—S—C angle which is 99.0 ± 0.7°. Table 6 lists a number of compounds of interest for comparative purposes. It can be seen that C—S—C angles are all in the range 93 to 100°, and that all C—S lengths are shorter than a C—S single-bond. Further, the tricyclic molecules which contain S are folded with a dihedral angle of approximately 140°.

The size of the C—S—C angles, the folding of the molecules, and the contraction of the C—S bonds in substituted anthracene-type molecules may possibly be explained in terms of the π–bonding molecular orbitals formed by the carbon atoms with the 3d orbitals of the sulfur atom. The

TABLE 6. Comparison of bond lengths and angles in heterocyclic compounds containing sulfur.

Compound	Chemical Formula	C–S–C (°)	C–S (Å)	C–N (Å)	Dihedral angle (°)	Reference
Thiophene		91±4 / 92.16±0.10	1.74 ±0.03 / 1.714±0.002	– / –	– / –	(a) (b) (c)
Thianthrene		100±0.5	1.76 ±0.015	–	128	(d) (e) (f)
Phenoxthionine		97.7±0.03	1.75±0.04	–	138	(d) (g) (h)
Phenothiazine		99.6±1.5	1.770±0.003	1.406±0.002	153.3	(d) (g) (i)
Chlorpromazine		97.3±0.3	1.75±0.01	1.41±0.01	139.4	(j)
Thiethylperazine		99.0±0.7	1.78±0.02	1.425±0.02	139.0	(k)

a) Schomaker & Pauling (1939).[29]
b) Longuet-Higgins (1949).[30]
c) Bak,Christensen, Hansen-Nygaard & Rastrup-Anderson (1961).[37]
d) Cullinane & Rees (1940).[18]
e) Lynton & Cox (1956).[15]
f) Rowe & Post (1958) [38]
g) Wood, McCale & Williams (1941).[19]
h) Hosoya (1966).[16]
i) Bell, Blount, Briscoe & Freeman (1968).[1]
j) McDowell (1969).[39]
k) McDowell (1970).[40]

suggestion that S in heterocyclic compounds can have a decet of electrons was first made by Schomaker and Pauling (29), and calculations of the molecular orbitals in thiophene were subsequently performed by Longuet-Higgins (30). In thiethylperazine it is possible that the $2p_z$ atomic orbitals of the C atoms conjugate with hybrid orbitals formed from linear combinations of the $3p_z$, $3d_{yz}$, and $3d_{xz}$ atomic orbitals of the S atom.

The best planes for the two benzene rings were calculated by the method of Schomaker et al. (17), with the program *LSPLANE* and are given by

$$-0.4453x + 0.1523y - 0.8824z = -0.6911 \text{ for C(1)—C(6)},$$
$$0.4963x + 0.5202y + 0.6950z = 8.0889 \text{ for C(7)—C(12)}.$$

The maximum deviation of the C atoms is 0.03 Å so that the benzene rings may be regarded as planar, within the limits of error. The S and N atoms, however, do not lie in both planes of the aromatic rings, as is also the case with phenothiazine and chlorpromazine. The dihedral angle between the planes is 139.0°, in close agreement with that in chlorpromazine but differing by 14° from that in phenothiazine.

Aliphatic Chains and Piperazine Ring

When the C(21)—C(22) bond is compared with a C—C single bond of 1.54 Å, the value obtained for $\delta l/\sigma$ is 3.3, which again is in the zone of probable significance. Double-bond character of a C—C bond in such a position would be most unusual, and it does seem more likely that the standard deviations in the positions of the two atoms with high thermal motion may have been underestimated.

The differences in the angles C(2)—C(1)—S(1) (121.5°) and C(6)—C(1)—S(1) (113.7°) are probably caused by steric hindrance between the hydrogen atoms attached to C(2) and C(21). The angles centered at N(1) are nearly trigonally symmetric, and the angles between the chain carbon atoms are quite close to the tetrahedral value (109°28′).

The average value of the six C—N bonds associated with the piperazine ring is 1.47 Å, which is close to the value given by Kennard (31) for three-covalent nitrogen (1.472 Å for sp^2–sp^3 bond type), but the individual bonds vary between 1.43 and 1.52 Å. It was shown by Kitajgorodskij (32) that the effects of intermolecular interaction on molecular shape are generally small, but that the packing can affect the molecular geometry in some cases. The atoms of the piperazine ring have a number of contacts shorter than 3.85 Å; also the distance between C(16) and benzene ring I of molecule (2) is 3.67 Å, and that between C(17) and benzene ring II is 3.73 Å. It seems possible that the slight distortions in the ring may be partly attributed to molecular close packing requirements. The piperazine ring has the chair configuration.

Molecular Packing

In Figs. 5 and 6 the packing in the crystal is viewed along the c and a axes, respectively. The molecules are arranged in parallel undulating layers perpendicular to the yz plane.

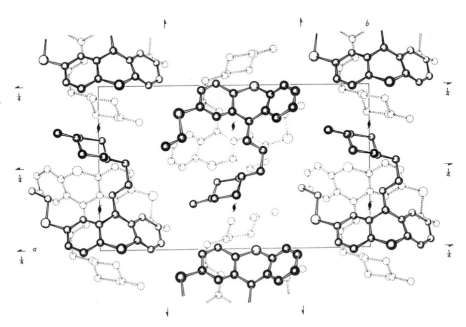

FIG. 5. The structure viewed down the c axis.

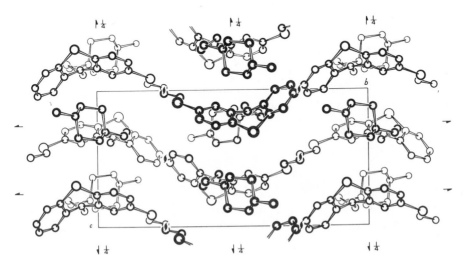

FIG. 6. The structure viewed down the a axis.

Unlike chlorpromazine, one enantiomorph only appears in the crystal. The molecular dissymmetry suggested the study of the optical activity of solutions of the compound. A 2.5% solution of powdered thiethylperazine in absolute alcohol was tested in the polarimeter using sodium *D* light and, as expected, was found to be optically inactive. Further experiments are in progress to investigate the optical activity of this material, and it is hoped to establish whether the crystals exhibit enantiomorphism.

Thermal Vibration Ellipsoids

The thermal vibration ellipsoids of chlorpromazine and thiethylperazine were calculated from the temperature factors in Tables 2 and 4 using Johnson's program *ORTEP*(33). The results are shown in Fig. 7.

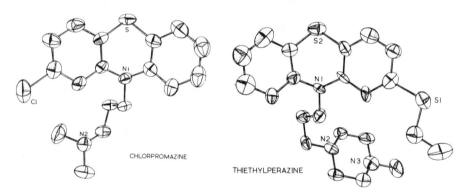

FIG. 7. Thermal vibration ellipsoids of chlorpromazine (left) and thiethylperazine (right).

Molecular Structure and Mechanism of Action

Although the phenothiazine derivatives form a vast class, the most useful ones have substituents at positions $2(R_1)$, and $10(R_2)$, and may be considered as consisting of two parts:

1. The R_2 Substituent

Effects on the higher centers of the nervous system only appear in earnest when the side chain consists of three carbon atoms in a row. It could be surmised that a substance of this molecular size fits best into the biological binding site (structure 1).

STRUCTURE 1.

The phenothiazine "nucleus" ($R_1 = R_2 = H$).

2. The Phenothiazine Nucleus and R_1 Substituent.

The phenothiazine nucleus consists of a system of conjugated double bonds having an extensive π pool of delocalized electrons and lone pairs of electrons on the N and S atoms. Chlorpromazine, thiethylperazine, and phenothiazine have closely similar structural features (Table 6) apart from the different dihedral angle in phenothiazine, which may possibly be of importance. The psychotropic potency is affected by the substituent forming all or part of R_1 in the ascending order H, S, Cl, F. It is of significance that this is in parallel with the order of increasing electronegativity of the atoms.

Although attempts to correlate molecular structure with biochemical action must be highly tentative owing, among other factors, to the complex nature of the action mechanism of the drugs (34), a suggestion has been made by Szent-Györgyi (22) which is of considerable interest and is compatible with the results of the present study. According to Szent-Györgyi, there are many factors tending to suggest that charge transfer is involved in biological activity, the drugs acting as electron donors or acceptors.

Using the LCAO approximation of the molecular orbital method, the energy levels of many molecules taking part in different biological reactions have been determined (35). Chlorpromazine was found (36) to have a most unusual antibonding highest-filled orbital in its normal, stable state, and is thus an exceedingly strong monovalent electron donor.

Thiethylperazine has little tranquilizing action, whereas prochlorperazine has five times, and trifluperazine 10 times the potency of chlorpromazine. The determination of the k values of these substances would be of considerable interest as it might lead to a direct relationship between potency and electron-donating properties, and provide further support for the theory that pharmacological action is due to a charge transfer.

The k values of phenothiazine have been determined and are found to be quite close to those of chlorpromazine. Since phenothiazine is *not* a psychotropically potent drug, it is therefore evident that the donor-acceptor properties must be combined with a suitable molecular complement, which it appears likely is provided by the R_2 substituent.

Szent-Györgyi brings forward some evidence in support of the fascinating suggestion that schizophrenia may be due to the presence of a strong electron acceptor in the blood (e.g., bilirubin, which inhibits production of hematoporphyrins and also inhibits oxidative phosphorylation). If such is the case, then the inactivation of this substance by a strong donor, such as chlorpromazine, affords the possible key to the mechanism of action. More exciting still, precise investigation of the nature of the electron acceptor causing the damage may lead eventually not only to permanent cure for the psychotically abnormal, but also to the prevention of this tragic disease.

SUMMARY

The molecular structure of *chlorpromazine* has been determined from three-dimensional X-ray diffraction data and refined by least-squares methods, using individual anisotropic temperature factors (structure 2). The space group is *Pbca* with $a = 23.50 \pm 0.04$ Å, $b = 15.20 \pm 0.02$ Å, $c = 9.23 \pm 0.01$ A. The molecule is folded about the S—N axis, and the angle between the best planes for the two benzene rings was found to be 139.4°. The C—S—C angle is $97.3 \pm 0.3°$; the C—S bonds are 1.75 ± 0.01 Å; and C—Cl is 1.74 ± 0.01 Å.

STRUCTURE 2.

The contraction of the C—S bond, the size of the C—S—C angle, and the folding of the molecule are characteristic of a number of related compounds, and can be explained by assuming the participation of d orbitals in the bonding of S.

The molecular structure of the phenothiazine derivative *thiethylperazine* has been determined from diffractometer data and refined with individual anisotropic thermal parameters by the least-squares methods to a final residual of 10.5% (structure 3). The space group is $P2_12_12_1$ with $a = 12.057 \pm 0.01$, $b = 19.953 \pm 0.01$, and $c = 9.215 \pm 0.01$ Å. The tricyclic group has a C—S—C angle of $99.0 \pm 0.7°$ and C—S bonds of 1.78 ± 0.02 Å, indicating the participation of d orbitals in the bonding of S. The dihedral angle between the two planes of the benzene rings is 139.0°. The piperazine ring has the chair configuration. A theory of charge transfer is discussed in connection with the action mechanism of the phenothiazines.

STRUCTURE 3.

ACKNOWLEDGMENTS

The author is indebted to the University Research Grants Committee, and to the Council for Scientific and Industrial Research for the use of their automatic diffractometer and for computing grants. Appreciation is recorded to Professor W. Schaffer and to Dr. M. H. Linck of the University of Cape Town for their interest and support. The author thanks the members of the crystallography division of the C.S.I.R., and gratefully acknowledges the generous assistance and skilled advice given by the head of the division, Dr. G. Gafner, who also organized the collection of the diffractometer data.

REFERENCES

1. Bell, J. D., Blount, J. F., Briscoe, O. V., and Freeman, H. C., *Chem. Comm., 1656*, (1968).
2. Delay, J., Deniker, P., and Harl, J. M., *Ann. Med. Psychol.*, **2**, 111 (1952).
3. *Colloque international chlorpromazine*, Doin et Cie, Paris, 1955.
4. Feil, D., Linck, M. H., and McDowell, J. J. H. *Nature*, **207**, 285 (1965).
5. Falkenberg, G., and Ringertz, H., *Acta Cryst.*, **23**, 1111 (1967).
6. Wilson, A. J. C., *Nature*, **150**, 151 (1942).
7. Berghuis, J., Haanappel, I. J. M., Potters, M., Loopstra, B. O., MacGillavry, C. H., and Veenendaal, A. L., *Acta Cryst.*, **8**, 478 (1955).
8. Busing, W. R., Martin, K. O., and Levy, H. A., USAEC Report ORNL-TM-305, Oak Ridge National Laboratory, Tennessee, 1962.
9. Hanson, H. P., Herman, F., Lea, J. D., and Skillman, S., *Acta Cryst.*, **17**, 1040 (1964).
10. Busing, W. R., Martin, K. O., and Levy, H. A., USAEC Report ORNL-TM-306, Oak Ridge National Laboratory, Tennessee, 1964.
11. Stoicheff, B. P., *Canad. J. Phys.*, **32**, 339 (1954).
12. Cox, E. G., Cruickshank, D. W. J., and Smith, J. A. S., *Proc. Roy. Soc.* **A247**, 1 (1958).
13. Sutton, L. E., *Tables of interatomic distances and configuration in molecules and ions*, Special Publication No. 18, The Chemical Society, London, 1965.
14. Palenik, G. H., Donohue, J., and Trueblood, K. N., *Acta Cryst.*, **B24**, 1139 (1968).
15. Lynton, H., and Cox, E. G., *J. Chem. Soc.*, 4886 (1956).
16. Hosoya, S., *Acta Cryst.*, **20**, 429 (1966).
17. Schomaker, V., Waser, J., Marsh, R. E. and Bergman, G., *Acta Cryst.* **12**, 600 (1959).
18. Cullinane, N. M., and Rees, W. T., *Trans. Faraday Soc.*, **36**, 507 (1940).

19. Wood, R. G., McCale, C. H., and Williams, G., *Phil. Mag.*, **31,** 71 (1941).
20. Hosoya, S., *Acta Cryst.*, **16,** 310 (1963).
21. Craig, D. P., and Magnusson, E. A., *J. Chem. Soc.*, 4895 (1965).
22. Szent-Györgyi, A., *Introduction to a submolecular biology*, Academic Press, New York, 1960.
23. Jacobson, R. A., Wunderlich, J. A., and Lipscomb, W. N., *Acta Cryst.*, **14,** 598 (1961).
24. Spencer, C. J., and Lipscomb, W. N., *Acta Cryst.*, **14,** 250 (1961).
25. Pauling, L., *The nature of the chemical bond*, Cornell Univ. Press, Ithaca, N.Y., 1960.
26. Cruickshank, D. W. J., *Acta Cryst.*, **2,** 65 (1949).
27. Cruickshank, D. W. J., *Acta Cryst.*, **13,** 774 (1960).
28. Abrahams, S. C., *Quart. Rev. Chem. Soc. London*, **10,** 407 (1956).
29. Schomaker, V., and Pauling, L. *J. Amer. Chem. Soc.*, **61,** 1769 (1939).
30. Longuet-Higgins, H. C., *Trans. Faraday Soc.*, **45,** 173 (1949).
31. Kennard, O., *International tables for x-ray crystallography*, Vol. III, Kynoch Press, Birmingham, 1962.
32. Kitajgorodskij, A. I., *Acta. Cryst.*, **18,** 585 (1965).
33. Johnson, C. K., ORNL-3794, Oak Ridge Laboratory, Oak Ridge, Tennessee, 1965.
34. *Scientific Basis of Drug Therapy in Psychiatry Symposium*, London, 1964.
35. Pullman, B., and Pullman, A., *Proc. Nat. Acad. Sci. Wash.*, **44,** 1197 (1958).
36. Karreman, G., Isenberg, I., and Szent-Györgyi, A., *Science*, **130,** 1191 (1959).
37. Bak, B., Christensen, D., Hansen-Nygaard, L., and Rastrup-Andersen, J., *J. Mol. Spect.*, **7,** 58 (1961).
38. Rowe, I., and Post, B., *Acta Cryst.*, **11,** 372 (1958).
39. McDowell, J. J. H., *Acta Cryst.*, **B25,** 2175 (1969).
40. McDowell, J. J. H., *Acta Cryst.*, **B26,** 954 (1970).

The Phenothiazines and Structurally Related Drugs, edited by I. S.
Forrest, C. J. Carr, and E. Usdin. Raven Press, New York © 1974.

Quantum Chemical and Other Theoretical Techniques for the Understanding of the Psychoactive Action of the Phenothiazines

Joyce J. Kaufman and Ellen Kerman*

*Division of Anesthesiology, Department of Surgery, The Johns Hopkins University
School of Medicine, Baltimore, Maryland 21205 and *Department of Chemistry,
The Johns Hopkins University, Baltimore, Maryland 21218*

INTRODUCTION

The neuroleptic drugs cover a wide and apparently diverse class of compounds, most of which have a similar mode of action. These molecules are quite large from the quantum chemical point of view, and one would like to focus on the conformational and electronic properties of the portions of the molecules vital for pharmacological action rather than have to analyze the quantum chemical results for the entire molecule. We started several concomitant paths of research.

One path was to perform quantum chemical computations on a series of neuroleptics [promazines, (1–4) perazines (1–4) and piperidopromazines (2–4)] to investigate their conformations and electronic distributions. By characterizing the electronic structures of these molecules, certain similar indices could point to a commonality. Molecules such as the perazines were larger than any previous compounds for which iterative molecular orbital calculations including even all valence electrons seemed ever to have been performed.

A second path of research was to set up the concepts of how topological and topographical analyses and systems analysis could be applied to unravel the mechanism of action of such drugs (2, 4, 5).

QUANTUM CHEMICAL CALCULATIONS

Theoretical Background

One of the major pieces of information that quantum chemical calculations can give is which possible low-energy conformations of a molecule are capable of existence. The crystal structure, when measured, is usually found among these, and some of the other permissible conformations may prove of importance in solution. However, one must use caution. The calculated lowest energy conformation may not correspond to the crystal structure, and it may not be possible from the crystallographic conformation to surmount the barriers to reach the calculated lowest energy conformation. We shall give examples of this.

Another major piece of information that quantum chemical calculations gives is the electronic charge distribution at each atom and between the atoms. This charge distribution is intimately connected to how a molecule behaves and what type of reactions and interactions it can undergo. The more closely the charge distributions of two related molecules resemble one another, the more probable it is that these molecules will interact in the same way. Semiempirical or semirigorous quantum chemical calculations have notable deficiencies in describing correctly the charge distributions at atoms, and certain of these methods have proven to be even less appropriate for describing the electron densities between atoms. The saving grace in such juxtapositions is that one makes comparisons between quantum chemical indices for reasonably related molecules calculated by the same theoretical technique.

Operationally, once a drug has reached its locus of action, there seem to be two main criteria governing whether or not it will be effective for a specific purpose. The first is the conformation of the drug — or at least of the vital part of it that is intimately connected to receptor site interaction. If the atoms are not in the correct spatial orientation, they will not fit into the receptor site and, thus, will be ineffective.

The second important factor is the electronic distribution on the atoms of a drug. In order to interact as an agonist with a receptor site, the drug must have a charge distribution compatible with the requirements of positive interaction with the receptor site. In cases where an effective drug has been found, then a related drug with a similar charge distribution in the part of the molecule vital for pharmacological action will have a reasonable probability of acting in the same way.

However, it is not justifiable to draw conclusions regarding *absolute* charge requirements of receptor sites from the mapping by the charge distributions of the biological or drug molecules calculated by semiempirical or semirigorous methods (or quantities derivable from these distributions). In cases where a drug is postulated to act by blocking the receptor site of an endogenous molecule, then the more closely the conformation (although perhaps less closely the electronic distribution) of the vital part of the drug resemble those of the endogenous molecule, the more probable it is that the drug will block the receptor site.

Calculational Techniques

Among the techniques available for all valence electron calculations are the following.

1. Semirigorous methods (6). These are iterative procedures where the Hamiltonian includes the nuclear–nuclear repulsion, the electron–nuclear attraction, and the electron–electron repulsion, however zero differential overlap approximations are made for certain of the charge distributions, which also affects the form of the equations to be solved, and the values of certain of the retained integrals are approximated. [The CNDO and INDO methods of Pople (7) are of this type.]

2. Semiempirical methods. These are noniterative procedures in which an effective one-electron Hamiltonian is used, the matrix elements are approximated from atomic properties, and electron–electron repulsion is neglected [the extended Hückel method (8, 9) is of this type].

For our quantum chemical calculations of the phenothiazines, some variant of a semirigorous method seemed the most expeditious manner by which to initiate our studies. Semirigorous calculations mimic to some degree the overall behavior of more rigorous calculations, and possible convergence problems inherent to certain molecules can often be ascertained from such calculations.

Chlorpromazine is known to have a low ionization potential and thus to give up electrons readily. An early hypothesis postulated that the pharmacological effectivity of chlorpromazine might be due to a positive free radical (10). Although this hypothesis is now somewhat in disrepute, nonetheless it stimulated research on the electron spin resonance (ESR) spectra of phenothiazine tranquilizers. In order to interpret ESR spectra, one needs to know the spin densities at the various atoms. The INDO method which retains all one-center integrals permits one to evaluate spin-spin coupling constants for systems with unpaired electrons. The CNDO method, which excludes one-center exchange integrals, does not permit such an evaluation. Due to a lack of atomic spectral data from which to evaluate the necessary parameters, the INDO method seemed only to have been derived and parametrized by Pople (7) for molecules containing first-row atoms. Hence we extended the INDO formulation by deriving the general INDO equations for d orbitals and obtaining the necessary parameters for second-row atoms (11).

All of the computational methods except the extended Hückel method are iterative SCF methods. We designed all of our computer programs to save all unchanged integrals from one molecule or conformation to another, to input whatever part of the density matrix or Fock matrix is applicable from another compound or conformation and thus cut down considerably on the computer time necessary to run a family of related molecules or conformations. The programs are designed to handle up to 200 basis functions and can be extended higher.

The question arises whether it is meaningful to use d orbitals on second-row atoms when only a minimal basis set of valence s and p orbitals is used. To assess the difference, CNDO/2 calculations were made for chlorpromazine both with and without the inclusion of such d functions on S and Cl (1). (Since CNDO/2 is a computational method in common usage, it will facilitate the reader in making comparisons.) The calculation was run for the crystallographically determined structure (12). The numbering system we used for chlorpromazine is shown in Fig. 1.

There are 110 valence electrons. An individual chlorpromazine calculation starting from scratch took about 400 sec on a CDC 6600. (We experienced none of the loss of precision in the matrix diagonalization and none of the convergence difficulties which others mentioned they sometimes obtained in such calculations on large systems, including this system. Part of our success may be due to the fact that we use crystallographically determined structures and then accurately make appropriate conformational changes. In lieu of an experimental crystal structure, we synthesize a structure using special computer programs that ensure such criteria as ring closure, etc. The standard model-builder programs often fail to meet these criteria and generate unphysical structures.) As we shall illustrate later, the calculations can oscillate for unphysical structures, but have always converged for us for physically reasonable structures. The electronic energy of chlorpromazine converged in 12 iterations without d functions to -1034.01051 a.u. ($E_{total} = -185.60805$ a.u.) and in 13 iterations with d functions to -1034.44056 a.u. ($E_{total} = -186.03811$ a.u.) (1 a.u. $= 27.20974$ eV). The drop in energy with addition of d functions is not necessarily illustrative of d orbital participation — but rather of adding any additional basis functions of appropriate symmetry.

The results below show a large gap between the E(HOMO) and E(LUMO):

	Orbital energy (a.u.)	
Orbital number	without d fns	with d fns
53	−0.4489	−0.4528
54	−0.4338	−0.4307
55 (HOMO)	−0.3662	−0.3673
56 (LUMO)	0.1274	0.0788
57	0.1355	0.0966
58	0.1375	0.1040

The inclusion of d functions has little effect on the energies of the occupied orbitals.

Examination of the electron densities even of the S, and C_5 and C_{10} adjacent to it, or of the Cl and C_2 adjacent to it shows that there is very little difference due to the addition of d orbitals.

As a result of the zero differential overlap approximation, there is nothing in the CNDO and INDO methods formally analogous to a total overlap

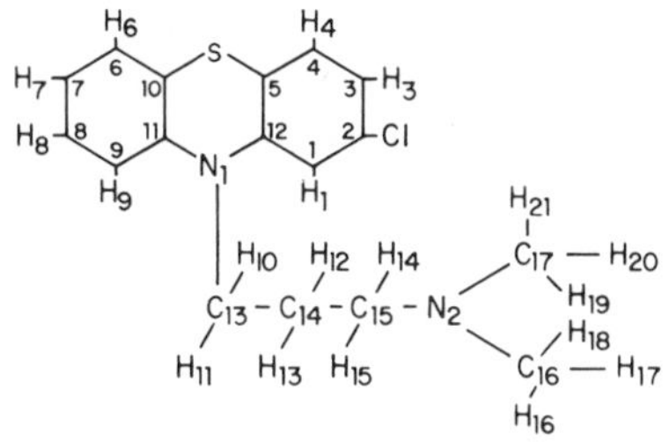

FIG. 1. Chlorpromazine—numbering system.

population. However, several years ago we showed by comparison with an *ab initio,* minimal STO basis LCAO-MO-SCF calculation that to within a scale factor of $\frac{1}{2}$ the off-diagonal density-matrix elements of the CNDO/ INDO methods connecting bonded atoms appear to mimic those from an *ab initio* calculation (13, 14). Thus, one can use these off-diagonal elements, scaled appropriately, in a Mulliken population analysis to obtain an approximation to total overlap populations between bonded atoms. TOP's between bonded atoms are large, of the order of 0.95 for C—C bonds or 0.7 for C to an external substituent atom. There was a fair sized increase in TOP's between C_5—S and between C_{10}—S and between C_2—Cl when *d* functions are added (without *d* functions: 0.6240, 0.6231, 0.5643; with *d* functions: 0.8318, 0.8330, 0.7219). Again, this may simply reflect the increase in the total number of basis functions on the second-row atoms. [TOP's between nonbonded atoms calculated in the same way are only of the order of 0.001. Our very recent research comparing the TOP's from large scale *ab initio* calculations on pyrrole and pyrazole (15) with TOP's derived from CNDO or INDO off-diagonal density-matrix elements (16, 17) showed that, while CNDO/INDO TOP's between bonded atoms were of reasonable magnitude, CNDO/INDO TOP's between nonbonded atoms were almost zero, instead of being large negative value for cross-ring atoms. Deorthogonalization which improves somewhat the atomic charge densities (18, 19) may be expected to ameliorate the TOP discrepancy to some extent.]

The question had been raised whether the highest occupied molecular orbital was localized on the sulfur atom. Examination of the coefficients of the HOMO showed that while the sulfur participated strongly, there were also significant contributions from all of the ring atoms except C_4 and C_6.

INDO calculations were performed for neutral chlorpromazine using both the unscaled theoretically calculated values for the *F* and *G* integrals and those scaled to match experimental values. In spite of the fact that the calculated and experimental *F* and *G* values differ by factors in the neighborhood of 1.5, the final INDO results are comparatively insensitive to whether scaled or unscaled *F* and *G* integrals are used. (*d* Orbitals were included for second-row atoms.) Using unscaled *F* and *G* values, the calculation converged smoothly in 17 iterations to $E_{\text{electronic}} = -1025.08541$ a.u.

($E_{total} = -176.68295$ a.u.). Using scaled F and G values, the calculation converged smoothly in 16 iterations to $E_{electronic} = -1027.97222$ a.u. ($E_{total} = -179.56976$ a.u.). These computations took on the order of 700 sec on a CDC 6600.

The relative energies of the HOMO's and LUMO's are in agreement from either calculation.

	Orbital energy (a.u.)	
Orbital number	Unscaled	Scaled
53	−0.4097	−0.4243
54	−0.3950	−0.4022
55 (HOMO)	−0.3280	−0.3349
56 (LUMO)	0.0589	0.0705
57	0.0661	0.0769
58	0.0838	0.0913

The overall pattern of the population analysis was very similar and the numerical differences between the two sets of INDO results are quite small. The molecular total overlap population (MTOP) using the scaled values is a bit higher (31.7823) than using the unscaled values (31.6918). The combination of a lower total energy and a higher MTOP suggests that the scaled values are more appropriate to use.

The similar overall behavior of the CNDO/2 and INDO results for chlorpromazine indicated that for the conformational studies of phenothiazine derivatives, the CNDO/2 method (which takes only about one-half as much computer time as the INDO method) would give very similar results to the INDO method.

Perazines are phenothiazine derivatives in which the alkyl nitrogen is contained as part of a piperazine ring and piperidopromazines have the alkyl nitrogen contained as part of a piperidine ring. Some results of CNDO/2 calculations on perazine and piperidopromazine and their Cl and CF_3 derivatives are presented for comparison between themselves and to the promazine, chlorpromazine, and triflupromazine results (d orbitals were included.) The calculations for perazines were performed for the structure as found in the crystallographic determination of thiethylperazine (20). The numbering system is shown in Fig. 2.

In lieu of any experimentally determined crystal structures, in the present study the geometries used for the piperidopromazines were similar to those of the perazines with C_{15} in the alkyl chain attached to N_2 in the piperidine ring. These compounds would be structural isomers of the piperidopromazines where C_{14} in the alkyl chain would be attached to C_{15} in the piperidine ring which could then be attached to N_2 (which would bear a CH_3 substitu-

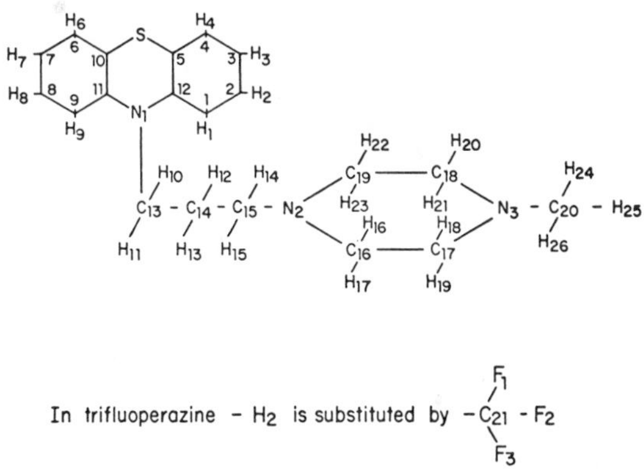

Fig. 2. Perazine and trifluoperazine — numbering system.

ent). Compounds 106, Ridazine, and 94, Piperidochlorpromazine (22) are of this type. One compound of the isomeric type we have calculated has been reported, SA-124 [Compound 112.2 in ref. (22), where it is noted, indeed, to be a major tranquilizer]. [We have a similar study underway at present on the other type of structural isomers of the piperidopromazines as exemplified by Compound 94; however, due to an absolute lack of crystallographic information, these geometrics have to be constructed synthetically.]

As an example of the results, perazine converged smoothly in 12 iterations to an $E_{electronic} = -1254.78930$ a.u. ($E_{total} = -207.67946$ a.u.) and required 700 sec on a CDC 6600. Trifluoperazine converged smoothly in 12 iterations to an $E_{electronic} = -1692.68759$ a.u. ($E_{total} = -297.32982$ a.u.) and required 1,000 sec on a CDC 6600. The energies of the HOMO's and LUMO's indicate that the lowest ionization potential of perazine would be expected to be about the same as that of chlorpromazine, and the lowest ionization potential of trifluoperazine would be expected to be slightly higher.

For comparison, the total energies and the several highest occupied and lowest unoccupied orbital energies for promazine, perazine, piperidopromazine, and their Cl and CF_3 derivatives in their crystallographic conformations are presented in Table 1. The highest occupied molecular orbital both in perazines and piperidopromazines has a sizable contribution from the S atom as well as significant contributions from all of the ring carbon atoms (with the exception of C_4 and C_6) and from the ring N atom. This is the same behavior as noted for chlorpromazine and other promazine derivatives.

From a comparison (Table 2) the electron density on N_2 appears somewhat larger in these perazines and piperidopromazines than in chlorpromazine. [N_2 is the N atom considered significant for neuroleptic activity (23).]

TABLE 1. Energies and orbital energies (a.u.)   CNDO/2

	Promazines			Perazines			Piperidopromazines		
	H	Cl	CF_3	H	Cl	CF_3	H	Cl	CF_3
Energy$_{Total}$	-170.61602	-186.03810	-260.28579	-207.67946	-223.10551	-297.32982	-195.21163	-210.64062	-284.88830
Orbital Energies									
3rd HOMO	-0.4471	-0.4528	-0.4583	-0.4460	-0.4512	-0.4476	-0.4466	-0.4536	-0.4565
2nd HOMO	-0.4246	-0.4307	-0.4385	-0.4257	-0.4359	-0.4403	-0.4257	-0.4355	-0.4377
HOMO	-0.3608	-0.3673	-0.3759	-0.3656	-0.3789	-0.3755	-0.3656	-0.3784	-0.3784
LUMO	0.1042	0.0788	0.0770	0.1034	0.0774	0.0721	0.1034	0.0758	0.0768
2nd LUMO	0.1058	0.0966	0.0932	0.1071	0.0955	0.0948	0.1071	0.0957	0.0947
3rd LUMO	0.1375	0.1040	0.1214	0.1349	0.1108	0.1191	0.1349	0.1179	0.1201

We have carried out a number of molecular orbital calculations to establish the conformational preferences of the side chains of promazine and its Cl and CF_3 derivatives, perazine, and its Cl and CF_3 derivatives, and piperidopromazine and its Cl and CF_3 derivatives. [The reference conformations were the crystallographically determined ones for chlorpromazine (12) and thiethylperazine (20) and a similar structure for piperidopromazine where C_{15} in the alkyl chain is attached to N_2 in the piperdine ring.] In each case for the vital rotation around the N_1—C_{13} bond (the one connecting the alkyl side chain to the phenothiazine ring), the lowest calculated total energy was at the crystallographic conformation.

As may be observed in the prototype (Fig. 3) (E_{total} versus N_1—C_{13} rotation angle for chlorpromazine), there are other low-lying possible conformations as well as some which are so high in energy as to be inaccessible. However, note that owing to the two high-energy barriers the low-lying conformation at 210° is *not* accessible from the crystallographic structures. This point merits emphasis because the crystallographic structure is not always the calculated lowest energy conformation, yet if it is energetically not possible to go from the crystallographic structure to the lower energy conformations, these conformations may not play an important role in the pharmacology. (Sometimes the route of synthesis determines the molecular conformation obtained.) Interestingly enough, this inability to reach the other permissible conformation may well be the genesis for the puzzling results that the identical medicinal compound obtained by two different synthetic routes can display a different pharmacological profile.

Promazine (Fig. 4) and triflupromazine (Fig. 5) show similar patterns for rotation around the N_1—C_{13} bond. Calculations at 15° increments for the rotation of the CF_3 group relative to the plane of the benzene molecule indicated the CF_3 to be a freely rotating group within the accuracy of the method. Similar calculations have been carried out for perazine (Fig. 6), prochlorperazine (Fig. 7), trifluoperazine (Fig. 8), piperidopromazine (Fig. 9), and its Cl derivative (Fig. 10) and CF_3 derivative. There is a great similarity in the rotational barriers for the piperazine derivatives (perazines) and the piperidine derivative (piperidopromazines). There is also a great similarity in the rotational barriers for the Cl and CF_3 derivatives in any series.

Calculations were carried out for 30° rotations around all subsequent bonds in the side chain. For promazines, rotation around the C_{13}—C_{14} bond gave a very slightly lower energy for 180° rotation than for the crystallographic structure; however, the lowest calculated energy conformation is probably not at all or just barely accessible from the crystallographic conformation. Structures with the bond rotated 90 to 120° led to unphysical structures where the quantum chemical calculations oscillated in spite of density-matrix averaging. Rotations around the C_{14}—C_{15} bond with the

TABLE 2. Atomic electron densities   CNDO/2

Atom Name	Promazines			Perazines			Piperidopromazines		
	H	Cl	CF₃	H	Cl	CF₃	H	Cl	CF₃
C 1	4.0595	4.0538	4.0386	4.0609	4.0546	4.0368	4.0611	4.0534	4.0379
C 2	3.9691	3.8968	4.0226	3.9604	3.8787	4.0219	3.9596	3.8782	4.0227
C 3	4.0297	4.0248	4.0056	4.0389	4.0231	4.0179	4.0390	4.0220	4.0189
C 4	3.9571	3.9583	3.9572	3.9493	3.9453	3.9533	3.9492	3.9460	3.9522
C 5	4.0348	4.0294	4.0280	4.0500	4.0483	4.0386	4.0500	4.0478	4.0397
C 6	3.9564	3.9567	3.9524	3.9676	3.9615	3.9660	3.9676	3.9615	3.9658
C 7	4.0303	4.0312	4.0248	4.0172	4.0101	4.0157	4.0172	4.0101	4.0157
C 8	3.9680	3.9683	3.9630	3.9733	3.9675	3.9714	3.9733	3.9675	3.9713
C 9	4.0589	4.0581	4.0574	4.0459	4.0447	4.0444	4.0458	4.0447	4.0445
C10	4.0348	4.0331	4.0371	4.0221	4.0248	4.0214	4.0221	4.0248	4.0215
C11	3.8394	3.8357	3.8464	3.8512	3.8613	3.8511	3.8512	3.8613	3.8511
C12	3.8381	3.8329	3.8464	3.8310	3.8414	3.8343	3.8308	3.8421	3.8335
S 1	6.1304	6.1240	6.1176	6.1296	6.1164	6.1186	6.1295	6.1164	6.1188
N 1	5.1616	5.1561	5.1709	5.1601	5.1728	5.1590	5.1600	5.1728	5.1597
C13	3.9056	3.9064	3.9046	3.8999	3.8988	3.9002	3.8998	3.8987	3.9000
C14	4.0196	4.0199	4.0194	4.0196	4.0186	4.0192	4.0196	4.0186	4.0192
C15	3.8903	3.8907	3.8898	3.8974	3.8963	3.8975	3.8971	3.8960	3.8972
C16	5.1488	5.1494	5.1506	5.1589	5.1596	5.1593	5.1635	5.1642	5.1639
N 2	3.9185	3.9184	3.9183	3.9123	3.9120	3.9121	3.8970	3.8967	3.8968
C17(C19)*	3.9295	3.9307	3.9340	3.9249	3.9250	3.9249	3.9075	3.9075	3.9073
H 1	0.9954	0.9798	0.9853	0.9946	0.9768	0.9845	0.9945	0.9774	0.9847
H 3	1.0042	0.9880	0.9904	0.9985	0.9827	0.9843	0.9984	0.9830	0.9835
H 4	1.0021	0.9955	0.9948	1.0080	1.0007	1.0010	1.0079	1.0008	1.0009
H 6	1.0023	1.0009	1.0000	0.9963	0.9947	0.9943	0.9963	0.9948	0.9943
H 7	1.0041	1.0021	1.0017	1.0074	1.0059	1.0049	1.0073	1.0059	1.0049
H 8	1.0056	1.0037	1.0030	1.0073	1.0055	1.0048	1.0072	1.0055	1.0048
H 9	.9983	0.9968	0.9954	0.9952	0.9929	0.9930	0.9951	0.9929	0.9929
H10	1.0112	1.0107	1.0095	1.0039	1.0017	1.0031	1.0182	1.0154	1.0163
H11	1.0047	1.0034	1.0017	1.0182	1.0154	1.0162	1.0040	1.0018	1.0031
H12	0.9902	0.9906	0.9913	0.9957	0.9957	0.9956	0.9915	0.9912	0.9910
H13	0.9951	0.9947	0.9945	0.9916	0.9913	0.9912	0.9958	0.9958	0.9958

Table 1

Atom	1	2	3	4	5	6	7	8	9
H14	1.0290	1.0281	1.0277	1.0284	1.0275	1.0274	1.0288	1.0279	1.0278
H15	1.0187	1.0187	1.0186	1.0166	1.0162	1.0161	1.0166	1.0162	1.0162
H16	1.0092	1.0098	1.0116	1.0169	1.0168	1.0167	1.0195	1.0195	1.0195
H17	1.0179	1.0177	1.0151	1.0193	1.0192	1.0192	1.0239	1.0237	1.0238
H18	1.0094	1.0082	1.0088						
H19(H22)*	1.0073	1.0067	1.0061	1.0104	1.0115	1.0116	1.0138	1.0149	1.0151
H20(H23)	1.0046	0.9998	0.9947	1.0117	1.0114	1.0115	1.0160	1.0157	1.0159
H21	1.0053	1.0060	1.0067						
H 2	1.0053			1.0164			1.0179		
Cl1	7.1641				7.1837			7.1844	
C18(C21)			3.3988			3.4113			3.4039
F 1			7.2218			7.2228			7.2251
F 2			7.2194			7.2282			7.2209
F 3			7.2186			7.2092			7.2200

Table 2

Atom	4	5	6	7	8	9
C17	3.9188	3.9190	3.9190	4.0029	4.0032	4.0032
C18	3.8997	3.8999	3.8999	3.9911	3.9914	3.9915
C20	3.9329	3.9330	3.9331	3.9923	.9919	3.9920
N 3	5.1487	5.1486	5.1488			
H18	1.0155	1.0145	1.0142	.9941	.9930	.9926
H19	1.0112	1.0107	1.0106	1.0108	1.0102	1.0102
H20	1.0247	1.0240	1.0241	.9972	.9963	.9957
H21	1.0177	1.0173	1.0174	1.0147	1.0143	1.0143
H24	1.0115	1.0103	1.0101	.9985	.9986	.9988
H25	1.0060	1.0058	1.0057	1.0048	1.0038	1.0035
H26	1.0067	1.0066	1.0066			

* In each case where there is a second atom name in parenthesis following the first, the first atom name refers to promazines and the second atom name refers to the corresponding atom in perazines or piperidopromazines.

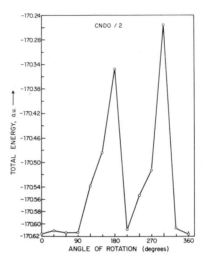

FIG. 3. Promazine–E_{total} versus rotation around N_1–C_{13} bond.

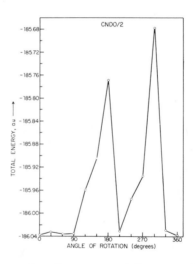

FIG. 4. Chlorpromazine–E_{total} versus rotation around N_1–C_{13} bond.

C_{13}–C_{14} bond as in the crystal structure, gave the crystal structure as the lowest energy conformation. Subsequent rotations of the C_{14}–C_{15} bond of promazine keeping the C_{13}–C_{14} bond at 180° from the crystallographic conformation (an energy minimum) led to a number of unphysical structures 60 to 180°, where the quantum chemical calculations oscillated in spite of density matrix averaging. The perazines and piperidopromazines showed a slightly lower minimum at 90° for rotation of the C_{13}–C_{14} bond than for the crystallographic conformation. (However, rotations from 120 to 240° led to the unphysical structures where the calculations oscillated.) A

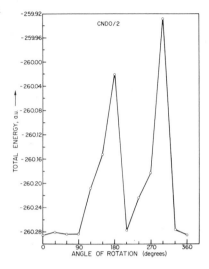

FIG. 5. Triflupromazine $-E_{total}$ versus rotation around N_1—C_{13} bond.

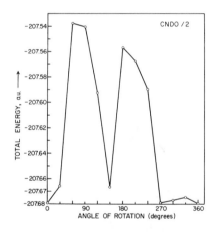

FIG. 6. Perazine $-E_{total}$ versus rotation around N_1—C_{13} bond.

number of subsequent rotations around the C_{14}—C_{15} bond (keeping the C_{13}—C_{14} bond at the 90° rotation) also led to unphysical structures, and the calculations oscillated for points 150 to 210° in spite of density-matrix averaging. Again, the lowest energy conformation could not be reached from the crystallographic conformation. Rotation around the C_{15}—N_2 bond for promazines and perazines (keeping the rest of the side chain in the crystallographic conformation) gave the crystallographic structure as the lowest energy conformation.

Molecular orbital energy levels, electron densities, and other calculated properties are available from the authors. Also, only the figures for the

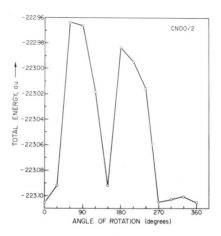

FIG. 7. Prochlorperazine $-E_{total}$ versus rotation around N_1—C_{13} bond.

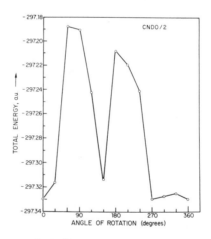

FIG. 8. Trifluoperazine $-E_{total}$ versus rotation around N_1—C_{13} bond.

energy versus rotation around the N_1—C_{13} bond are included here because of space limitations. A more complete set of figures for the calculated energies as a function of rotation around the subsequent bonds is available upon request.

Similar calculations have been carried out for the butyrophenones and other psychoactive drugs.

TOPOLOGICAL AND TOPOGRAPHICAL CONFORMATIONAL SIMILARITIES AMONG NEUROLEPTIC DRUGS AND THEIR POSSIBLE RELATIONSHIPS TO BIOGENIC AMINES

Topological analysis deals with which atoms are connected to which other atoms. Often a common topological pattern of atoms is buried within

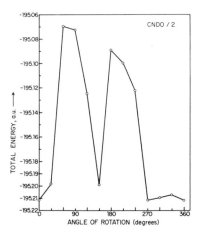

FIG. 9. Piperidopromazine $-E_{\text{total}}$ versus rotation around N_1—C_{13} bond.

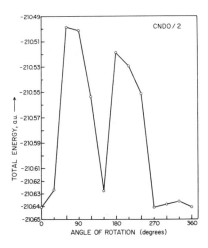

FIG. 10. Piperidochlorpromazine $-E_{\text{total}}$ versus rotation around N_1—C_{13} bond.

a series of much larger molecules. Topographical analysis deals with patterns of atoms which are in the same spatial positions relative to one another (although not necessarily topologically related).

The very recent reference *Orthomolecular Psychiatry* by Pauling (24) states that all antipsychotics produce a postsynaptic dopamine receptor blockade leading to stabilization of the membrane at the receptor site.

It had been hypothesized previously that dopamine may be superimposable upon a portion (the *a* ring bearing the Cl substituent) of the known X-ray structure of chlorpromazine (25). It also seemed to us that while there could be involvement of the *a* ring as invoked by Snyder, it is perhaps equally probable that the opposite *c* ring is also involved at some point interfering in the dopamine pathway. Many phenothiazines with very bulky substituents in the 2-position are effective tranquilizers (21), yet the *a* ring bearing these substituents could scarcely fit into any receptor sites that would be conformationally appropriate for dopamine. (It is quite possibly involvement of the *c* ring of chlorpromazine which causes a number of the well-defined side effects.)

In order to see most vividly the conformational similarities, space-filling CPK molecular models were constructed for chlorpromazine, perazine, and the biogenic amines. Using a technique developed previously by another member of our group (26), we mounted the models in a frame and photographed them from all sides relative to a fixed point. These transparencies would then be projected superimposed to show the similarities. Only one face of the chlorpromazine could superimpose on the dopamine.

Janssen had proposed originally in 1964 (27) that the fundamental structure necessary for neuroleptic action was as shown in structure 1.

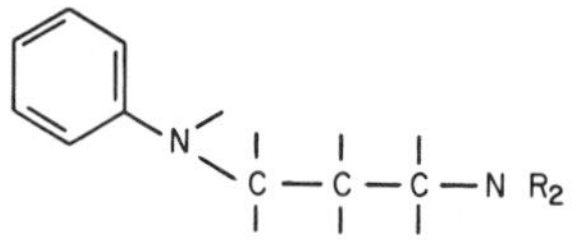

STRUCTURE 1.

This proposal was criticized by Julou in 1965 (28) on the grounds that it did not include such classes as tetrabenazine, the piperazinic derivatives of indole (which, however, are more closely related structurally to reserpine), and dibenzothiazepines (structures 2).

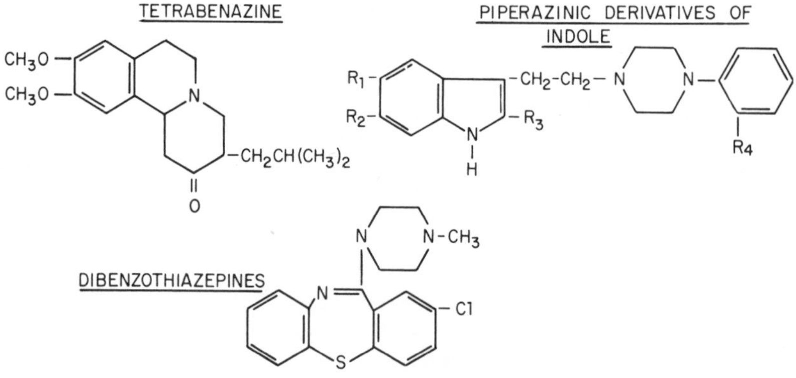

STRUCTURES 2.

Janssen later reexamined these classes and other effective neuroleptics and in 1969 (29) postulated that all that seems necessary is the fundamental structure shown in structure 3. This fundamental structure alone can

STRUCTURE 3.

correlate the antipsychotic activity of the three major classes of neuroleptics: 4-phenylbutylamines (such as the butyrophenones), 3-anilinopropy-
lamines (such as the phenothiazines), and 3-phenoxypropylamines (such as
spiramide). All neuroleptics of these three classes seem to be able to adopt
only one S-shaped common conformation, and Janssen expected, therefore,
that it is in this conformational state that they interact with receptor molecules (23).

Our topological examination indicated that the dibenzothiazepines (structure 4) do fit into the customary classification.

STRUCTURE 4.

Janssen indicated there were exceptions such as the ethylaminoindoles,
which could have a three-carbon chain or benzoquinolizines which could
have a two-carbon chain. However, our careful examination of the stereo-
topology of the ethylaminoindoles (which are topologically related to
Rauwolfia alkaloids) indicates that the three-carbon chain is probably
not effective of itself but rather because the three carbon atoms and the
attached nitrogen are sitting where they would have had there been an extra
carbon between them and the first aromatic ring (structure 5).

STRUCTURE 5.

The tetrabenzazines do not fit the general pattern. In this particular
case, because of the rigidity of the structure, the N must be in an orientation
relative to the ring closely resembling that of the biogenic amines which
have only a two-carbon chain. They thus resemble reserpine.

Interestingly enough, just the pattern recognition of this type made us question [J. Levine, D. H. Efron, and J. J. Kaufman, *private communication*, 1971] the correctness of the structure sketched for Compound 55, piperidochlorpromazine in the book [Usdin and Efron (21)], which as drawn showed a pattern (structure 6).

(with four carbon attached to the ring N atom)

STRUCTURE 6.

Upon examination of the original data it was found that this structure contained a misprint and that the structure should really be structure 7,

STRUCTURE 7.

which does meet the necessary topological requisites. (This misprint had already been caught on straight proofreading for the second edition of the book. [E. Usdin, *private communication*, 1971.])

Chemically, the nitrogen of the phenothiazine ring is not a vital part of the structure. Rather, what is important is that being a part of a ring it is conformationally rigid and, thus, at least at the position of attachment holds the

side chain in a specific position relative to the ring. This hypothesis then explains the effectiveness of the thioxanthene class of antipsychotic drugs. The C—C linkage is conformationally rigid and serves the same purpose

as the $\diagdown\!\!\mathrm{N}\!\!\diagup$ in attaching the side chain in a certain conformational position

relative to the ring.

We also set up a systems analysis approach to facilitate an understanding of the mechanism of action of the neuroleptics, both their major tranquilizing action and their almost bizarre side effects (2, 4, 5). It became obvious that although the neuroleptics were acting as tranquilizers by blocking the postsynaptic dopamine receptors, they were also mimicking other normal neurotransmitters and becoming involved to a lesser extent in both the norepinephrine and serotonin pathways. Examination of the space-filling models indicated the probable face of the neuroleptics which was involved in blockade of the dopamine receptor. Rather detailed discussions of this approach have been presented previously (2, 4, 5). A more complete manuscript of this systems analysis discussion of the present article is available from the authors since space restrictions prevented its inclusion here.

CONCLUSION

CNDO/2 calculations have been performed for promazines, perazines, piperidopromazines, and their Cl and CF_3 derivatives. Calculations as a function of the rotation of the side chain indicate that the crystallographic conformations are the lowest or among the lowest in energy. Some other low-energy conformers cannot be reached from the crystallographic conformations due to very high-energy barriers. This has pharmacological implications. Comparison of the calculated electron densities on the alkyl N atom (which is involved in the neuroleptic activity) shows a slightly higher electron density on this nitrogen in perazines (5,1509) and piperidopromazines (5.1635) than in promazines (5.1488). [It is interesting to note that our comparable CNDO/2 calculations on haloperidol and spiroperidol (J. J. Kaufman and E. Kerman, *unpublished results*) in their crystallographic conformations indicate that for these compounds the nitrogen atoms involved in neuroleptic activity have almost identical electron densities (haloperidol 5.1604, and spiroperidol 5.1614) to those of the comparable N atoms in the perazines or piperidopromazines.] We have also carried out successful INDO calculations on chlorpromazine using our previously derived extension of the INDO method to include *d* orbitals and the necessary parameters for second-row elements.

It is significant to note that when we originally picked a hitherto unknown structural isomer for piperidopromazines, which was analogous to that of the crystallographic structure for perazines, there were no reported neuroleptic drugs of this structure. Our quantum calculations indicated that compounds of this type should be effective neuroleptics. In the interim, a piperidopromazine of the structural type we chose has been reported (22) and is, indeed, a major tranquilizer.

Furthermore, topological and topographical considerations led us to question the correctness of the structure for piperidochlorpromazine in the original edition of the Usdin and Efron book (21), which as drawn showed four carbon atoms from the nitrogen of the phenothiazine ring to the nitrogen in the piperidine ring; whereas the analysis indicated there should only be three carbon atoms if it were to be an effective neuroleptic. This incorrect structure turned out to be a typesetting error which was corrected for ed. 2. The significance of our questioning the incorrect structure is that if a medicinal chemist proposed to synthesize that particular structure for an effective neuroleptic, we would have suggested synthesizing the alternative structure with three carbon atoms between the two nitrogens.

ACKNOWLEDGMENTS

In part, this research was supported by N.I.M.H. Psychopharmacology Branch under grant No. RO1 MH18967 and performed in collaboration with them. We especially acknowledge the inspiration of the late Dr. Daniel H. Efron and the stimulating discussions with Drs. Jerome Levine, Albert A. Manian, and Earl Usdin of NIMH.

Special thanks to the U.S. Air Force Office of Scientific Research, Energetics Division and to Dr. Joseph Masi, Chief, Energetics Division, for their long-time support of our theoretical research, which led to the understanding and computational methods necessary to formulate this problem.

The calculations were carried out on CDC 6600 computers. The preliminary calculations were carried out at CDC Rockville and we thank R. W. Hansen and B. Feely of CDC for arranging our use of the computer and the Rockville staff for their cooperation.

REFERENCES

1. Kaufman, J. J., and Kerman, E., *Int. J. Quantum Chem.*, **6S,** 319 (1972).
2. Kaufman, J. J., Plenary Lecture presented at Collegium Internationale Neuro-Psychopharmacologicum Meeting, Copenhagen, Denmark, August, 1972; in press in the proceedings of the meeting.
3. Kaufman, J. J., and Kerman, E., *Abstract MEDI 008*, 164th National American Chemical Society Meeting, 1972.
4. Kaufman, J. J., and Kerman, E., invited lecture presented at the International Symposium on Chemical and Biochemical Reactivity, Jerusalem, Israel, April 9–13, 1973; in press in the proceedings of the meeting.
5. Kaufman, J. J., and Manian, A. A., *Int. J. Quantum Chem.*, **6S,** 375 (1972).
6. Kaufman, J. J., *J. Chem. Phys.*, **43,** S152 (1965).
7. Pople, J. A., and Beveridge, D. L., *Approximate Molecular Orbital Theory*, McGraw-Hill Book Company, New York, 1970.
8. Wolfsberg, M., and Helmholz, L., *J. Chem. Phys.*, **29,** 837 (1952).
9. Hoffman, R., *J. Chem. Phys.*, **39,** 1397 (1963).
10. Szent-Gyorgi, A. E., Isenberg, I., and Karreman, G., *Science*, **130,** 1191 (1959).
11. Kaufman, J. J., and Predney, R., *Int. J. Quantum Chem.*, **6S,** 231 (1972).
12. McDowell, J. J. H., *Acta Cryst.*, **B25,** 2175 (1969).
13. Kaufman, J. J., *Int. J. Quantum Chem.*, **4S,** 205 (1971).
14. Kaufman, J. J., *Int. J. Quantum Chem.*, **1S,** 485 (1967).
15. Preston, H. J. T., and Kaufman, J. J., presented at the International Symposium on Atomic, Molecular and Solid-State Theory and Quantum Biology, Sanibel Island, Florida, January, 1973, *Int. J. Quantum Chem.*, in press, Symp. issue.

16. Kaufman, J. J., Preston, H. J. T., and Kerman, E., presented at the International Symposium on Atomic, Molecular and Solid-State Theory and Quantum Biology, Sanibel Island, Florida, January, 1973, *Int. J. Quantum Chem.*, in press, Symp. issue.
17. Kaufman, J. J., Preston, H. J. T., Kerman, E., and Cusachs, L. C., *Int. J. Quantum Chem.*, to be published.
18. Giessner-Prethe, C., and Pullman, A., *Theor. chim. Acta*, **11**, 159 (1968).
19. Shillady, D. D., Billingsley, II, F. P., and Bloor, J. E., *Theor. chim. Acta*, **21**, 1 (1971).
20. McDowell, J. J. H., *Acta Cryst.*, **B26**, 954 (1970).
21. Usdin, E., and Efron, D. H., *Psychotropic Drugs and Related Compounds*, U.S. Public Health Service, Department of Health, Education and Welfare, 1967.
22. Usdin, E., and Efron, D. H., *Psychotropic Drugs and Related Compounds*, 2nd edition, U.S. Public Health Service, Department of Health, Education and Welfare, 1972.
23. Janssen, P. A. J., *The Neuroleptics*, Bobon, D. P., Janssen, P. A. J., and Obon, J. B., eds., S. Karger, Basel, 1970, p. 33.
24. Hawkins, D., and Pauling, L., ed., *Orthomolecular Psychiatry*, W. H. Freeman and Company, San Francisco, 1973.
25. Horn, A., and Snyder, S., *Proc. Natl. Acad. Sci.*, **68**, 2325 (1971).
26. Wilson, K., *Abstract #23*, 144th ACS National Meeting, Division of Chem. Education, 1963.
27. Janssen, P. A. J., IVe Reunion du College International de Neuro-Psychopharmacology, Birmingham, 31/8–3/9/64.
28. Julou, L., Ducrot, R., and Fouche, J., Atti Convegni Farmitalia, *Agiornamento in Psiconeurofarmacologia*, Milano, November 1965, p. 20.
29. Janssen, P. A. J., *Abstract MEDI 36*, 158th National Meeting of the American Chemical Society, September 1969.

The Phenothiazines and Structurally Related Drugs, edited by I. S. Forrest, C. J. Carr, and E. Usdin. Raven Press, New York © 1974.

Tentative Correlations Between Some Spectroscopic and Biological Properties of Phenothiazine and Parafluorobutyrophenone Derivatives

François Leterrier and *Corinne Thiery

*Centre de Recherches du Service de Santé des Armées, Division de Biophysique, 92140, Clarmart, France and *Département de Biologie, C. E. N. Saclay, B. P. No. 2, 91190 Gif sur Yvette, France*

INTRODUCTION

Phenothiazine and parafluorobutyrophenone derivatives are two large groups of very active pharmacological compounds. In each of them, slight modifications of the chemical structure are followed by important changes in the biological properties. For many years we have been interested in the spectroscopic properties of both classes of compounds (1–6). By correlating results obtained by absorption, fluorescence, phosphorescence, and electron spin resonance (ESR) spectroscopies, it is possible to get some information on the probable conformations of these molecules in solution. On the other hand, numerous studies have been made on the membrane properties of these drugs. We have observed their action on the microsomal and synaptic membranes (7–9). This report will correlate our spectroscopic results with the principal observations we have made on biological membranes.

MATERIAL AND METHODS

Compounds Studied

Phenothiazine derivatives. We have studied 20 derivatives. Their formulas are given in Table 1. They are classified according to (a) the nature of the substituent in position 3 (Beilstein numbering) on the tricyclic nucleus, (b) the structure of the side chain.

"Butyrophenone" derivatives. We have studied a series of 19 compounds designated as AB and obtained from parafluorobutyrophenone (A) by replacement of one hydrogen atom of the methyl group by various heterocyclic

77

TABLE 1. *Effect of phenothiazine derivatives on NADH cytochrome c reductase and on the fluorescence of microsome-bound ANS*

Phenothiazine skeleton: ring positions 1–9, with N (position 10) bearing R_2 and the ring bearing R_1; S at the central position.

$R_1 = H$ / CF_3 / $O{-}CH_3$ / $C{\equiv}N$

R_2	NADH[a]	ANS[b]
$R_1 = H$		
$-(CH_2)_3-NH_2$	115	90
$-(CH_2)_3-NHCH_3$	60	45
$-(CH_2)_3-N(CH_3)_2$	17	10
$-CH_2-CH(CH_3)-N(CH_3)_2$	-15	0
$-CH_2-CH(CH_3)-CH_2-N(CH_3)_2$	-18	0
$R_1 = CF_3$		
$-(CH_2)_3-N\langle\text{piperazine}\rangle-CH_2-CH_2OH$	100	100
$R_1 = O-CH_3$		
$CH_2-CH(CH_3)-CH_2-N(CH_3)_2$	24	15
$R_1 = C{\equiv}N$		

$R_1 = Cl$

R_2	NADH[a]	ANS[b]
$-(CH_2)_3-NH_2$	140	100
$-(CH_2)_3-NHCH_3$	103	
$-(CH_2)_3-N(CH_3)_2$ (CPZ)	85	100
$-(CH_2)_3-NH(C_2H_5)$	130	120
$-(CH_2)_3-N(C_2H_5)_2$	43	80
$-(CH_2)-CH(CH_3)-CH_2-N(CH_3)_2$	-19	0
$-(CH_2)_4-N(CH_3)_2$	38	
$-(CH_2)_3-N\langle\text{piperazine}\rangle N(CH_2)_2OH$	85	100
CPZ Sulfoxide	0	0
$-(CH_2)_3-N(CH_3)_2 {\rightarrow} O$	0	8

$-(CH_2)_3-N$⟩$-OH$	80	45	(CPZ N oxide)
$R_1 = SO_2-N(CH_3)_2$		CPZ N oxide, sulfoxide	0	0	0
$-(CH_2)_2-N$⟩$-CH_3$	16		

[a] Percent activation or inhibition of NADH cytochrome c reductase in presence of 4×10^{-5} M drug concentration.
[b] Relative increase in ANS fluorescence intensity CPZ = 100 at 3×10^{-5} M drug concentration.

TABLE 2. Structures of butyrophenone derivatives

Haloperidol group

	X	R₁	R₂
		R_1	R_2
Name:			
Haloperidol	—(CH₂)₃—	H	Cl
Methylperidol	"	H	CH₃
Triperidol	"	CF₃	H
Seperol	"	CF₃	Cl
Haloperidol cis		H	Cl
Haloperidol trans		H	Cl
Phenothiazine analogue of haloperidol			

Spiroperidol group

Spiroperidol	$-\overset{O}{\underset{\parallel}{C}}-(CH_2)_{3}-$

and two derivatives: —CO—(CH₂)₂— and CO—(CH₂)—

S_1 —(CH₂)₄—

S_2 $-\underset{CH_3}{\overset{}{C}}=CH-CH_3$

Other derivatives

Droperidol	double bond Δ4–5
Benperidol	H
Pipamperone	CO—NH₂
Propyperone	CO—CH₂—CH₃
Aceperone	CH₂—NH—CO—CH₃

Fluanisone

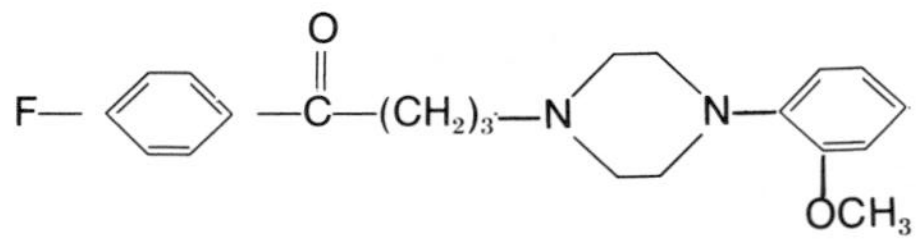

Benperidol
analogue

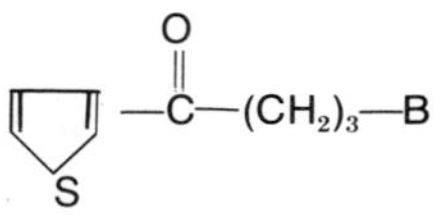

groups (B) differing from each other in their steric properties and their degree of conjugation. Some A derivatives are isosteric of parafluorobutyro-phenone (PFBP). In other compounds, the aliphatic chain binding parts A and B has a variable length or hindered flexibility. Their formulas are presented in Table 2.

Preparation of samples. For spectroscopic studies, all compounds were sufficiently soluble in ethanol. For the studies with biological membranes, they were solubilized with 1% dimethylsulfoxide in pH 7 phosphate buffer. It was verified that dimethylsulfoxide does not change the enzymatic and fluorescence properties of the membranes (9).

Reagents and Solvents

Alcohols (methanol, ethanol) were analytical grade (Rhône-Poulenc) and the other solvents of spectroscopic grade (Merck). They were used without further purification, but all spectroscopic studies were preceded by preliminary studies of the solvent alone as blank. All other chemicals were of commercially available analytical grade.

Spectroscopic Techniques

Absorption. Absorption spectra were recorded at room temperature with a Cary 15 spectrophotometer, in quartz cells of different pathlengths (1, 5, and 10 cm).

Luminescence. Luminescence spectra were measured with an Aminco-Bowman spectrophosphofluorometer equipped with a Hewlett Packard *X-Y* recorder. The spectra were not corrected for the variations of lamp emission and photomultiplier sensitivity. Fluorescence spectra were recorded in 1×1 cm quartz cells thermostated at +25°C. Phosphorescence measurements were carried out with 3-mm sample tubes in liquid nitrogen. The lifetime τ was determined with a Polaroid camera adapted to a Hewlett-Packard 140 A oscilloscope.

Electron spin resonance. The paramagnetic triplet state was studied with a Varian V 4502–13 spectrometer equipped with an Osram HBO 200w high-pressure mercury lamp. Interpretation of the spectra was carried out as previously described (5, 6).

Spectra of phenothiazine free radicals were recorded with a Varian E 3 spectrometer at room temperature. Radicals were produced in 75% H_3PO_4 in the presence of 10^{-4} M parabenzoquinone (1, 2, 10) or by electrolysis in dimethylformamide-HCl (1:9 v/v) (4).

Preparation and Study of Biological Membranes

Rat liver microsomes were isolated by ultracentrifugation of post-mitochondrial supernatant at 105,000 g for 60 min in 0.25 M sucrose (Spinco L 2 50 B). Proteins were measured by the method of Lowry et al. (11). NADH and NADPH cytochrome c reductases activities were measured at 28°C in microsomes added to a system containing the drug to be studied at concentrations ranging between 10^{-5} and 2×10^{-4} M, 0.1 mM NADH or NADPH, 0.05 mM cytochrome c, and 0.3 mM KCN in *tris* HCl (50 mM) pH 7.5 buffer, in a final volume of 1 ml (12). The reduction of cytochrome c was followed at 550 nm with a Perkin-Elmer model 402 spectrophotometer. Enzymatic activities were expressed as μmoles of cytochrome c reduced per min per mg protein. A value of 18.5×10^3 l mole^{-1} cm^{-1} was used for the extinction coefficient of reduced minus oxidized cytochrome c at 550 nm (13).

Rat brain synaptic membranes were prepared according to Whittaker (14). Binding of ANS (8 anilinonaphtalene sulfonate) on these membranes and on microsomes is measured by spectrofluorometry in a system containing *tris* HCl 20 mM pH 7.4 buffer, 0.225 M mannitol, 0.075 M saccharose, 10^{-5} M ANS, the drug to be studied at a concentration ranging between 5×10^{-6} and 10^{-4} M and membranes at a concentration ranging between 0.025 and 0.5 mg/ml protein in a final volume of 2ml.

RESULTS

Spectroscopic Study

Phenothiazine derivatives. Absorption, fluorescence, phosphorescence, and triplet state ESR spectra of phenothiazine derivatives have been reported in numerous studies (1–4, 6, 16, 17). Their characteristics depend principally on the substitution in the position 3 of the nucleus (Beilstein numbering). The presence of a lateral chain on the N atom is followed by an increase in the energy level of the triplet state and by a decrease in the value of the D^* parameter in ESR (4). But the nature of this side chain (either linear or branched, ending in a primary, secondary, or tertiary amine or in a piperidine or piperazine nucleus) does not significantly influence the spectra.

Free radicals of phenothiazine drugs are obtained without difficulty by numerous methods (3, 4). Spectra of radicals of N-unsubstituted derivatives are well resolved (17). The presence of a side chain generally induces a considerable loss of spectral resolution; however, it is possible to distinguish two groups of compounds. Derivatives with linear side chains show very poorly resolved spectra, whereas compounds with a β-substituted side chain give spectra where the lines of the unsubstituted parent compound are superimposed on a less resolved structure (Fig. 1). The same results are obtained with all the typical methods used for producing the free radicals.

Butyrophenone derivatives. The spectroscopic study of these molecules was performed in three steps: (a) the spectral characteristics of parts A and

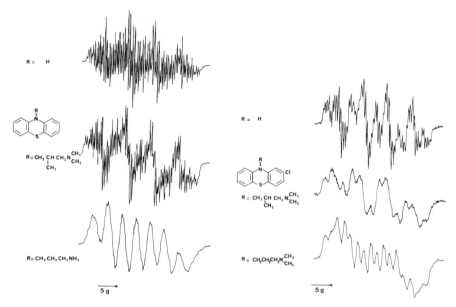

FIG. 1. ESR spectra of phenothiazine and chlorophenothiazine free radicals with either unbranched or β-branched side chains.

B were recorded separately, (b) they were compared with the spectra of the equimolar mixture of both constituents in order to reveal some *inter*molecular interactions between A and B, (c) finally, the spectral properties of the entire molecule AB were studied. The difference observed between AB and A + B can thus be attributed to *intra*molecular interactions.

In this study of 19 compounds, we confirmed and refined the first results previously obtained on only five derivatives (5).

(a) General results observed for all butyrophenone derivatives at wavelengths shorter than 300 nm.

– Absorption: spectra of AB and A + B are identical with the spectra obtained by adding the absorbancies of A and B measured separately.

– Fluorescence: fraction A (PFBP) is not fluorescent. Fractions B are generally strongly fluorescent, except when they do not possess any conjugated structure (pipamperone and propyperone). Emission of AB is qualitatively identical with emission of B, but quantitatively its intensity is quenched about 80 to 90%.

– Triplet state: fraction A is highly phosphorescent with an emission maximum at 415 nm. The lifetime of this emission ($\tau = 0.004$ sec) (18) is not measurable in our experimental conditions. No ESR signal is observed in pure ethanol. A weak signal is observed in the mixture methanol, ethanol, water (55:25:20 v/v) of high dielectric constant (19) ($H_{min} = 1385$ Gauss). When they are conjugated, fractions B are phosphorescent with their emission maximum below 415 ñm, and they show a strong ESR signal. All AB derivatives possess a phosphorescence emission at 415 nm with a lifetime shorter than 0.1 sec and no ESR signal can be observed (except in the case of haloperidol).

(b) Influence of the structure of the compounds on these general characteristics.

—Absorption: absorption spectrum of the compound formed with the phenothiazine nucleus and part B of haloperidol is the sum of the spectra of both components. When fraction A does not contain the ketone function (spiroperidol analogues S1 and S2), one observes a slight decrease in the spectral resolution when comparing the spectrum with that of A + B.

—Fluorescence: when part A is not PFBP, it does fluoresce. In the whole compounds AB (S1, S2, benperidol derivative) this emission is strongly quenched. In compounds where the length of the aliphatic chain is modified, the quenching of the B emission varies in the following order: $n = 2$: 75%, $n = 3$: 80% and $n = 1$: 90% (n is the number of CH_2 between A and B). The partial rigidification of this chain (haloperidol derivatives) is followed by a complete quenching of the B fluorescence.

—Triplet state: parts A of both spiroperidol derivatives S1 and S2 do not phosphoresce. In S1, the phosphorescence of fraction B is recorded without modification, whereas in S2 it is completely quenched. When the aliphatic chain is formed from two methylene bridges (instead of 3:spiroperidol), the phosphorescence emissions of neither A nor B are recorded. When only one methylene links A and B, it is no longer possible to know the origin of the weak phosphorescence observed. The modification of flexibility in the haloperidol chain is followed by a complete quenching of phosphorescence.

All these results are summarized in Table 3.

(c) Spectra of the compounds at wavelengths longer than 300 nm. With compounds where fraction A is PFBP and only in these compounds, new spectroscopic characteristics are observed at wavelengths longer than 300 nm by comparison with the equimolar mixture of A + B.

—Absorption: Fig. 2 shows the differential spectra obtained between AB derivatives and the corresponding mixture of A + B. For all derivatives, a new band is observed, which is large, without structure and which expands from 300 to about 380 nm. This band varies with the nature of part B (Fig. 2B). Marked differences are observed in the case of the haloperidol group (Fig. 2A) and with the length and flexibility of the aliphatic chain (Figs. 2C and 2A).

—Phosphorescence: for each compound, excitation in this absorption band is followed by a weak phosphorescence emission at about 450 nm (lifetime 0.5 sec), and by a new ESR triplet state signal ($D^* = 0.096$).

All these results are summarized in Table 4.

TABLE 3. Spectroscopic properties of butyrophenone derivatives for wavelength shorter than 300 nm

Compound	Absorption	Fluorescence			Phosphorescence				RPE D^*
		exc.	em.	I rel.	exc.	em.	I rel.	τ (s)	
PFBP	242 (312)	—	—	—	250 (370)	415	100	<0.1	—
Haloperidol group									
Fraction B	220, 225, 272	290	352	100	250, 270	425	10	~0.1	0.107
A + B	220, 225, 242, 272 (312)	290	352	100	250, 270	420	100	~0.1	0.107
Haloperidol	220, 225, 242, 272	297	360	10	250, 270	415	100	<0.1	0.107
Seperol	222, 243, 267, 278	—	—	—	245, 270	415		<0.1	—
Halop. *cis*	247.5	—	—	—	252, 285	415	100	<0.1	—
Halop. *trans*	244	—	—	—	248, 275	415	100	<0.1	—
Spiroperidol group									
Fraction B	250, 293	265, 300	332	100	270 (310)	390	100	2.5	0.127
Spiroperidol $n = 3$	247, 293	265, 300	332	20	240, 285	415	250	<0.1	—
" $n = 2$	247, 293 (hypochrom)	265, 300	332	25	240, 285	415	140	<0.1 (2.5)	0.127
" $n = 1$	247, 292 (hypochrom)	265, 300	332	10	240, 285	415	60	<0.1	—
Compound S$_1$									
Fraction A	253, 261, 266, 272	275	290		—	—	—	—	—
AB	253, 266, 272 (293)	265, 275	330		270 (310)	390	100	2.5	0.127
Compound S$_2$									
Fraction A	247, 273, (282) (291)	270	310		—	—	—	—	—
AB	250(257), 290, (302)	270 (300)	330		—	—	—	—	—
Benperidol									
Fraction B	230, 282	285	325	100	290	385	130	3.3	0.133
AB	233 (240), 282	285	325	10	255, 295	415	250	<0.1	—
Benperidol derivative									
Fraction A	260, 283 (290)	240 (295)	330	4	290	485	175	<0.1	0.143
AB	232, 260, 283 (290)	290	325	1	285	485	165	<0.1	0.143
		305	330	20	290	385	5	3.3	0.133

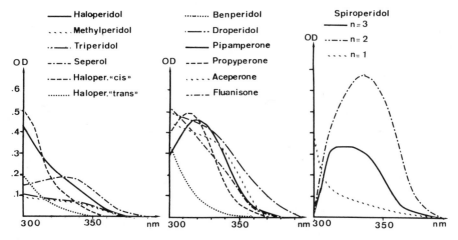

FIG. 2. Differential absorption spectra of butyrophenone derivatives for wavelength longer than 300 nm. The reference cuvette contains an equimolar concentration of parafluoro-butyrophenone and of the molecule corresponding to part B of the whole compound studied. This latter compound is dissolved at the same concentration in the other cuvette. Concentrations are 2×10^{-4} M in ethanol, with an optical path length of 10 cm.

TABLE 4. *Correlations between the spectroscopic data obtained at wavelength longer than 300 nm and the membrane effects of butyrophenone derivatives*

Compounds	Absorption λ max (a)	ε (b)	Phosphorescence λ exc. nm	λ em. nm	NADH cyt. c reduct. (c)	ANS fluor. (d)
Haloperidol group						
Haloperidol	*	120	350	460	90	27
Methylperidol	*	34	320	450–500	24	12
Triperidol	*	34	350	445	28	12
Seperol	330	85	320, 330	458	147	35
Haloperidol *cis*	*	120	300	460	75	30
Haloperidol *trans*	*	55	300	460	23	20
Phenothiazine analogue	–	–	–	–	210	60
Spiroperidol group						
Spiroperidol $n = 3$	325	165	332	452	19	10
" $n = 2$	330	335	337	462	35	15
" $n = 1$	*	50	–	–	0	0
Compound S1	–	–	–	–	39	
Compound S2	–	–	–	–	73	
Other derivatives						
Droperidol	325	220	328	454	17	10
Benperidol	*	30	–	–	0	0
Pipamperone	320	240	330	455	47	30
Aceperone	335	200	334	460	37	0
Propyperone	315	250	330	452	40	15
Fluanisone	*	165	325	455	12	0

[a] Maxima determined on the differential spectra as indicated on Fig. 2. Symbol * indicates that no defined maximum exists.

[b] l mole^{-1} cm^{-1}.

[c] Percent activation in presence of 10^{-4}M drug.

[d] Percent increase of ANS fluorescence intensity in presence of 4×10^{-5}M drug (microsome concentration 0.15 mg/ml protein)

Results on Membranes

The actions of both series of drugs on biological membranes can be evidenced by their effects on the activity of microsomal bound enzymes NADH and NADPH cytochrome c reductases (7) and by their influence on the binding capacity of the fluorescent dye ANS (8, 20, 21).

Effects of drugs on NADH and NADPH cytochrome c reductases.

(a) Phenothiazine derivatives. NADPH cytochrome c reductase activity is not modified by these drugs, even at very high concentration (3×10^{-3} M chlorpromazine: CPZ). On the other hand, NADH cytochrome c reductase is often strongly activated. Figure 3 shows the variations of this enzymatic activity as a function of concentration of various phenothiazine derivatives. Oxidized chlorpromazine derivatives (CPZ sulfoxide and N-oxide) are inactive. Compounds ended by a primary or a secondary amine are as active as those which possess a tertiary amine. It is interesting to note that a slight inhibition is observed when the lateral chain is β-branched, except in the case of the methoxy-3 derivative (levomepromazine). In Table 1 are given the percent activation or inhibition of NADH cytochrome c reductase observed at a concentration of 4×10^{-5} M for the 19 derivatives studied.

(b) Butyrophenone derivatives. As in the preceding case, NADPH cytochrome c reductase activity is not modified by these compounds, even in the presence of a 10^{-2} M concentration of the highly soluble derivative pipamperone.

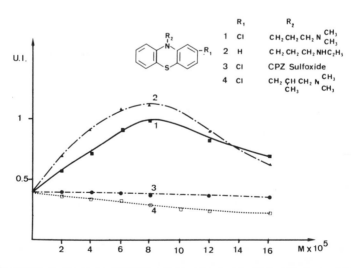

FIG. 3. Variation of microsomal NADH cytochrome c reductase activity as a function of phenothiazine concentration. One international unit (I.U.) corresponds to one micromole of cytochrome c reduced per min per mg protein.

NADH cytochrome c reductase is activated by butyrophenone derivatives, but to a lesser extent than in the case of phenothiazines. Very important variations are observed from compound to compound. Results
are given in Table 4, at a concentration of 10^{-4} M.

Effects of drugs on ANS binding by membranes.

(a) Phenothiazine derivatives. The effect of this series of drugs was
studied on increasing concentrations of membranes (0.025 to 0.5 mg/ml
protein) in the presence of 10^{-5} M ANS and of 0 to 10^{-4} M drug concentrations. At these concentrations, phenothiazine derivatives do not influence the dye fluorescence in the absence of membranes. In their presence,
ANS fluorescence is often strongly increased. Figure 4 shows these variations as a function of the concentration of various compounds in the presence of either liver microsomes or rat synaptic membranes. In Table 1 the
relative variations of fluorescence intensity measured for the other phenothiazines studied at a concentration of 3×10^{-5} M and in the presence of
0.15 mg/ml membrane proteins are given.

We observed that oxidized derivatives of CPZ and compounds with β-
branched side chains are very weakly active or more often inactive; the
other drugs have about the same action.

Another observation is the following: at the same concentrations of
membrane protein and ANS, the enhancement of dye fluorescence intensity

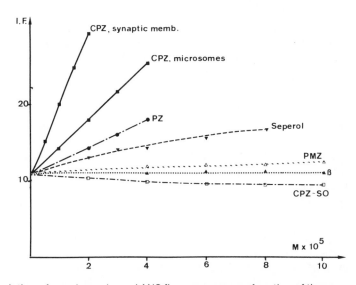

FIG. 4. Variation of membrane bound ANS fluorescence as a function of the concentration
of various drugs. Protein: 0.15 mg/ml, ANS: 10^{-5} M ; CPZ: chlorpromazine, PZ: promazine,
PMZ: promethazine, β: β-branched phenothiazine derivatives, CPZ-SO: chlorpromazine
sulfoxide. All measurements are made on microsomal membranes, except in the case indicated on the figure (synaptic membranes).

in the presence of increasing CPZ concentrations is about three times greater with synaptic membranes than with microsomes.

(b) Butyrophenone derivatives. In the presence of these drugs, one observes also an enhancement of the membrane-bound ANS fluorescence intensity (Fig. 4). However, this effect is less important than with the phenothiazines. In Table 4, the relative variations observed with the principal butyrophenone derivatives studied are given.

DISCUSSION

Spectroscopic Results

Phenothiazine derivatives. The spectroscopic data we have obtained show that there is no observable interaction between the phenothiazine nucleus and the amine side chain. This conclusion has been obtained also in a magnetic resonance study (22) of a similar series of derivatives. These results agree with the configuration predicted by quantum mechanical calculations (23, 24) made on the phenothiazine molecule and its N-substituted derivatives. It would possess a bent configuration along the nitrogen-sulfur axis. In the case of an unsubstituted derivative, the N-10 proton would be in an equatorial position, whereas the amine side chain would be in an axial position.

The theory predicts also that the side chain β-methylene group is in proximity with one of the benzene rings. In the case of β-branched side chain, the mobility of the α-methylene protons would therefore be hindered. The hypothesis could be made that the coupling constant of one of these two protons would be about the same as the coupling constant of the N-unsubstituted phenothiazine proton in order to account for the close similarities observed in the ESR spectra of the β-substituted and of the corresponding unsubstituted phenothiazine free radicals (Fig. 1).

Butyrophenone derivatives. The principal results obtained at wavelengths shorter than 300 nm have been discussed in a previous report (5). They are confirmed by the present study on a wider series of compounds. They can be summarized as follows:

— In compounds where part A is PFBP, one observes: (i) a partial singlet-singlet energy transfer (however it must be emphasized that the fluorescence quenching of part B can be due principally to a nonradioactive deactivation process), (ii) a total triplet–triplet energy transfer, in each case where it is energetically possible.

— When part A is not PFBP, energy transfers and nonradioactive deactivation processes are also observed (compounds S1, S2, and benperidol derivative). When the length of the chain binding A to B varies, or when its flexibility is reduced, the interactions between A and B are not suppressed, but the triplet–triplet energy transfer is no longer complete.

It is more difficult to interpret the new absorption band observed with all PFBP derivatives at wavelength longer than 300 nm. We have previously eliminated the possibility of a systematic impurity, of the formation of aggregates, or of a trivial photochemical degradation of the whole molecule (5, 6). The hypothesis of an excitonic delocalization (25) is not probable, because some preliminary experiments made with magnetic circular dichroism (6) demonstrate the existence of a true new band and thus eliminate the possibility of a shift of a preexisting band.

Intramolecular charge transfer complexes have been reported in numerous cases (26–28) between two conjugated parts of the same molecule. This interpretation is difficult to accept in the butyrophenone series, because pipamperone and propyperone, which have an unconjugated B fraction, show also a relatively intense long wavelength absorption band.

Another possibility is that this absorption band could be due to a partial interpenetration of the n π^* orbitals of the PFBP carbonyl and of the piperidine nitrogen (29). If this be the case, it is no longer necessary for part B to be conjugated.

The lifetime of the new phosphorescence emission and the corresponding ESR signal ($D^* = 0.096$) are characteristic of a $\pi\pi^*$ triplet state. Triplet states of intermolecular charge-transfer complexes have been reported (30), but not, as far as we know, in the case of intramolecular complexes. Thus in the compounds we have studied, this phosphorescence emission could be due to a new molecular species resulting from a rapid intramolecular photochemical reaction. It may be recalled that the PFBP ketone is highly reactive in its n π^* excited triplet state. (31, 32).

Whatever the hypothesis, the observed variations of these spectral characteristics with the nature of the compounds are probably due to variations in the stereochemistry of the derivatives as a function of the nature of the substitutents and of the length of the chain linking A with B.

Triplet–triplet energy transfers are possible only by an exchange mechanism (33, 34). This implies an overlapping of the orbitals of the two chromophores, and therefore their close spatial proximity (necessarily less than 10 Å). Molecular models show that butyrophenone molecules are able to assume numerous spatial configurations. However, one of the most probable, which is compatible with both triplet and singlet energy transfers, is represented in Fig. 5A, in the case of spiroperidol. In the configurations represented on Fig. 5B, both chromophores are too far from each other to explain the energy transfers. The model shown in Fig. 5A is a limiting case and shows that the PFBP and the B phenyl nuclei can be as close as 4.3 Å. This distance increases, when the number of CH_2's linking A with B is diminished (about 5 Å when $n = 2$ and more than 8 Å when $n = 1$). This "closed" configuration is completely compatible with the results obtained at wavelengths longer than 300 nm, and can be explained by any of the three mechanisms suggested above, i.e., a charge-transfer complex, an

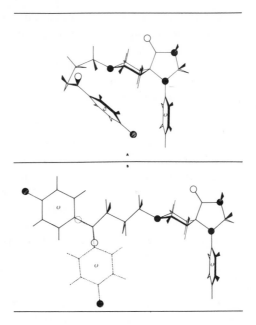

FIG. 5. Schematic representations of two limit configurations of the spiroperidol molecule. A: "closed" configuration, B: "open" configuration. ○: oxygen, ●: nitrogen ⌀: fluorine.

interaction between the PFBP carbonyl and the piperidine nitrogen, or a possible intramolecular photochemical reaction.

Membrane Results

NADH and NADPH cytochrome c reductases. NADH and NADPH cytochrome *c* reductases are enzymes tightly bound to the microsomal membrane (13). They can be solubilized by various methods, particularly by detergents (35, 36). Phenothiazine and butyrophenone derivatives are tensioactive compounds as powerful as true detergents (37). However, with a detergent such as deoxycholate, one observes only a slight activation of NADH cytochrome *c* reductase (20% maximum) preceding a rapid loss of microsomal enzyme activity at concentrations higher than 2.5×10^{-3} M. Solubilization by sodium dodecylsulfate begins abruptly at a concentration of 7×10^{-4} M and no activation is observed at lower concentrations (7). Thus the mechanism of enzyme activation by psychoactive drugs is not due to a trivial detergent-like action.

NADH cytochrome *c* reductase cannot reduce cytochrome *c* directly. The presence of cytochrome b_5 is necessary. On the other hand NADPH cytochrome *c* reductase reduces cytochrome *c* without an intermediary compound, and it may be recalled that the latter enzyme is not activated by the drugs we have studied. Both microsomal enzymes directly reduce dichlorophenolindophenol (DCPIP) (38). Experiments actually performed in our laboratory show that phenothiazine and butyrophenone derivatives do not activate NADH cytochrome c reductase, when DCPIP is used as substrate in place of cytochrome c. Thus we think that the observed activation process could be explained by a modification of the membrane protein structure under the action of the drugs which would increase the accessibility of cytochrome b_5 to cytochrome c.

Fluorescence of Membrane Bound ANS. Analysis of the fluorescence results by the method of Klotz (15, 20) has shown that in the presence of chlorpromazine or promazine the number of binding sites is decreased (4.5×10^{-5} mole ANS/g protein without drug and 1.2 and 1.6×10^{-5} mole/g respectively in the presence of 4×10^{-5} M CPZ or PZ) whereas the affinity constant (K association) is increased (from 0.35×10^5 in the absence of drug to 5.9×10^5 and 2.6×10^5 l mole^{-1} in presence of 4×10^{-5} M CPZ or PZ). With a detergent such as deoxycholate, the number of sites did not change but the affinity constant decreased (0.23×10^5 l mole^{-1} in presence of 2×10^{-4} M DOC). Since butyrophenone effects are less intense, it is difficult to obtain significant measurements by the method of Klotz. We conclude, however, that in the case of the phenothiazines, these drugs provoke a rigidification of the membrane (decrease in the number of ANS binding sites) and an increase in its hydrophobic character (increase of the affinity constant).

These observed membrane actions are perhaps unspecific and without correlation with the psychopharmacological properties of the studied drugs. However, it is interesting to note, that both groups of compounds, structurally different but pharmacologically related, possess similar activities on membranes, and that synaptic membranes are three times more sensitive than microsomes in the fluorescence experiment. This result can be correlated with the observation we have made in a spin-label study of both erythrocytes and synaptosomes that butyrophenone compounds are active only on the latter type of membranes (9).

Correlations between Spectroscopic and Membrane Results

Phenothiazine derivatives. The membrane effects we have measured do not depend strongly on the nature of substitution in position 2. The chemical structure of the amine part of the side chain is also without marked influence (secondary amines are the most active compounds). Oxidation of the tricyclic nucleus (CPZ sulfoxide) or of the side chain (CPZ N-oxide) is followed by a loss of activity. Thus the fact that β-branched derivatives — with their different free radical spectra — are inhibitory or inactive is an indication for the importance of the stereochemical structure of these compounds in their mode of interaction with biological membranes.

Butyrophenone derivatives. In this series of drugs, we can correlate the measured membrane effects with the intensity of the absorption band observed at wavelengths longer than 300 nm. This correlation is made separately in the three families of compounds studied.

— "Spiroperidol $n = 2$" has the most intense absorption band and is twice as active as "spiroperidol $n = 3$," whereas "spiroperidol $n = 1$" shows a weak band and is inactive.

— Haloperidol and its *"cis"* derivative have about the same membrane actions and the same spectra. Haloperidol *"trans"* shows a weak absorption band and is much less active. This is also the case for methylperidol and triperidol. Seperol is the most membrane active compound. Its molecular extinction coefficient value at 320 nm is weaker than that of haloperidol, but its spectrum shows a defined maximum at 335 nm and extends to longer wavelengths.

— The third group of compounds is not as homogeneous: it is interesting to note the large differences in absorption spectra and membrane actions of droperidol and benperidol which differ only by a double bond in part B.

— The existence of this absorption band is not necessary to observe the membrane effects, since compounds S1 and S2 also activate NADH cytochrome c reductase, but they are not true parafluorobutyrophenone derivatives.

Thus, in the light of our preceding conclusions concerning the spectroscopic properties of the PFBP derivatives, the correlations observed are another strong indication of the intimate relationship between the stereochemistry and the membrane action of these drugs.

We plan to measure the variations of this absorption band in the presence of membrane suspension and of the enzyme glutamic dehydrogenase, which has been shown to be strongly inhibited by haloperidol and the phenothiazine derivatives (39–41).

SUMMARY

We have studied the absorption, fluorescence, phosphorescence, and electron spin resonance spectra of 20 phenothiazine and 19 parafluorobutyrophenone derivatives. In a parallel study, we have measured the activity of microsomal NADH and NADPH cytochrome c reductases and the variation of fluorescence intensity of membrane-bound anilinonaphtalenesulfonate (ANS) in the presence of both series of drugs.

The majority of the phenothiazine and butyrophenone derivatives activate NADH cytochrome c reductase and enhance the fluorescence of membrane bound ANS. However, β-branched phenothiazines show ESR free radical spectra different from those of the corresponding unbranched compounds, inhibit the enzyme slightly, and have no effect on the ANS fluorescence.

Butyrophenone derivatives are generally less active than phenothiazines in both types of membrane tests studied. Their spectral properties, however, indicate that they could possess a "closed" stereochemical configuration. Reasonable correlations are found between these spectral characteristics and their action on the membrane.

ACKNOWLEDGMENTS

The major part of this work was carried out at the Institut de Biologie Physico-Chimique, 13 rue Pierre et Marie Curie, Paris(5) France. The authors wish to thank Prof. P. Douzou and Dr. C. Balny for several helpful discussions, as well as J. F. Mariaud and Mrs. A. Faguer for their valuable technical assistance. The authors gratefully acknowledge the help of Dr. S. Lecolier, who synthesized numerous butyrophenone compounds, and thank Laboratoires Specia(Rhône-Poulenc) for the gift of numerous phenothiazines. The work was supported by the following research organizations: DRME (convention No.: 68.34.217.00.480.75.01), INSERM and CRSSA.

REFERENCES

1. Meunier J., Viossat B., Leterrier, F., and Douzou P., *Ann. Pharm. Françaises,* **25,** 683 (1967).
2. Meunier, J., and Leterrier, F., *C. R. Acad. Sc; Paris,* **265,** 1034 (1967).
3. Meunier, J., Leterrier, F., Viossat, B., Capette, J., and Douzou, P., in *2nd International Symposium on Phenothiazines and Related Compounds, Agressologie,* **9,** 1 (1968).
4. Thiery, C., Capette, J., Meunier, J., and Leterrier, F., *J. Chim. Phys,* **66,** 134 (1969).
5. Thiery, C., *Mol. Photochem.,* **2,** 1 (1970).
6. Thiery, C., *Thesis,* University Paris VI, 1972.
7. Leterrier, F., Canva, J., and Mariaud, J. F., *C. R. Acad. Sc. Paris,* **273,** 2668 série D (1971).
8. Leterrier, F., Canva, J., Mariaud, J. F., and Calloud, J. M., *C. R. Acad. Sc. Paris,* **274,** 2094 série D (1972).
9. Leterrier, F., Rieger, F., and Mariaud, J. F., *J. Pharmacology and Exp. Ther.,* **186,** 609 (1973).
10. Meunier, J., *Thesis,* Faculté de Pharmacie, Paris, 1970.
11. Lowry, O. H., Rosebrough, N. J., Farr, A. L., and Randall, R. S., *J. Biol. Chem.,* **193,** 265 (1951).
12. Ernster, L., Siekewitz, P., and Palade, G., *J. Cell Biol.,* **15,** 541 (1962).
13. Omura, T., Siekewitz, P., and Palade, G. E., *J. Biol. Chem.,* **242,** 2389 (1967).
14. Whittaker, V. P., Michaelson, I. A., and Kirkland, R. J. A., *Biochem. J.,* **90,** 293 (1964).
15. Klotz, I., *Chem. Rev.,* **41,** 373 (1947).
16. Piette, L. H., and Forrest, I. S., *Biochim. Biophys. Acta,* **57,** 419 (1962).
17. Lhoste, J. M., and Tonnard, F., *J. Chim. Phys.,* **63,** 678 (1966).
18. Calvert, J. G., and Pitts, J. N., Jr., *Photochemistry,* vol. 1, Wiley, New York, 1966, p. 383.
19. Travers, F., and Douzou, P., *J. Phys. Chem.,* **74,** 2243 (1970).
20. Rubacalva, B., de Munoz, D. M., and Gitler, C., *Biochemistry,* **8,** 2742 (1969).
21. Flanagan, M. T., and Hesketh, T. R., *Biochim. Biophys. Acta,* **298,** 535 (1973).
22. Azzaro, M., Cambon, A., Gouezo, F., and Guedj, R., *Bull. Soc. Chim. France,* 1977 (1967).
23. Malrieu, J. P., and Pullman, B., *Theoret. Chim. Acta,* **2,** 293 (1964).
24. Coubeils, J. L., and Pullman, B., *Theoret. Chim. Acta,* **24,** 35 (1972).
25. Lamola, A. A., Leermakers, P. A., Byers, G. W., and Hammonds, G. S., *J. Am. Chem. Soc.,* **87,** 2322 (1965).

26. Shifrin, S., *Molecular Associations in Biology*, Pullman, B., (ed.) Paris, 1967, p. 323.
27. Foster, R., *Organic Charge Transfer Complexes*, vol. 1 Academic, London, 1969.
28. Oki, M., and Mutai, K., *Tetrahedron*, **26**, 1181 (1970).
29. Prout, C. K., and Castellano, E. E., *J. Chem. Soc. A.*, **2775** (1970).
30. Hayashi, H., Iwata, S., and Nagakura, S., *J. Chem. Phys.*, **50**, 993 (1969).
31. Barltrop, J. A., and Coyle, J. D., *J. Am. Chem. Soc.*, **90**, 2246 (1968).
32. Pitts, J. N., Burley, D. R., Mani, J. C., and Broadbent, A. D., *J. Am. Chem. Soc.*, **90**, 5902 (1968).
33. Terenin, A., and Ermolaev, V., *Dokl. Akad. Nauk SSSR*, **85**, 547 (1952).
34. Dexter, D. L., *J. Chem. Phys.*, **21**, 836 (1953).
35. Sato, R., Mihara, K., and Okuda, T., in *2nd International Symposium on Oxidases and Related Oxidation Reduction Systems*, Memphis, Tenn., 1971.
36. Spatz, L., and Strittmatter, P., *Proc. Nat. Acad. Sc. USA.*, **68**, 1042 (1971).
37. Seeman, P. M., and Bialy, H. S., *Biochem. Pharm*, **12**, 1181 (1963).
38. Strittmatter, P., and Velick, S. F., *J. Biol. Chem.*, **221**, 277 (1956).
39. Fahien, L. A., and Shemisa, O. A., *Mol. Pharm.*, **6**, 156 (1970).
40. Shemisa, O. A., and Fahien, L. A., *Mol. Pharm.*, **7**, 8 (1971).
41. Lees, H., *Biochem. Pharm.*, **20**, 173 (1971).

The Phenothiazines and Structurally Related Drugs, edited by I. S. Forrest, C. J. Carr, and E. Usdin. Raven Press, New York © 1974.

Isolation and Characterization of Phenothiazine-Copper Complexes

Ping C. Huang and Sabit Gabay

Biochemical Research Laboratory, Veterans Administration Hospital, Brockton, Massachusetts 02401 and Harvard School of Dental Medicine, Boston, Massachusetts 02115

INTRODUCTION

The interaction between chlorpromazine (CPZ) and cupric ion in solution has been studied as a model for trace metal participation in drug binding and metabolic processes. A number of observations led us to believe that there are unique interactions between cupric ion and CPZ. (a) The fluorescence of CPZ was found to be quenched by a series of metal ions such as Fe^{3+}, Cr^{3+}, Cu^{2+}, Ni^{2+}, Co^{2+}, and Ag^+, whereas Sn^{4+}, Al^{3+}, Mn^{2+}, Cd^{2+}, Na^+, and K^+ had no effect. However, an analysis of the fluorescence excitation spectra of CPZ revealed that only in the presence of cupric ion was the excitation band at the 270 nm region completely quenched, and a red shift of about 20 nm of the second excitation band at 315 nm region was observed (1). (b) From nuclear magnetic resonance (NMR) spectroscopy studies, a preferential broadening of the proton resonance of the first methylene group attached to the phenothiazine ring nitrogen of CPZ was detected only with cupric ion (2), suggesting a specific interaction with the ring. (c) Oxidation of CPZ with H_2O_2 at pH above 1.5 proceeds without color development yielding CPZ sulfoxide as the end product. In the presence of $CuCl_2$, however, the reaction would turn reddish and show absorption maxima at 495 and 535 nm (2). The formation and lifetime profile of this red intermediate was different from the enzymic oxidation of CPZ with peroxidase and catalase (3). The interaction of cupric ion with CPZ was found to be much stronger in nonaqueous media. Consequently, for the first time, a well-defined 1:1 CPZ-copper complex was isolated in pure crystalline form in ethanol. The isolation as well as the physical and chemical properties of the CPZ-copper complex are the main subjects of the present study.

MATERIALS AND METHODS

All reagents used were of analytical or spectro grade. CPZ hydrochloride and CPZ sulfoxide hydrochloride were kindly supplied by Smith, Kline and

French Laboratories, promazine hydrochloride by Wyeth Laboratories, fluphenazine dihydrochloride by Squibb, Inc., and imipramine by Geigy Pharmaceuticals. The perchlorate salt of the free radical of CPZ was prepared according to Felmeister (4). Prepurified nitrogen (Matheson Co., Inc.) was used for deaeration.

A pH Meter 25 (Radiometer, Copenhagen) was provided with a glass electrode and a calomel-saturated KCl reference electrode for pH measurements. Quantitative microanalyses were performed by both Galbraith Laboratories, Inc. (Knoxville, Tenn.) and Werby Laboratories, Inc. (Boston, Mass.). A Buchler-Cotlove Automatic Chloridometer from Buchler Instruments, Inc. (Fort Lee, N.J.) and standard $AgNO_3$ titration were used for the determination of ionizable chloride ion.

Ultraviolet (UV) and visible absorption spectra were recorded on a Cary 15 spectrophotometer. Infrared (IR) spectra were taken in solid KCl sample plates with a Perkin Elmer Infracord 137B Grating Infrared spectrophotometer. The electron spin resonance (ESR) was measured with a Varian V-4500 X-band spectrometer, utilizing 100-KHz modulation and Field-Dial regulation of the magnetic field. The mass spectra were obtained on a Finnigan 1015 quadrupole mass spectrometer with probe temperature at 125 or 190°C, 200 μA, 70 eV.

For kinetic studies, approximately 1 mg of the complex crystals was weighed into an amber-colored 50-ml volumetric flask to which a buffer solution pre-equilibrated and deaerated at 25°C was added. After the crystals went into solution, a 3-ml portion was immediately transferred into a rectangular absorption cell with ground-glass joint stopper under nitrogen and placed into the sample compartment of the spectrophotometer. In unbuffered cases, the sample solutions were adjusted to the desired pH with 0.05 N HCl under nitrogen in the dark. The concentration of the solution was determined at 525 nm on the basis of the molar extinction coefficient (ϵ) of the CPZ free radical perchlorate salt being 8.4×10^3 (5); that of the CPZ-copper complex was found to be 9.55×10^3.

RESULTS

Isolation and Characterization of the CPZ-Copper Complex

Various solvent systems were tried as medium to prepare, isolate, and purify the CPZ-copper complex in crystalline form. Ethanol was the first solvent to be used, as it readily dissolves both the free base and hydrochloride of CPZ as well as $CuCl_2$. Neither a change of color nor formation of a complex was obtained by combining CPZ free base and $CuCl_2$ at various molar ratios in ethanol, and thus the reaction mixture remained unchanged.

When a 2:1 equivalent mole of CPZ-HCl and $CuCl_2$ in ethanol at room temperature (71 mg/6 ml + 13.5 mg/3 ml, respectively) was mixed, the reaction mixture turned into a clear, light brownish-red solution which, when kept at 4°C overnight in the dark, yielded a precipitate of long red prisms. The crystalline product (31 mg) was collected on a filter, washed with ethanol (10 ml), and vacuum dried (m.p. 147 to 148°C, with decomposition). Microanalysis showed the product to be a 1-to-1 complex. Calculated for $CPZ \cdot CuCl_2 \cdot 2HCl = C_{12}H_{21}N_2SCl_5Cu$ was: C, 38.80; H, 4.02; N, 5.32; Cl, 33.69. Actually found was: C, 39.03; H, 3.70; N, 5.43; Cl, 33.97. Acid-base and chlorine titration studies showed it contained two equivalents of hydrogen ions and four ionizable chloride ions.

Microanalysis of the 1:1 complex showed that it contained 2 moles of HCl, obviously derived from the extra mole of CPZ-HCl used. Subsequently, the same product was obtained from the reaction of 1:1 equivalent mole of CPZ-HCl and $CuCl_2$ mixture, in the presence of small amounts of concentrated HCl (0.1 ml). The formation of 1:1 complex could also be achieved in many other organic solvents, although ethanol seemed to be the best. Similar results were obtained for promazine, which gave a brownish 1:1 copper complex containing 2 moles of HCl: $C_{17}H_{20}N_2S \cdot CuCl_2 \cdot 2HCl$ (m.p. 153 to 154°C, with decomposition), whereas CPZ sulfoxide yielded an orange-colored 1:1 copper complex containing only 1 mole of HCl: $C_{17}H_{19}N_2ClSO \cdot CuCl_2 \cdot HCl$ (m.p. 200 to 203°C, with decomposition). Fluphenazine gave a brownish copper complex (m.p. 146 to 147°C, with decomposition), whereas imipramine yielded an orange-colored complex (m.p. 132 to 133°C, with decomposition).

Absorption Spectra

The spectroscopic properties of the complex were examined in various solvents in the UV and visible regions. Nine solvent systems (water, 95% ethanol, acetonitrile, methanol, ethylene glycol, propylene glycol, dimethylformamide, dimethylsulfoxide, and dimethylacetamide) were used. The complex was readily soluble in water to give a reddish solution. It was more stable in an acidic medium; in strong acid such as 6 N H_2SO_4, the solution remained unchanged for several months.

Figure 1 illustrates the UV spectrum of the freshly prepared CPZ-copper complex and that of the starting material, CPZ-HCl, in water. As can be seen, the absorption maximum of CPZ-HCl solution at 254 nm shifted to a twin peak at 268 nm and 274 nm. The absorption maximum of CPZ-HCl at 306 nm also showed a hyperchromic shift of approximately 20 nm to 325 nm for the complex. Variable shifts were observed in other organic solvent systems. The absorption maxima of the CPZ-copper complex in various solvents studied are summarized in Table 1. The spectral properties of the solid complex in water solution are unique, particularly the red visible peak at 523 nm (Fig. 1C). Only in methanol and ethylene glycol, the solutions showed maximum absorption at 523 and 525 nm, respectively; however,

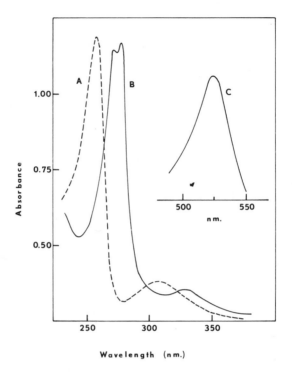

FIG. 1. Absorption spectra in aqueous solution. (A) CPZ-HCl 43.1 μM; (B) CPZ-copper complex 26.4 μM; (C) visible region of the CPZ-copper complex 50 μM.

these peaks were transient in nature and quickly disappeared within 1 min. The absorption maxima of several phenothiazines and imipramine and their copper complexes in aqueous solution are listed in Table 2.

The IR Spectra

The IR spectra of CPZ hydrochloride and the CPZ-copper complex were obtained from standard KCl pellets and are shown in Fig. 2. One of the characteristics of the CPZ hydrochloride is the strong absorption of the tertiary amine hydrochloride at the 2,500 to 2,700 cm^{-1} region. The IR spectrum of the CPZ-copper complex (Fig. 2A) showed no strong absorption in this region, although we knew from microanalysis and titration data that there were 2 moles of HCl in the molecule. Other regions of the spectrum of the complex showed marked differences when compared to the starting material. Some changes have been observed in the 1,500 to 1,600 cm^{-1} region of the phenothiazine ring (6). The new peak seen at 1,630 cm^{-1} in the CPZ-copper complex indicates an increase of the double-bond character of the N—C stretching, whereas in the complex the 1,460 cm^{-1} region

TABLE 1. *Absorption maxima of CPZ-copper complex and CPZ-HCl in various solvents*

Solvent	CPZ-HCl (nm)	CPZ-copper complex (nm)
Water	254, 306	268, 274, 325, 523
Ethanol	256, 310	255, 300
Methanol	256, 310	255, 300, 340 (sh), 523*
Acetonitrile	256, 310	256, 300
Ethylene glycol	258, 310	258, 276 (sh), 310, 525*
Propylene glycol	256, 308	256, 300, 340 (sh)
Dimethy sulfoxide	312	302
Dimethylformamide	312	300, 340 (sh)
Dimethylacetamide	312	300, 340 (sh)

* Metastable (ca. 60 sec).
(sh) = shoulder.

TABLE 2. *Absorption maxima of some phenothiazines and imipramine and their copper complexes in aqueous solution*

Compound	HCl salts (nm)	Copper-complexes (nm)
Promazine	253, 309	267, 272, 320, 511
CPZ	254, 306	268, 274, 325, 523
Fluphenazine	256, 308	260, 273, 300, 350, 495
CPZ sulfoxide	239, 272, 298, 341	239, 272, 298, 341
Imipramine	250	250

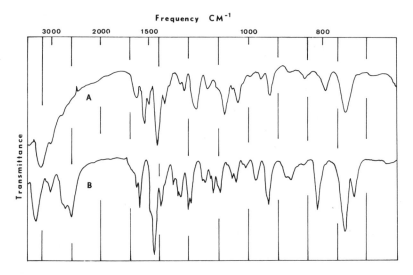

FIG. 2. Infrared spectra. (A) CPZ-copper complex; (B) CPZ-HCl.

of the alkyl C—H bondings were lower than that of CPZ-HCl. Changes were also observed in the 1,030 cm^{-1} region of the phenyl-S stretching. Although peak assignments would be difficult to interpret, the spectral differences did suggest that the complex is relatively rigid-bonded with specific orientations of the groups involved.

The ESR Spectrum

The ESR spectrum (100 gauss) of the CPZ-copper complex in aqueous solution is shown in Fig. 3. The spectrum thus recorded is very similar to the ESR spectra of the CPZ free radical generated electrochemically (7), enzymatically (8), or by chemical means (9, 10). No ESR signal was observed from the complex in solid form.

Mass Spectrometry

The mass spectrum of the CPZ-copper complex is shown in Fig. 4. No molecular ion peak or fragments containing copper could be detected. The base peak at m/e 36 is characteristic for HCl in hydrochloride salts. The other base peak at m/e 58 is characteristic for β-elimination of the CPZ side chain $[CH_2 = \overset{+}{N}—(CH_3)_2]$. Other significant ions in the fragmentation patterns occur as follows: at m/e 86 $[\overset{+}{C}H_2CH_2CH_2N(CH_3)_2]$, m/e 46 $[(CH_3)_2 \overset{+}{N}H_2]$, m/e 318 $[CPZ = C_{17}H_{19}N_2SCl]$, m/e 232 $[CPZ-86]$, and m/e 272 $[CPZ-46]$. The most striking feature of the mass spectrum is the clusters of ions beginning at m/e 352 and at 386 which indicate that two additional chlorine atoms have been incorporated into the basic CPZ unit (m/e 318). The fragmentation pattern shows significant ions at m/e 266 (352–86), 272 (353–46), 300 (386–86), and 340 (386–46), which indicates that the side chain is intact and, therefore, the chlorines have replaced hydrogens on the phenothiazine nucleus.

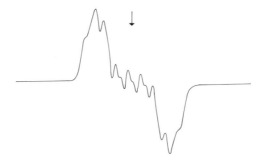

FIG. 3. ESR spectrum in aqueous solution. Module 1.0, gain 6.4×10^{-2}, 100 gauss (courtesy of Dr. Piette).

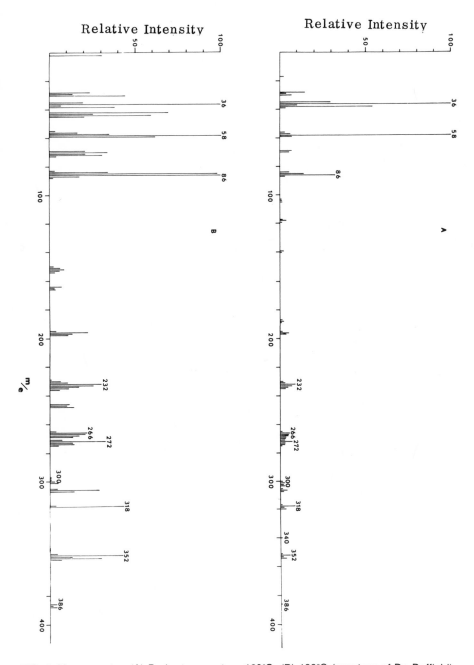

FIG. 4. Mass spectra. (A) Probe temperature 120°C; (B) 190°C (courtesy of Dr. Duffield).

Kinetic Studies of the Dismutation of the CPZ-Copper Complex in Aqueous Solution

By absorption and ESR spectroscopy we have shown that in the CPZ-copper complex, dissolved in water, the spectral properties resemble those of the CPZ free radical. It is known that the CPZ free radical in water undergoes dismutation to give CPZ and CPZ sulfoxide (11) as follows:

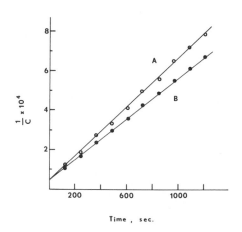

$$R = CH_2CH_2CH_2N(CH_3)_2$$

Thus, the dismutation of CPZ free radical should follow second-order kinetics.

It has been reported that a solid form of the CPZ free radical was isolated from the perchlorate salt (4), and its dismutation in aqueous solution indeed followed second-order kinetics (5). In the present study, the decay of the CPZ-copper complex and the CPZ free radical perchlorate salt in aqueous solution were compared under identical experimental conditions. Two different buffer systems and pH values were used. The dismutation of the CPZ complex in aqueous solution was also found to follow second-order kinetics, as shown in Fig. 5. The observed second-order rate constant k_{obs} for the

FIG. 5. Second-order dismutation kinetic plots. (A) CPZ free radical perchlorate salt; (B) CPZ-copper complex in 0.04 M sodium acetate buffer, pH 3.8 at 25°C.

CPZ-copper complex and for the CPZ free radical perchlorate salt at two different pH values are listed in Table 3. The k_{obs} in water for the CPZ free radical perchlorate salt was consistently higher than the CPZ-copper complex in all the conditions studied.

TABLE 3. *Experimental rate constants for the dismutation of CPZ-copper and CPZ free radical perchlorate salt*

	k_{obs} (l · mole^{-1} sec^{-1})	
pH	CPZ-copper complex	CPZ free radical perchlorate salt
2.2[a]	5.52	5.90
2.2[b]	4.08	4.36
3.8[a]	52.5	62.6
3.8[c]	11.9	15.0

[a] pH was adjusted with 0.05 N HCl (unbuffered).
[b] In 0.05 M KCl-HCl buffer.
[c] In 0.05 M Na acetate buffer.

DISCUSSION

The electron energy levels of many molecules of biological interest have been determined using the linear combination of atomic orbitals (LCAO) approximation of the molecular orbital method (12, 13). CPZ has been reported (14, 15) to have a most unusual, antibonding, highest filled molecular orbital in its ordinary stable state and is thus an exceedingly strong monovalent electron donor. On the other hand, cupric ion, by virtue of its unfilled third orbitals, is a good electron acceptor. The interaction between CPZ and $CuCl_2$ would thus fit into the general donor-acceptor type reaction. Although a series of transition metal ions of biological interest have been shown (2) to interact with CPZ, the CPZ-copper complex is the first complex to be isolated in pure crystalline form so that its properties could be studied in detail.

The absorption spectroscopic properties of the CPZ complex in water are unique in that they resemble CPZ free radical solution generated by other means (8, 10). On the other hand, the spectra of the complex in many organic solvents are generally quite similar. For example, a blue shift of about 10 nm from the long wavelength absorption band of CPZ · HCl at approximately 310 nm to approximately 300 nm for the complex was observed in nearly all cases. This is probably due to the $\pi \rightarrow \pi^*$ transition involving the phenothiazine ring electrons. A higher electron energy is required to excite the molecule, which is consistent with the fact that now the ring of the complex becomes relatively electron deficient as the result of the charge transfer.

In methanol or ethylene glycol, transient free radicals with a characteristic absorption peak near 523 nm were formed, but which disappeared within 1 min. Initial formation of some free radicals appeared to inhibit further generation of the species since the complex was recovered after evaporation of solvent. The absorption maxima of promazine and fluphenazine complexes in aqueous solution showed characteristics similar to those of the CPZ-copper complex. Whereas the absorption peaks at 511 and 495 nm for promazine and fluphenazine, respectively, showed the generation of free radical species (Table 2), the copper complexes of CPZ sulfoxide and imipramine yielded spectra in aqueous solution identical to those of their hydrochloride salts. It can thus be concluded that these latter compounds form complexes of a completely different nature. In contrast to promazine, CPZ, and fluphenazine, no free radical species have been generated in these instances.

Comparison of the IR spectra of CPZ-HCl and the CPZ-copper complex revealed that the most distinguishing feature seemed to be the strong absorption of the tertiary amine hydrochloride in the 2,500 to 2,700 cm^{-1} region which disappeared in the complex. This is a strong indication that copper has replaced the tertiary amine hydrochloride to form a direct bond with the terminal nitrogen. It has been reported from IR and other spectroscopic studies that the complex formation between copper and other ligands (e.g., amino acids and polypeptides) generally involved the displacement of the dissociable hydrogen in the molecule (16–18). Our previous NMR studies (2) had already shown a preferential broadening of the proton resonance of the first methylene group attached to the phenothiazine ring nitrogen (N-10) of the CPZ by CuCl$_2$. This could be due to free radical for the spin density is very high on the first CH$_2$.

The ESR spectrum of the crystalline CPZ-copper complex did not show any signal either from the complex itself or the cupric ion which constitutes part of the complex (25% CuCl$_2$). This might be an indication that the CPZ-copper complex is not, in a strict sense, a free radical species, and as such it more likely suggests complete two-electron transfer.

However, Piette et al. (8) showed that the color at 520 nm is due to free radicals. It should also be noted that some mixed valence copper chelates, for example, the penicillamine-copper complex (19), are red (its aqueous solution has an absorption peak at 520 nm). It was postulated (20) that the red color in that instance probably arose from charge-transfer transitions of the oligomeric forms of copper (I) and copper (II).

The changes that occur in the CPZ-copper complex molecule are manifested in the mass spectrometric studies. As seen in Fig. 4, upon electron impact pure samples of CPZ-copper complex generated dichlorpromazine and trichlorpromazine. Since no promazine fragmentation pattern was found, disproportionation did not occur, and the extra chlorine incorporated into the phenothiazine nucleus had to come from the chloride ligands of the complex. Formation of the CPZ-copper complex involved transferring an electron from the phenothiazine nucleus to a d-orbital of the cupric ion or, more strictly, to a molecular orbital which was largely concentrated on the metal. The phenothiazine ring thus becomes relatively electron deficient. Actually, in the mass spectrometer, where more electrons are knocked out, the ring becomes even more electron deficient. Thus, the electrophilic character of the phenothiazine ring may become so prominent that intra-molecular nucleophilic substitution by a chloride ion nearby in the matrix may occur.

The decay of the CPZ-copper complex in aqueous solution followed second-order kinetics. Its behavior was very similar to that of the so-called CPZ free radical perchlorate salt, further proving that CPZ free radicals were indeed generated in the solution. The difference in the observed second-order rate constants in buffered or unbuffered media within the same pH ranges showed that the hydrolysis of the phenazothionium ion (see Eq. 2 in the reaction scheme) still influences the rate of dismutation. The rate would increase as hydrogen ions are removed in a buffer solution. In un-buffered media, the final pH of the solution decreased (about 0.3 of a pH unit) after the reaction. In extreme cases, i.e., in a strong acidic medium, Eq. 2 could be reversible, and this is indeed the principle at generating CPZ free radical from CPZ and CPZ sulfoxide in strong acids (11, 21). The observed second-order rate constant for the CPZ-copper complex in aqueous medium showed consistently lower values than the CPZ free radi-cal perchlorate salt in all of the conditions studied. This probably reflects the influence of copper (I) ion as a result of the electron transfer. Whether the copper (I) ions are complexed with the CPZ free radical cannot be re-solved at this time.

A proposed structure for the 1:1 CPZ-copper complex which would best accommodate all the analytical and spectroscopic findings is shown in Fig. 6. The central copper atom is coordinated with both nitrogens in the CPZ molecule. In a three-dimensional model, carbons at each end of the three-carbon side chain, the two nitrogens, the central copper atom, and the two chloride ligands in the molecule form a plane, which bisects the slightly

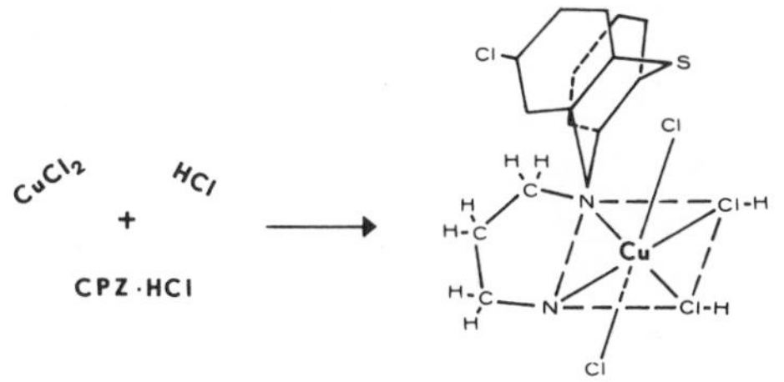

FIG. 6. Proposed molecular structure for the CPZ-copper complex.

folded phenothiazine nucleus. The other two chloride ligands are in the proximity of the two benzoid rings of the phenothiazine nucleus.

The relatively weak interaction between CPZ and cupric ion in aqueous solution (1), as manifested by the high concentration required, seemed to preclude any role that cupric ion might play in the pharmacological action of the widely used antipsychotic CPZ at the molecular level. However, studies in nonaqueous media and the actual isolation of the CPZ-copper complex indicate that strong interaction could take place in an organic biophase. Previous studies (22–25) have shown significant hydrophobic behavior for CPZ and other phenothiazines which appears to be related to their pharmacological activity (26). Strong binding between CPZ and different enzyme systems (27–29), membranes (30–32), and proteins (33–35) has been observed. Conceivably, cupric ion could play a role in such systems, especially in those with high affinity for, or actually containing, copper. Very recently ternary complexes containing copper, protein, and other active ingredients have been reported (20, 27). The cupric ion may form a complex with donor atoms of either the enzyme protein or CPZ and thereby enhance their reactivities. For instance, it may serve as a bridge by means of coordination, thus bringing the enzyme and CPZ into proximity, and it may provide a chemical activating influence as well. The cupric ion coordinated to either the enzyme or CPZ may appropriately orient groups and thereby facilitate reaction. Studies involving such possible roles of cupric ion in the interaction between CPZ and its congeners and proteins are currently in progress.

SUMMARY

CPZ and cupric chloride formed a 1:1 complex in nonaqueous organic solvents which could be isolated in pure crystalline form. The physical and chemical properties of the complex have been recorded by UV, visible, IR, ESR and mass spectrometry; kinetic studies have also been carried out. Nine different solvent systems have been used for the spectroscopic absorption studies. The IR spectrum of the complex showed that copper has replaced the tertiary amine hydrochloride to form a direct bond with the terminal nitrogen of CPZ. Whereas no ESR signal was observed from the complex in solid form, the complex dissociated into free radical species in aqueous solution. The decay of the complex in water was pH dependent and followed second-order kinetics. The mass spectrum of the complex showed fragmentation patterns of CPZ accompanied by that of dichlorpromazine and trichlorpromazine, indicating that a unique intramolecular nucleophilic substitution might have taken place. A molecular structure for the complex which involves copper ion coordinating with the two nitrogen atoms of CPZ and four other chloride ligands is proposed. The copper complexes of promazine, fluphenazine, CPZ sulfoxide, and imipramine have also been prepared under similar conditions, and the properties are discussed in comparison with the CPZ-copper complex.

ACKNOWLEDGMENTS

The authors are indebted to Dr. Lawrence Piette of the University of Hawaii, Department of Biophysics and Biochemistry, for the ESR experiments and for reading the manuscript and offering helpful comments. Many thanks are also due to Dr. Allan Duffield of Stanford University, Department of Genetics, for carrying out the mass-spectroscopy experiments.

REFERENCES

1. Huang, P. C., and Gabay, S., *The Pharmacologist,* **13,** 270 (1971).
2. Huang, P. C., and Gabay, S., *Federation Proc.,* **30,** 629 (1971).
3. Cavanaugh, D. J., *Science,* **125,** 1040 (1957).
4. Merkle, F. H., Discher, C. A., and Felmeister, A., *J. Pharm. Sci.,* **53,** 965 (1964).
5. Felmeister, A., Schaubman, R., and Howe, H., *J. Pharm. Sci.,* **54,** 1589 (1965).
6. Warren, R. J., Eisdorfer, I. B., Thompson, W. G., and Zarembo, J. E., *J. Pharm. Sci.,* **55,** 144 (1966).
7. Piette, L. H., Ludwig, P., and Adams, R. N., *Anal. Chem.,* **34,** 916 (1962).
8. Piette, L. H., Bulow, G., and Yamazaki, I., *Biochim. Biophys. Acta,* **88,** 120 (1964).
9. Lagercrantz, C., *Acta Chem. Scand.,* **15,** 1545 (1961).
10. Piette, L. H., and Forrest, I. S., *Biochim. Biophys. Acta,* **57,** 419 (1962).
11. Borg, D. C., and Cotzias, G. C., *Proc. Nat. Acad. Sci. U.S.A.,* **48,** 643 (1962).
12. Pullman, B., and Pullman, A., *Proc. Nat. Acad. Sci. U.S.A.,* **44,** 1197 (1958).
13. Pullman, B., and Pullman, A., in *Quantum Biochemistry,* Interscience, New York, 1963.
14. Karreman, G., Isenberg, I., and Szent-Gyorgyi, A., *Science,* **130,** 1191 (1959).
15. Pullman, B., and Pullman, A., *Biochim. Biophys. Acta,* **35,** 535 (1959).
16. Kim, M. K., and Martell, A. E., *Biochemistry,* **3,** 1169 (1964).
17. Carlson, R. H., and Brown, T. L., *Inorg. Chem.,* **5,** 268 (1966).
18. Rosenberg, A., *Acta Chem. Scand.,* **11,** 1390 (1957).
19. Sugiura, Y., and Tanaka, H., *Chem. Pharm. Bull. (Japan),* **18,** 368 (1970).
20. Sugiura, Y., and Tanaka, H., *Mol. Pharmacol.,* **8,** 249 (1972).
21. Felmeister, A., and Discher, C. A., *J. Pharm. Sci.,* **53,** 756 (1964).
22. Murthy, K. S. and Zografi, G., *J. Pharm. Sci.,* **59,** 1281 (1970).
23. Domino, E. F., Hudson, R. H., and Zografi, G., in *Drugs Affecting the Central Nervous System,* Vol. 2, Burger, A. (ed.), Marcel Dekker, New York, 1968.
24. Florence, A. T., *Adv. Colloid Interface Sci.,* **2,** 115 (1968).
25. Reese, D. R., Irwin, G. M., Dittert, L. W., Chong, C. W., and Swintosky, J. V., *J. Pharm. Sci.,* **53,** 591 (1964).
26. Hansch, C. and Dunn, W. J., *J. Pharm. Sci.,* **61,** 2 (1972).
27. Seghatchian, M. J., *Biochem. Pharmacol.,* **20,** 683 (1971).
28. Levine, R. J. C., Teller, D. N. and Denber, H. C. B., *Mol. Pharmacol.,* **4,** 435 (1968).
29. Gabay, S. and Harris, S. R., in *Topics in Medicinal Chemistry,* Vol. 3, Rabinowitz, J. L., and Myerson, R. M. (eds.), Wiley Interscience, New York, 1970, pp. 57–89.
30. Holmes, D. E., and Piette, L. H., *J. Pharmacol. Exptl. Therap.,* **173,** 78 (1970).
31. Guth, P. S. and Spirtes, M. A., in *International Review in Neurobiology,* Vol. 7, Academic Press, New York, 1965, pp. 231–253.
32. Doluisio, J. T., Growthamel, W. G., Tan, G. H., Swintosky, J. V., and Dittert, L. W., *J. Pharm. Sci.,* **59,** 72 (1970).
33. Krieglstein J., Lier, F., and Michaelis, J., *Naunyn-Schmiedeberg's Arch. Pharmacol.,* **272,** 121 (1972).
34. Krieglstein, J., Meiler, W., and Staab, J., *Biochem. Pharmacol.,* **21,** 985 (1972).
35. Huang, P. C. and Gabay, S. *Biochem. Pharmacol. (in press).*

The Phenothiazines and Structurally Related Drugs, edited by I. S.
Forrest, C. J. Carr, and E. Usdin. Raven Press, New York © 1974.

The Use of Mass Spectrometry for the Identification of Metabolites of Phenothiazines

A. M. Duffield

Department of Genetics, Stanford University Medical Center, Stanford, California 94305

During a study (1) of the *in vitro* metabolism by sheep-liver microsomes of chlorpromazine (I), we recorded the mass spectrum of chlorpromazine sulfoxide (II) and 7-hydroxychlorpromazine sulfoxide (III). The mass spectra of the sulfoxides (II and III) contain an ion of mass $84(C_5H_{10}N^+)$, which is absent from the mass spectra of the analogous compounds lacking the sulfoxide group. The ion in question corresponds to the dimethylamino-propyl side-chain less two hydrogen atoms. In order to define which two hydrogen atoms were lost in this fragmentation process, we initiated a synthesis of promazine sulfoxide (IV) labeled specifically at each side-chain atom with deuterium. In addition we decided to investigate the mass spectrometric fragmentation process of similarly labeled promazine (V) to confirm or deny the fragmentation processes previously suggested (2–7) for this heterocyclic system, without the confirmatory evidence of deuterium labeling.

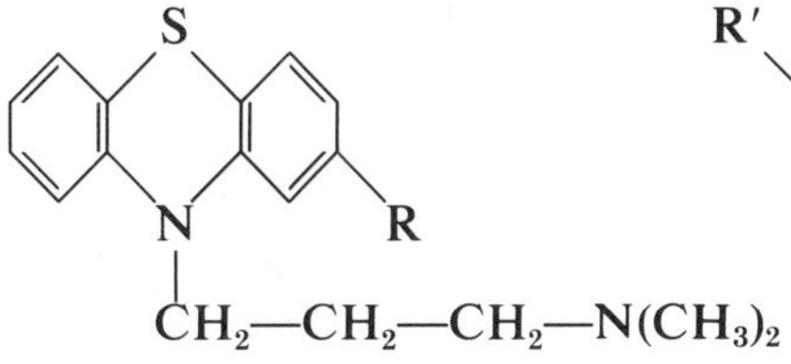

I, R=Cl
V, R=H

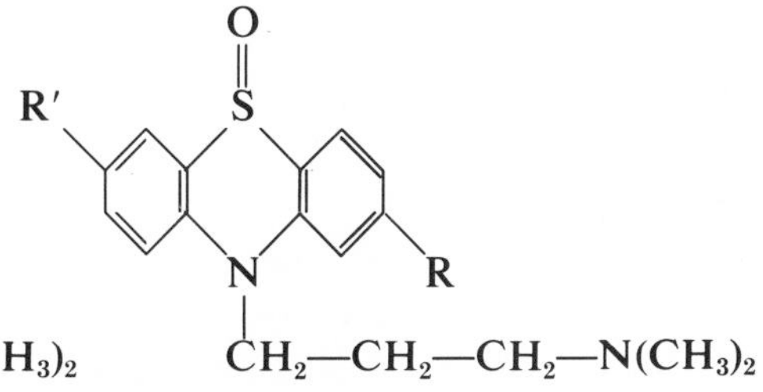

II, R=Cl, R=H
III, R=Cl, R'=OH
IV, R=R'=H

SYNTHESIS OF DEUTERATED PROMAZINE SULFOXIDES (IVa–d) AND PROMAZINES (Va–d)

The desired deuterated promazines were conveniently synthesized from condensation of phenothiazine (VI) with the appropriately deuterated tosyl-

111

ate derivative according to the method of Kaiser et al. (8). Oxidation (periodic acid) (9) then yielded the corresponding sulfoxides (IVa–d).

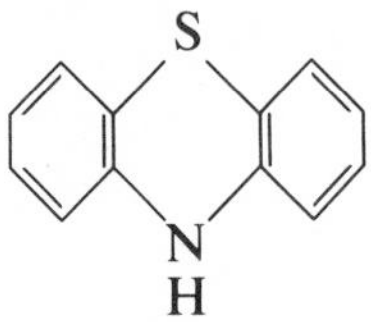

VI

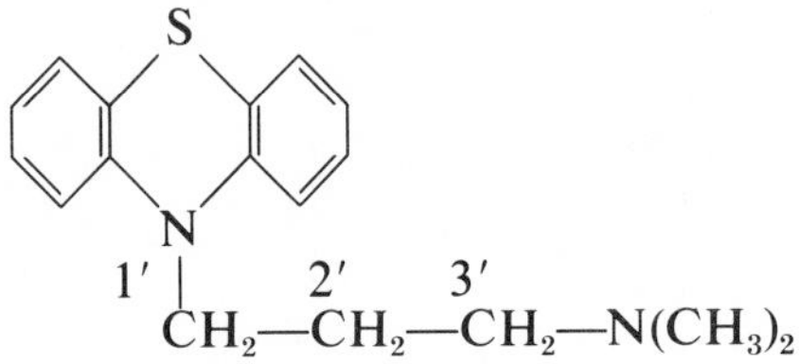

Va, 1′,1′-d₂
b, 2′,2′-d₂
c, 3′,3′-d₂
d, N(CD₃)₂

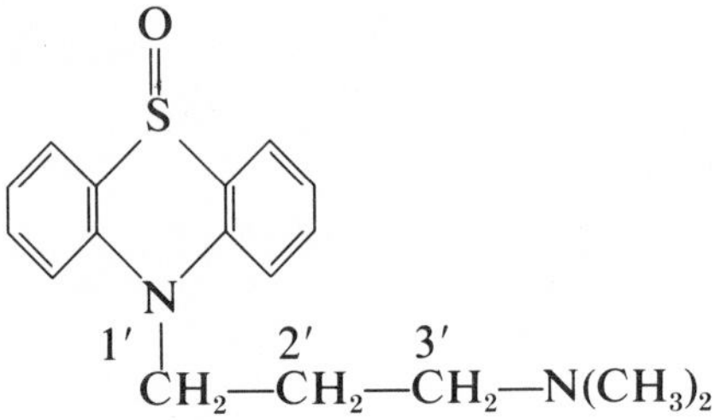

IVa, 1′, 1′-d₂
b, 2′,2′-d₂
c, 3′,3′-d₂
d, N(CD₃)₂

The synthesis of each of the four possible specifically deuterated 3-dimethylaminoprop-1-yl-p-toluenesulfonates (VIIa–d) was accomplished as indicated in Scheme 1. Precise experimental details are available (10).

DISCUSSION OF MASS SPECTRA

Ions Originating from the Side-Chains of Promazine Sulfoxide (IV) and Promazine (V)

m/e 84. This ion is prominent in the mass spectrum (Fig. 1) of promazine sulfoxide (IV), and deuterium labeling indicated that the two hydrogen atoms eliminated from the side-chain in its origin arose from C-2′ (0.75 H), C-3′ (0.30 H), and 1.0 H from the terminal dimethyl amino group. Thus one representation for 75% of this ion's yield is *a,* which by a 1,3-hydrogen shift could yield the more stable ion *a′.*

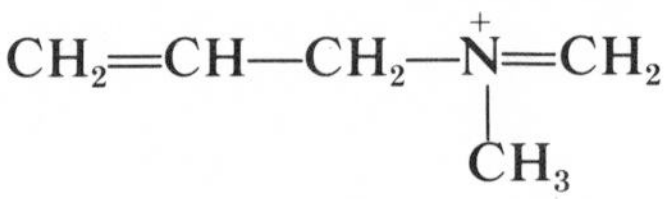

$$CH_2{=}CH{-}CH_2{-}\overset{+}{N}{=}CH_2 \qquad CH_2{=}CH{-}CH{=}\overset{+}{N}{-}CH_3$$
$$\underset{CH_3}{|} \qquad\qquad\qquad\qquad \underset{CH_3}{|}$$

a; m/e 84 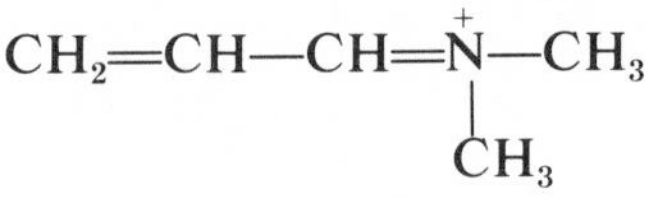   *a′; m/e* 84

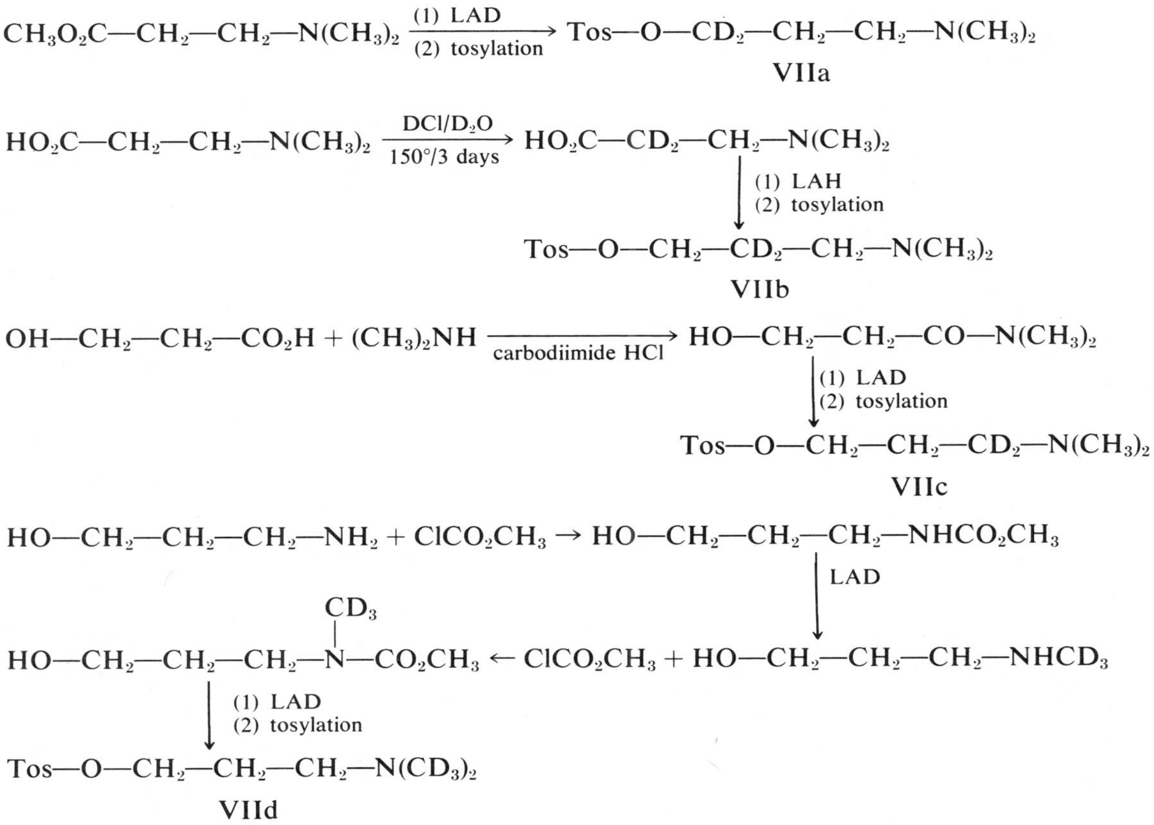

$$CH_3O_2C-CH_2-CH_2-N(CH_3)_2 \xrightarrow[\text{(2) tosylation}]{\text{(1) LAD}} Tos-O-CD_2-CH_2-CH_2-N(CH_3)_2$$

VIIa

$$HO_2C-CH_2-CH_2-N(CH_3)_2 \xrightarrow[150°/3 \text{ days}]{DCl/D_2O} HO_2C-CD_2-CH_2-N(CH_3)_2$$

$$\xrightarrow[\text{(2) tosylation}]{\text{(1) LAH}} Tos-O-CH_2-CD_2-CH_2-N(CH_3)_2$$

VIIb

$$OH-CH_2-CH_2-CO_2H + (CH_3)_2NH \xrightarrow[\text{carbodiimide HCl}]{} HO-CH_2-CH_2-CO-N(CH_3)_2$$

$$\xrightarrow[\text{(2) tosylation}]{\text{(1) LAD}} Tos-O-CH_2-CH_2-CD_2-N(CH_3)_2$$

VIIc

$$HO-CH_2-CH_2-CH_2-NH_2 + ClCO_2CH_3 \rightarrow HO-CH_2-CH_2-CH_2-NHCO_2CH_3$$

$$\downarrow \text{LAD}$$

$$HO-CH_2-CH_2-CH_2-N-CO_2CH_3 \leftarrow ClCO_2CH_3 + HO-CH_2-CH_2-CH_2-NHCD_3$$

$$\overset{\displaystyle CD_3}{|}$$

$$\xrightarrow[\text{(2) tosylation}]{\text{(1) LAD}} Tos-O-CH_2-CH_2-CH_2-N(CD_3)_2$$

VIId

SCHEME 1. Synthesis of specifically deuterated 3-dimethylaminoprop-1-yl-p-toluenesulfonates (VIIa–d). LAD = lithium aluminum deuteride; LAH = lithium aluminum hydride; Tos = p-toluenesulfonyl.

m/e 86. This ion is of low yield in the mass spectrum of the sulfoxide (IV) and is more conspicuous in the mass spectrum (Fig. 2) of promazine (V). The empirical composition of this ion ($C_5H_{12}N^+$) was established by high-resolution mass spectrometry and corresponds to the intact side chain of IV and V. This leads to the assignment of the linear structure *b* to this ion, but, as explained below, the cyclic structure *b'* must also contribute to the ion yield of mass 86 in Figs. 1 and 2.

m/e 58. The most abundant ion in the mass spectrum of IV and V is *c*, *m/e* 58, the product from ethylene ($CH_2=CH_2$) expulsion from *b*, *m/e* 86. Although this route accounts for the major fraction (60–70%) of the ion current of mass 86 in the mass spectrum (Fig. 1) of IV, another mode of formation is utilized. This was apparent from the examination of the mass spectra of the deuterated analogues (IVa and IVc). Thus in the mass spectrum of promazine sulfoxide-3,3-d$_2$ (IVc), the ion of mass 58 was distributed between *m/e* 60 (75%) and *m/e* 58 (25%), while in the spectrum of promazine sulfoxide-1,1-d$_2$ (IVa) a distribution between *m/e* 60 (15%),

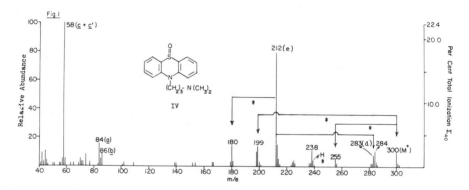

FIG. 1. Mass spectrum (70 eV) of promazine sulfoxide (IV).

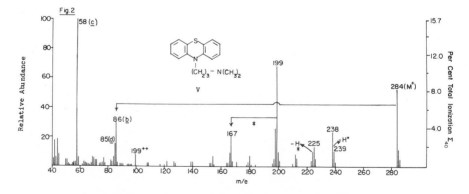

FIG. 2. Mass spectrum (70 eV) of promazine (V).

m/e 59 (25%), and *m/e* 58 (60%) was recorded. Hence it is attractive to consider a cyclic species such as *b'*, *m/e* 86 as being responsible for a portion (30–40%) of this ion's yield in Fig. 1. Note that the ion *b'* is symmetrical with respect to ethylene loss from C-1', C-2', and C-3', C-2', thereby requiring that equal amounts of *c* and *c'* should originate from *b'*. Similar reasoning, after examination of the mass spectra of the deuterated promazines (Va and Vc), leads to the conclusion that approximately 20 to 30% of the ion of mass 86 must exist in the ring form *b'* with the remainder having the linear structure *b*.

$$\overset{\bullet}{C}H_2\text{---}CH_2\text{---}CD_2\text{---}\overset{+}{N}(CH_3)_2$$
$$1' \qquad 2' \qquad 3'$$

b; m/e 88

$$\begin{array}{c} 1' \quad 2' \\ \text{---}CH_2\text{=-}CH_2 \end{array}$$

$$\begin{array}{c} 2' \quad 3' \\ \text{---}CH_2\text{=-}CD_2 \end{array}$$

$$\begin{array}{c} 1' \quad 2' \\ \text{---}CH_2\text{=-}CH_2 \end{array}$$

$$CH_2\text{=-}\overset{+}{N}(CH_3)_2 \longleftarrow$$

$$\text{D}\text{---}\overset{+}{N}\text{---}CH_3$$

$$CD_2\text{=-}\overset{+}{N}(CH_3)_2$$

c'; m/e 58

$$\text{D} \quad \overset{|}{C}H_3$$

c; m/e 60

b'; m/e 88

Ions Originating from the Ring Systems of Promazine Sulfoxide (IV) and Promazine (V)

m/e 284 in IV. Loss of an oxygen atom from the molecular ion of IV may well involve thermal, rather than electron-impact-directed, fragmentation in view of the documented examples of thermal elimination of oxygen from the molecular ions of N-oxides (11) and the known loss of oxygen from the molecular ion of phenothiazine sulfoxide (12).

m/e 212 in IV. This ion is prominent in the mass spectrum (Fig. 1) of promazine sulfoxide, and it is formed by loss of a hydroxyl radical from the molecular ion (*d, m/e* 283) followed by α-cleavage to the ring nitrogen with production of a species which can be represented by *e, m/e* 212.

$$\xrightarrow{\overset{\bullet}{-}CH_2\text{---}CHN(CH_3)_2}$$

$$CH_2\text{---}CH_2\text{---}CH\text{=-}\overset{+}{N}(CH_3)_2$$

$$\overset{+}{C}H_2$$

d, m/e 283

e, m/e 212

m/e 199 in V. This ion in Fig. 2 has its origin from elimination of the dimethylaminopropyl side-chain less one hydrogen atom from the molecular ion of promazine (V). The sources of the hydrogen atom transferred were shown from the mass spectra of the deuterated promazine derivatives to be C-3' (60%), C-1' (10%), and the dimethylamino function (10%).

SUMMARY

In conclusion, this study demonstrated that the mass spectral fragmentation processes of promazine sulfoxide and promazine are complex from the point of view of the number of different locations from which hydrogen atoms are transferred in the rearrangement processes. This state of affairs would not have been elucidated without the aid of specifically deuterated analogues of promazine and its sulfoxide and shows the danger of postulating modes of ion formation (2–7) without confirmatory evidence obtained from deuterated analogues.

The synthetic methods used to introduce deuterium into the dimethylaminopropyl side-chain of promazine should be applicable to the synthesis of chlorpromazine and its metabolites (13) specifically deuterated in any position of the side-chain. If these deuterated compounds were synthesized they would find ready application as internal standards in the quantitation of chlorpromazine and its metabolites by mass fragmentography (14). In view of the recent development of quadrupole mass fragmentography for the simultaneous quantitation of up to 12 compounds (15), it would seem possible, if the deuterated analogues were available, to quantitate for chlorpromazine and its metabolites below the nanogram level in a single analysis.

ACKNOWLEDGMENT

The author is grateful to the National Aeronautics and Space Administration (Grant No. NGR–05–020–004) for financial support.

REFERENCES

1. Brookes, L. G., Holmes, M. A., Forrest, I. S., Bacon, V. A., Duffield, A. M., and Solomon, M. D., *Agressologie*, **12**, 333 (1971).
2. Duffield, A. M., Craig, J. C., and Kray, L. R., *Tetrahedron*, **24**, 4267 (1968).
3. Audier, L., Azzaro, M., Cambon, A., and Guedj, R., *Bull. Soc. Chim. Fr.*, 1013 (1968).
4. Guedj, R., Cambon, A., Audier, L., and Azzaro, M., *Bull. Soc. Chim. Fr.* 1021 (1968).
5. Audier, L., Cambon, A., Guedj, R., and Azzaro, M., *J. Heterocycl. Chem.*, **5**, 393 (1968).
6. Mital, R. L., Jain, S. K., Azzaro, M., Cambon, A., and Rosset, J. P., *Bull. Soc. Chim. Fr.*, 2195 (1970).
7. Forrest, I. S., Rose, S. D., Brookes, L. G., Halpern, B., Bacon, V., and Silberg, I. A., *Aggresologie*, **11**, 127 (1970).
8. Kaiser, C., Tedeschi, D. H., Fowler, P. J., Pavloff, A. M., Lester, B. M., and Zirkle, C. L., *J. Med. Chem.*, **14**, 179 (1971).
9. Leonard, N. J., and Johnson, C. R., *J. Org. Chem.*, **27**, 282 (1962).
10. Solomon, M. D., Summons, R., Pereira, W., and Duffield, A. M., *Austral. J. Chem.*, **26**, 325 (1973).

11. Duffield, A. M., Buchardt, O., *Acta Chem. Scand.*, **26,** 2423 (1972).
12. Heiss, J., and Zeller, K.-P., *Org. Mass Spectrom.*, **2,** 819 (1969).
13. Cymerman-Craig, J., and Kray, L. R., *Aggresologie*, **IX,** 55 (1968).
14. Hammar, C.-G., Holmstedt, B., and Ryhage, R., *Anal. Biochem.*, **25,** 532 (1968).
15. Pereira, W. E., Hoyano, Y., Reynolds, W. E., Summons, R. E., and Duffield, A. M., *Anal. Biochem.*, **55,** 236 (1973).

The Phenothiazines and Structurally Related Drugs, edited by I. S. Forrest, C. J. Carr, and E. Usdin. Raven Press, New York © 1974.

Direct, Multiple Ion Detection of Chlorpromazine by Mass Fragmentography

Donald E. Green

Stanford University School of Medicine and Biochemical Research Laboratory, Veterans Administration Hospital, Palo Alto, California 94304

BACKGROUND

The application of mass spectrometry or combined gas-liquid chromatography/mass spectrometry to the analysis of drugs and their metabolites has been hindered by the fact that mass spectrometry, as it is usually applied, is not a separative technique. Because it is such an extremely sensitive technique, the presence of impurities causes great interferences and necessitates rigorous purification of the sample or, alternatively, introduction of the sample via a gas-liquid chromatograph (GLC) in order to achieve the required isolation of the pure material. Both of these alternatives are slow and troublesome and require highly skilled personnel for their accomplishment.

Another detractant is that mass spectrometry is not ordinarily considered to be a quantitative technique except when operated in conjunction with an internal standard (such as the target drug labeled with stable isotopes). Lastly, mass-spectrometry instrumentation has a reputation for being very bulky, costly, and temperamental (out of service more often than not), and requiring a doctorate in mass spectrometry as an operator. These shortcomings have been largely eliminated by a new instrument whose operation will be described in this chapter.

Identification of specific compounds by means of mass spectrum interpretation relies upon the principle of pattern recognition. That is, most compounds have a unique "fingerprint" composed of characteristic masses of fragment ions and relative abundances of those ions. Mass fragmentography (MF) is a form of mass spectrometry (MS) consisting of a group of techniques in which one or more characteristic fragment ions are simultaneously monitored, rather than scanning the total ion spectrum as in conventional mass spectrometry (1). In using MS as an identifying technique, it is of utmost importance to understand that there is a very significant difference between the two questions: "is chlorpromazine (CP) present in this particular sample?" and "what is this unknown material (which happens to contain CP)?" Thus, if CP *is* present, *all* of the specific ions in the CP mass spectrum *must* be present although some of their relative abundances may be enhanced due to contamination by impurities. Extraneous ions due to the impurities may also be present.

In order to minimize this type of contamination, MF is almost always performed in conjunction with GLC/MS. An additional advantage of that procedure is that one more independent physical parameter (GLC retention time) is generated to aid in the identification of a complete unknown. Moreover, single-ion detection (SID) MF in the form of a "mass chromatogram" usually extends the detection limit of the GLC method, often by a factor in excess of 1,000.

Multiple-ion detection (MID) mass fragmentography, especially if the relative abundances of the ions are considered, is capable of greatly increasing the specificity of the method with only a minimal sacrifice in sensitivity. However, as the technique has most often been applied to date, only two to four fragment ions within a span of 10 to 20% of the mass range are monitored simultaneously (2), and no attempts are made to exploit the information potential of the relative abundances of significant masses. Such a combination of MID with a consideration of relative abundances of the ions and GLC retention times — coupled with the sample purification aspect of GLC — would constitute without doubt the most powerful analytical procedure, from the standpoint of both specificity and sensitivity, that is possible with present-day instrumentation.

In spite of its advantages of sensitivity and specificity, the use of MID has not become widespread and little of its true potential has been realized. One reason for this is attributable to inherent difficulties in instrumentation because most mass spectrometers operate on the principle of magnetic focusing and cannot jump rapidly and accurately from one mass to another noncontiguous mass (3).

Data in a recent publication (4) suggested a particularly useful application of MID mass fragmentography and gave impetus to the work being described today. For a list of nearly 100 commonly abused drugs, it was reported that the mere presence of five abundant specific ions — without regard to their relative abundances and without any retention time data — was sufficient information by which to identify each of the drugs (including CP). Although five ions might be sufficient, a greater number of ions and/or relative abundance criteria will increase the certainty of identification (just as more points of similarity increase the certainty of fingerprint identification). Therefore the capability of monitoring a large number of ions and comparing their relative abundances was established as a desired feature of the new instrument.

Another major disadvantage of all existing MF instruments, either SID or MID, is the slowness inherent in the method because of the time required for the sample to make its way through the GLC column. A method which could eliminate this GLC "waiting time" would be much faster than ordinary MF but could still be approximately comparable to mass chromatography in specificity if it did possess the capability of monitoring the two independent parameters — MID and relative abundance criteria.

However, monitoring a large number of ions from the mass spectrum of a compound and simultaneously observing the relative abundances of each ion, i.e., rapidly monitoring an entire mass spectrum, is a technique that has not hitherto been possible. With the advent of modern computer technology, it has now become practical to achieve these objectives.

EXPERIMENTAL

Methods and Materials

All drugs analyzed in this work were available in the Biochemical Research Laboratory of the V.A. Hospital, Palo Alto, or were extracted from pharmaceutical dosage forms obtained commercially.

The urine specimen was obtained from a psychiatric patient at the V.A. Hospital, Palo Alto, who had been on chronic CP therapy (1,200 mg per day) for several years. The urine was hydrolyzed with 6 N NaOH by boiling under reflux for 30 min and then, after saturating the aqueous phase with NaCl, was extracted into tetrahydrofuran (THF). The THF extract was concentrated to a volume equal to 1% of the original urine volume. Aliquots (0.5 μl) of the extract were taken for analysis.

All samples were analyzed without derivatization.

Instrumentation

The automated, direct MF instrument (Olfax 7000)[1] is a conventional quadrupole mass spectrometer to which a unique inlet system, including a two-stage, semipermeable-membrane molecular separator, is attached and the operation of which is totally controlled by a specifically designed, dedicated microcomputer.

For GLC/MS operation, this instrument was integrated with a modified Varian Aerograph 204–1B gas chromatograph equipped with flame-ionization detectors, an isokinetic 10:1 column effluent splitter, and a sampling gate. Integration was effected by coupling the $\frac{1}{8}$-in sampling gate effluent line to the Olfax inlet by a $\frac{1}{4}$-in Swagelok fitting with a special reducing ferrule.

---

[1] Developed by Universal Monitor Corporation, 430 No. Halstead Street, Pasadena, Calif. 91107.

A 6-ft glass spiral column ($1/4$-in OD, 2 mm ID) packed with 1.5% OV-17 on H.P. Chromasorb G was used for all chromatography.

The Algorithms

Computer routines controlling the manner in which MID is applied and interpreted are called algorithms. Operational algorithms used in the Olfax may be written in many different ways, from very simple (a small number of ions with all ions recorded at a single, fixed gain and without intensity thresholds or subtraction of background) to very sophisticated (more than 20 ions with each ion observed at an independent gain and each ion's abundance compared with all other ions in the algorithm, with any contaminated ions rejected from consideration, with background subtraction), with only the minimum number of ions monitored as are needed to give a predetermined "confidence index," and with averaging of normalized spectral intensities in order to provide quantitation.

RESULTS AND DISCUSSION

GLC/MS Operation

One approach this system uses for obtaining mass-spectral data in the minimum time is to avoid a typical scan of a mass spectrum such as depicted for CP in Fig. 1. Assuming a scanning rate of 100 amu/sec, which is quite respectable, it would require 2.8 sec to scan from m/e 40 to m/e 320. Note all the "empty" space between major lines. Thus much time is wasted looking at portions of the spectrum where there is no information. If, on the other hand, a number of the most significant ions from the entire spectrum are selected, much time can be saved by skipping directly from one significant ion to another. A typical "contracted" spectrum for CP is shown in Fig. 2 for which a single cycle "sweep" time (at 10 msec per ion — i.e., the same nominal 100 mass numbers per sec as above) is only 0.1 sec. Thus, in this example the Olfax can look at CP 28 times in the same elapsed time that ordinary mass spectrometers could look once.

By selecting characteristic entities from a mass spectrum, algorithms can be written which are highly specific (as depicted for CP in Fig. 2) or which are representative of a general class of molecules. An example of the latter is an MID algorithm for the 2-chlorophenothiazine (2-Cl-PTZ) moiety — m/e 154, 166, 198, 214, and 233 (most of which are present at <2% of the abundance of the base peak) — which is useful for detecting the entire series of side-chain CP metabolites.

In the GLC/MS examples, the effluent gas stream from the GLC column was split — one part going to a normal flame ionization detector (FID) and the remainder to the ion source of the mass analyzer by means of a two-stage

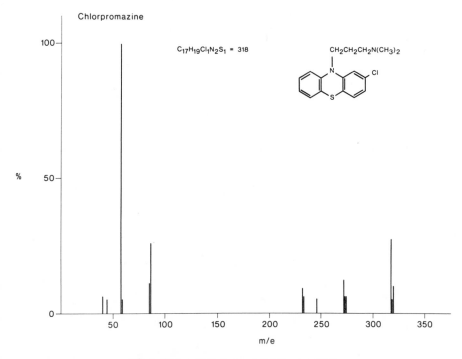

FIG. 1. Conventional mass spectrum of CP.

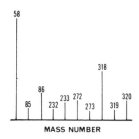

FIG. 2. "Contracted" mass spectrum of CP.

semipermeable-membrane molecular separator. The group of five ions in this simple algorithm is swept repetitively at about 1.5-sec intervals, and the ion current of each ion is monitored (5). Figure 3 shows the results obtained using this algorithm on a mixture of synthetic drugs — GLC peaks (from the left): solvent, methadone metabolite, methadone, meperidine, cannabidiol, "impurity," oxyphenbutazone, and CP. The upper record is an FID GLC record. The lower record is a simultaneous recording of the 2-Cl-PTZ algorithm, repeated at approximately 1.5-sec intervals. Note that the impurity has several of the ions in the 2-Cl-PTZ algorithm, but not all five. Hence, it

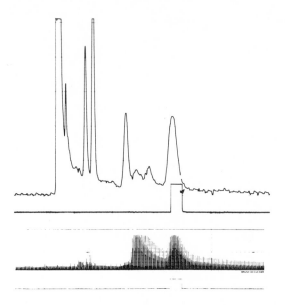

FIG. 3. GLC/MS of mixture of synthetic drugs. *Top:* FID gas chromatogram of (from left) methadone metabolite, methadone, meperidine, cannabidiol, impurity, oxyphenbutazone, and chlorpromazine. *Bottom:* MID mass fragmentogram using a 2-Cl-PTZ algorithm. *Center:* Event marker indicating computer identification of a molecule containing 2-Cl-PTZ (i.e., CP).

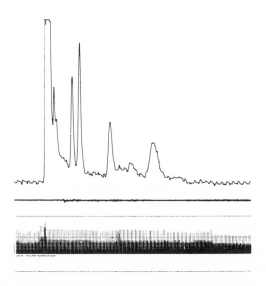

FIG. 4. Same as Fig. 3 but using a tetrahydrocannabinol algorithm.

is probably some decomposition product of CP. In the middle, between these two records, is an event marker trace, which shows when the computer in the Olfax has sensed all five ions above the required threshold and hence has "identified" the presence of CP (as 2-Cl-PTZ) (5).

The results obtained when the same sample was run against a tetrahydrocannabinol algorithm (*m/e* 231, 243, 271, 299, and 314) show clearly (Fig. 4) that very few of any of those ions are present in any of the constituents of this mixture.

A THF extract of a base-hydrolyzed urine of a patient on chronic CP therapy was chromatographed in a similar manner to give the results shown in Fig. 5. Note that the 2-Cl-PTZ algorithm (bottom) shows that several of the ions are present in three GLC peaks, but only two small GLC peaks have all five of the required ions and hence only those two may be considered to be CP metabolites.

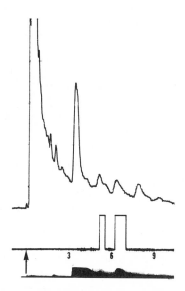

FIG. 5. GLC/MS of extract of urine from human subject on long-term CP therapy. *Top:* FID gas chromatogram. *Bottom:* MID mass fragmentogram using a 2-Cl-PTZ algorithm. *Center:* Event marker indicating detection of two metabolites possessing 2-Cl-PTZ moiety.

Direct Mass Fragmentography Operation

The elimination of the GLC in order to make the method very fast (6–9) and the application of a more complex algorithm in direct, MID MF are shown in the next example. The typical 10-ion CP pattern of Fig. 2 was used, with background subtraction and relative abundance consideration, on direct injections (i.e., without GLC separation). In this algorithm, each ion was monitored as an individual, independent entity, with its amplitude measured by autoranging the gain of each ion in each cycle with appropriate changes in filter constant and scan time. (When more material is present, less gain is required which in turn requires less filtering and allows faster scan speeds.) Figure 6 shows the results obtained when 50 ng of CP is injected and the algorithm is cycled repeatedly. Note that the maximum ion currents are obtained in a little over 2 sec and that from the maximum currents onward the relative abundances remain essentially constant.

Figure 7 is a different way of presenting the same data as shown in Fig. 6; it shows more clearly that each of the 10 ions peaks at exactly the same time and that each is present at the correct relative abundance (as represented by the reference bars which are constructed from data obtained by a slow, constant introduction of CP). This experiment shows clearly that good identification can easily be obtained in less than 5 sec.

The average intensity of all of these ions, referred to their expected values, gives a good measure of the quantity of material present. A calibration curve which was constructed in this manner is shown in Fig. 8. The deviation from linearity at the top of the range (>5 μg) is an artifact produced because only the points of maximum ion current were plotted, rather than integrating the area under the curve. More recent experiments have shown that the deviation shown at 10 ng was an experimental error and that linearity continues to below 5 ng. Each concentration on the calibration curve is the result of triplicate determinations with the maximum and minimum values as indicated.

In a similar manner, a 10-ion algorithm for 7-hydroxychlorpromazine was selected (m/e 86, 140, 184, 219, 248, 249, 275, 288, 334, and 336). When the same THF extract of the base-hydrolyzed human urine as was run by GLC/MS (Fig. 5) was injected, only three of these ions proved to be uncontaminated. A plot of those ions (m/e 288, 334, and 336) is shown in Fig. 9 along with reference bars which indicate the theoretical relative abundances.

Work was completed recently at Universal Monitor Corporation, the makers of the Olfax, on an algorithm which automatically selects uncontaminated ions from an array of up to 20 ions, calculates a confidence index to describe the goodness of fit, and averages the intensity of the utilized ions with respect to their theoretical relative abundances (i.e., quantitation). All of these activities, as well as monitoring and adjustment of system parameters such as mass calibration, multiplier gain, critical temperatures, analyzer pressure, etc., are completely under the control of the dedicated computer, which can conduct searches for up to 16 different compounds simultaneously in a single injection of as little as 0.1 μl of sample in less than 10 sec. For most substances the detection limit is approximately 50 ng and the time required to achieve both qualitative and quantitative analyses is less than 5 sec. As a consequence, totally unskilled personnel can produce reliable analyses if they are able to handle a microsyringe properly. These

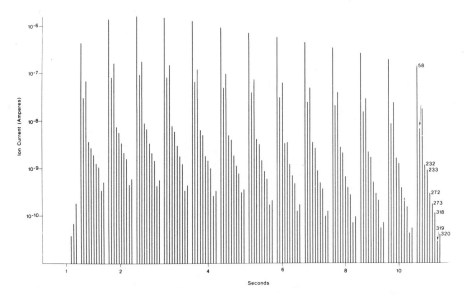

FIG. 6. Direct injection mass fragmentogram using 10-ion algorithm produced by injecting 50 ng of CP. Data presented in cyclic mode as actually collected.

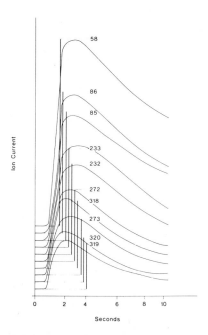

FIG. 7. Same data as Fig. 6 but with each individual ion plotted as a separate curve. Reference bars indicate the theoretical relative intensity values.

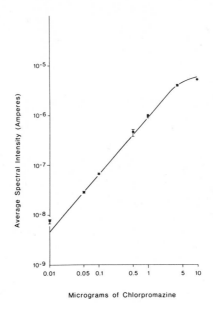

FIG. 8. Calibration curve for CP by direct injection, MID MF.

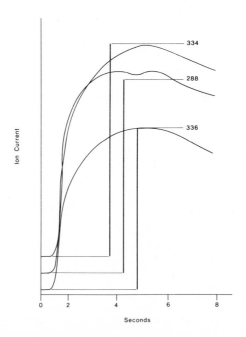

FIG. 9. Direct-injection mass fragmentogram of extract of urine from human subject on long-term CP therapy. Three individual ions (out of a 10-ion algorithm) plotted as separate curves. Reference bars indicate the theoretical relative intensity values.

attributes indicate clearly that this MID MF is the forerunner of analytical instrumentation of the future.

SUMMARY

Automated specific molecule detection by means of multiple-ion detection mass fragmentography using a specifically designed dedicated microcomputer to control the operation of, and to retrieve and analyze the data from, a unique mass-analyzer system is described. Utilization of this powerful new tool for the study of drug disposition in a somewhat conventional manner in conjunction with a gas chromatograph is described.

Examples of direct mass fragmentography (i.e., without the use of a gas chromatograph) demonstrate the ability of this novel system to detect and quantitate chlorpromazine and its metabolites at levels from 10 ng to 10 μg in a few seconds in complex biological specimens.

ACKNOWLEDGMENTS

This study was supported in part by U.S. Public Health Service grants MH 18190 and MH 20094.

REFERENCES

1. Gordon, A. E., and Frigerio, A., *J. Chromatog.,* **73,** 401 (1972).
2. Hammar, C.-G., and Hessling, R., *Anal. Chem.,* **43,** 298 (1971).
3. Holland, J. F., Sweeley, C. C., Thrush, R. E., Teets, R. E., and Bieber, M. A., *Anal. Chem.,* **45,** 308 (1973).
4. Law, N. C., Aandahl, V., Fales, H. M., and Milne, G. W. A., *Clin. Chim. Acta,* **32,** 221 (1971).
5. Green, D. E., and Littlejohn, D. P., *Proc. Western Pharmacol. Soc.,* **16,** 226 (1973).
6. Green, D. E., *Proc. Western Pharmacol. Soc.,* **12,** 50 (1969).
7. Green, D. E., *Intra-Sci. Chem. Rep.,* **4,** 211 (1970).
8. Green, D. E., Rose, S. D., and Forrest, I. S., *Proc. Western Pharmacol. Soc.,* **14,** 187 (1971).
9. Green, D. E., *Proc. Western Pharmacol. Soc.,* **15,** 74 (1972).

The Phenothiazines and Structurally Related Drugs, edited by I. S. Forrest, C. J. Carr, and E. Usdin. Raven Press, New York © 1974.

Discussion

Donald J. Jenden

I would like to try and bring together several points raised in Dr. Carr's opening remarks and in the last two papers concerning the analytical applications of mass spectrometry to the study of phenothiazines and related drugs.

Dr. Carr indicated that two analytical approaches now under development were likely to have a substantial impact on our knowledge of phenothiazines: immunochemical assays and mass spectrometry. The former, represented, for example, by a radioimmunoassay, is extremely sensitive and very specific. Mass spectrometry at its present state of development is about equally sensitive and considerably more specific. The specificity of the information provided is so great that it is frequently sufficient to identify an unknown compound unequivocally, and it is therefore of obvious value in tracing the metabolic pathways of drugs.

Applications of mass spectrometry to pharmacology and medicine now utilize most commonly an instrumental system in which a gas chromatograph is coupled to a mass spectrometer, which continuously monitors its effluent. Such a system can provide a prodigious amount of information, frequently exceeding that which can be conveniently analyzed. In such a powerful and versatile system, it is not surprising that some of its features are often sacrificed to enhance others. Two such trade-offs are illustrated in the papers just presented and in others which will be presented later.

When the aim is to identify an unknown compound unequivocally, it is necessary to collect as much information as possible about the compound with the greatest possible accuracy. This requires a relatively large quantity—generally in the range 10 ng to 1 μg. On the other hand, when the compound and its mass spectrum are known and the objective is detection or quantitation, much of the multivariate information needed for identification can be sacrificed, and much greater sensitivity can be achieved by focusing the instrument on a few masses or on a single mass which is characteristic of the compound to be measured. This commonly enhances the sensitivity up to 1,000-fold, so that it becomes quite possible to detect as little as 10 pg. With some of the newer experimental systems providing higher ion-source efficiency, sensitivities in the femtogram (1 femtogram = 10^{-15} g) range are being discussed (1, 2).

Another kind of trade-off, exemplified in the system described by Dr. Green, is the sacrifice of both sensitivity and specificity in order to simplify the sample preparation. Because the mass spectrum of most compounds is so highly specific, it may be possible to detect the characteristic relative abundance of a few selected ions even when a grossly impure sample—even raw urine—is introduced into the ion source through the special membrane separator he described. But when a sample is introduced without either preliminary extraction or separation in a gas chromatograph, hundreds of other compounds are also likely to be present simultaneously, most of them in very much larger quantities than the compound to be analyzed. They will produce a large background spectrum containing essentially all masses up to several hundred a.m.u., against which it is difficult or impossible to recognize the specific pattern of the compound one seeks to detect with any degree of confidence. Another difficulty which is likely to be encountered in this simplified system with labile compounds such as chlorpromazine and its metabolites is partial or complete loss as a result of reaction with other components of the sample (e.g., urine or a crude extract of it) when this is flash-vaporized. These are inevitable trade-offs in a system in which sample preparation is inadequate, and obviously cannot be compensated for by manipulation of the data, no matter how sophisticated the algorithm may be. On the other hand, if the compounds to be analyzed are first separated, even incompletely, by a suitable extraction procedure or, more powerfully, by a gas chromatograph, a variety of algorithms may be used to recognize and measure them, many of which have been published (3–5). The relative merits of the algorithms used in the "Olfax" cannot be adequately assessed until they also are available in published form.

Dr. Duffield described an elegant use of deuterium substitution in interpreting the fragmentation patterns of phenothiazines and their sulfoxides following electron-impact ionization. Two other uses of stable isotopes may be mentioned in this context. One is the use of a stable isotope label (generally deuterium) to provide an internal standard for the quantitative analysis of chlorpromazine and other compounds—a procedure we have followed. This is now a widely used approach in quantitative gas chromatography/mass spectrometry (6, 7), and depends upon the ability of the mass spectrometer to discriminate between two isotopic variants of the same compound on the basis of their difference in mass. The analysis is an isotope dilution method, the accuracy of which is not much affected by the troublesome variable losses in workup which plague the field of chlorpromazine metabolite analysis.

Another application of stable isotope labeling in this field, which has not so far been extensively used, is for tracer studies in clinical pharmacology (8). Here one is free of the hazards of radioisotopic tracers, but comparable sensitivity is achievable.

In summary, mass spectrometry provides a variety of powerful analytical capabilities in studying the metabolism and pharmacokinetics of phenothiazines, particularly when used in conjunction with gas chromatography. Some of the most promising of these involve the use of stable isotope labels for accurate quantitation and tracer studies.

REFERENCES

1. Horning, E. C., Horning, M. G., Carroll, D. I., Dzidic, I., and Stillwell, R. N., *Anal. Chem.*, **45**, 936 (1973).
2. Horning, M. G., Stillwell, W. G., Stillwell, R. N., Zion, T. E., and Hill, R. M., in *Proceedings of First International Symposium on Stable Isotopes in Chemistry, Biology, and Medicine*, Klein, P. D. (Ed.), Argonne National Laboratories, 1973.
3. Grotch, S. L., *Anal. Chem.*, **43**, 1362 (1971).
4. Hertz, H. S., Hites, R. A., and Biemann, K., *Anal. Chem.*, **43**, 681 (1971).
5. Reynolds, W. E., Bacon, V. A., Bridges, J. C., Coburn, T. C., Halpern, B., Lederberg, J., Levinthal, E. C., Steed, E., and Tucker, R. B., *Anal. Chem.*, **42**, 1122 (1970).
6. Jenden, D. J., and Cho., A. K., *Ann. Rev. Pharmacol.*, **13**, 371 (1973).
7. Gordon, A. E., and Frigerio, A., *J. Chromatog.*, **73**, 401 (1972).
8. Knapp, D. R., and Gaffney, T. E., *Clin. Pharmacol. Therap.*, **13**, 307 (1972).

The Phenothiazines and Structurally Related Drugs, edited by I. S. Forrest, C. J. Carr, and E. Usdin. Raven Press, New York © 1974.

Session I: Discussion

Reporter: J. C. Craig

1. *H. Fenner*

Q. Piette: Is the redox potential important in the biological activity of the substituted phenothiazines?

A. These drugs have very similar redox potentials. It seems to be more the electron density which determines the relative ease of biological hydroxylation.

Q. Gutmann: What is the relative activation energy of the two forms of the tricyclic compounds?

A. The more stable form at high temperature is the *exo* form, i.e., that in which there is less steric hindrance to rotation.

2. *F. Gutmann*

Q. F. Forrest: Has the charge-transfer complex between 6-hydroxy-dopamine and melanin been measured?

A. This has not been done so far. There would be problems due to the insolubility of melanin.

Q. Stern: Have you tried histamine?

A. It has been done by Dr. Slifkin.

Q. Jenden: Have you tried interaction of acetylcholine with phenothiazines?

A. Yes, phenothiazine itself also gives a charge-transfer complex.

Q. Fenner: The donor molecule must be in a planar transition state to form a complex. The drug reacting must be in free base form, as suggested by the low pK_a of Alimemazine® (pK_a 6.9).

Q. Seeman: At what concentrations were these interactions obtained?

A. At 10^{-3} molar.

Q. Piette: Do you feel that the charge-transfer complex was the binding mechanism?

A. The CPZ-membrane complex may dissociate to give a CPZ-6-hydroxydopamine charge-transfer complex, in which the dative bond may eventually change to a shorter covalent bond.

Q. Conway: Is the nature of this chemical adduct known?

A. It is not known yet.

3. *J. J. Kaufman*

Q. Conway: Were the models used available?

A. Yes, they were constructed from commercially available CPK (Corey-Pauling-Kolton) molecular models.

Q. Kaul: How do the structures calculated by quantum chemical and electron density methods change at the biophase, where there may be induced conformational changes? Can the quantum calculations be correlated with clinical or pharmacological activity of CPZ-type drugs?

A. One can only make calculations for both CPZ and the biogenic amine receptor, and then compare these.

Q. Piette: Have the electron densities been calculated for the hydroxy-CPZ metabolites?

A. Not so far, but it can be predicted that the important part is the electron density at the side chain. The conformation of the drug would not be changed by a hydroxy substituent on the ring. The hydroxy-CPZ is also known to turn over dopamine at the same rate as CPZ does (reported by Sjoquist at Karolinska).

Q. Gabay: Can the total *energy* of the molecule be related to its clinical efficacy?

A. No—the total molecular energy is only related to the total number of electrons in the molecule. The important quantity to calculate is the energy *level* of the electrons.

5. *F. Leterrier*

Q. Wollemann: How could NADPH-cytochrome C reductase activity be measured, knowing that CPZ can react directly with both of these?

A. At the low CPZ concentration used (10^{-5} M), there is no change in absorption and no interference with direct oxidation.

Q. Gabay: Are mitochondria present in the enzyme preparation?

A. There is only a very low contamination of the enzyme by mitochondria.

6. *A. Duffield*

Q. Walkenstein: What equipment was used, and has any quantitation been done?

A. An MS-9 and a Finnigan Quadrupole mass spectrometer were used. No quantitation has been done.

7. *D. E. Green*

Q. Walkenstein: Is the "Olfax" adaptable to other compounds?

A. Yes—algorithms for "Olfax" can be written for any compounds which are volatile enough at temperatures below 275°, i.e., those which can be chromatographed by GC.

Session II

Mode of Action and Metabolism

Chairmen: John W. Gorrod and Philip Seeman

The Phenothiazines and Structurally Related Drugs, edited by I. S. Forrest, C. J. Carr, and E. Usdin. Raven Press, New York © 1974.

The Membrane Actions of Tranquilizers in Relation to Neuroleptic-Induced Parkinsonism and Tardive Dyskinesia

P. Seeman, A. Staiman, T. Lee, and M. Chau-Wong

Pharmacology Department, University of Toronto, Toronto, Ontario, Canada

INTRODUCTION

This chapter considers how some of the fundamental actions of neuroleptics on biological membranes may help our understanding of the main clinical tranquilizing actions as well as the important side effects brought on by the neuroleptic drugs (e.g., parkinsonism and tardive dyskinesia).

THE GENERAL ACTIONS OF TRANQUILIZERS ON MEMBRANES

Membrane Expansion

It is known that biological membranes are expanded by neuroleptics (1, 2). An example of neuroleptic-induced expansion of erythrocyte ghost membranes is shown in Fig. 1B. The membrane area of the spherical erythrocyte ghosts progressively expands up to a maximum of 5% (at the concentration of 2×10^{-5} M), at which point the cell "buckles inward" (3, 4).

This phenomenon of membrane expansion underlies the antihemolytic action of neuroleptics. This is shown in Fig. 1A, where the value of 1.0 represents approximately 60% hypotonic hemolysis of human erythrocytes (4). Low concentrations of chlorpromazine are effective in protecting the erythrocytes from hypotonic hemolysis because they increase the area/volume ratio of the erythrocytes (5–7). Membrane expansion may result from membrane occupation by drug, from membrane lipid fluidization, from membrane protein expansion, and from displacement of membrane Ca^{++} by neuroleptics.

Volume Occupation of the Membrane by the Neuroleptic

The simplest factor contributing to neuroleptic-induced membrane expansion is the membrane-occupying volume of the neuroleptic molecules

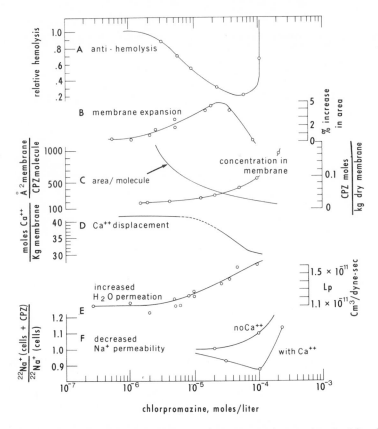

FIG. 1. Some effects of chlorpromazine on erythrocyte membranes (see text for details).

themselves. As analyzed elsewhere (1), the actual membrane-occupying volume is only about 10% of the total amount of membrane expansion. Figure 1C shows that the chlorpromazine concentration in the membrane is 0.016 moles/kg of membrane (or 16 nmolal) when the external chlorpromazine concentration is 10^{-5} M. Since the molecular volume of chlorpromazine is 164 ml/mole, the membrane-occupying volume of chlorpromazine is 2.6 ml/kg of membrane, or 0.26% (v/v). This occupying volume of 0.26% is approximately 10% of the observed membrane expansion of 2% (see Fig. 1B).

Fluidization of Membrane Lipid by Neuroleptics

On the basis that anesthetics (including the neuroleptics) expand and fluidize (i.e., loosen) lipid films at an air/water interface (8–10), it appears that membrane fluidization or expansion of membrane lipid regions can occur in the presence of neuroleptics. The expansion of such hydrocarbon regions, on the other hand, appears to be no more than expected on the basis of the occupying volume of the drug (1, 11). The fluidization of membrane lipid, therefore, cannot account for more than 10% of the overall expansion of the membrane.

Expansion and Distortion of Membrane Proteins

Anesthetics and tranquilizers readily adsorb to proteins, changing the conformation of these proteins [see references in (1)]. Since proteins and membrane globule-associated proteins (12) account for approximately 50% of the membrane mass, and since conformational changes in proteins can be rather large, it appears that neuroleptic-induced alterations in protein conformation could account for the observed membrane expansion. A diagram of this is depicted in Fig. 2, where chlorpromazine molecules are expanding membrane proteins, distorting facilitated diffusion channels (13), and distorting the Na^+-conductance channels (14). Figure 1F summarizes results [modified from (15)] illustrating that chlorpromazine reduces the resting passive influx of Na^+ in erythrocytes.

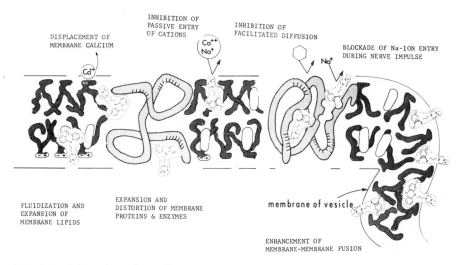

FIG. 2. Depicting the various effects of prochlorperazine on a biological membrane (see text for details).

Displacement of Membrane Ca^{++} by Neuroleptics

Neuroleptics, as with other tertiary amine local anesthetics, readily displace membrane-associated Ca^{++}. An example of this for erythrocyte membranes is shown in Fig. 1D [adapted from (16)]. Such displacement of membrane Ca^{++} might reduce the contracted state of postulated contractile proteins in the membrane (17), or might reduce the distance between lipid molecules normally crosslinked by Ca^{++} [see (18)]. These effects may partly contribute to neuroleptic-induced membrane expansion.

Membrane-Membrane Fusion

A wide variety of lipid-soluble anesthetics and tranquilizers increase the frequency of miniature end-plate potentials (mepp) [(19); further references in (1)]. This is thought to result from the drug's fluidizing action on both the presynaptic membrane and the vesicle membrane, since it is known that a wide variety of membranes are fluidized by these drugs (20). Figure 2 depicts the possible molecular pharmacology of this phenomenon, the significance of which is considered in the next section.

THE MEMBRANE ACTIONS OF TRANQUILIZERS IN RELATION TO THE CLINICAL EFFECTS

There are two types of theories explaining the main tranquilizing actions and side effects of antipsychotic drugs.

Receptor-Blockade Theory

The receptor-blockade theory of neuroleptic action generally states that the neuroleptic drugs specifically attach to dopamine receptors in the nervous system, such as in the caudate nucleus and the pituitary (21–27).

Since caudate neurons are usually inhibited by dopamine (27–29), the blockade of these dopamine receptors by neuroleptics, therefore, would activate the caudate neurons. This activation would in turn also activate the cell bodies of the dopaminergic neurons.

The net result of the activating neuronal feedback would be to increase the frequency of firing of the dopaminergic neurons (30–32) and to increase the impulse-triggered secretion of dopamine, as sketched in Fig. 3 (24, 33–36).

The increased neurosecretion of dopamine would in turn be associated with an increased synthesis of dopamine, since tyrosine hydroxylase would be disinhibited by the removal of end-product inhibition (37, 38).

Impulse-Blockade Theory

The impulse-blockade theory of neuroleptic action acknowledges that the neuroleptic drugs are potent impulse-blocking or impulse-modulating drugs (1, 14, 39–49), and can thus act as local anesthetics in the "schizophrenogenic" regions of the brain, wherever these unknown regions may be (50, 51). The resultant clinical specificity of the neuroleptics is thought

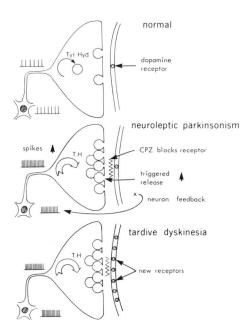

FIG. 3. The receptor-blockade theory of neuroleptic-induced Parkinsonism and tardive dyskinesia. Normally there is a resting spontaneous release of dopamine, as well as an impulse-triggered release of dopamine, from the neuron coming from the substantia nigra. The dopamine receptor-blockade theory states that the neuroleptic blocks the dopamine receptor, thus increasing the impulse frequency by neuron feedback. Parkinsonism in this theory is explained by receptor occupation; tardive dyskinesia would have to be explained by receptor synthesis or receptor supersensitivity.

to reside in the particular distribution pattern of the drugs to different brain regions (1, 23, 50–58).

The reduction in the frequency of impulses or in the impulse amplitude in the presynaptic terminal of the nigral neuron is thought to result in a reduction in the impulse-triggered release of neurotransmitter (19, 59), as shown in Fig. 4.

Concomitant with impulse-blockade presynaptically, the neuroleptics are thought to "fluidize" membranes [see (1)], thus promoting fusion between the neurovesicle membrane and the presynaptic membrane. This membrane-membrane fusion would thus lead to an increased *spontaneous secretion,* unrelated to the frequency of impulses arriving at the terminal [*cf.* (19)].

The increased spontaneous neurosecretion would in turn result in disinhibition of tyrosine hydroxylase; dopamine turnover would increase.

In effect, therefore, the receptor-blockade theory advocates that the extrapyramidal disturbances, and possibly the antipsychotic actions, produced by the neuroleptics can be attributed to the blockade of dopamine receptors. The impulse-blockade theory, on the other hand, attributes the extra-

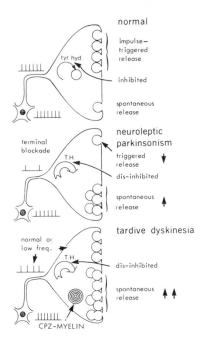

FIG. 4. The presynaptic or impulse-blockade theory of neuroleptic action states that the neuroleptic reduces the frequency or amplitude (5% or less, before complete blockade) of the presynaptic impulses; impulse-triggered release is thus reduced and parkinsonism ensues. The membrane-fluidizing action, however, enhances spontaneous neurosecretion, and this may underly tardive dyskinesia; tyrosine hydroxylase is disinhibited, thus increasing dopamine synthesis and turnover.

pyramidal effects to the diminution in impulse-triggered release of dopamine.

In order to test these two hypotheses, we determined the nerve-blocking concentrations of neuroleptic drugs on nerves having neurons of different diameters, and we obtained the dopamine-releasing potencies of the neuroleptics on rat caudate synaptosomes.

CORRELATION BETWEEN CLINICAL ANTIPSYCHOTIC DOSAGES AND THE NEURON-BLOCKING POTENCIES OF THE NEUROLEPTICS

The results in Fig. 5 indicate that the neuroleptics are very potent impulse-blocking drugs, having potencies in the nanomolar to micromolar range [rat phrenic nerve, 22°C; see (60)]. Figure 6 illustrates that these nerve impulse-blocking concentrations correlate with the clinical dosages used to control acute schizophrenia. The correlation shown in Fig. 6 suggests, therefore, that imipramine and promethazine might also be useful in treating acute schizophrenia, but at massive doses of 10^5 and 10^6 micromoles per day. Since such enormous doses would either be lethal or cause extensive

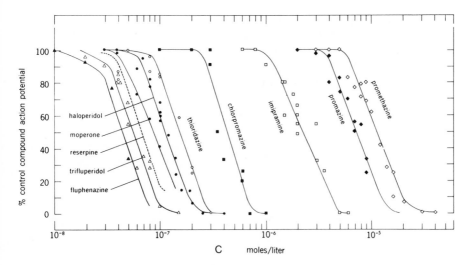

FIG. 5. Phrenic nerve block by neuroleptics. Dose-response data for neuroleptics and minor tranquilizers and antidepressants. Rat phrenic nerve (22°). Each point represents an equilibrium value. There are from two to 10 nerves per drug.

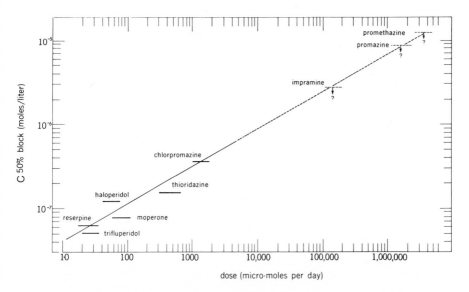

FIG. 6. Correlation between the phrenic nerve impulse-blocking potencies of the neuroleptics with their clinical efficacy in controlling acute schizophrenia. [From (61)]

side effects (62), there is no way of testing this prediction. The correlation suggests, however, that the blockade of nerve impulses may be a factor in the clinical action of these drugs.

RELATION BETWEEN *IN VIVO* AND *IN VITRO* NEUROLEPTIC CONCENTRATIONS

The question arises as to whether the blocking concentrations of the neuroleptics are the same as those found in the serum of patients. The threshold concentrations (for the onset of blockade of impulse conduction) for chlorpromazine and haloperidol are 2.5×10^{-7} and 5×10^{-8} M, respectively (see Fig. 5). Patients receiving 600 mg of chlorpromazine per day would have a plasma water molarity of approximately 3×10^{-7} M (63–65). Patients receiving 9 to 15 mg of haloperidol per day would have a plasma water molarity of about 6×10^{-8} M (66). As shown in Fig. 7, the nerve impulse-blocking concentrations for smaller fibers in the nervous system would be expected to be even lower than those found for the phrenic nerve in Fig. 5. Hence, the nerve impulse-blocking concentrations found *in vitro* are of the same order as those found clinically *in vivo*.

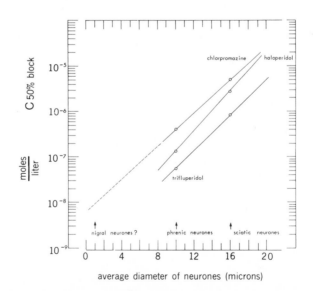

FIG. 7. Fiber-size dependence of neuron blockade by neuroleptics, showing that smaller diameter neurons are more sensitive to impulse-blockade by the neuroleptics (rat phrenic and frog sciatic nerve). The data for frog and rat sciatic nerve were the same. If this relation holds down to small fibers (0.8 μ) found in the nigral pathway, then these fibers might be blocked by the neuroleptics.

THE "SPECIFICITY" OF BUTYROPHENONES
FOR THE SODIUM CHANNEL

It has been shown by Seeman (1) that the nerve impulse-blocking concentrations for a wide range of drugs correlate with the membrane/buffer partition coefficients. The phenothiazines fit this correlation (see Fig. 8). The data in Fig. 8 also show, however, that the butyrophenones are much more potent impulse-blocking drugs than would be expected from their low membrane/buffer partition coefficients. This exception for the butyrophenones (haloperidol, trifluperidol, and moperone) suggests that these drugs may be relatively specific in blocking the sodium conductance channel in the neurolemma.

The phenothiazines, while also blocking the sodium conductance channel (14, 47), would not be considered specific in this context since the membrane concentrations of these drugs fit the classical Meyer-Overton rule of local anesthesia (1, 67).

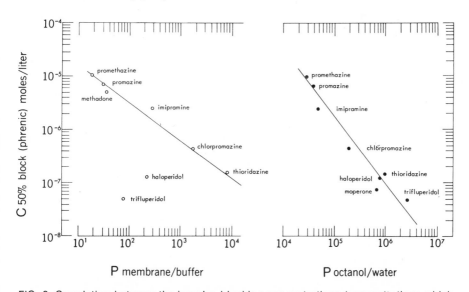

FIG. 8. Correlation between the impulse-blocking concentrations (concentrations which produce 50% blockade) and the octanol/water, as well as the membrane/buffer, partition coefficients. The butyrophenones (haloperidol and trifluperidol) do not fit the correlation on the left, and this suggests that they may be relatively specific for the sodium conductance channel.

THE DOPAMINE-RELEASING ACTIONS OF NEUROLEPTICS

The neuroleptics are potent dopamine-releasing drugs, as shown in Fig. 9 for haloperidol acting directly on rat caudate synaptosomes. The most

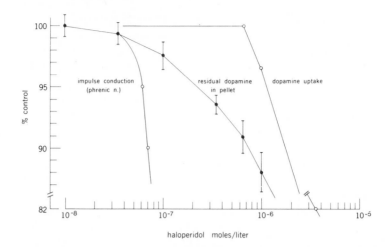

FIG. 9. Effect of haloperidol on release and uptake of dopamine, showing that haloperidol releases dopamine from rat caudate synaptosomes at concentrations which are about 10 to 20 times less than those required for inhibiting dopamine uptake. The impulse-blocking data are taken from Fig. 5.

plausible explanation for this releasing action is that the neuroleptics potentiate exocytosis (1) in the dopaminergic system in the same way as they do in the cholinergic system (19). It is known that these drugs are potent membrane expanders and membrane fluidizers, in addition to their electrical stabilizing actions (1). It is possible that the increased membrane fluidization can lead to an increased fusion rate between the vesicle membrane and the presynaptic membrane.

These effects might lead to an increased *spontaneous* neurosecretion of dopamine *in vivo*, in analogy to the increase in spontaneous neurosecretion found by Quastel et al. (19) for acetylcholine. The increased spontaneous release would disinhibit tyrosine hydroxylase (37, 38) in the presynaptic nerve terminal, thus triggering more dopamine synthesis (68) locally and intraneuronally (69, 70).

ARE THE NEUROLEPTICS ANTIDOPAMINERGIC? NEUROLEPTIC PARKINSONISM AND TARDIVE DYSKINESIA

As mentioned earlier, there are indications that the neuroleptics may specifically block dopamine receptors. There are, however no *in vitro* results where this has been properly tested using controlled dose-response procedures. Current work in this laboratory indicates that dopamine and the neuroleptics are additive rather than antagonistic in inhibiting the smooth muscle contractions of the ileum. Dopamine receptors in the ileum nerve plexus, however, may differ from those in the brain, although it is known that both tissues contain identical narcotic receptor properties (71).

This chapter thus indicates that it is possible to explain many of the neuroleptic actions and side effects on a presynaptic basis, without invoking a specific dopamine receptor blockade hypothesis. As outlined in Fig. 4, parkinsonism induced by neuroleptics would be attributed to the decrease in impulse-triggered release of dopamine. In addition, tardive dyskinesia (72, 73) can be attributed to the increase in spontaneous neurosecretion of dopamine. Dopamine neurosecretion could even persist for long periods after discontinuing use of neuroleptics, since these drugs produce membrane-drug organelles ("myelin figures") which can serve as long-term storage sites of the neuroleptic (74).

ACKNOWLEDGMENTS

This work was supported by the Ontario Mental Health Foundation and Grant MT-2951 (from the Medical Research Council of Canada).

REFERENCES

 1. Seeman, P., *Pharmacol. Rev.*, **24**, 583 (1972).
 2. Seeman, P., Kwant, W. O., and Sauks, T., *Biochim. Biophys. Acta*, **183**, 499 (1969).
 3. Seeman, P., in Deutsch, E., Gerlach, E., and Moser, K., (Eds.) *Metabolism and Membrane Permeability of Erythrocytes and Thrombocytes*, Georg Thieme Verlag, Stuttgart, 1968, p. 384.
 4. Seeman, P., *Biochem. Pharmacol.*, **15**, 1753 (1966).
 5. van Steveninck, J., Gjösünd, W. K., and Booij, H. L., *Biochem. Pharmacol.*, **16**, 837 (1967).
 6. Seeman, P., and Kwant, W. O., *Biochim. Biophys. Acta*, **183**, 512 (1969).
 7. Kwant, W. O., and van Steveninck, J., *Biochem. Pharmacol.*, **17**, 2215 (1968).
 8. Deenen, L. L. M. van, and Demel, R. A., *Biochim. Biophys. Acta*, **94**, 312 (1965).
 9. Demel, R. A., and van Deenen, L. L. M., *Chem. Phys. Lipids*, **1**, 68 (1966).
10. Sears, D. F., and Brandes, K. K., *Agents and Actions*, **1**, 28 (1969).
11. Sears, D. F., and Fuller, E. L., *Resp. Physiol.*, **5**, 175 (1968).
12. MacLennan, D. H., Seeman, P., Iles, G. H., and Yip, C. C., *J. Biol. Chem.*, **246**, 2702 (1971).
13. Hunter, F. R., George, J., and Ospina, B., *J. Cell. Comp. Physiol.*, **65**, 299 (1965).
14. Gruener, R., and Narahashi, T., *J. Pharmacol. Exp. Ther.*, **181**, 161 (1972).
15. Seeman, P., Kwant, W. O., Goldberg, M., and Chau-Wong, M., *Biochim. Biophys. Acta*, **241**, 349 (1971).
16. Kwant, W. O., and Seeman, P., *Biochim. Biophys. Acta*, **193**, 338 (1969).
17. Wins, P., and Schoffeniels, E., *Arch. Int. Physiol. Biochim.*, **74**, 812 (1966).
18. Hauser, H., and Dawson, R. M. C., *Biochem. J.*, **109**, 909 (1968).
19. Quastel, D. M. J., Hackett, J. T., and Okamoto, K., *Can. J. Physiol. Pharmacol.*, **50**, 279 (1972).
20. Metcalfe, J. C., and Burgen, A. S. V., *Nature*, **220**, 587 (1968).
21. Kebabian, J. W., Petzold, G. L., and Greengard, P., *Proc. Nat. Acad. Sci., U.S.A.*, **69**, 2145 (1972).
22. Horn, A. S., and Snyder, S. H., *Proc. Nat. Acad. Sci., U.S.A.*, **68**, 2325 (1971).
23. Janssen, P. A. J., and Allewijn, F. T. N., *Arzneim.-Forsch.*, **19**, 199 (1969).
24. Andén, N.-E., Corrodi, H., Fuxe, K., and Ungerstedt, U., *Europ. J. Pharmacol.*, **15**, 193 (1971).
25. Bieger, D., Larochelle, L., and Hornykiewicz, O., *Europ. J. Pharmacol.*, **18**, 128 (1972).
26. Hornykiewicz, O., *Pharmacol. Rev.*, **18**, 925 (1966).
27. York, D. H., *Brain Res.*, **37**, 91 (1972).
28. MacLennan, H., and York, D. H., *J. Physiol.*, **189**, 393 (1967).

29. Connor, J. D., *J. Physiol.*, **208**, 691 (1970).
30. Bunney, B. S., Aghajanian, G. K., and Roth, R. H., *Fed. Proc.*, **32**, 247A (1973).
31. Bunney, B. S., Walters, J. R., Roth, R. H., and Aghajanian, G. K., *J. Pharmacol. Exp. Ther. (in press)*, cited by Ref. 32.
32. Roth, R. H., *Brit. J. Pharmacol.*, **47**, 408 (1973).
33. Andén, N.-E., Butcher, S. G., Corrodi, H., Fuxe, K., and Ungerstedt, U., *Europ. J. Pharmacol.*, **11**, 303 (1970).
34. Da Prada, M., and Pletscher, A., *Experientia*, **22**, 465 (1966).
35. Nybäck, H., *Acta Physiol. Scand.*, **84**, 54 (1972).
36. Kehr, W., Carlsson, A., Lindqvist, M., Magnusson, T., and Atack, C., *J. Pharm. Pharmacol.*, **24**, 744 (1972).
37. Spector, S., Gordon, R., Sjoerdsma, A., and Udenfriend, S., *Mol. Pharmacol.*, **3**, 549 (1967).
38. Javoy, F., Agid, Y., Bouvet, D., and Glowinski, J., *J. Pharmacol. Exp. Ther.*, **182**, 454 (1972).
39. Courvoisier, S., Fournel, J., Ducrot, R., Kolsky, M., and Koetschet, P., *Arch. Int. Pharmacodyn. Thér.*, **92**, 305 (1953).
40. Halpern, B. N., Perrin, G., and Dews, P. B., *J. Physiol. (Paris)*, **40**, 210A (1948).
41. Rosenberg, P., and Ehrenpreis, S., *Biochem. Pharmacol.*, **8**, 192 (1961).
42. Balzer, H., and Hellenbrecht, D., *Naunyn-Schmiedeberg's Arch. Pharmakol.*, **264**, 129 (1969).
43. Elliott, R. C., and Quilliam, J. P., *Brit. J. Pharmacol.*, **23**, 222 (1964).
44. Rosenberg, P., and Bartels, E., *J. Pharmacol. Exp. Ther.*, **155**, 532 (1967).
45. Ritchie, J. M., and Greengard, P., *J. Pharmacol. Exp. Ther.*, **133**, 241 (1961).
46. Sabelli, H. C., Marks, R., and Toman, J. E. P., *Fed. Proc.*, **22**, 1374 (1963).
47. Hille, B., *Nature (London)*, **210**, 1220 (1966).
48. Pruett, M. K., and Williams, B. B., *J. Pharmaceut. Sci.*, **55**, 1139 (1966).
49. Hellenbrecht, D., *Naunyn-Schmiedeberg's Arch. Pharmakol.*, **271**, 125 (1971).
50. Seeman, P., *Int. Rev. Neurobiol.*, **9**, 145 (1966).
51. Kwant, W. O., and Seeman, P., *Biochem. Pharmacol.*, **20**, 2089 (1971).
52. Janssen, P. A. J., Soudijn, W., van Wigngaarden, I., and Dresse, A., *Arzneim.-Forsch.*, **18**, 282 (1969).
53. Lindqvist, N. G., *Arch. Int. Pharmacodyn. Thér.*, **200**, 190 (1972).
54. Cassano, G. B., Sjöstrand, S. E., and Hansson, E., *Arch. Int. Pharmacodyn. Thér.*, **156**, 48 (1965).
55. Eckert, H., and Hopf, A., *Int. Pharmacopsychiat.*, **4**, 98 (1970).
56. Guth, P. S., and Amaro, J., *Biochem. Pharmacol.*, **14**, 67 (1965).
57. De Jaramillo, G. A. V., and Guth, P. S., Biochem. Pharmacol., **12**, 525 (1963).
58. Fog, R. L., Randrup, A., and Pakkenberg, H., *Psychopharmacologia (Berl.)*, **12**, 428 (1968).
59. Takeuchi, A., and Takeuchi, N., *J. Gen. Physiol.*, **45**, 1181 (1962).
60. Seeman, P., Chau-Wong, M., and Moyyen, S., *Can. J. Physiol. Pharmacol.*, **50**, 1181 (1972).
61. Seeman, P., and Bialy, H. S., *Biochem. Pharmacol.*, **12**, 1181 (1963).
62. Gallant, D. M., and Bishop, M. P., *Curr. Ther. Res.*, **9**, 309 (1967).
63. Curry, S. H., *J. Pharm. Pharmacol.*, **22**, 753 (1970).
64. Sakalis, G., Curry, S. H., Mould, G. P., and Lader, M. H., *Clin. Pharmacol. Ther.*, **13**, 931 (1972).
65. Cooper, S. F., Albert, J.-M. Hillel, J., and Caille, G., *Curr. Ther. Res.*, **15**, 73 (1973).
66. Zingales, I. A., *J. Chromatog.*, **54**, 15 (1972).
67. Kwant, W., and Seeman, P., *Biochim. Biophys. Acta*, **183**, 530 (1969).
68. Matthysse, S., *Fed. Proc.*, **32**, 200 (1973).
69. Farnebo, L.-O., and Hamberger, B., *Acta Physiol. Scand., Suppl.*, **371**, 35 (1971).
70. Farnebo, L.-O., and Hamberger, B., *Proc. 5th Int. Pharmacol. Congr.*, 1972, p. 66.
71. Pert, C., and Snyder, S. H., *Science*, **179**, 1011 (1973).
72. Kazamatsuri, H., Chien, C.-P., and Cole, J. O., *Arch. Gen. Psychiat.*, **27**, 491 (1972).
73. Schiele, B. C., Gallant, D., Simpson, G., Gardner, E. A., Cole, J., Crane, G., Chase, T., Ayd, F., Levine, J., and Ochota, L., *Arch. Gen. Psychiat.*, **28**, 463 (1973).
74. Tousimis, A. J., and Barron, C. N., *Exp. Mol. Pathol.*, **13**, 89 (1970).

The Phenothiazines and Structurally Related Drugs, edited by I. S.
Forrest, C. J. Carr, and E. Usdin. Raven Press, New York © 1974.

Red Blood Cell Drug Binding as a Possible Mechanism for Tranquilization

Albert A. Manian, Lawrence H. Piette,* Deena Holland,*
Thomas Grover,* and François Leterrier**

National Institute of Mental Health, Rockville, Maryland;* Department of Biochemistry and
Biophysics, School of Medicine, University of Hawaii, Honolulu, Hawaii;** and Institut de
Biologie et Physico Chimique, Paris, France

INTRODUCTION

In the course of developing a radioassay procedure for measuring chlorpromazine (CPZ) and some of its metabolites in the plasma of schizophrenic
patients Efron et al. (1, 2) found that 50% of added hydroxylated chlorpromazine (OH-CPZ) derivatives was accountable in the aqueous fraction
after a heptane extraction. Further attempts by these investigators to
establish a reliable and reproducible means for measuring the hydroxylated
compounds were pursued but never completed. During these studies,
however, it was learned that 7-OH-CPZ and 8-OH-CPZ were also bound
to the erythrocytes. Early studies by Freeman and Spirtes (3, 4) showed
adsorption to and changes in the red blood cells (RBC) occurred with the
administration of various concentrations of CPZ. Turano et al. (5) recently
performed qualitative and quantitative analyses of plasma, erythrocyte
washings, and hemolysates of schizophrenics on long-term CPZ therapy.
In the hemolysates 7-OH-CPZ, its mono- and didesmethylated derivatives
and their sulfoxides were identified in the free form; whereas, CPZ was
present both free and conjugated with glucuronic acid. The erythrocyte
washings yielded free CPZ; 7-OH-CPZ, its sulfoxide, and desmethylated
derivatives were found as glucuronides.

Using a unique electron spin resonance (ESR), nitroxide spin-label probe
technique to detect the interactions between various phenothiazine derivatives and bovine erythrocyte ghosts, Holmes and Piette found drug-induced
changes in ESR spectra from the spin-labeled membranes (6). At the same
concentration of 3.0×10^{-4} M, 7-OH-CPZ demonstrated greater activity
than CPZ in inducing such alterations. These changes suggested that the
phenothiazines induce a protein conformational change at one of at least
three surface membrane sulfhydryl (SH) sites which can be spin labeled.
With increased drug concentration, this conformational alteration in the

149

protein structure is reflected by a change in the environment of the spin label in that some of the membrane surface SH sites are converted to SH sites buried within the membrane. It was later shown by Piette that the degree of antipsychotic activity exhibited by phenothiazine drugs correlated well with the degree of drug adsorption to rat RBC ghosts and brain synaptosomes.[1]

The 7-hydroxy metabolite of CPZ has been shown to possess biological activity in animals most similar to the parent compound but no significant pharmacological effects were elicited by 8-OH-CPZ (7). Further investigations on these two metabolites demonstrated that they are able to cross the blood–brain barrier and localize in the central nervous system (8–10).

From these above developments, the possibility has been considered that the two metabolites, as well as CPZ, are transported to the brain by means of the erythrocytes and are possibly released there by a subsequent transfer mechanism to initiate pharmacological activity. To test this hypothesis we have undertaken these preliminary studies in which attempts are made (a) to investigate the binding properties of these compounds on the membranes of rat RBC and brain synaptosomes, (b) to observe if tranquilization occurs in rats after i.v. injection of RBC bound with either CPZ or one of the metabolites, and (c) to compare levels of the administered compounds in the erythrocytes, plasma, and brain of rats. We, also, have included for study a dihydroxylated metabolite of CPZ, 7,8-dihydroxychlorpromazine (7,8-diOH-CPZ), recently identified in biological samples taken from chronic schizophrenic patients solely on CPZ therapy (11).

EXPERIMENTAL

Materials

Randomly tritiated 7-OH-CPZ (0.332 mCi/mg), 8-OH-CPZ (0.212 mCi/mg), 7,8-diOH-CPZ (0.616 mCi/mg), and didesmethylchlorpromazine (Nor$_2$-CPZ) hydrochloride were obtained from the Psychopharmacology Research Branch, N.I.M.H. CPZ-[3]H(9) hydrochloride (0.164 mCi/mg) was kindly provided by Dr. Alfred R. Maass of the Smith Kline and French Laboratories, Inc.

Preparation of Spin-Labeled Nor$_2$-CPZ

The acid chloride of 3-carboxy-2,2,5,5,-tetramethylpyrroline-1-oxyl was prepared by the method of Rozantsev (12) and recrystallized to constant melting point (211 to 212°) before use. It was synthesized by adding under

---

[1] Piette, L. H., *Progress report to National Institute of Mental Health*, Grant MH–12952–05, June 1971.

dry conditions (2.9 mmoles) thionyl chloride to a benzene solution (10 ml) of the acid (2.84 mmoles) containing pyridine (3.0 mmoles). After stirring one hour, the solution was decanted from the solid pyridinium hydrochloride into a benzene solution (10 ml) of Nor_2-CPZ (2.84 mmoles) at 60° and stirred in the dark for one hour. The stirring was continued at room temperature for one day. The solvent was removed at reduced pressure and the residue extracted with 40 ml chloroform, the chloroform solution quickly washed with 5% hydrochloric acid, then with water, dried, and solvent removed to yield a yellow oil. This was chromatographed on a column of 60–100 mesh Fluorisil (70 g) using ether and ether-methanol to develop. Four bands in all were present. The spin-labeled Nor_2-CPZ (0.701 g, 1.53 mmoles, 54% overall yield) eluted as the third band gave a yellow glass. The molecular weight of spin-labeled Nor_2-CPZ was 456 (calc. 456 for mono spin-labeled compound) as determined by low-resolution mass spectrometry and by ESR.

Preparation of RBC

Red blood cells were freshly prepared from blood withdrawn by heart puncture from adult Holtzman rats into heparinized tubes. They were separated from plasma by centrifugation and washed with five volumes of phosphate buffer (0.15 M, pH 7.2) a total of four times. The washed RBC were then routinely resuspended to a volume equal to the initial blood sample and aliquots taken for binding experiments.

Preparation of Synaptosomes

Synaptosomes were prepared from brains of Holtzman rats (20 to 30 day old) on discontinuous Ficoll gradients by the method of Abdel-Latif (13) as modified by Autilio et al. (14). A Packard Tri-carb liquid scintillation counter and Varian E-4 spectrometer were used in the counting and ESR experiments.

METHODS AND RESULTS

Binding Affinities to RBC and Synaptosomes

A considerable number of studies have been made on the measurement of phenothiazine drug levels in blood of humans and animals. Measurements have been made on levels in serum, plasma, and intact erythrocytes as well as in hemolysates of erythrocyte suspensions (5). In addition, a great deal of attention has been given to the effect of these drugs on cell membranes (3, 4, 15), demonstrating for RBC at least, that the phenothiazines are capable of protection against hemolysis at low concentrations but induce hemolysis at higher concentrations and produce local anesthesia at even higher concentrations, all of which suggest membrane alterations. In most of the studies reported, however, the measurements of drug levels or membrane effects have been by indirect physical or chemical methods, i.e., where the blood is either fractionated or hemolyzed and the drug subsequently removed by extraction and analyzed by chromatographic or other techniques, or in the case of the membrane studies, cell volume or hemolysis is measured as a function of drug concentration.

We have used two different direct methods to compare the relative binding capacity of the phenothiazine drugs as well as their distribution in blood and brain tissues. The two methods are an isotope-labeling technique and an ESR spin-labeling method.

Isotope-labeling technique. Tritiated drug derivatives are incubated with varying concentrations of freshly harvested RBC either alone, or in the presence of other drugs as in the case of competition studies, for a fixed time after which the cells are spun down and counts are taken of the supernatant. The amount of drug bound is reflected by the difference in counts between the total added and that found in the supernatant. A similar method was also used in which instead of centrifuging the cells and counting the supernatant, the radioactive drug was allowed to equilibrate itself in a dialysis apparatus consisting of two chambers: one containing RBC, the other buffer separated by a dialysis membrane.

For assessing the relative similarities in the binding of CPZ, 7-OH-CPZ, 8-OH-CPZ, and 7,8-diOH-CPZ to RBC, duplicate samples with equal aliquots of washed RBC were incubated with unlabeled compound (5×10^{-6} M) for 5 min at 4°C followed by the addition of CPZ-^{3}H(9) (5×10^{-6} M) and further incubation at 4°C for 60 min. The samples were then centrifuged to remove RBC and 0.1 ml aliquots of the supernatant placed in 10 ml of Bray's solution for counting on a Packard Tri-carb liquid scintillation counter. The results are given in Table 1.

Relative binding affinities of CPZ, 7-OH-CPZ, and 7,8-diOH-CPZ were

TABLE 1. *Comparison of the relative affinity of CPZ-^{3}H(9)*
(5×10^{-6} M) for rat RBC alone and in the presence of
added CPZ, 7-OH-CPZ, 8-OH-CPZ, or 7,8-diOH-CPZ

Sample[a]	CPZ-^{3}H(9) in supernatant	
	n moles	% of total
1. CPZ-^{3}H(9)	2.2	44
2. CPZ + CPZ-^{3}H(9)	2.6	52
3. 7-OH-CPZ + CPZ-^{3}H(9)	2.6	52
4. 8-OH-CPZ + CPZ-^{3}H(9)	2.5	50
5. 7,8-diOH-CPZ + CPZ-^{3}H(9)	2.6	52

[a] All compounds are at 5×10^{-6} M conc.

determined by incubating the particular phenothiazine at 1×10^{-5} M with varying numbers of washed RBC from 1×10^8 to 3×10^9 cells/ml at 4°C for 60 min. The samples were then centrifuged and 0.1 ml of supernatant removed and counted as mentioned previously.

In Fig. 1, Klotz plots (16) are presented, which clearly show the differences in binding between CPZ and the hydroxylated metabolites. A binding constant K of 2.5×10^5 M^{-1} and number of binding sites $n = 4 \times 10^6$ molecules/RBC were calculated for CPZ; the metabolite binding however is too weak to allow for similar calculations.

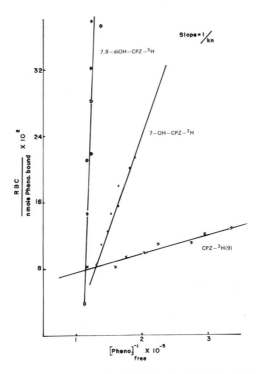

FIG. 1. Klotz plots of the binding of CPZ-³H(9), 7-OH-CPZ-³H, and 7,8-diOH-CPZ-³H at 1×10^{-5} M to varying quantities of rat RBC (1×10^8 to 3×10^9 cells/ml).

ESR spin-labeling method. A modified drug with the spin-label attached to the side chain via an amide linkage such as the one presented in Fig. 2 is added directly in varying concentrations to a fixed number of RBC or synaptosomes. The characteristics of the ESR spectrum for this spin label is such that when the molecule is bound to a large macromolecule, such as a protein, either hydrophobically or covalently, the spectrum changes dramatically from a sharp three-line spectrum for the free label to a very broad anisotropic spectrum for the bound label (Fig. 3A and B). By measuring the relative intensities of the free spectrum to that of the bound, an approximate binding constant can be extracted directly. Similarly, com-

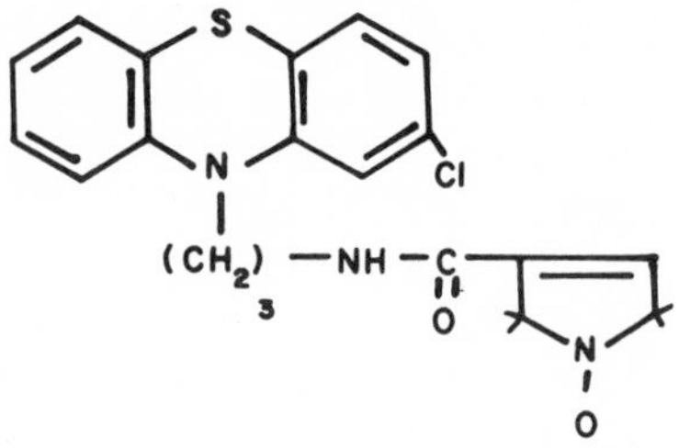

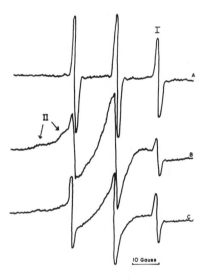

FIG. 2. Structure of spin-labeled Nor$_2$-CPZ (CPZ-SL).

FIG. 3. ESR spectra of CPZ spin label at 1.0-Gauss modulation amplitude: (A) CPZ-SL (8×10^{-6} M) in aqueous solution, (B) CPZ-SL (1×10^{-4} M) with rat RBC, (C) CPZ-SL (5×10^{-5} M) with rat brain synaptosomes.

petitive binding studies can be made by displacing the bound spin-labeled derivative with an unlabeled derivative. Upon displacement from the membrane, the bound spectrum reverts to the sharp three-lined free spectrum.

The spin-label shown above was dissolved in dimethyl sulfoxide at a concentration of 10^{-3} M. Aliquots were added to freshly harvested RBC or synaptosomes and ESR spectra recorded. Figure 3 shows typical spectra obtained (A) for the drug spin-label in the absence of red blood cells and (B) in the presence of 10^9 RBC/ml. Figure 3C shows similar spectra obtained with synaptosomes. The peak amplitude of the free spin-label spectrum peak I is directly proportional to the concentration of unbound label. The difference between this peak amplitude and that of a control sample without RBC gives the concentration of bound spin-label. Figure 4

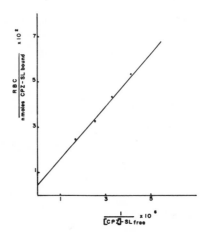

FIG. 4. Klotz plot of the binding of CPZ-SL at 1×10^{-5} M to varying quantities of rat RBC (3×10^8 to 6×10^9 RBC/ml).

shows a typical Klotz plot using this spin-label data from which the binding constant K and number of binding sites for the spin-labeled drug with RBC membranes can be extracted.

The question arises as to whether or not the binding affinities obtained for the spin-labeled drug are the same as the unlabeled parent compound. In Fig. 5, we have compared the ESR spin-label method with the isotope-labeling method using a Klotz plot in which the slope of the line is equal to the product of the binding constant and the number of sites. Were the lines superimposable, the two parameters would be the same. If the slopes differed and the intercepts were the same, only the binding constants would differ.

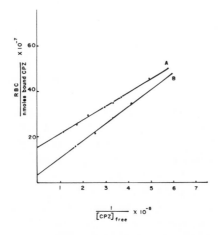

FIG. 5. Klotz plot comparing the binding affinities for rat RBC of: (A) CPZ-^{3}H(9) (1×10^{-5} M), (B) (1×10^{-5} M) spin-labeled Nor$_2$-CPZ (CPZ-SL).

In this case, it can be seen that the slopes are very similar but the intercepts are different, indicating slightly different binding constants and binding number as might be expected. The fact that the lines are close together, however, indicates the differences are small.

Tranquilization via RBC Drug Transport

The initial intent of these membrane studies was to see if in fact drug transport via the RBC was a possible mechanism for tranquilization. To demonstrate this possibility, some direct attempts were made to observe tranquilization qualitatively in animals in which drug was administered only through binding to their RBC. CPZ, 7-OH-CPZ, 8-OH-CPZ, and 7,8-diOH-CPZ were tested for tranquilization effects.

Three adult male Holtzman rats of 200 to 300 g body weight were used in testing each compound. Four milliters of whole blood was removed by heart puncture and the RBC spun down. Two milliters of saline was added to the packed cells, which were then labeled with 0.4 mg drug/ml packed RBC (0.8 mg total added) at room temperature for 1 hr. The cells were washed once with 10 ml saline, which removed 20 to 50% of the added compound depending on the derivative being tested, and then 1 ml saline was added to bring the cells to volume and injected into the tail vein of the donating rat. Care was taken to ensure that the cells did not hemolyze. Tranquilization was determined only by observation of the rats overall behavior. The rats received no anesthesia during the entire procedure. Marked tranquilization was seen almost immediately with CPZ and 7-OH-CPZ, but no tranquilization for 8-OH-CPZ and 7,8-diOH-CPZ could be observed.

Drug Distribution Studies

Since we were able to show binding to RBC and tranquilization by RBC binding, it was necessary then to see how the drug is distributed once the drug-treated erythrocytes are injected in the rat. Drug distribution was monitored as a function of time in the plasma, RBC, and brain using tritiated drug derivatives.

Adult male Holtzman rats were used of around 250 g body weight. Two milliliters of whole blood was removed by heart puncture into heparinized centrifuge tubes and the RBC spun down. The plasma was removed and 1 ml 0.85% saline was added to the packed RBC. Then, 0.2 ml of tritiated drug was added (0.4 to 0.5 mg/ml in equal volumes of 10 mM HCl and 0.85% saline) and allowed to stand at room temperature for one hour with periodic mixing. The RBC were then washed with 5×10 ml 0.85% saline (washes counted). After the last wash, 0.1 ml of packed RBC was removed from the sample and added to 0.9 ml distilled water and 0.1 ml of this solution was taken for counting (equivalent to 10 μl RBC). To the remaining 0.9 ml

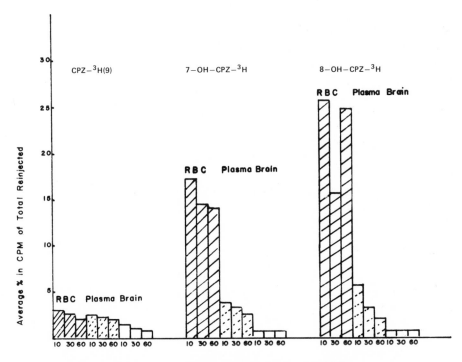

FIG. 6. Histogram comparing the percentage of injected tritiated CPZ, 7-OH-CPZ, and 8-OH-CPZ that appear in rat plasma, brain, and on RBC following injection of these compounds adsorbed on RBC.

packed RBC was added 0.5 ml saline and this was injected into the tail vein of the donating rat. (No anesthesia was used in this procedure.) Rats were sacrificed by rapid stunning and decapitation at various times after the injection. Blood was collected and RBC spun down. Ten microliters of RBC and 0.1 ml plasma were counted. The brains were removed and washed and as much external membrane and blood vessels as possible were removed. Brains were weighed and then homogenized with an equal volume of distilled water, and 0.1 ml of the brain homogenate was counted.

If Fig. 6, we have plotted our results in terms of the percentage in counts per minute of the initial activity on the RBC found in the animal's plasma, RBC, and brain as a function of fixed times.

DISCUSSION

The results presented here clearly indicate that all the phenothiazine drugs have an affinity for the RBC membrane. It appears in addition from the two drugs studied to date, i.e., CPZ and perphenazine spin label, that the same type of binding is present with rat brain synaptosomes. This binding to the RBC could very well be an important mechanism by which the drug is transported to possible receptor sites in the brain. Qualitatively, the results suggest that the binding affinities vary depending upon the drug structure, being greater for the nonhydroxylated derivative (Fig. 1). This difference in binding, however, does not seem to account for the higher percentage of injected drug found on the cells for the hydroxylated derivatives compared to CPZ as shown in Fig. 6. This difference may merely reflect the fact that the hydroxylation reaction itself, whether it occurs in the liver microsomal system or elsewhere, is a driving force for drug displacement from the cell membrane. The exchange to the brain however does seem to parallel the binding-constant differences. Qualitatively, it appears also that the binding constants for the RBC and synaptosomes are similar but that the total number of sites may be different, being greater in the synaptosomes than the RBC. It is difficult to compare these two systems quantitatively since in the case of RBC, binding is in terms of number of cells, and in synaptosomes protein content. Additional studies are underway to make them more directly comparable so as to demonstrate whether or not thermodynamic exchange from the RBC to the brain is favored, thereby supporting a drug RBC transportation and tranquilization mechanism.

Although the data presented in Fig. 1 clearly show differences in the binding constants between the hydroxylated derivatives and CPZ, there does not appear to be a unique binding site for these metabolites. This fact is borne out in an analysis of the isotope-labeling data that was presented in Table 1. The amount of free label in the supernatant of the control RBC, which when exposed only to tritium-labeled CPZ prior to centrifugation, is $\sim 10\%$ lower than those that had been previously incubated with the same concentration of either cold CPZ or hydroxy metabolite prior to addition of the same amount of hot CPZ as in the control. These later samples did in fact all yield the same level in the supernatant, indicating that the binding sites for CPZ and the metabolites are similar.

Although previous studies involving spin-labeled protein SH sites on RBC membranes and synaptosomes (6) clearly suggested drug interaction with the protein of the membrane and not the lipid, the evidence is indirect.

In preliminary experiments to provide more direct evidence for a protein interaction, we have compared the effects of CPZ on spin labels that are known to intercalate into the lipid such as a C_{12} stearic acid spin label where the nitroxide label is attached at the C_{12} carbon position. These labels are only slightly soluble in water but very soluble in lipid.

Figure 7A shows the ESR spectrum obtained for the stearate label intercalated into RBC membranes. Figure 7B shows the spectrum after titration with 10^{-4} M CPZ. Very little change in the basic structure of the spectrum occurs upon addition of CPZ with the exception that the sharp peak "I" identified as free label in solution disappears, indicating a change in the

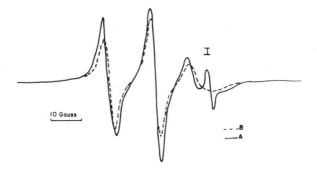

FIG. 7. ESR spectra of 12-dimethyl oxazolidine stearate (12 NS) with rat RBC: (A) _____
___ without CPZ, (B) _ _ _ _ _ _ _ in the presence of 1 × 10⁻⁴ м CPZ.

partitioning of the label between solvent and membrane. If CPZ did in fact
localize in the lipid of the membrane, we would have expected a gross
change in the spectrum as was the case with the protein labels (6). A second
piece of evidence for interaction at the membrane protein is shown in Fig.
8A where we have employed a spin label which covalently binds to the
active site of the enzyme cholinestearase (17) in synaptosome membranes.
It is well known that this enzyme is in the protein fraction of the membrane
rather than the lipid. Figure 8B shows the change that occurs in the spectrum
upon titration with 10⁻⁴ м CPZ. The original spectrum consists of five lines

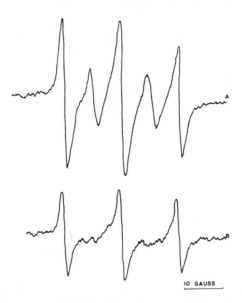

FIG. 8. ESR spectra of di-(2,2,6,6-tetramethylpiperidine-1-oxyl) fluorophosphate bound to
acetylcholinesterase in rat brain synaptosomes: (A) without CPZ, (B) in the presence of
1 × 10⁻⁴ м CPZ.

instead of three as for the previous labels, since this particular label contains two nitroxides which can exchange with each other. Upon reaction with CPZ the exchange is interrupted and only a three-lined spectrum indicative of no exchange is observed. This change in the labeled enzyme with added CPZ and the fact that the enzyme is in the protein fraction again strongly suggest that CPZ is acting at the protein level of the membrane and not the lipid.

Our finding that drug-binding transport and subsequent transfer via the RBC to the brain take place could provide significant insights into the overall mode of action of CPZ. It is possible that drug-RBC binding (affinity) serves as an important step in the activity and therapeutic effectiveness, i.e., the difference between psychotic responders versus nonresponders to the drug. A decrease in drug binding by the RBC could indicate (a) a reduction in accessibility of drug to brain receptor sites of nonresponders, and also (b) these patients lack the ability to catalyze specific biotransformation(s) required for drug expression. With CPZ, this could involve hydroxylation to 7-OH-CPZ. On the other hand, the lack of response could be a result of stronger affinity for the RBC. If the binding affinity to the RBC is many fold higher than binding of the same drug molecule to the receptor site in the brain, then transfer in the brain would be thermodynamically unfavorable and leads then to a "no response" on the part of the patient. With these points of consideration, a simple assay procedure could be devised reflecting the ability of a psychotic patient to respond to drug treatment. In addition, it is conceivable that such an assay could be utilized to titer a patient as to the threshold amount of drug necessary for therapeutic maintenance and efficacy, with a possible reduction in the occurrence of side effects.

SUMMARY

Chlorpromazine (CPZ) and its hydroxylated metabolites were compared as to: (1) their relative binding affinity to rat erythrocytes, (2) the degree to which tranquilization can be induced when the cells with bound drug are reinjected into the animals, and (3) the distribution of drug in plasma, RBC, and brain after drug-bound erythrocytes are reinjected in animals. Binding affinity to rat erythrocytes parallel the degree of hydroxylation, CPZ having the greatest affinity ($K_d = 4 \times 10^{-6}$ M) followed by its monohydroxy and lastly the dihydroxy derivatives. Binding sites in rat erythrocytes appear to be similar for CPZ and the metabolites tested. Injection into rats of drug-bound erythrocytes produced marked tranquilization with CPZ and 7-OH-CPZ but no tranquilization for 8-OH-CPZ and 7,8-diOH-CPZ could be detected. Distribution of CPZ and its hydroxylated metabolites from drug-bound erythrocytes to the whole rat brain qualitatively parallels the binding constant differences. Results obtained from the interaction of CPZ with a hydrophobic fatty acid spin label and a covalent protein spin label strongly suggest CPZ is acting at the protein level of membranes rather than the lipid. An interesting mechanism which may control therapeutic effectiveness is discussed.

ACKNOWLEDGMENT

This work was supported by funds from Psychopharmacology Research Branch, National Institute of Mental Health, under contract No. HSM–42–71–1 and from Grant MH–12952–07 (from the National Institute of Mental Health).

REFERENCES

1. Efron, D. H., Gaudette, L. E., and Harris, S. R., *Agressologie,* **9,** 103 (1968).
2. Efron, D. H., Harris, S. R., Manian, A. A., and Gaudette, L. E., *Psychopharmacologia (Berlin),* **19,** 207 (1971).
3. Freeman, A. R., and Spirtes, M. A., *Biochem. Pharmacol.,* **11,** 161 (1962).
4. Freeman, A. R., and Spirtes, M. A., *Biochem. Pharmacol.,* **12,** 47 (1963).
5. Turano, P., March, J. E., Turner, W. J., and Merlis, S., *J. Med. (Basel),* **3,** 109 (1972).
6. Holmes, D. E., and Piette, L. H., *J. Pharmacol. Exp. Ther.,* **173,** 78 (1969).
7. Manian, A. A., Efron, D. H., and Goldberg, M. E., *Life Sci.,* **4,** 2425 (1965).
8. Brookes, L. G., Holmes, M. A., Serra, M. T., and Forrest, I. S., *Proc. West. Pharmacol. Soc.,* **13,** 127 (1970).
9. Maickel, R. P., Potter, W. Z., and Manian, A. A., *Fed. Proc.,* **30,** 336 (1971).
10. Manian, A. A., Efron, D. H., and Harris, S. R., *Life Sci.,* **10,** Part I, 679 (1971).
11. Turano, P., Turner, W. J., and Manian, A. A., *J. Chromat.,* **75,** 277 (1973).
12. Rozantsev, E. G., *Free Nitroxyl Radicals,* Plenum Press, New York, 1970, p. 206.
13. Abdel-Latif, A. A., *Biochim. Biophys. Acta,* **121,** 403 (1966).
14. Autilio, L. A., Appel, S. H., Pettis, P., and Gambetti, P., *Biochemistry,* **7,** 2615 (1968).
15. Seeman, P., Bolis, L., Katchalsky, A., Keynes, R. D., Loewenstein, W. R., and Pethica, B. A., *Permeability and Function of Biological Membranes,* Holland Publishers, Amsterdam, 1970, pp. 40–56.
16. Hughes, T. R., and Klotz, I. M., *Methods Biochem. Analysis,* **3,** 284 (1956).
17. Hsia, J. C., Kosman, D. J., and Piette, L. H., *Biochem. Biophys. Res. Comm.,* **36,** 75 (1969).

The Phenothiazines and Structurally Related Drugs, edited by I. S.
Forrest, C. J. Carr, and E. Usdin. Raven Press, New York © 1974.

Binding of Phenothiazines and Related Compounds to Tissues and Cell Constituents

M. H. Bickel

Medizinisch-chemisches Institut, University of Berne, Berne, Switzerland

INTRODUCTION

Tricyclic drugs such as phenothiazines or dibenzazepines are proto-
types of basic lipophilic drugs. They are known to show high apparent
volumes of distribution, i.e., high tissue/plasma concentration ratios. As an
example, rapid tissue uptake and accumulation of imipramine or desipramine
have been shown in rats *in vivo* (1), in the isolated perfused rat liver (2, 3),
and in liver slices (4). This type of distribution, extremely in favor of the
intracellular space, can only be explained by both penetration through the
cell membranes and intracellular fixation. The tissues thereby assume a
depot function, which seems to largely govern the pharmacokinetics of this
type of drug, particularly the availability for the sites of action, metabolism,
and excretion. It is surprising, therefore, that so much effort has been devoted to the study of drug binding to serum proteins rather than to tissues.
Since most tricyclic drugs are also bound to serum proteins (5–8), the overall drug distribution may be governed by a competition between the two sites
of binding, or else binding to serum proteins may be without pharmacokinetic consequences. The aim of the present study was to examine the
intracellular localization of the binding sites, the type of binding and structural features influencing it, and to quantitate the binding of various drugs
in terms of affinity and capacity values.

EXPERIMENTAL DATA

Studies on the binding of drugs to tissue preparations were performed
using the techniques of centrifugal sedimentation (9) and/or equilibrium
dialysis (7). Total drug concentrations were varied in the 1 to 1,600 μM
range; protein concentrations of the tissue fractions of 1, 2, or 4 mg/ml were
used. All binding experiments were carried out in a medium of KCl/phosphate
buffer pH 7.4, ionic strength 0.17, at 37°C. Free and bound ligand concen-

163

trations $[c_{L(f)}$ and $c_{L(b)}$ respectively] were determined by spectrophoto-fluorometry, UV spectrophotometry, or by using ^{14}C-labeled drugs. The data obtained from 3 to 11 experiments were analyzed by computer using the modified Scatchard plot $c_{L(b)}/c_{L(f)}$ versus $c_{L(b)}$ in order to obtain the apparent association constants K_i and the binding capacities C_i for individual classes of binding sites i.

Experiments aiming at localization and quantitation of the binding of chlorpromazine and imipramine to rat-liver tissue are summarized in Table 1. The binding of both compounds to purified nuclei, mitochondria, microsomes, and cytosol fraction are of the Scatchard type. With all cell fractions, a low-affinity, high-capacity binding site with an association constant of about 2×10^3 M^{-1} is occupied. With microsomes and mitochondria, an additional high-affinity, low-capacity site ($K_1 = 1.4 \times 10^5$ M^{-1} for chlorpromazine) is revealed. For both drugs the total binding capacity C_{1+2} is in the range of 300 to 1,000 nmoles or 100 to 350 $\mu g/mg$ protein.

TABLE 1. *Binding of chlorpromazine and imipramine to rat-liver fractions*

		Affinity		Capacity	
Drug	Fraction	K_1	K_2 (M^{-1})	C_1 (nmoles/mg)	C_{1+2}
Chlorpromazine	Nuclei	1.5×10^3		545	
	Mitochondria	5.8×10^4	1.9×10^3	211	978
	Microsomes	1.4×10^5	3.9×10^3	161	715
	Cytosol	4.0×10^2		617	
Imipramine	Nuclei	1.9×10^3		188	
	Mitochondria	2.2×10^4	3.2×10^3	88	307
	Microsomes	2.0×10^4	3.3×10^3	79	380
	Cytosol	2.4×10^3		59	

The binding values of chlorpromazine and imipramine with microsomal fractions from extrahepatic tissues were also determined (Table 2). The two drugs show the same Scatchard-type binding with two classes of binding sites as with liver microsomes. Quantitatively the K_i and C_i values were comparable to microsomal fractions from liver, lung, kidney, brain, and skeletal muscle.

Table 3 compares binding parameters of the tricyclic drugs chlorpromazine, imipramine, 3-chloroimipramine, and 10-ketoimipramine. With all these drugs, both association constants for the high-affinity site and total capacity values are higher than the corresponding values of bovine serum albumin. Methadone, another basic lipophilic drug, although structurally very different, shows similar binding characteristics as do tricyclic drugs. On the other hand, acidic drugs such as phenylbutazone, sulfadimethoxine, and salicylic acid show little or negligible binding to tissue fractions but strong binding to serum albumin.

TABLE 2. *Binding of chlorpromazine and imipramine to rat-tissue microsomes*

Drug	Tissue	Affinity K_1 (M^{-1})	K_2	Capacity C_1 (nmoles/mg)	C_{1+2}
Chlorpromazine	Liver	1.4×10^5	3.9×10^3	161	715
	Lung	2.2×10^4	2.2×10^3	272	1015
	Kidney	9.7×10^4	2.1×10^3	223	930
	Brain	2.2×10^4	2.9×10^3	225	730
	Sk. muscle	1.7×10^4	1.8×10^3	262	954
Imipramine	Liver	2.0×10^4	3.3×10^3	79	380
	Lung	3.9×10^4	2.0×10^3	70	230
	Kidney	5.2×10^4	3.9×10^3	80	280
	Brain	1.8×10^4	2.0×10^3	100	260
	Sk. muscle	3.9×10^4	2.7×10^3	70	290

TABLE 3. *Binding of basic tricyclic drugs to rat-liver microsomes (RLM) and to bovine serum albumin (BSA)*

	K_1 (M^{-1}) RLM	BSA	C_{1+2} (nmoles/mg) RLM	BSA
Chlorpromazine	1.4×10^5	2.1×10^4 [a]	715	15
Imipramine	2.0×10^4	6.3×10^3	380	93
3-Cl-imipramine	2.6×10^4	2.2×10^4	840	93
10-ketoimipramine	1.7×10^3	negligible [b]	140	negl.

[a] cf. (8).
[b] H. J. Weder (*unpublished results*).

SUMMARY

Chlorpromazine, imipramine, and other basic lipophilic drugs are strongly bound to rat-liver microsomes and mitochondria, whereas the binding to nuclei and soluble cell constituents is much weaker. With microsomes, the drug interaction is a regular Scatchard-type reversible binding to two independent classes of binding sites with association constants of 10^4 to 10^5 M^{-1} and 10^3 M^{-1}, respectively. The total binding capacity is in the range of 300 to 1,000 nmoles/mg microsomal protein. Liver mitochondria and microsomal fractions from extrahepatic tissues reveal comparable binding characteristics both qualitatively and quantitatively. These results help explain the high tissue/plasma concentration ratios observed with these drugs in various biological systems by demonstrating an intracellular binding with considerable affinity and capacity. In addition, the data suggest that much more than the well-known binding to cytochrome P-450 is involved, *viz.,* binding to lipids and/or proteins of cytomembranes. Pharmaco-kinetically, the fact that the values of binding affinity and capacity to microsomes are much higher than those to serum albumin, would suggest that in a competition for the binding sites the intracellular ones would be strongly favored. It must therefore be assumed that with certain types of drugs, binding to tissue constituents is much more important in determining overall pharmacokinetics than is binding to plasma proteins. Precisely which binding parameters are decisive remains to be elucidated.

ACKNOWLEDGMENT

This study has been supported by grants of the Swiss National Foundation.

REFERENCES

1. Bickel, M. H., and Weder, H. J., *Arch. int. Pharmacodyn. Thérap.,* **173,** 433 (1968).
2. Bickel, M. H., and Minder, R., *Biochem. Pharmacol.,* **19,** 2425 (1970).
3. Von Bahr, C., and Borga, O., *Acta pharmacol. toxicol.,* **29,** 359 (1971).
4. Bickel, M. H., and Gigon, P. L., *Xenobiotica,* **1,** 631 (1971).
5. Borga, O., Azarnoff, D. L., Forshell, G. P., and Sjoqvist, F., *Biochem. Pharmacol.,* **18,** 1251 (1969).
6. Weder, H. J., and Bickel, M. H., *J. pharm. Sci.,* **59,** 1505 (1970).
7. Weder, H. J., and Bickel, M. H., *J. pharm. Sci.,* **59,** 1563 (1970).
8. Krieglstein, J., Lier, F., and Michaelis, J., *Arch. Pharmacol.,* **272,** 121 (1972).
9. Ernster, L., and Orrenius, S., *Fed. Proc.,* **24,** 1190 (1965).

The Phenothiazines and Structurally Related Drugs, edited by I. S. Forrest, C. J. Carr, and E. Usdin. Raven Press, New York © 1974.

Tissue Accumulation of Metabolites During Chronic Administration of Piperazine-Substituted Phenothiazine Drugs

Ursula Breyer and Hans Jörg Gaertner

Institut für Toxikologie der Universität Tübingen, D-7400 Tübingen, West Germany

INTRODUCTION

Studies on the metabolism of antipsychotic drugs seem to be particularly relevant for clinico-pharmacological considerations when they are carried out during chronic treatment. The demonstration of changes in the metabolite pattern in the organism with time might give a clue to the understanding of such phenomena as the delayed onset of therapeutic effect and the delayed relapse after discontinuation of medication.

Investigations on tissue metabolites of the piperazine-substituted phenothiazine drug perazine have led to the detection of a biotransformation product that accounted for a small fraction of a single dose only. However, due to its long half-life in parenchymatous organs, it accumulated upon repeated administration of sufficiently high perazine doses in the absence of accumulation of perazine or of another precursor (1). The structural elucidation showed that this product resulted from degradation of the piperazine ring to ethylenediamine (2). A further metabolite, which was present in low concentrations, could be identified as the primary amine formed by complete degradation of the piperazine ring. This compound is also produced from the corresponding dimethylamino-substituted phenothiazine drug promazine (3) and thus represents the product of a metabolic convergence in two series of drugs.

The questions to be studied subsequently were whether an analogous biodegradation could be demonstrated using piperazine-substituted phenothiazines that contain a chloro- or a trifluoromethyl substituent in the aromatic nucleus and whether the same pathway was operative in man.

EXPERIMENTAL

Male Wistar rats weighing 280 to 350 g were given daily doses of aqueous solutions of the drugs by gavage. The doses were increased slowly over several weeks (trifluoperazine 5 to 40 mg/kg, fluphenazine 2 to 40 mg/kg, prochlorperazine 10 to 50 mg/kg, and perphenazine 2 to 50 mg/kg). A female beagle was given fluphenazine dihydrochloride in gelatine capsules, 10 or 20 mg/kg. Urine collection in rats was performed as described previously (4). Dog urine was obtained by catheterization following a 6-hr period in a metabolic cage during which time no urine was voided.

Twenty-four-hr urine samples were obtained from psychiatric inpatients receiving perazine (200 to 600 mg daily) or fluphenazine (18 or 36 mg daily). In addition, urine was collected from patients withdrawn from perazine.

The extraction of tissues (1) and urine (4) and the isolation and purification of metabolites by thin-layer chromatography (1, 4, 5) have been described previously. The chromatographic properties of the tissue metabolites are given in Table 1.

Synthetic analogues of the metabolites were prepared by reacting γ-(2-trifluoromethyl-phenothiazinyl-10)-propylchloride or the 2-chloro compound (6) with ethylenediamine, N-methyl-ethylenediamine, or N-(β-hydroxyethyl)-ethylenediamine (Breyer et al., *to be published*). The structures of the compounds and the identity of metabolites and synthetic products

TABLE 1. R_F values of piperazine-substituted phenothiazine drugs and of their tissue metabolites in thin-layer chromatography on silica gel GF_{254}

	R_F value in solvent[a]	
Compound	S_I	S_{II}
Trifluoperazine	0.86	0.81
N-[γ-(2-trifluoromethyl-phenothiazinyl-10)-propyl]-piperazine (CF$_3$-PPP)	0.44	0.50
N-[γ-(2-trifluoromethyl-phenothiazinyl-10)-propyl]-N'-methyl-ethylenediamine (CF$_3$-PPMED)	0.20	0.49
N-[γ-(2-trifluoromethyl-phenothiazinyl-10)-propyl]-ethylenediamine (CF$_3$-PPED)	0.20	0.70
Fluphenazine	0.76	0.90
N-[γ-(2-trifluoromethyl-phenothiazinyl-10)-propyl]-N'-(β-hydroxyethyl)-ethylenediamine (CF$_3$-PPHED)	0.20	0.54
Prochlorperazine	0.86	0.81
N-[γ-(2-chloro-phenothiazinyl-10)-propyl]-piperazine (Cl-PPP)	0.42	0.43
N-[γ-(2-chloro-phenothiazinyl-10)-propyl]-N'-methyl-ethylenediamine (Cl-PPMED)	0.15	0.42
N-[γ-(2-chloro-phenothiazinyl-10)-propyl]-ethylenediamine (Cl-PPED)	0.15	0.63
Perphenazine	0.76	0.90
N-[γ-(2-chloro-phenothiazinyl-10)-propyl]-N'-(β-hydroxyethyl)-ethylenediamine (Cl-PPHED)	0.15	0.47

[a] S_I isopropanol/chloroform/25% ammonia/water (32 : 16 : 2 : 1). S_{II} acetone/isopropanol/1 N ammonia (27 : 21 : 12). Plates containing tissue extracts were washed with chloroform/isopropanol (10 : 1) prior to development with solvent S_I. Mixtures of CF$_3$-PPMED + CF$_3$-PPED or of CF$_3$-PPHED + CF$_3$-PPED or of the corresponding Cl-substituted compounds were subsequently separated in solvent S_{II}.

were proven by mass spectrometry using a MS 902 S-DS 30 instrument (AEI, Manchester, England).

RESULTS

Tissue Metabolites in Rats

By means of thin-layer chromatographic and mass spectrometric identification of the resulting compounds, it could be demonstrated that the piperazine ring in the neuroleptic drugs trifluoperazine, fluphenazine, prochlorperazine, and perphenazine underwent cleavage *in vivo* to ethylenediamine derivatives (Fig. 1). This degradation took place with or without removal of the alkyl groups on the terminal nitrogen atom. Thus, two ethylenediamine metabolites were formed from each drug, for instance, CF_3-PPMED and CF_3-PPED from trifluoperazine.

When animals were killed 12 or 24 hr after administration of the last drug dose, the parent compounds and the N-dealkylated metabolites CF_3-PPP or Cl-PPP, respectively, were also present. Investigations after longer intervals following termination of treatment, revealed that the ethylenediamine derivatives were eliminated more slowly than were the compounds with an intact piperazine ring. As an example, the quantities of trifluoperazine metabolites are given in Table 2. Similar results were obtained by treat-

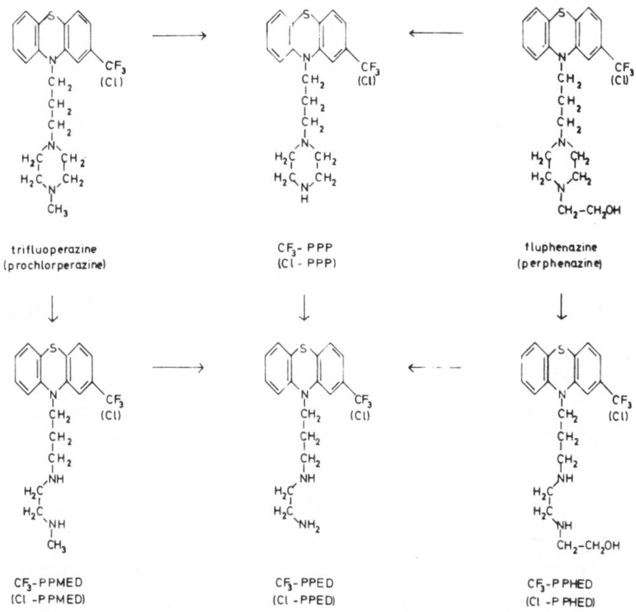

FIG. 1. Structures of trifluoperazine, fluphenazine, prochlorperazine, perphenazine, and their tissue metabolites

TABLE 2. *Concentrations of trifluoperazine and its metabolites in organs of rats following treatment with increasing drug doses*

Organ	Time after last dose (days)	Metabolite concentration $(\mu g/g)^a$			
		Trifluoperazine	CF$_3$-PPP	CF$_3$-PPMED	CF$_3$-PPED
Liver	1	13 ± 2	40 ± 5	14 ± 1	31 ± 3
	4	n. d.^{b}	n. d.	6 ± 2	23 ± 5
	7	n. d.	n. d.	n. d.	7 ± 0.5
	14	n. d.	n. d.	n. d.	n. d.
Kidney	1	11 ± 2	43 ± 6	11 ± 0.5	20 ± 2
	4	n. d.	n. d.	9.5 ± 0.5	20 ± 3
	7	n. d.	n. d.	11 ± 2	11 ± 2
	14	n. d.	n. d.	n. d.	2 ± 0.3
Brain	1	3.5 ± 1	9 ± 0.5	n. d.	n. d.

^{a} Mean $\pm$ S.E.M.
^{b} n. d. = not detectable.
Male rats received 5, 10, 15, 20, 25, 30, and 35 mg/kg trifluoperazine for 3 days each and 40 mg/kg for 6 days. Five grams of liver, one pair of kidneys or the pooled brains of two animals were extracted (1). The values are corrected for recoveries of metabolites.

ing rats with prochlorperazine. As with perazine (1), the minimal dose required for accumulation of measurable levels of ethylenediamine derivatives was 25 mg/kg daily.

Urinary Metabolites in Animals

When small doses (10 mg/kg) of the piperazine-substituted phenothiazine drugs were given to rats, the only metabolites detected in urine were the sulfoxides of the drugs and of the N-dealkylated metabolites. After administration of higher doses (25 or 50 mg/kg) or during chronic application of 10 or 20 mg/kg a further biotransformation product was consistently present. It could be identified as γ-(2-trifluoromethyl-phenothiazinyl-10)-propylamine sulfoxide (CF$_3$-PPA-SO) when trifluoperazine or fluphenazine had been administered, and as the 2-chloro analogue Cl-PPA-SO in rats treated with prochlorperazine or perphenazine (Fig. 2). Identical metabolites were obtained when rats were given trifluopromazine or chlorpromazine, respectively, in accordance with reports in the literature (7). Analogously, perazine was degraded to PPA-SO (4), which is known to be a promazine metabolite (3).

The metabolites containing a partially degraded piperazine ring can serve as precursors of the propylamines. Administration of N-[γ-(phenothiazinyl-10)-propyl]-ethylenediamine (PPED, IV: $R_1 = H$, Fig. 2) to rats resulted in the excretion of PPA-SO, and Cl-PPED (IV: $R_1 = Cl$) and Cl-PPMED (III: $R_1 = Cl$, $R_2 = CH_3$) were metabolized to Cl-PPA-SO.

The time course of the excretion of the primary amine sulfoxide was

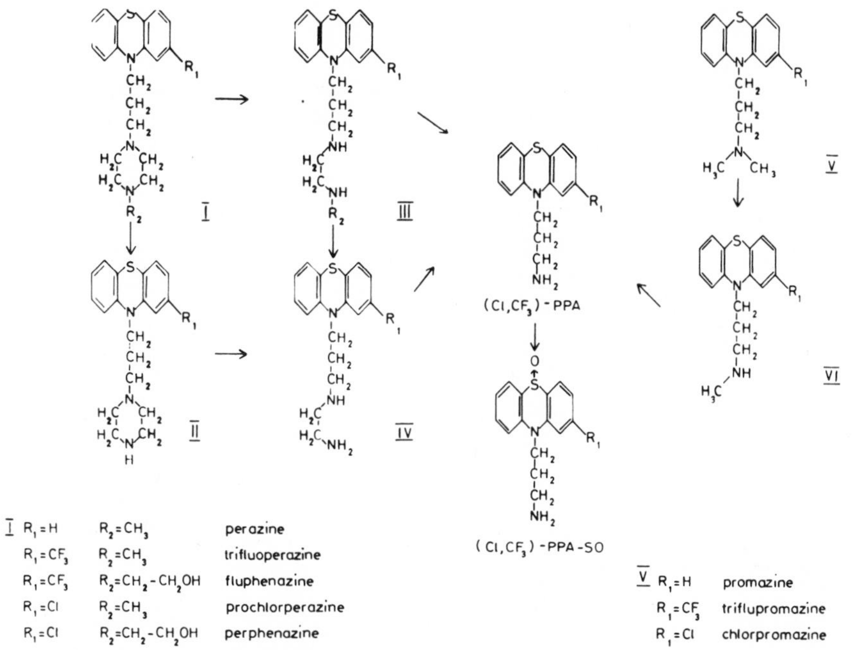

FIG. 2. Metabolic pathways in piperazine- and dimethylamino-substituted phenothiazine drugs leading to identical metabolites.

followed in a female dog that received 10 mg/kg fluphenazine on days 1 to 6 and 20 mg/kg on days 7 to 17. CF_3-PPA-SO was consistently present in urine, and its quantity amounted to 5% of the quantity of fluphenazine sulfoxide on day 2, to 15% on day 11, and to 27 to 30% on days 13 and 16. Analyses on the days following termination of treatment revealed that fluphenazine sulfoxide had disappeared on day 19 and CF_3-PPP-SO on day 20, but CF_3-PPA-SO declined slowly, and traces were still detected on day 23.

Urinary Metabolites in Man

In contrast to rats, humans ingesting perazine (200 to 600 mg per day) excreted not only the product of complete piperazine ring degradation PPA-SO but also measurable quantities of the sulfoxides of the intermediates PPED and PPMED (III: $R_1 = H$, $R_2 = CH_3$, Fig. 2). When drug administration was stopped in two patients, PPA-SO, PPED-SO, and PPMED-SO continued to be excreted in nearly constant quantities for 18 and 31 days, respectively (4), which points to the presence of slowly eliminated tissue stores probably containing PPED and PPMED. In a third patient, small quantities of PPA-SO were detected in urine 3 months after discontinuation of perazine medication (final dose 900 mg).

Two patients medicated with fluphenazine (18 and 36 mg per day) were found to excrete CF_3-PPA-SO regularly. In terms of percentage of the dose, the quantity was small (around 0.4%). However, in relation to fluphenazine sulfoxide, the quantity was remarkably high since it amounted to around 70% of the fluphenazine sulfoxide quantity in the patient receiving 18 mg and to 34 to 40% in the one treated with 36 mg. In the latter patient's urine, minor quantities of the sulfoxide of CF_3-PPED were also demonstrable. Intermittent discontinuation of medication in this patient for 2 days led to a disappearance of fluphenazine sulfoxide from the urine on the second drug-free day, to a marked reduction of the quantity of CF_3-PPP-SO and to a lesser decline in the CF_3-PPA-SO quantity.

DISCUSSION

Whether or not the reported findings are relevant to the therapeutic action of the drugs studied is not easy to decide. The pharmacological investigation of the ethylenediamine derivatives is problematical because of their slow distribution within the organism (1). Nonetheless, in chronic treatment of rats with perazine, PPED could be measured in the brain, and the elimination proceeded more slowly than from other tissues (1).

Another possible importance of the ethylenediamines may be seen in their ability to serve as precursors of the primary amines. The increase in the CF_3-PPA-SO excretion with time in the dog receiving fluphenazine was probably caused by continued accumulation of CF_3-PPHED and CF_3-PPED. The sustained excretion of PPA-SO or CF_3-PPA-SO after withdrawal of patients from perazine or fluphenazine, respectively, probably reflected the presence of ethylenediamines in tissues that had accumulated during the period of treatment. In patients having received perazine, this was confirmed by the observation that PPED-SO and PPMED-SO excretion followed the same time course as that of PPA-SO (4).

The primary amines resulting from complete biodegradation of the piperazine ring deserve special attention because of their formation from piperazine-substituted as well as from dimethylamino-substituted phenothiazine drugs. The pharmacological properties of the Cl-containing compound (nor$_2$-chlorpromazine) only have been investigated. Whereas in behavioral studies it did not exhibit appreciable activity (8–10), it proved to be comparable to chlorpromazine in influencing cerebral dopamine metabolism (11, 12). A finding which should prompt more intensive investigations of this compound and its analogues is the observation that patients receiving chlorpromazine had higher plasma levels of Cl-PPA than of chlorpromazine or any other metabolite (13). This result, however, is at variance with that of measurements using a different method (14).

SUMMARY

Chronic oral treatment of rats with trifluoperazine, fluphenazine, pro-chlorperazine, or perphenazine in doses of 25 mg/kg daily or more resulted in the accumulation in tissues of ethylenediamine derivatives formed by partial degradation of the piperazine ring in the side chain. Under the same conditions, the animals excreted primary amines as sulfoxides in which the piperazine ring had been completely degraded, leaving an amino group only. A dog receiving repeated oral doses of fluphenazine (10 and 20 mg/kg) excreted the primary amine sulfoxide in quantities increasing with time and finally reaching 30% of the quantity of fluphenazine sulfoxide.

In patients medicated with fluphenazine (18 or 36 mg daily) the primary amine sulfoxide was consistently present in urine and amounted to 34 to 70% of the fluphenazine sulfoxide excreted during the same period. Patients under treatment with perazine (200 to 600 mg daily) excreted the sulfoxides of the ethylenediamine metabolites, as well as phenothiazinyl–propylamine sulfoxide. All three compounds continued to be present in unchanged quantities for several weeks after termination of drug administration.

ACKNOWLEDGMENTS

We wish to thank Dr. R. Bertele for preparation of part of the compounds and Dr. A. Prox, Thomae GmbH, Biberach/Riss, for carrying out the mass spectrometry. Thanks are due to Miss G. Liomin and to Mr. G. Joachim for technical assistance. The work was supported by Deutsche Forschungs-gemeinschaft.

REFERENCES

1. Breyer, U., *Biochem. Pharmac.*, **21**, 1419 (1972).
2. Breyer, U., Krauss, D., and Jochims, J. C., *Experientia*, **28**, 312 (1972).
3. Goldenberg, H., Fishman, V., Heaton, A., and Burnett, R., *Proc. Soc. exp. Biol. Med.*, **115**, 1044 (1964).
4. Breyer, U., and Gaertner, H. J., in: *Review and Preview in Toxicology. Proceedings of the European Society for the Study of Drug Toxicity*, Excerpta Medica Int. Congr. Series **288**, 59 (1973).
5. Breyer, U., *Biochem. Pharmac.*, **18**, 777 (1969).
6. Sherlock, M. H., and Sperber, N., U.S. Pat. 2,860,138 (1958) [*C.A.* **53**, P 7212, 1959].
7. Goldenberg, H., and Fishman, V., *Proc. Soc. exp. Biol. Med.*, **108**, 178 (1961).
8. Brune, G. G., Kohl, H. H., Steiner, W. G., and Himwich, H. E., *Biochem. Pharmac.*, **12**, 679 (1963).
9. Kohl, H. H., Brune, G. G., and Himwich, H. E., *Biochem. Pharmac.*, **13**, 539 (1964).
10. Lal, S., and Sourkes, T. L., *Eur. J. Pharmac.*, **17**, 283 (1972).
11. Nybäck, N., and Sedvall, G., *Psychopharmacologia*, **26**, 155 (1972).
12. Dailey, J., Sedvall, G., and Sjoquist, B., *J. Pharm. Pharmac.*, **24**, 580 (1972).
13. Turano, P., March, J. E., Turner, W. J., and Merlis, S., *J. Med.*, **3**, 109 (1972).
14. Curry, S. H., and Marshall, J. H., *Life Sci.*, **7**, 9 (1968).

The Phenothiazines and Structurally Related Drugs, edited by I. S. Forrest, C. J. Carr, and E. Usdin. Raven Press, New York © 1974.

The Binding Behavior of Phenothiazines and Structurally Related Compounds to Albumin from Several Species

Sabit Gabay and Ping C. Huang

Biochemical Research Laboratory, Veterans Administration Hospital, Brockton, Massachusetts 02401, and Harvard School of Dental Medicine, Boston, Massachusetts 02115

INTRODUCTION

Species differences in the responses of animals to drugs are known to exist in many drugs. These differences probably arise from the nature of the tissue receptor sites with which the drugs interact or from differences in the physiological mechanisms involved (1). On the other hand, it has been shown that identical plasma levels of certain drugs produce similar pharmacological effects in various species so that extrapolation from one species to another can be facilitated by comparing effects produced by similar plasma levels (2). The binding behavior of a series of phenothiazines and structurally related compounds to serum albumin from several species including human, bovine, dog, rat, rabbit, pig, horse, sheep, goat, and chicken has been systematically studied using ultraviolet (UV) difference spectrophotometry and intrinsic protein fluorescence quenching methods. Only purified crystallized or fraction V albumins were used in the present *in vitro* studies, and emphasis will be on the structural requirements, common mode of action, and factors influencing the binding.

MATERIALS AND METHODS

All crystalline or fraction V albumin preparations were obtained from Research Division, Miles Laboratories, Inc. Fatty acids were removed from the albumin by the charcoal treatment method of Chen (3) at acidic pH. The activated charcoal (Mallinckrodt) was washed with distilled water, filtered, and dried prior to its use. Chlorpromazine (CPZ) hydrochloride, CPZ sulfoxide hydrochloride, trifluoperazine dihydrochloride, and trimeprazine tartrate were kindly supplied by Smith, Kline, and French Laboratories; promazine hydrochloride and promethazine hydrochloride by Wyeth Laboratories; fluphenazine dihydrochloride and triflupromazine hydrochloride by Squibb Inc.; perphenazine and acetophazine maleate by Schering Corp.; imipramine by Geigy Pharmaceuticals; and chlorprothixene hydrochloride by Hoffmann-LaRoche Inc. Samples of 2-bromopromazine, 6-hydroxychlorpromazine, 7-hydrochlorpromazine, 8-hydroxychlorproma-zine, 7-methoxychlorpromazine hydrochloride, 7,8-dimethoxychlorpro-mazine hydrochloride, 3,7-dimethoxychlorpromazine hydrochloride, 7-hydroxychlorpromazine sulfoxide, chlorpromazine N-oxide-2H$_2$O, and 3,7-dichlorpromazine were kindly provided by Dr. A. A. Manian (National Institute of Mental Health, Psychopharmacology Research Branch). The compounds were used without further purification. Aqueous solution of the samples was prepared by first dissolving the sample in small amounts of doubly glass-distilled water or, in the case of free base, in 0.1 N hydro-chloride, then made up with appropriate buffer. Solutions were always freshly prepared prior to their use and screened from exposure to direct light at all times.

Ultraviolet absorption spectra were recorded on a Cary 15 spectro-photometer. Difference absorption spectra were obtained by using a pair of split-compartment tandem mixing cells (4) with 2×4 mm light path and 1 ml volume in each compartment (Pyrocell 5014). Solutions of albumin and drugs were placed separately in each compartment in both the sample and reference cell. Since the contents of both cells were equal, a straight baseline was obtained. The albumin and drug solution in the sample cell were then mixed (after the cell was covered with a small piece of parafilm paper) and inverted several times. The difference spectra thus recorded are expressed in terms of difference absorbance (ΔA). The solvent perturba-tion difference spectra of drugs were obtained using regular 10 mm light path rectangular cells. Calculated amounts of drugs were first dissolved in 95% ethanol; equal portions of 0.01 ml were placed in each of the sample and reference cells. The solvents were carefully evaporated to dryness under a stream of nitrogen and the reference cell was then filled with 2 ml of buffer; the sample cell was filled with 2 ml of the perturbing solvent used.

A custom-made spectrofluorometer was used for all fluorescence quench-ing studies. It consisted of a d.c. operated 450 watt Osram xenon arc lamp as light source, a 600-line-per-mm grating-unit excitation monochromator (Bausch and Lomb) equipped with a Servo motor-driven wavelength drum, a thermostatically controlled cell compartment, a 1,200-line-per-mm grating-unit emission monochromator (Bausch and Lomb) also equipped with a servo-motoring wavelength drum, an EMI 9601 photomultiplier tube, a 414 amplifier and microammeter by Keithley Instruments, and an HR-97 X-Y recorder from Houston Instruments. The intrinsic tryptophyl fluorescence of the albumins was monitored at 340 nm with excitation at 295 nm.

RESULTS

The difference absorption spectrum for the interaction of human serum albumin (HSA) and CPZ in phosphate buffer, pH 7.4, as presented in Fig. 1A, is characterized by two positive (263 and 335 nm) and two negative (248 and 294 nm) absorption peaks. Figure 1 also shows the difference spectra of three structurally related compounds under identical conditions—they are (1) CPZ sulfoxide, a major metabolite of CPZ, (2) imipramine, an iminodibenzyl derivative and an antidepressant, and (3) chlorprothixene, a thioxanthene derivative. It is noteworthy that the last three compounds showed an absorption pattern entirely different from that of CPZ.

7-Hydroxychlorpromazine sulfoxide showed a difference spectrum similar to the parent compound, CPZ sulfoxide. Acetophenazine with an acetyl group at carbon-2 and a slightly different side chain at N-10, showed one positive peak at 275 nm and two negative peaks at 236 nm and 264 nm with very weak intensities (about the same as those of CPZ sulfoxide), whereas perphenazine, a 2-chloro derivative showed a spectrum nearly identical to that obtained from CPZ. When all of the above compounds were interacted with various albumins from different species, the characteristics of the

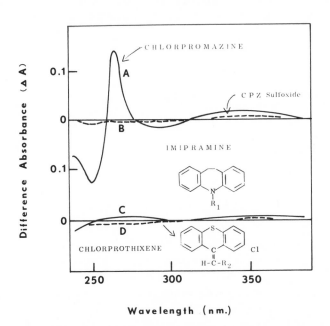

Wavelength (nm.)

FIG. 1. Difference spectra of the interaction of HSA with CPZ and structurally related compounds. [HSA] = 1.8×10^{-5} M and [Drug] = 5×10^{-5} M in 0.05 M phosphate buffer at pH 7.4, 25°. Curve A, CPZ; B, CPZ sulfoxide; C, imipramine [R_1: $(CH_2)_3$—$N(CH_3)_2$]; D, chlorprothixene [R_2: $(CH_2)_2$—$N(CH_3)_2$].

difference spectra were the same, with regard to maxima and shape, and only the absorption intensities were different with different albumins.

The difference absorption spectra resulting from the interaction between albumins and phenothiazine derivatives were markedly influenced by the substitutions at the carbon-2 position of the phenothiazine nuclei as shown in Fig. 2 with HSA. The absorption intensities increased from promazine to CPZ and to triflupromazine, and at the same time this was accompanied by a slight red shift of the absorption maxima. Different side-chain substitution at the N-10 position of the phenothiazine nucleus slightly changed the peak intensities, but the maxima remained essentially the same. Such substituent effects were observed for all the albumins studied.

The generation of the difference absorption peaks could be attributed either to the perturbation of the phenothiazine absorption bands by a different environment at the protein-binding sites or to the perturbation of the protein aromatic amino-acid residues as the result of the interaction or a combination of both. The solvent-perturbation difference spectra between cyclohexane and buffer of CPZ, as well as the three structurally related compounds are shown in Fig. 3. It is evident that the solvent-perturbation difference spectrum of CPZ was quite similar to the HSA and CPZ difference spectrum in buffer, particularly in the 260 nm region. This distinguishing feature was observed in serum albumin of all species used.

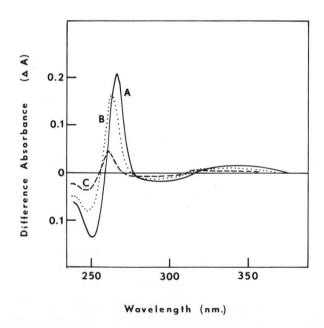

FIG. 2. The effect of substitution on the difference spectra of HSA and phenothiazines. $[HSA] = 1.8 \times 10^{-5}$ M and $[Drug] = 5 \times 10^{-5}$ M phosphate buffer at pH 7.4, 25°, Curve A, triflupromazine; B, CPZ; and C, promazine.

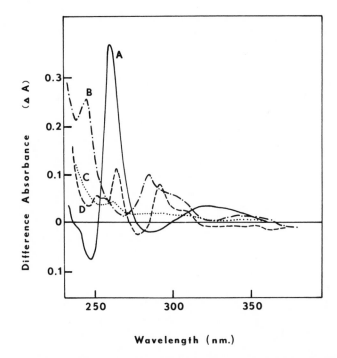

Wavelength (nm.)

FIG. 3. Solvent perturbation spectra in cyclohexane versus 0.05 M phosphate buffer, pH 7.4. Curve A (——) chlorpromazine; B ($- \cdot - \cdot -$), chlorprothixene; C ($\cdots$), imipramine; and D ($---$), chlorpromazine sulfoxide. The concentration used was 2.5×10^{-5} M throughout.

On the other hand, similar comparison of CPZ sulfoxide, imipramine, and chlorprothixene between their protein interaction difference spectra under identical conditions revealed entirely different peaks and intensities.

In order to have a better understanding of the functional groups and regions of the phenothiazine molecule involved in the interaction and binding to albumins, with HSA and bovine serum albumin (BSA) as representative, the difference spectra of a series of phenothiazine with HSA and BSA were thoroughly examined. Some of their relevant properties are listed in Tables 1 and 2. Of the 17 phenothiazine derivatives tested under identical conditions as described in the legends to Tables 1 and 2, all exhibited the same characteristics, i.e., two positive and two negative peaks as with CPZ. The positive peaks at the 260 nm region being the predominant ones, they were used as the basis for comparison. The intensities of the difference absorption peaks being a good indication of the degree of interaction or the binding processes for various phenothiazine derivatives, they were expressed in terms of difference absorbance (ΔA) and difference relative oscillator strength ($\Delta \int \epsilon d\lambda$). The latter parameter was obtained by integrating the whole area under the difference absorption

TABLE 1. *Comparison of albumin binding of various phenothiazine derivatives from difference spectra data*[a]

Compound	Human serum albumin			Bovine serum albumin		
	$\Delta\lambda$max[b]	ΔA[c]	$\Delta\int\epsilon d\lambda$[d]	$\Delta\lambda$max[b]	ΔA[c]	$\Delta\int\epsilon d\lambda$[d]
Chlorpromazine	263	100	100	263	100	100
Promazine	259	29.4	25.2	258	42.8	45.5
Promethazine	259	35.3	37.6	258	65.9	71.7
Trimeprazine	260	42.6	46.6	259	69.2	82.2
Perphenazine	263	96.5	95.9	263	83.6	87.7
Triflupromazine	267	141	130	266	126	126
Fluphenazine	267	106	101	267	94.5	94.8
Trifluoperazine	267	112	120	267	108	110

[a] Conditions: temperature = 25°, 0.05 M phosphate buffer, pH 7.4, albumin [1.8×10^{-5} M] + phenothiazines [5.0×10^{-5} M].

[b] The positive absorption maximum of the difference spectra used for comparison.

[c] Normalized difference absorbance at $\Delta\lambda$max against CPZ as 100.

[d] Normalized relative oscillator strength for the difference absorption peak $\Delta\lambda$max against CPZ as 100.

peak. All data were averaged from three runs (mean ± S.E. 2%) and were normalized against CPZ as the standard (100) for comparison. Similarly, the degrees of interaction as expressed in terms of normalized ΔA at the maxima of the difference absorption peak (260 region) between serum albumin of various species and phenothiazine derivatives at pH 7.4 are listed in Table 3.

The binding of phenothiazines to albumins of the ten species used was

TABLE 2. *Comparison of the effects of various substitutions on the phenothiazine ring towards albumin binding from difference spectra data*[a]

Compound	Human serum albumin			Bovine serum albumin		
	$\Delta\lambda$max[b]	ΔA[c]	$\Delta\int\epsilon d\lambda$[d]	$\Delta\lambda$max[b]	ΔA[c]	$\Delta\int\epsilon d\lambda$[d]
Chlorpromazine	263	100	100	263	100	100
2-Bromopromazine	263	120	122	263	115	118
3,7-dichlorpromazine	265	135	132	265	138	130
6-hydroxychlorpromazine	270	76.2	82.3	269	85.1	87.4
7-hydroxychlorpromazine	266	37.8	50.0	265	47.6	48.1
8-hydroxychlorpromazine	268	62.6	71.6	266	54.9	61.8
7-methoxychlorpromazine	266	35.2	40.3	266	42.5	39.9
3,7-dimethoxychlorpromazine	264	53.3	54.8	264	35.0	37.1
7,8-dimethoxychlorpromazine	267	59.1	62.0	266	31.8	34.0
Chlorpromazine N-oxide	263	41.2	44.5	263	40.1	43.4

[a] Conditions: temperature = 25°, 0.05 M phosphate buffer, pH 7.4, albumin [1.8×10^{-5} M] + phenothiazines [5.0×10^{-5} M].

[b] The positive absorption maximum of the difference spectra used for comparison.

[c] Normalized difference absorbance at $\Delta\lambda$ max against CPZ as 100.

[d] Normalized relative oscillator strength for the difference absorption peak $\Delta\lambda$ max against CPZ as 100.

TABLE 3. *Relative binding between serum albumins of various species and different phenothiazine derivatives*[a]

Species	PMZ	PRO	TMZ	CPZ	PPZ	TFP	FLU	TFZ
Human	29.4	35.3	42.6	100	96.5	141	106	112
Bovine	42.8	65.9	69.2	100	83.6	126	94.5	108
Rat	27.5	24.6	36.4	100	97.4	112	122	100
Rabbit	45.7	71.7	68.3	100	104	118	114	107
Dog	34.6	67.6	45.0	100	101	132	109	103
Chicken	43.9	44.5	59.7	100	153	100	110	95.5
Goat	35.9	80.9	55.0	100	113	112	112	105
Horse	60.5	46.8	60.5	100	112	121	117	120
Sheep	36.8	77.5	50.4	100	98.3	124	117	110
Pig	36.0	74.6	59.3	100	131	144	151	106

[a] Relative binding is expressed in terms of normalized difference absorbance (ΔA) at the maxima of the difference absorption peak (260 region) against CPZ as 100 of the same species. [Albumin] $= 1.8 \times 10^{-5}$ M. [Phenothiazine] $= 5.0 \times 10^{-5}$ M in 0.05 M phosphate buffer, pH 7.4, 25°.

Abbreviations: PMZ = Promazine, PRO = Promethazine, TMZ = Trimeprazine, CPZ = Chlorpromazine, PPZ = Perphenazine, TFP = Triflupromazine, FLU = Fluphenazine, TFZ = Trifluoperazine.

highly pH dependent. The relative binding between serum albumin of various species and CPZ at different pH's are listed in Table 4 in terms of normalized ΔA. At pH 7.4, the degree of binding was highest in rat, followed by bovine, rabbit, horse, dog, goat, man, sheep, pig, and chicken. It should be noted that the binding of CPZ to rat albumin is nearly 80% higher than to human. Generally, binding improved at higher pH's. At pH 7.9, binding between CPZ and albumins of different species was relatively similar

TABLE 4. *Relative binding between serum albumin of various species and chlorpromazine at different pH's*[a]

Species	pH			
	5.8	6.5	7.4	7.9
Human	10.2	22.0	100	224
Bovine	4.03	19.3	143	208
Dog	23.1	38.3	121	235
Rat	84.3	111	178	271
Rabbit	37.5	82.5	133	215
Sheep	14.0	24.2	90	246
Horse	13.5	30.8	125	240
Pig	9.38	20.9	78	217
Chicken	25.5	41.6	72	144
Goat	18.8	29.7	118	251

[a] Relative binding is expressed in terms of normalized difference absorbance (ΔA) at the maxima of the difference absorption peak (260 region) against CPZ as 100 of the same species. [Albumin] $= 1.8 \times 10^{-5}$ M. [Phenothiazine] $= 5.0 \times 10^{-5}$ M in 0.05 phosphate buffer, 25°.

(within 25%), while at pH 6.5, rat albumin was five-times higher than human and eight-times higher than human at pH 5.8.

The binding equilibrium between albumin (P) with a single binding site and phenothiazine (C) can be expressed as follows:

$$P + C \rightleftharpoons PC.$$

The association constant (k) relates the concentration of the components at equilibrium

$$k = \frac{[PC]}{[P][C]}.$$

Let ϕ be the fractional saturation of the albumin,

$$\phi = \frac{\text{mole of phenothiazine bound}}{\text{mole of total albumin}} = \frac{[PC]}{[P_0]} = \frac{[PC]}{[P] + [PC]} = \frac{k[P][C]}{[P] + k[P][C]},$$

or

$$\phi = \frac{kC}{1 + kC},$$

where C is the molar concentration of the unbound phenothiazine. In the difference spectrophotometric study of the binding, the difference absorption peaks derive only from the perturbation of PC (5, 6). Thus,

$$\phi = \frac{\Delta A}{\Delta A_{\max}}, \tag{1}$$

where $\Delta A_{\max}$ is the maximum difference absorbance at P. In the fluorescence quenching study of the binding, ϕ is related to the quenching of the albumin fluorescence (7).

$$\phi = \frac{F_f - F}{F_f - F_b}, \tag{2}$$

where F_f is the fluorescence of the free albumin, F is the corrected fluorescence (8) of the albumin-phenothiazine mixture, F_b is the fluorescence of the fully bound albumin which is obtained in the presence of a large excess of phenothiazine. If the albumin had N independent binding sites for phenothiazine,

$$r = \phi N, \tag{3}$$

or

$$= \frac{NkC}{1 + kC}, \tag{4}$$

where r is the average number of binding sites bound and N is the stoichiometry of the binding, and

$$C = C_0 - rP_0. \tag{5}$$

Equation (4) could be rearranged to the familiar

Klotz' equation: $1/r = 1/N + 1/Nk \times 1/C,$

or

Scatchard's equation: $r/C = kN - kr.$

A typical binding equilibrium study using difference spectrophotometry method for the binding between HSA and triflupromazine is shown in Fig. 4. The stoichiometry *(N)* was obtained from a plot of ΔA versus C_0. The data were then compiled from Eqs. (1), (3), and (5) and subjected to Scatchard's plot. The association constant *(k)* was thus obtained. Similar binding equilibrium studies with a few representative phenothiazines were carried out; results are listed in Table 5. A typical binding equilibrium study using the fluorescence quenching method for the binding between HSA and CPZ is shown in Fig. 5. The data could be compiled from Eqs. (2), (3), and (5) and again subjected to Scatchard's plot. The effect of protein concentration on the binding of CPZ is shown in Table 6. The fluorescence quenching behavior of BSA was very similar to HSA. The stoichiometry is the same as

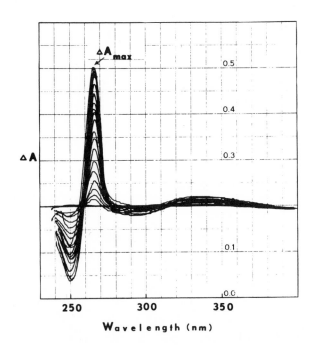

FIG. 4. Difference spectrophotometric study of the binding between HSA and triflupromazine. [HSA] $= 1.8 \times 10^{-5}$ M; [Triflupromazine] $= 3.6 \times 10^{-6}$ to 1.5×10^{-4} M in 0.05 M phosphate buffer, pH 7.4, 25°.

TABLE 5. *Binding of several phenothiazine derivatives to human serum albumin from difference spectra data[a]*

Compound(s)	ΔA[b]	N[c]	k[d] $\times 10^4$ 1/M	$-\Delta F^{\circ e}$
Chlorpromazine	100	4	4.2	6270
Triflupromazine	141	4	5.5	6430
6-Hydroxychlorpromazine	76.2	4	3.0	6080
3,7-Dimethoxychlorpromazine	53.3	4	2.2	5890

[a] Temperature = 25°, 0.05 M phosphate buffer, pH 7.4. HSA [1.8×10^{-5} M].
[b] Normalized difference absorbance taken from Tables 2 and 3.
[c] Stoichiometry of drug binding sites per albumin molecule.
[d] Binding association constant.
[e] Binding free energy calculated from $\Delta F^{\circ} = -RT \ln k$.

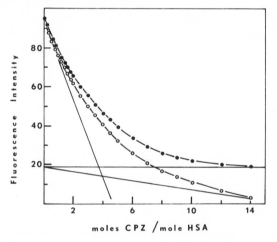

FIG. 5. Fluorometric quenching titration of HSA with CPZ. [HSA] = 1.8×10^{-5} M, [CPZ] = 3.6×10^{-6} to 2.5×10^{-4} M in 0.05 M phosphate buffer, pH 7.4, 25°. Excitation wavelength = 295 nm, fluorescence wavelength = 340 nm.

TABLE 6. *Effect of protein concentration on the binding of chlorpromazine to human serum albumin and bovine serum albumin from fluorescence quenching studies[a]*

Protein concentration (M)	Human Serum Albumin		Bovine Serum Albumin	
	N[b]	k[c] $\times 10^4$ 1/M	N[b]	k[c] $\times 10^4$ 1/M
3.6×10^{-5}	3	6.2	3	8.3
1.8×10^{-5}	4	6.1	4	8.1
9.0×10^{-6}	6	6.1	6	8.2
4.5×10^{-6}	13	6.4	13	8.5

[a] Temperature = 25°, 0.05 M phosphate buffer, pH 7.4.
[b] Stoichiometry of drug binding sites per albumin molecule.
[c] Binding association constant.

HSA with the same concentration; the equilibrium constants could be obtained in similar ways.

DISCUSSION

The difference spectra for the interaction between various albumin and a series of phenothiazine derivatives revealed consistently, as with CPZ, two positive and two negative absorption peaks. In contrast, several of the structurally related compounds, such as imipramine, chlorprothixene, and CPZ sulfoxide, failed to show this characteristic pattern. Comparison of the difference spectra of the interaction between albumins and CPZ with the solvent-perturbation difference spectra of CPZ in cyclohexane versus buffer showed close similarities, which is a direct indication of the existence of a hydrophobic environment around the albumin-binding sites. Imipramine, chlorprothixene, and CPZ sulfoxide have nevertheless been shown (9, 10) to bind albumin from data derived from gel filtration and equilibrium dialysis techniques; in fact, chlorprothixene was found to bind albumin even stronger than CPZ (9). The negligible appearance of their difference spectra with albumin and the large discrepancy between the solvent-perturbation difference spectra indicates that their binding sites on albumin are quite different from those of the phenothiazines. Accordingly, their binding sites are most likely not in a hydrophobic environment, and only very weak perturbation could be observed between the absorption chromophores of these molecules and the protein.

The increase in the intensity of the difference spectra for the interaction of albumin with promazine, CPZ, and triflupromazine is consistent with the increase of the hydrophobic character of the substitutions at the C-2 position of these molecules. Similar conclusions attributable to the hydrophobic binding had been obtained through the comparison of other parameters from gel filtration and equilibrium dialysis (11, 12). In keeping with the same rationale, in our studies, 2-bromopromazine was found to bind albumin stronger than CPZ, and 3,7-dichlorpromazine was stronger than either CPZ or 2-bromopromazine. On the other hand, the presence of any hydrophilic groups on the phenothiazine molecule, either on the nucleus or the side chain, caused considerable reduction in the magnitude of the difference spectra. For example, CPZ-N-oxide was bound to albumin less than half compared to CPZ. However, the substituent effect of a hydroxyl group appears to vary according to the site in the nucleus, the 6-position being least sensitive, while the 7-position had the greatest effect. Introduction of a methoxyl group into the phenothiazine ring moiety also resulted in lowering the binding ability to albumin. The effect of the 7-methoxyl group was quite similar to that of the 7-hydroxyl group. However, by introducing a second methoxyl group, such as in 3,7- or 7,8-dimethoxyl CPZ, a significant difference between the two species was observed.

While the serum albumin of all ten species interacts with phenothiazines generally in a similar fashion, i.e., they all are involved in a hydrophobic binding area, affinity towards various phenothiazine derivatives showed a wide spectrum among the albumins of different species. These differences probably reflect small alterations of the amino-acid sequence near the binding sites. Also, the difference spectra were very sensitive to pH changes, as shown in Table 4. It is evident that although hydrophobic bonding was the predominant factor, ionic interaction could not be ignored. Since the pK_a of CPZ is about 9.3, most of the species are protonated in aqueous buffered solution below pH 7.9. The ionization of the amino-acid residues in the binding sites might be of major importance if some weakly acidic groups, which were only partially ionized at pH 7.4, were involved. These should be the binding region for the charged side-chain dimethylamino group. The drastic reduction of binding in some of the species at slightly higher pH's might not be completely due to the conformational changes of the protein, and charge repulsion might have also occurred from the protonation of the acidic groups. It appears that the binding sites of some of the albumins less sensitive to pH changes, such as those of rat, rabbit, chicken, and dog, might have different and stronger acidic groups.

While numerous studies on the binding of acidic drugs to plasma protein have been reported (13), publication on basic drugs are relatively scanty. It is generally assumed that albumin has different binding sites for acidic and basic drugs (14). While some acidic drugs could displace another acidic drug from a particular binding site, basic drugs never replace acidic drugs in the same site (15). Recent papers (11, 16) have proposed that only one of the benzene rings of the phenothiazine nucleus is involved in albumin binding. The base for this conclusion was that simple aromatic substances, such as benzoic acid or acetylsalicylic acid, were able to displace CPZ from its albumin binding, and competition occurred between single benzene rings, which were integral parts of the structure of all substances used. From the present studies, the ability of various substituents (particularly in the 6-, 7-, and 8-positions) on the phenothiazine ring to give rise to marked differences in the degree of binding and the inability to do so of some of the structurally related compounds (which all contain benzene rings) strongly suggested that all three rings of the phenothiazine nucleus are essential to the binding of CPZ and its congeners to the hydrophobic sites in all the albumins studied.

The three-dimensional crystalline and molecular structure of CPZ has been resolved (17). The molecule is folded about the S-N axis and the angle between the best planes for the two benzene rings was found to be 139.4°. The folding of the molecule enables the sulfur atom to retain its natural valency angle. For the same reason, the formation of the phenothiazine ring in solution would probably remain the same, it would fit in some hollowed contour area as indicated by the binding sites in the hydrophobic region of the albumins. Any alteration of this geometric requirement, as in the case of CPZ sulfoxide, imipramine, or chlorprothixene, excluded such molecules from this particular albumin binding site.

From difference spectroscopic studies, it appears that these phenothiazine binding sites are quite specific and generally quite similar in all the albumins studied. This is somewhat different with regard to albumin binding of some acidic drugs. The binding equilibrium studies of a few selected phenothiazines towards HSA indicated that the binding constants obtained from Scatchard plots corresponded quite well to the normalized difference absorbances (ΔAs). It is evident that under identical experimental conditions, the intensities of the difference absorption peaks are good indicators of the degree of the interaction and that various phenothiazines studied involve a common binding mechanism. Studies of various other species of albumin showed that the binding behavior was very similar and comparable.

The fluorescence quenching of the intrinsic protein tryptophan residue by CPZ has been studied with both HSA and BSA. HSA contains only one tryptophan residue and previous studies (18) have suggested that it is in a binding area of the protein especially active for small anions. The amino acid sequences around this lone tryptophan site have been elucidated and indeed show a very favorable environment for binding of small anions. The quenching of the tryptophan fluorescence by the basic phenothiazine drugs probably is not due directly to this binding site but to an adjacent site, either due to a slight structural transformation of the protein or due to Forster's energy-transfer mechanism. The fluorescence-quenching behavior of BSA by CPZ was very similar to that of HSA. Although BSA is known to contain two tryptophan residues, the similarity between HSA and BSA is probably due to the fact that the two tryptophans in the BSA molecule are relatively far apart and only one of them is involved. Recent studies (19) on the quenching by cupric ion have shown that this is indeed the case, one of the tryptophans being located deep in the center of the BSA molecule. The stoichiometry for the binding of phenothiazine to albumin has been reported as BSA and HSA values ranging from 1 to 23 (15, 20, 21). It is evident that the stoichiometric relation depends on the albumin concentration, as is shown by the fluorescence quenching studies.

It thus becomes evident that the UV difference spectrophotometry and fluorescence-quenching methods are very useful tools in studying the interaction between albumins and phenothiazines. Their advantages include rapid handling and convenience and they require only small amounts of albumins (in the mg range). There are differences between the direct methods such as equilibrium dialysis of gel filtration which measures directly the concentration of the unbound drugs, and indirect spectroscopic methods such as difference spectrophotometry or fluorescence, which correlates the concentration of the bound drug to spectral changes. This concentration is the same as the complex, which in turn depends on the environment, conformations of the binding sites, etc. Such information is generally not available from the direct methods. It is thus proposed that difference spectrophotometry and fluorescence quenching are complementary methods providing additional insight into the stoichiometry and affinity of the binding mechanism unavailable from the widely used equilibrium dialysis or gel filtration techniques.

SUMMARY

The serum albumin's binding of various phenothiazines has been studied in human, bovine, dog, rat, rabbit, pig, horse, sheep, goat, and chicken using UV difference spectrophotometry and intrinsic protein fluorescence quenching methods. The difference spectra of their interaction showed characteristically two positive and two negative peaks at the 260, 330 and 250, 290 nm region, respectively. From solvent perturbation difference spectrophotometry studies, it has been shown that the difference spectra between albumins and phenothiazines arise mostly from the perturbation of the phenothiazine absorption bands by a hydrophobic environment at the albumin binding sites. The characters and shapes of the difference spectra of all the albumin interactions were almost identical, indicating the overall binding site environment of the ten species were quite similar. On the other hand, three structurally similar compounds, chlorpromazine sulfoxide, imipramine, and chlorprothixene gave entirely different patterns of much weaker absorption in all species. This might be taken as evidence that the latter compounds were bound at sites on the albumin surface quite different from those of the phenothiazines.

The degree of different albumins binding with chlorpromazine varied at pH 7.4 as well as towards different phenothiazines. All the phenothiazine bindings of the ten species were highly pH dependent. Generally, binding improved at higher pHs. The results obtained from fluorescence quenching studies corroborated the UV difference spectrophotometry method.

ACKNOWLEDGMENTS

This work was supported by the Veterans Administration Research Program.

REFERENCES

1. Vogt, M., in *Comparative Neurochemistry*, Richter, D. (ed.), Pergamon Press, Oxford, 1964, p. 387.
2. Brodie, B. B., *J. Amer. Med. Assoc.*, **202**, 606 (1967).
3. Chen, R. F., *J. Biol. Chem.*, **242**, 173 (1967).
4. Yankeelov, J. A., *Anal. Biochem.*, **6**, 287 (1963).

5. Hermans, J., Jr., Donovan, J. W., and Scheraga, H. A., *J. Biol. Chem.*, **235**, 91 (1960).
6. Suelter, C. H., and Melander, W., *J. Biol. Chem.*, **238**, 4108 (1963).
7. Davenport, D., in *Fluorescence Spectroscopy*, Pesce, A. J., Rosen, C. G., and Pasby, T. L. (eds.), Marcel Dekker, New York, 1971, chap. 7, pp. 203–233.
8. Valick, S. F., Parker, L. W., and Eisen, H. N., *Proc. Nat. Acad. Sci. U.S.A.*, **46**, 1470 (1960).
9. Stephan, Y., Welin, L., and Mainard, F., *C. R. Acad. Sci. Paris*, **272**, 1451 (Series D) (1971).
10. Franz, J. W., Jahnchen, E., and Krieglstein, J., *Naunyn-Schmiedeberg's Arch. Pharmak. Exp. Path.*, **264**, 462 (1969).
11. Krieglstein, J., Meiler, W., and Staab, J., *Biochem. Pharmacol.*, **21**, 985 (1972).
12. Krieglstein, J., and Kuschinsky, G., *Naunyn-Schmiedeberg's Arch. Pharmak. Exp. Path.*, **262**, 1 (1969).
13. Meyer, M. C., and Guttman, D. E., *J. Pharmacol. Sci.*, **57**, 895 (1968).
14. Brodie, B. B., in *Transport Function of Plasma Proteins*, Desgrez, P. and De Traverse, P. M. (eds.), Elsevier Press, Amsterdam, 1966, pp. 137–145.
15. Brodie, B. B., *Proc. Roy. Soc. Med.*, **58**, 946 (1965).
16. Jahnchen, E., Krieglstein, J., and Kuschinsky, G., *Naunyn-Schmiedeberg's Arch. Pharmak. Exp. Path.*, **263**, 375 (1969).
17. McDowell, J. J. H., *Acta Cryst.*, **25**, 2175 (1969).
18. Swaney, J. B., and Klotz, I. M., *Biochemistry*, **9**, 2570 (1970).
19. Luk, C. K., *Biopolymers*, **10**, 1229 (1971).
20. Krieglstein, J., Lier, F., and Michaelis, J., *Naunyn-Schmiedeberg's Arch. Pharmac.*, **272**, 121 (1972).
21. Naval, J. J., and Mao, T. S. S., *Bull. Inst. Chem., Acad. Sinica*, **18**, 82 (1970).

The Phenothiazines and Structurally Related Drugs, edited by I. S. Forrest, C. J. Carr, and E. Usdin. Raven Press, New York © 1974.

Some Aspects of the *In Vitro* Oxidation of ^{35}S-Chlorpromazine

J. W. Gorrod, C. R. Lazarus, and A. H. Beckett

Department of Pharmacy, Chelsea College, University of London, S.W.3., London, England

INTRODUCTION

Following the introduction of chlorpromazine (CPZ)[1] into human therapy, numerous studies on the metabolic fate of this and related phenothiazines have been undertaken in both man and experimental animals and have been adequately reviewed (1–4). Results from these studies indicate that the principle routes of oxidative metabolism of CPZ involve attack on the sulfur or side-chain nitrogen to produce the corresponding oxides or attack on the carbon of the N-methyl group or the aromatic ring of the phenothiazine nucleus. These metabolic processes lead to N-oxidation, S-oxidation, N-dealkylation, and 7-hydroxylation as the primary metabolic routes. Recently Beckett and Essien (5) have recognized N-hydroxylation of the demethyl-ated product, to yield the hydroxylamine as a secondary metabolite (6).

It is the purpose of this chapter to present details of studies done to dif-ferentiate the enzymic processes by which these metabolic reactions are mediated.

MATERIALS AND METHODS

Chemicals

^{35}S-CPZ HCl was purchased from the Radiochemical Centre (Amer-sham). Unlabeled CPZ, HCl (Largactil) was obtained from May and Baker Ltd., (Dagenham). Samples of D · CPZ, D · D · CPZ, and their sulfoxides, CPZ · SO, CPZ · SO$_2$, were obtained from Smith, Kline, and French Lab-oratories (Philadelphia). 7-OH · CPZ was a gift from Dr. A. A. Manian (Pharmacology Section, National Institute of Mental Health). CPZ · NO

---

[1] Abbreviations used in this paper are as follows: CPZ = chlorpromazine; D · CPZ = mono-desmethylchlorpromazine; CPZ · SO = chlorpromazine sulfoxide; 7-OH · CPZ = 7-hydroxy-chlorpromazine; CPZ · NO = chlorpromazine N-oxides; NADP = nicotinamide adenine dinucleotide phosphate; NADPH = reduced NADP.

and CPZ · NO · SO were obtained from Rhone-Poulenc (Paris). 1,4-Dioxan (A.R.) was obtained from Hopkins and Williams (England); methanol (A.R.) from B.D.H. Ltd., (Dorset, England). Ethylene glycol (Extrapure) from B.D.H., and diethylamine from May and Baker. All chemicals for liquid scintillation counting were obtained from the Packard Instrument Co. (Illinois).

Biochemicals and Enzymes

NADP, NADPH, glucose-6-phosphate (G-6-P), and glucose-6-phosphate dehydrogenase (G-6-P · D) were obtained from Boehringer Mannheim (London). Nicotinamide and $MgCl_2$ were obtained from B.D.H. Ltd. (Poole, England).

Animals and Tissue Preparation

Male albino Wistar rats, each weighing 300 to 450 g (aged 10 to 14 weeks), were used, and fed on normal laboratory diet [Diet 86, E. Dixon and Sons (Ware) Ltd.]; albino guinea pigs 350 to 450 g; albino New Zealand White rabbits approximately 3 kg; mice, 30 to 40 g. The animals were stunned and decapitated, and the tissues immediately removed into ice-cold Tris KCl buffer, pH 7.4. The tissues were homogenized (1 g of liver with 2 ml of Tris KCl buffer) using a Teflon glass tissue grinder (Arthur H. Thomas size B) for three 1-min passes. The homogenate was centrifuged at $10,000 \times g$ for 20 min in a Sorvall RC2-B refrigerated centrifuge. Liver microsomes were sedimented by centrifuging the $10,000 \times g$ supernatant at $140,000 \times g$ for 60 min in an M.S.E. Superspeed "40" centrifuge. The microsomal pellet was resuspended in Tris KCl buffer to give the equivalent of 1 g of original liver per 2 ml of suspension. All the above operations were carried out below 4°C.

For experiments involving the induction of hepatic microsomal enzymes, female rats were pretreated with appropriate substances as described below.

Incubations

Incubates contained tissue (equivalent to 0.5 g wet weight of original tissue as microsomes or homogenate as appropriate), NADP, 2 μmoles; G-6-P 25 μmoles, G-6-P · D · 3 units; nicotinamide, 20 μmoles; $MgCl_2$, 25μmoles; all were suspended in 0.1 M phosphate buffer, pH 7.4, to 4 ml. Incubations were performed in 25-ml open Erhlenmeyer flasks in a Gallenkamp shaking incubator at 37°C. Light was excluded during incubation. All glassware was washed in, and all solutions prepared in double glass-distilled water to eliminate trace metals.

Extraction of CPZ and Metabolites and Concentration of Extracts

The incubates were transferred to 50-ml stoppered polyethylene centrifuge tubes and 20 ml of n-butanol added, together with 3 ml of aqueous washings from the incubation flasks. Ammonium hydroxide 2.5 ml (S.G. 0.88) was added, and the centrifuge tubes were shaken on a Griffin flask shaker for 1 min. The emulsions which formed were separated by centrifugation at 10,000 rpm for 10 min. The organic phase was removed and the aqueous phase reextracted with a further 2×20 ml of *n*-butanol. During extraction, exposure of the solutions to light was minimized. Extracts were stored under nitrogen.

The butanol extracts were concentrated under vacuum in the absence of light, using a rotary film evaporator, at 55°C. After evaporation almost to dryness, the flask was filled with nitrogen (oxygen-free, British Oxygen Co.), and 0.5 ml methanol (A.R.) was added to the extract to facilitate application to thin-layer plates and subsequent drying.

Thin-Layer Chromatography

Thin-layer chromatography was carried out on glass plates spread with 0.5 mm silica gel MN-Kieselgel G/UV 254 (Machery Nagel & Co). The plates were activated at 100°C for 45 min. During chromatography, the temperature was maintained at $23° \pm 1°C$; development involved benzene-dioxane-diethylamine-water (70:17.5:7.5:1 by volume) in the dark.

Phenothiazine-positive material was located by viewing with a Hanovia portable ultraviolet (UV) lamp (CHI/294).

The area of silica gel containing ^{35}S-CPZ or a radioactive metabolite corresponding to the R_f value of the authentic substance was removed from the chromatogram and transferred to a counting vial. One ml of methanol (A.R.) was added and the vial sealed and shaken vigorously to elute the labeled product from the silica gel. Scintillant (10 ml), consisting of naphthalene 60 g; 2,5-diphenyloxazole (PPO) 4 g; 1,4-*bis*-2-(4-methyl-5-phenyloxazolyl-1)-benzene (dimethyl POPOP) 0.2 g; methanol (A.R.) 100 ml; toluene (A.R.) 100 ml; ethylene glycol (extra pure) 20 ml, and dioxan (A.R.) to 1 liter, was added. Duplicate determinations were performed and each sample was counted in a Packard Tricarb Liquid Scintillation Spectrometer (Model 314 EX). All counts were corrected for background, control samples for background being prepared similarly to the corresponding experimental samples, but omitting the radioactive drug.

RESULTS

The Influence of Various Potential Inhibitors on the *In Vitro* Metabolism of ^{35}S-CPZ

Results obtained on the inhibition of the various routes of CPZ metabolism, by the incorporation of various compounds into the incubation media using guinea pig hepatic microsomal system, are presented in Table 1. Clear evidence for the differentiation of the various metabolic pathways is obtained. Thus, 1,10-phenanthroline, SKF 525A, and imidazole, all compounds known to interact with microsomal cytochromes to give either type I or type II spectra, inhibited the two routes of carbon oxidation while leaving the N-oxidative pathway unaffected. However, ring hydroxylation was generally less sensitive to inhibition than demethylation. Similar results were found when incubation was carried out in an atmosphere containing CO, although a slight inhibition of N-oxidation was observed. Considerable inhibition of sulfoxidation was also found with all these compounds.

The antioxidant propyl gallate, previously shown by Torrielli and Slater (7) to inhibit microsomal NADPH cytochrome c reductase, inhibited the carbon-oxidative routes, leaving hetero-atom oxidation unaffected. In a similar manner, the two substances which are known to react with protein sulfhydryl groups, N-ethylmaleimide and *p*-chloromercuribenzoate, had a dramatic effect on the two carbon-oxidative pathways, but again left the N-oxidation pathway unaffected. Unlike propyl gallate however, these latter two reagents also inhibited sulfoxidation.

The failure of catalase to substantially inhibit any route of metabolism is in agreement with other findings that these oxidative processes are not mediated by microsomal hydrogen-peroxide formation.

Cysteamine and dithiothreitol, previously shown to specifically inhibit the N-oxidation of nicotine (8) and normethadone (9) whereas they leave the carbon-oxidative route unaffected, showed a similar influence on the *in vitro* hepatic metabolism of CPZ.

Initial experiments had indicated that failure to use multiple glass-distilled water often led to poor reproducibility of results. This was considered to be due to the presence of trace metals as contaminants; deliberate addition of either Cu^{++} or Hg^{++} to the incubation system led to inhibition of demethylation and 7-hydroxylation with a concomitant increase of N-oxidation.

The Influence of "Aging" and Deoxycholate Pretreatment on the *In Vitro* Metabolism and Cytochrome P450 Levels

The influence of "aging" of guinea pig microsomes by storage at 0°C for periods of up to 14 days is shown in Fig. 1. With the exception of N-oxida-

TABLE 1. *The effect of compounds on the in vitro metabolism of ^{35}S-CPZ using hepatic microsomes from male guinea pigs*

	Concentration	Demethylation	Sulfoxidation	7-Hydroxylation	N-Oxidation
SKF525A[a]	10^{-3} M	75 ± 11	51 ± 2	74 ± 8	118 ± 2
1,10-Phenanthroline	10^{-3} M	20 ± 0	74 ± 1	67 ± 4	101 ± 5
Imidazole	10^{-3} M	59 ± 0	56 ± 6	73 ± 4	104 ± 8
CO[b]	—	44 ± 3	59 ± 8	49 ± 7	76 ± 6
Propyl gallate	10^{-3} M	45 ± 1	112 ± 3	48 ± 7	104 ± 1
N-ethylmaleimide	10^{-3} M	33 ± 7	77 ± 24	51 ± 6	98 ± 8
p-Chloromercuribenzoate	10^{-3} M	9 ± 0	21 ± 1	44 ± 11	134 ± 7
Catalase	2000 units	90 ± 3	93 ± 7	82 ± 4	96 ± 2
Cysteamine	10^{-2} M	84 ± 3	114 ± 6	93 ± 3	47 ± 4
Dithiothreitol	10^{-2} M	86 ± 4	97 ± 2	88 ± 3	74 ± 1
CuCl$_2$	10^{-4} M	27 ± 3	122 ± 7	89 ± 4	134 ± 2
HgCl$_2$	10^{-4} M	29 ± 3	70 ± 7	70 ± 6	154 ± 7

Results are expressed as percentage activity of identical incubates without the addition of the compound and are mean values ± experimental variation obtained from two or more animals. Incubation conditions are as described in the text, and were carried out for 10 min. [a] 2-Diethylaminoethyl-2,2-diphenylvalerate hydrochloride. [b] N_2:O_2:CO = 4:1:5 by volume.

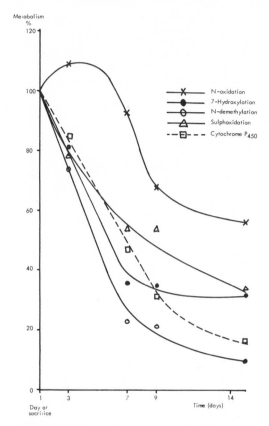

FIG. 1. The effect of "aging" of guinea pig liver microsomes on the *in vitro* metabolism of ^{35}S-CPZ and cytochrome P_{450} levels.

tion, the oxidative routes of CPZ metabolism decay at a rate very similar to that of cytochrome P450. N-oxidation, however, shows an increase in activity during the first few days of "aging" before the decay in N-oxidative activity begins. Similarly, when guinea pig microsomes are preincubated at 0°C for 1 hr with low concentrations of deoxycholate, the N-oxidation is increased, whereas the other pathways show an immediate decline which is paralleled by the decline in cytochrome P450 levels (Fig. 2).

The Effect of Animal Pretreatments on the *In Vitro* Metabolism of ^{35}S-CPZ

Following the pretreatment of female rats with a variety of potential inducing agents, the *in vitro* hepatic metabolism of CPZ was examined. The results (Table 2) indicate that the classical inducing agents phenobarbital and 3-methylcholanthrene enhanced the demethylation and 7-hydroxylation

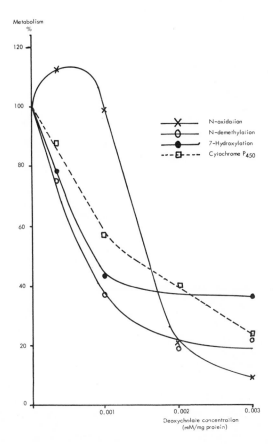

FIG. 2. The effect of deoxycholate treated microsomes on the *in vitro* metabolism of ^{35}S-CPZ and cytochrome P_{450} levels.

routes, but were without effect on the N-oxidative pathway. Of the other compounds tested, only the insecticides DDT, aldrin, and dieldrin significantly increased carbon oxidation, and only in the case of aldrin was any significant increase in the N-oxidative pathway observed.

The Extrahepatic Distribution of Oxidative Routes of CPZ Metabolism
In Vitro

Further evidence as to the heterogeneity of the various oxidative pathways of CPZ metabolism was obtained when these activities were examined in various extrahepatic tissues. Because of the differing sedimentation characteristics of the endoplasmic reticulum from various tissues, no attempt was made to prepare the microsomal fractions; instead, the whole-tissue homogenates were used as the enzyme source. The results are shown in Table 3.

TABLE 2. *Effect of animal pretreatments on the* in vitro *metabolism of* [35]*S-CPZ*

Compound administered and dose	Demethylation	Sulfoxidation	7-Hydroxylation	N-Oxidation
Phenobarbital (80 mg/kg × 3)	212	137	367	96
3-Methylcholanthrene (25 mg/kg × 3)	174	118	142	88
o.p. DDT (25 mg/kg × 3)	166	104	135	80
pp. DDT (25 mg/kg × 3)	125	87	120	86
Naphthylthiourea (5 mg/kg × 3)	117	79	136	96
Azobenzene (25 mg/kg × 3)	130	116	131	115
Aldrin (25 mg/kg × 3)	178	123	191	123
Dieldrin (25 mg/kg × 3)	169	145	176	101

Results are expressed as percentage activity of identical incubates using hepatic microsomes from untreated female rats, and are mean values obtained from two or more animals. Incubation conditions are as described in the text, and carried out for 10 min.

TABLE 3. *The extrahepatic distribution of oxidative routes of CPZ metabolism in vitro by various organs from four animal species*

Species	Tissue	Route of metabolism			
		Demethylation	Sulfoxidation	7-Hydroxylation	N-Oxidation
Guinea Pig	Brain	6	16	32	9
	Kidney	8	21	34	20
	Lung	8	21	35	10
Rat	Brain	24	118	37	24
	Kidney	21	55	21	44
	Lung	24	98	25	35
Rabbit	Brain	3	35	5	16
	Kidney	3	31	7	23
	Lung	6	78	8	15
Mouse	Brain	24	136	16	16
	Kidney	28	92	38	68
	Lung	39	268	52	55

Results are expressed as the activity of the whole organ homogenate as a percentage of whole liver homogenate. Incubation conditions are as described in the text, and carried out for 10 min.

While all the tissues examined had the ability to carry out all the metabolic routes to some extent, a wide variation both in organ and species distribution of activity was found. Whole brain, kidney, and lung homogenates from the mouse and rat appeared to be generally more efficient at metabolizing CPZ by the routes examined than were the same organs from the guinea pig and rabbit.

In many of the tissues examined, sulfoxidation approached, and in some cases exceeded, that formed by the equivalent weight of hepatic homogenate. The other routes of metabolism usually occurred to a much smaller extent than that obtained from the hepatic system, with N-demethylation being relatively less than ring hydroxylation. In kidney and lung tissue of both the mouse and rat, the N-oxidative route was about half that found in the corresponding hepatic preparation.

DISCUSSION

The results reported herein clearly indicate that the various routes of CPZ metabolism are not mediated by the same enzyme systems. Present evidence suggests that the two routes of C-oxidation studied, that is demethylation and ring hydroxylation, occur through the involvement of the microsomal cytochrome P450 system. In contrast, the oxidation of the basic tertiary nitrogen, while still occurring in the microsomes, seems to be oxidized independently of cytochrome P450, and this probably involves a flavo-protein enzyme system (10, 11).

The oxidation of the heterosulfur atom does not parallel either of the other routes; it is of interest that this route is uninhibited by propyl gallate, although affected by reagents attacking cytochrome P450, suggesting the involvement of a NADPH-linked system differing from the usual primary reductase.

Although the extrapolation of *in vitro* data to the *in vivo* situation must be interpreted with caution, it is of interest that these experiments have revealed that extrahepatic tissues have considerable drug-metabolizing potential.

The specific finding that brain tissue has drug metabolic activity will have to be considered now in the pharmacology of psychoactive drugs. Further, when it is considered that patients on therapy with this group of drugs receive large doses over long periods, the possibility that extrahepatic metabolism may play some role in the etiology of the side effects produced must not be overlooked.

SUMMARY

CPZ is metabolized *in vitro* by microsomal systems of various species by four major metabolic routes, i.e., N-oxidation, N-demethylation, ring hydroxylation, and S-oxidation. The object of the present work was to attempt to differentiate these various routes.

CPZ and its metabolites were quantified by a method based on solvent extraction, thin-layer chromatography, and liquid scintillation counting. Incorporation of potential inhibitors into the incubation media allowed differentiation of the various pathways of metabolism by rabbit-liver microsomal preparations. Thus, although reagents which primarily react with sulfhydryl groups of proteins usually inhibited both demethylation and ring hydroxylation, they were without effect on N-oxide formation. This inhibitory effect on routes which are thought to involve cytochrome P450 were also observed with SKF 525A, 1:10 phenanthroline, imidazole, and certain metal ions. Conversely, the N-oxidative pathway was inhibited by cysteamine, leaving the other pathways relatively unaffected.

Pretreatment of female rats with a variety of inducing agents produced an increase in demethylation and ring hydroxylation of CPZ, but were without effect on the N-oxidation.

Storage of guinea pig microsomal suspensions of 0°C, or treatment with deoxycholate prior to metabolic oxidation of CPZ, caused demethylation and ring hydroxylation to decay at a rate similar to that of cytochrome P450, whereas neither of these treatments affected the N-oxidative route.

Further evidence for the heterogeneity of the various enzymic processes involved have been obtained by a study of the *in vitro* extrahepatic metabolism of CPZ with tissue homogenates from various species.

All the tissues examined were able to carry out these oxidative routes, but at a much lower level than obtained with the corresponding hepatic system. In most species, CPZ sulfoxide was the major metabolite detected using extrahepatic tissues, but using guinea pig tissue, ring hydroxylation predominated.

REFERENCES

1. Anon., *Psychopharmacol. Bull.*, **6**, 44 (1970).
2. Usdin, E., *Critical Reviews in Clinical Laboratory Sciences*, 347 (1971).
3. Forrest, I. S., Bolt, A. G., and Aber, R. C., *Agressologie*, **9**, 259 (1968).
4. Brookes, L. G., and Forrest, I. S., *Pharmacologist*, **11**, 273 (1969).
5. Beckett, A. H., Essien, E., *J. Pharm. Pharmac.*, **25**, 188 (1973).
6. Beckett, A. H., van Dyk, J. M., Chissick, H. H., and Gorrod, J. W., *J. Pharm. Pharmac.*, **23**, 809 (1971).
7. Torrielli, M. V. and Slater, T. F., *Biochem. Pharmac.*, **20**, 2027 (1971).
8. Gorrod, J. W., Jenner, P., Keysell, G., and Beckett, A. H., *Chem-Biol. Interactions*, **3**, 269 (1971).
9. Beckett, A. H., Mitchard, M., and Shihab, A. A., *J. Pharm. Pharmac.*, **23**, 347 (1971).
10. Ziegler, D. M., Mitchell, C. H., and Jollow, D., in *Microsomes and Drug Oxidations*, Gillette, J. R., Conney, A. H., Cosmides, G. J., Estabrook, R. W., Fouts, J. R., and Mannering, G. J. (eds.), Academic Press, New York, 1969, p. 173.
11. Gorrod, J. W. *Chem-Biol. Interactions*, **7**, 289 (1973).

The Phenothiazines and Structurally Related Drugs, edited by I. S.
Forrest, C. J. Carr, and E. Usdin. Raven Press, New York © 1974.

Imipramine and Chlorpromazine in Hepatic Microsomal Systems

J. M. Perel, L. O'Brien, N. B. Black, G. D. Bellward,
and P. G. Dayton

*New York State Psychiatric Institute and Department of Psychiatry, Columbia University,
New York, New York 10032 and Clinical Pharmacology Program, Emory University
School of Medicine, Atlanta, Georgia 30322*

INTRODUCTION

Imipramine and chlorpromazine have been shown to be extensively metabolized to a variety of compounds, some of which are as pharmacologically active as their respective parent drugs (1–3). These metabolites represent diverse enzymatic reactions such as aromatic hydroxylation, N-demethylation, sulfoxidation and N-oxidation, the latter yielding both N-oxides and hydroxylamines (4, 5). With the possible exception of N-oxidation, the *in vitro* metabolism of imipramine and chlorpromazine involves a microsomal enzyme system requiring $NADPH_2$ and oxygen (6, 7). The formation of a large number of products has led to the suggestion that these psychotropic agents may be metabolized by independent pathways (8).

The plasma of patients chronically treated with either of these agents contains appreciable amounts of metabolites (9, 10) and, it is feasible that drug interactions are occurring between the metabolites and parent drugs leading to additional variability in response. Furthermore, it has been previously shown (11, 12) that methylphenidate, a microsomal enzyme inhibitor, causes a rise in imipramine plasma levels. Similar findings have been reported in clinical studies showing that neuroleptics inhibit the metabolism of tricyclic antidepressants (13). On the other hand, pretreatment with phenobarbital decreased steady-state plasma levels of tricyclic antidepressants (14) and increased the urinary excretion of chlorpromazine metabolites (15).

The present studies were undertaken, therefore, to reexamine the relationships of the various metabolic transformations in rat liver and, further, to determine the involvement of these possible pathways in imipramine and chlorpromazine metabolism. We have also attempted to obtain mechanistic information on the reactions of the parent compounds after pretreatment with the respective metabolites or drug-metabolism modifying agents. The possible role of the cytochrome P-450 system has also been investigated.

MATERIALS AND METHODS

In Vitro Studies with Imipramine

Imipramine labeled with ^{14}C in the 10 and 11 positions of the central ring of the molecule was obtained [N-(3-Dimethylaminopropyl) iminodibenzyl (methylene-C-14) hydrochloride] from Amersham/Searle (5.8 mCi/mmole). Purity was established by thin-layer chromatography by the vendor and ourselves. Male Wistar rats (200 to 250 g) were purchased from the Camm Research Institute (Wayne, N.J.) and fed *ad libitum* with Purina chow. The rats were stunned by a blow on the head and bled by decapitation. The livers were immediately removed and 25% (w/v) homogenates were prepared in cold (0 to 5°) pH 7.5 buffer consisting of 7.6 g triethanolamine, 15 ml of 2 N HCl and 2.0 g of disodium EDTA per liter (16). One ml of the 9,000 × *g* supernatant obtained from the homogenate was used in each incubation (equivalent to 250 mg of whole liver).

The microsomal protein concentrations in all the incubation systems were determined by the method of Sutherland et al. (17) as modified by Robson et al. (18) with bovine serum albumin as standard. The cofactor mixture was the same as previously described by Bickel and Baggiolini (6) with the omission of semicarbazide hydrochloride; the total final volume of each incubation, including cofactors, inhibitor, or H_2O, substrate, and 9,000 × *g* supernatant, was 5 ml. The reaction mixtures were incubated in air with shaking at 1 cps at 37°C in a metabolic water-bath shaker (New Brunswick Scientific Co.) for 10 min. These reactions were stopped by the addition of 1 ml of 10 N NaOH. At least five substrate concentrations ranging from 6.3 × 10^{-6} to 3.8 × 10^{-4} M were used. The inhibitor to be tested was present in concentrations ranging from 6 × 10^{-5} to 1 × 10^{-3} M.

The analytical techniques are based on the method previously described by Moody et al. (19). After the reactions were terminated, the entire incubation mixtures were extracted with 6 ml of an organic solvent consisting of 3% isoamyl alcohol (v/v) in *n*-heptane. All of the imipramine and the principal metabolite desmethylimipramine were coextracted. The organic layer was separated; a 0.5-ml aliquot was counted; 4 ml of the organic layer was transferred into clean and oven-dried tubes. Four to six drops of fresh acetic anhydride (Fisher) was added after mixing in a Vortex apparatus for 2 min, 5 ml of 0.1 N H_2SO_4 was added and the tubes again shaken. The sulfuric acid removes only the imipramine because the drug cannot be acetylated and is basic enough for removal by the acid. The desmethylimipramine was acetylated and remained in the organic layer. The procedure was shown to be quantitative by analyzing control mixtures of imipramine and desmethylimipramine, and 1.0 ml of the organic layer (desmethylimipramine alone) was counted after acid extraction. A suitable aliquot of the sulfuric acid layer (imipramine alone) was also counted after neutralization with equal volumes of 0.1 N NaOH. The incubation mixture remaining after organic solvent extraction was in turn extracted with 10 ml of dichloromethane at 4°C. This portion was shown to be mostly the polar metabolites (hydroxylated) of imipramine, desmethylimipramine, and the corresponding imipramine N-oxide. The outline of the overall procedure is described in Table 1.

TABLE 1. *Procedure for the analyses of imipramine metabolites*

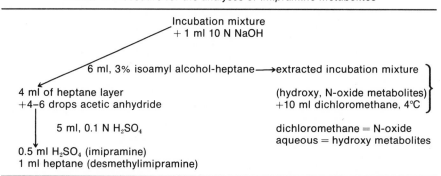

The specificity of this methodology has been demonstrated by thin-layer chromatography (TLC) techniques. The solvent system found to be most effective is chloroform:*n*-propanol:sat. ammonium hydroxide (100:100:2) on silica gel G of 0.25 mm thickness. The visualizing diazo reagent was made up of 0.5 g *p*-nitroaniline in 50 ml 1 N HCl + 0.5 g $NaNO_2$ in 50 ml water + 0.5 g sulfanilic acid in 50 ml water. The initial diazo spray was superimposed with another spray of concentrated HCl. In this system, the R_f values for imipramine, desmethylimipramine, 2-OH-imipramine, and 2-OH-desmethylimipramine are: 0.67, 0.40, 0.50, and 0.17, respectively. Bickel and Baggiolini (6) had previously established that other metabolites such as iminodibenzyl were formed in negligible amounts by this *in vitro* system. In the specificity experiments, incubations containing 600 and 100 μg of ^{14}C-imipramine were extracted in a similar manner as described above. Aliquots from the organic and sulfuric acid phases were evaporated under N_2 and studied by means of the TLC system described above. After visualization followed by drying at 45°C, the appropriate silica gel areas were scraped and added to vials containing scintillation cocktail.

The incubation mixture left after organic extraction was saturated with NaCl, pH adjusted to 5 with concentrated acetic acid and extracted with three portions of ethyl acetate (25 ml each); only 5 to 10% of the radioactivity was recovered in the pooled extracts. The pH was then adjusted to 12 and three more extractions with a mixture of tetrahydrofuran:isoamyl alcohol (1:1, 10 ml each time) were done. After pooling the extracts, washing with 5 ml of 0.1 N NaOH and evaporating to dryness under vacuum at 70°C, the residues were redissolved with methanol and chromatographed in the same TLC system. Measurements of ^{14}C were made with a scintillation solution prepared as follows: to 1 l of toluene, 7 g of PPO, 0.36 g POPOP, and 200 ml Bio-Solv BBS-3 (Beckman) were added. In all experiments 18 ml of solution was used.

In Vitro Studies with Chlorpromazine

A 25% (w/v) rat-liver homogenate was prepared with cold (0 to 5°) pH 7.4, 0.2 M Sorensen buffer. Two ml of the $9,000 \times g$ supernatant was used in each incubation mixture (equivalent to 500 mg of tissue). The cofactor mixture was the same as previously described for diphenylhydantoin by Kutt and Verebely (20), the final volume also being 5 ml. The incubation mixtures were reacted in air with shaking for 15 min, at which point 0.5 ml of 2.5 N NaOH was added to terminate the reactions. A minimum of five substrate concentrations ranging from 1×10^{-6} to 2×10^{-4} M were used. The inhibitor to be studied was present in concentrations ranging from 6×10^{-5} to 1×10^{-3} M.

For these studies, chlorpromazine-ring-^{14}C · HCl with a specific activity of 30.5 mCi/mmole was obtained from Applied Science Laboratories, Inc. Purity was established by TLC.

The analytical procedure utilized the entire incubation mixture. The pH was adjusted to between 9 and 10 by adding 50% acetic acid to each sample. Serial extractions, using 15 ml of dichloromethane each time, removed essentially all the radioactivity from the incubation mixture. The organic extracts were pooled and dried over anhydrous Na_2SO_4. Fifty-μl aliquots of the pooled extracts were spotted onto silica gel H (Merck) plates for quantitative analysis by TLC. The solvent systems routinely applied are based on those of Forrest and associates (21) except that, for solvent system B, we used methanol-diethylamine-benzene (7:9:84). Although all the chlorpromazine metabolites are completely separated by these procedures, for the purpose of this study we report them as sulfoxide, phenolic, and demethylated compounds. The reference standards were obtained through the courtesy of Dr. A. A. Manian (Psychopharmacology Research Branch, NIMH). Individual spots were measured by scraping off the plates and placing into vials containing the same scintillation mixtures as described for imipramine.

Studies with Microsomal Enzyme Inhibitors and Stimulators

The effects of threo-methylphenidate (Ritalin®) and ethylphenidate on the metabolism of chlorpromazine and imipramine were studied in the microsomal in vitro preparations. These compounds were obtained through the courtesy of Ciba-Geigy. In addition, SKF 525A was also compared in the same systems. In these studies, several concentrations (1×10^{-6} to 1×10^{-3} M) of the compound were added to the incubation mixtures containing either chlorpromazine or imipramine. The enzyme kinetics were first examined by means of Lineweaver-Burk plots and the constants K_m, V_{max} were determined by the use of Hofstee-type graphs. The values of K_i were graphically obtained from Dixon-type plots.

The effect of drug pretreatment was also studied with rats. Methylphenidate was administered i.p. to several sets of animals, each set receiving a different dosage; 10, 15, 20, 25, 30, and 50 mg/kg. Rats were sacrificed at 30 and 60 min after injection, livers removed and kinetics were obtained with the microsomal preparations in a similar manner as previously described both for imipramine and chlorpromazine.

Pretreatment effects were also investigated in rats with phenobarbital, which was administered i.p. 80 mg/kg for 5 days. The animals were sacrificed at least 48 hr after the last injection, livers removed, and hepatic microsomal kinetic studies done using imipramine as the substrate. The addition of several concentrations of methylphenidate to the microsomal preparations obtained from the phenobarbital-pretreated rats was also kinetically examined.

Doses, routes, and periods of administration of other compounds were: SKF 525A in 0.9% saline — 40 mg/kg, intraperitoneally, 24 hr before rats were sacrificed; cobalt chloride in distilled water — 60 mg/kg, subcutaneously, 48 and 24 hr before sacrifice; 3-methylcholanthrene in corn oil — 20 mg/kg, subcutaneously, on a daily basis for 10 days; Nor_2CPZ and CPZ-SO in ethanolic solution — 30 mg/kg, intraperitoneally, daily for 3 days, the last injection 6 hr before sacrifice.

Spectral Studies

The spectral changes produced by addition of various substances to the microsomal suspensions were recorded with an Aminco-Chance dual-wavelength/split-beam recording spectrophotometer (courtesy of Dr. James R. Gillette). Each cuvette contained microsomes (3 mg protein/ml), 50 mM phosphate buffer (pH 7.4), and 15 mM KCl in 3 ml. The substance under study was dissolved in water (0.1 to 2 mM) and added to the sample cuvette. An equivalent amount of water was added to the reference cuvette. The type I and II microsomal differences were obtained by scanning over a wavelength range from 350 to 500 nm. The ΔA for the type I response was calculated from the difference in absorbance between the peak at 390 nm and the trough at 425 nm, and the ΔA for the type II response between the trough at 395 nm and the peak at 435 nm. The following ligands or substances were used: imidazole (1 mM), SKF-525A (0.1 mM), hexobarbital (1 mM), methylphenidate (1 and 2 mM), and Nor_2CPZ (0.5 mM).

Cytochrome P-450 was determined according to the method of Sladek and Mannering (22). NADPH cytochrome C reductase was measured by the technique of Masters et al. (23).

RESULTS

In Vitro Enzyme Systems

The kinetic studies with both psychotropic agents indicate that the formation of metabolites is linear for at least 15 min. The velocity of the imipramine reaction was a linear function of protein content up to 15 mg, whereas chlorpromazine showed linearity to 45 mg.

Although desmethylimipramine was the major metabolite formed from imipramine, there was considerable aromatic hydroxylation, mostly in the form of 2-hydroxyimipramine with a small amount of 2-hydroxydesmethyl-imipramine. In addition, a fairly small but significant amount of imipramine-N-oxide was measured in this microsomal system. These data confirm the previous reports (1, 6) that the rat metabolized imipramine in an analogous manner to the human liver systems (24). The analytical procedure was consistently quantitative; we were able to account for at least 96% of the starting ^{14}C-imipramine in terms of metabolites and apparently unchanged substrate concentrations, so that the kinetic values reported herein are those obtained after suitable correction for the apparent substrate inhibition.

The monodemethylation of imipramine is inhibited by fairly large concentrations of methylphenidate (Table 2), the K_i values being about 1.3×10^{-3} M. Ethylphenidate, an analogue with lesser central nervous system activity, showed equipotent metabolic inhibitory action.

TABLE 2. *The inhibition of the monodemethylation of imipramine by rat liver $9,000 \times g$ supernatant*[a]

Inhibitor	V_{max} μmole/g-min	K_i (M $\times 10^{-3}$)
[b] —	0.148 ± 0.01	—
Methylphenidate[c]	0.151 ± 0.02	1.3 ± 0.2
Ethylphenidate[c]	0.156 ± 0.02	1.1 ± 0.1

[a] Data expressed as mean ± S.E. are the results of five experiments. Concentrations of imipramine used (M): 6.32 $\times 10^{-6}$; 1.26×10^{-5}; 3.16×10^{-5}; 6.3×10^{-5}; 1.26×10^{-4}; 1.89×10^{-4} and 3.78×10^{-4}.

[b] K_m for control system: $6.7 \times 10^{-5} \pm 0.4$.

[c] Inhibitor concentrations (M): 6×10^{-5}; 6×10^{-4}; 1×10^{-3}.

In contrast, the aromatic hydroxylation is inhibited to a substantially greater extent (Table 3); the K_i values were 7×10^{-4} M. As in the mono-demethylation, ethyl- and methylphenidates gave similar kinetic constants.

TABLE 3. *The inhibition of hydroxylation of imipramine by rat liver 9000 × g supernatant[a]*

Inhibitor	Vmax μmol/g-min ($\times 10^{-3}$)	K_i ($M \times 10^{-4}$)
[b] —	13.8 ± 1.2	—
Methylphenidate[c]	14.6 ± 1.1	7.1 ± 0.2
Ethylphenidate[c]	14.8 ± 1.2	5.1 ± 0.1

[a] Data expressed as mean ± S.E. are the results of four experiments. Concentrations of imipramine used (M): 6.3×10^{-6}; 1.26×10^{-5}; 3.16×10^{-5}; 6.3×10^{-5}; 1.89×10^{-4} and 3.78×10^{-4}.

[b] K_m for control system: 5.6×10^{-5} M ± 0.5.

[c] Inhibitor concentrations (M): 6×10^{-5}; 6×10^{-4}; 1×10^{-3}.

The relatively low K_m values for monodemethylation and hydroxylation, 6.7 and 5.6×10^{-5} M, respectively, suggest a relatively strong affinity between imipramine and the microsomal enzyme systems. Nevertheless, the observed inhibition by the phenidates was competitive. Similar results were observed with SKF 525A and imipramine when they were simultaneously introduced into the medium to minimize the extent of N-dealkylation of the inhibitor (25, 26). The observed retardation of hydroxylation was competitive with a K_i of 8×10^{-5} M, whereas demethylation was affected to a much lesser extent, about 7×10^{-4} M.

Chlorpromazine ($K_m = 3 \times 10^{-5}$ M for overall metabolism) also showed a relatively strong affinity for its respective microsomal system. Methylphenidate inhibited the hydroxylation reaction in a competitive manner with a K_i of 8×10^{-5} M, which is the same as for imipramine. In contrast, SKF 525A was a strong noncompetitive inhibitor of hydroxylation, $K_i = 2 \times 10^{-6}$ M. Both compounds had a slight effect on demethylation. The inhibitory constant appears to rule out the possibility that SKF 525A acts as an alternative substrate in this system because its metabolism has a $K_m = 3.6 \times 10^{-5}$ M (27). As with imipramine, the analytical procedure is essentially quantitative; at least 90% of the starting ^{14}C-chlorpromazine is accounted for by metabolites and unreacted substrate.

Pretreatment Studies

There appears to be selectivity both in the stimulation and inhibition of imipramine and chlorpromazine metabolism. Pretreatment with phenobarbital led to increases in hydroxylation and demethylation of imipramine, whereas N-oxidation diminished (Table 4). These studies were done with relatively low concentrations of substrate in order to prevent substrate inhibition effects. In contrast, SKF 525A caused a sharp decrease in hydroxy metabolite production, no change in demethylation, and a sharp increase in

TABLE 4. *Effect of drug pretreatment on metabolism of ^{14}C-imipramine by liver microsomal enzymes*

Drug pretreatment	Concentration of metabolite			
	Percent of control			
	Hydroxy	DMI	N-Oxide	P-450
Phenobarbital	180	130	70	140
SKF-525-A	20	102	140	95
3-Methylcholanthrene	110	90	92	—
Cobalt chloride	77	109	93	70
Phenobarbital + methylphenidate	140	110	90	110
Phenobarbital + cobalt chloride	120	130	80	80

N-oxide formation. Thus, pretreatment of imipramine metabolism with these two agents, shows that their effects on hydroxylation are opposite to those observed with N-oxidation.

The concentration of cytochrome P-450 followed the course of demethylation and appeared to have no obvious relationship with hydroxylation or N-oxidation. However, cobalt chloride pretreatment, which decreases P-450 synthesis, caused only a decrease in hydroxylation and no significant change in the other two reactions. Thus, the rise of P-450 levels with phenobarbital pretreatment may only be coincidental with the increase of demethylation. This is further confirmed when phenobarbital and cobalt chloride were jointly administered. A partial cancellation of the hydroxylation increase was seen, but no changes were observed in the other reactions.

Additional proof for the lack of correspondence between P-450 changes and imipramine metabolism was obtained from the SKF 525A effects, which markedly reduced hydroxylation with no significant decrease of the cytochrome levels. Pretreatment by subcutaneous administration of 3-methylcholanthrene (28) did not cause any significant changes in the amounts of metabolites. The *in vitro* addition of methylphenidate to phenobarbital-pretreated microsomal fractions caused a partial return to control values of all the metabolic products. Pretreatment with methylphenidate caused a partial cancellation of the higher P-450 levels obtained from phenobarbital-induced rats.

Methylphenidate and SKF 525A pretreatment of chlorpromazine metabolism led to an overall increase in product formation. As with imipramine, there was a marked decrease in phenolic metabolites. Simultaneously, a large increase in sulfoxide synthesis and a moderate rise in demethylation were also noted. It is quite possible that some of the chlorpromazine, which is inhibited from forming hydroxylated metabolites, is diverted to the other pathways (Table 5).

The administration of CPZ-SO also produced an overall stimulation of substrate metabolism, particularly, a very large increase in demethylated

TABLE 5. *Effect of pretreatment on the in vitro metabolism of chlorpromazine*

Drug pretreatment	Percent metabolism		
	Sulfoxides	Phenolic	Demethylated
Control	9	8	10
Methylphenidate[a]	22	3	12
SKF-525-A[b]	25	1	14
CPZ-SO	15	4	24
Nor$_2$CPZ	10	8	5

K_m based on CPZ overall metabolism $= 3 \times 10^{-5}$ M.
[a] Competitive inhibition, $K_i = 8 \times 10^{-5}$ M.
[b] Noncompetitive inhibition, $K_i = 2 \times 10^{-6}$ M.

and sulfoxylated metabolites. Again, the aromatic hydroxylation showed a marked decrease. In contrast, pretreatment of Nor$_2$CPZ[1] caused a moderate decrease in overall metabolism; most of the change occurred in the demethylation.

Spectral Results

Methylphenidate exhibited a type-I spectral change when added to suspensions of rat liver microsomes. On the other hand, Nor$_2$CPZ gave rise to type-II spectral changes. The reference ligands showed the same spectral changes previously reported in the literature. NADPH cytochrome C reductase was not significantly changed in the livers of animals pretreated with methylphenidate.

DISCUSSION

The results demonstrate the independence of the metabolic pathways of imipramine caused by demethylation, aromatic hydroxylation, and N-oxidation. Both the *in vitro* and *in vivo* studies provide evidence for the concept that the responsible enzymes are separate entities, since they were affected differently by drugs. These investigations have been made possible by the development of sensitive and accurate assays which measure the rates of appearance of several types of metabolic transformations in the self-same incubation mixtures.

Aromatic hydroxylation, the slowest metabolic pathway, showed the most response to stimulation and inhibition of metabolism. There appears to be an inverse relationship between aromatic hydroxylation and N-oxidation.

---

[1] Preliminary studies with lung microsomal systems indicate that Nor$_2$CPZ causes a marked inhibition of the demethylation reaction and is, in turn, remethylated to Nor$_1$-chlorpromazine and chlorpromazine to a considerable extent.

Thus, a simple increase in substrate concentration due to inhibition of hydroxylation led to a simultaneous rise in N-oxidation and, to a slight extent, demethylation. The opposite trends were observed upon stimulation of hydroxy metabolites. It is also quite clear that, although the changes in cytochrome P-450 levels parallel the metabolic effects of stimulation and inhibition, no causal relationships were found between the cytochrome levels and the pathways of metabolism.

Contrary to previous reports (29), the demethylation pathway was found to be insensitive to SKF 525A pretreatment. This apparent discrepancy is probably due to significant substrate inhibition. Thus, prior investigations have utilized 2 μmoles of imipramine in the incubation systems, whereas we have corrected with initial kinetic studies or by using much smaller amounts of substrate (50 nmoles). As a result of substrate inhibition, very different data will be obtained depending on the concentration of imipramine. Higher concentrations of imipramine will decrease the apparent effects of inducing agents, and increase the apparent effects of inhibitors on imipramine metabolism.

The effects on chlorpromazine metabolism also illustrate the independence of pathways. Although there is a net stimulation of overall metabolism by SKF 525A and methylphenidate pretreatment, the production of phenolic metabolites is sharply inhibited, so that additional substrate becomes available for the other metabolic routes.

The effect of Nor_2CPZ on the metabolism of chlorpromazine is significant because it relates to some clinical situations. The inhibition of demethylation is quite pronounced without any effect on the other routes. In analogy to the work of Bahr and Orrenius (30) with didesmethylimipramine, it is quite possible that, at the concentrations employed, by interacting with the heme prosthetic group, Nor_2CPZ saturates the type-II binding site without affecting the type-I site that is evidently involved in the other reactions. Similarly, the noncompetitive inhibition by SKF 525A may be due to the metabolism of the inhibitor to its primary amine, which also gives a type-II spectral response (25). Thus the chronic variability in response in patients is to be expected and, indeed, is observed. At present, we are examining other possible interactions between chlorpromazine and its metabolites in liver and lung microsomal systems.

SUMMARY

The metabolism of imipramine in rat-liver microsomal preparations was evaluated with a new specific and quantitative assay system that measures the simultaneous rate of appearance of the products in the self-same incubation mixtures. The demethylation, N-oxidation, and aromatic hydroxylation reactions are independent pathways and the responsible enzymes may be separate entities, since they were affected differently by drug metabolism enzyme stimulators and inhibitors. Aromatic hydroxylation was the pathway most influenced by pretreatment and the amount of the observed changes was inversely related to N-oxidation. Methylphenidate and phenobarbital inhibited and stimulated, respectively, the formation of hydroxy- and demethylated products, whereas SKF 525A was found mostly to inhibit the hydroxylation. These inhibitors acted in a competitive manner. The induction and decrease of cytochrome P-450 levels do not appear to be responsible for the changes in rate of the various metabolic pathways.

The kinetics of chlorpromazine metabolism was also investigated by an assay system that simultaneously measures the various metabolites. Although methylphenidate competitively and SKF 525A noncompetitively are inhibitors of the hydroxylation pathway, the overall rate of metabolism increases. Pretreatment with Nor_2CPZ, a type-II binding metabolite, inhibits the demethylation of chlorpromazine.

ACKNOWLEDGMENTS

This work was supported by Public Health Service grants MH-17044 (from the National Institute of Mental Health) and GM-14270 (from the National Institute of General Medical Sciences).

We thank Dr. Albert A. Manian of the Psychopharmacology Research Branch, National Institute of Mental Health, for the various chlorpromazine metabolites.

REFERENCES

1. Dingell, J. V., Sulser, F., and Gillette, J. R., J. Pharmacol. Exp. Ther., 143, 14 (1964).
2. Christiansen, J., Gram, L. F., Kofod, B., and Rafaelsen, O. J., Psychopharmacologia (Berlin), 11, 255 (1967).
3. Forrest, I. S., Bolt, A. G., and Aber, R. C., Agressologie, 9 (2), 259 (1968).
4. Bickel, M. H., Weder, H. J., and Aebi, H., Biochem. Biophys. Res. Commun., 33, 1012 (1968).
5. Beckett, A. H., and Al-Sarraj, S., J. Pharma. Pharmac., 25, 336 (1973).
6. Bickel, M. H., and Baggiolini, M., Biochem. Pharmacol., 15, 1155 (1966).
7. Forrest, I. S., Brookes, L. G., and Barth, R., Proc. Western Pharmacol. Soc., 13, 1 (1970).
8. Nakazawa, K., Biochem. Pharmacol., 19, 1363 (1970).
9. Crammer, J. R., Woods, H., and Rolfe, B., Psychopharmacologia (Berlin), 12, 263 (1968).
10. Wechsler, M. B., Wharton, R. N., Tanaka, E., and Malitz, S., J. Psychiat. Res., 5, 327 (1967).
11. Perel, J. M., Black, N., Wharton, R. N., and Malitz, S., Fed. Proc., 28, 418 (1969).
12. Cooper, T. B., and Simpson, G. M., Am. J. Psychiatry, 130, 721 (1973).
13. Gram, L. F., and Oveeø, K. F., Brit. J. Psychiat., 1, 463 (1972).
14. Sjoqvist, F., Hammer, W., Idestrom, C. M., Lind, M., Tuck, D., and Asberg, M., in Proc. Europ. Soc. Study Drug Toxicity, de C. Baker, S. B., Boissier, J. R., and Koll, W. (Eds.), 9, 246, Excerpta Medica, Amsterdam, 1968.
15. Forrest, F. M., Forrest, I. S., and Serra, M. T., Biol. Psychiat., 2, 53 (1970).
16. Beisenherz, G., Boltze, H. J., Bucher, T., Czok, R., Garbade, K. H., Meyer-Arendt, E., and Pfeideler, G., Z. Naturforsch, 80, 555 (1953).

17. Sutherland, E. W., Cori, C. F., Haynes, R., and Olsen, N. S., *J. Biol. Chem.,* **180,** 825 (1949).
18. Robson, R. M., Goll, D. E., and Temple, M. L., *Anal. Biochem.,* **24,** 339 (1968).
19. Moody, J. P., Tait, A. C., and Todrick, A., *Brit. J. Psychiat.,* **113,** 183 (1967).
20. Kutt, H., and Verebely, K., *Biochem. Pharmacol.,* **19,** 675 (1970).
21. Forrest, I. S., Bolt, A. G., and Serra, M. T., *Biochem. Pharmacol.,* **17,** 2061 (1968).
22. Sladek, N. E., and Mannering, G. J., *Biochem. Biophys. Res. Commun.,* **24,** 668 (1966).
23. Masters, B. S. S., Williams, C. H., and Kamin, H., *Methods in Enzymology,* **10,** 565 (1967).
24. Wharton, R. N., Perel, J. M., Dayton, P. G., and Malitz, S., *Am. J. Psychiat.,* **127,** 1619 (1971).
25. Schenkman, J. B., Wilson, B. J., and Cinti, D. L., *Biochem. Pharmacol.,* **21,** 2373 (1972).
26. Anders, M. W., Alvares, A. P., and Mannering, G. J., *Mol. Pharmacol.,* **2,** 328 (1966).
27. Anders, M. W., and Mannering, G. J., *Mol. Pharmacol.,* **2,** 319 (1966).
28. Dayton, P. G., Vrindten, P., and Perel, J. M., *Biochem. Pharmacol.,* **13,** 145 (1964).
29. Bickel, M. H., and Weder, H. J., *Life Sci.,* **7,** 1223 (1968).
30. Bahr, C. V., and Orrenius, S., *Xenobiotica,* **1,** 69 (1971).

The Phenothiazines and Structurally Related Drugs, edited by I. S. Forrest, C. J. Carr, and E. Usdin. Raven Press, New York © 1974.

Pharmacokinetics of ^{14}C-Dimethothiazine: Part I—Distribution and Excretion Following Oral Administration in the Dog and Rat

Owen R. W. Lewellen and Richard Templeton

Drug Metabolism Division, Pharmacological Research Laboratories, May and Baker Ltd., Dagenham, Essex, RM10 7XS, England

INTRODUCTION

Dimethothiazine [10-(2-dimethylaminopropyl)-2-dimethylsulfamoylphenothiazine] mesylate (Fig. 1) has been used for several years in antihistamine therapy. In addition, it abolishes decerebrate rigidity in the cat, has weak sedative properties (1,2), and reduces fusimotor activity in human volunteers (3). Dimethothiazine has proved to be of some value in the relief of spasticity in man (4, 5) and the compound is currently undergoing therapeutic trials. Only limited information, however, is available on the pharmacokinetics of dimethothiazine. Populaire et al. (6) presented data on the levels in plasma and excreta of the dog and rabbit, and Crawley et al. (3) measured the plasma levels in human volunteers, both following oral administration. The preliminary data of a detailed pharmacokinetic study of dimethothiazine in animals and man are presented here.

MATERIALS AND METHODS

Materials

Solvents and chemicals were "Pronalys" grade (May and Baker Ltd.) or equivalent, or reagent grade. Neomycin sulfate, glucose-6-phosphate, and NADP were obtained from Sigma Chemical Co. Solvents used for extraction were purified to remove peroxides and stored under oxygen-free nitrogen. Beagle dogs (5 to 10 kg) and Charles River strain rats (170 to 220 g) were used.

[Propyl-2-^{14}C] dimethothiazine mesylate (Fig. 1) (specific activity 5.2 mCi/mmole) was kindly provided by our colleagues in Service des Recherches Nucléaires of the Société des Usines Chimiques Rhône-Poulenc.

213

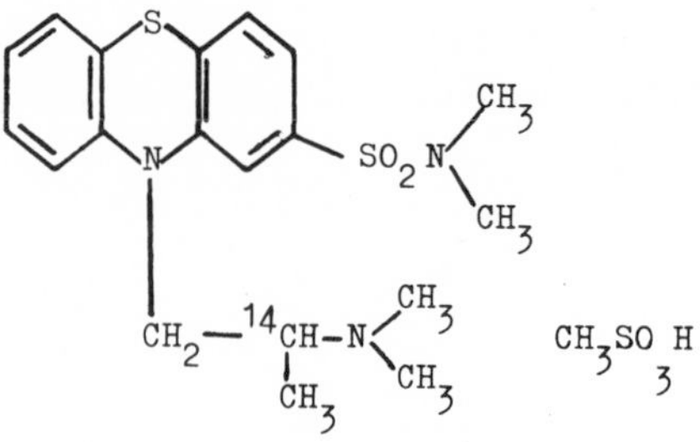

FIG. 1. [Propyl-2-¹⁴C] dimethothiazine mesylate.

The radiochemical purity of this material was determined by two-dimensional thin-layer chromatography to be $98.0 \pm 0.5\%$, the main impurities being dimethothiazine sulfoxide [10-(2-dimethylaminopropyl)-2-dimethylsulfamoylphenothiazine-5-oxide] and desmethyldimethothiazine [10-(2-methylaminopropyl)-2-dimethylsulfamoylphenothiazine], which together amounted to $1.4 \pm 0.4\%$. For oral administration in capsules to dogs, the material was formulated as: ¹⁴C-dimethothiazine mesylate -6.67% (w/w), lactose B.P. -44.4% (w/w), starch maize B.P. -42.8% (w/w), French chalk powder -5.9% (w/w), and "Aerosil" -0.29% (w/w). Similarly unlabeled material was formulated as: dimethothiazine mesylate -20.8% (w/w), lactose B.P. -36.35% (w/w), starch maize B.P. -37.6% (w/w), French chalk powder -5.0% (w/w), and "Aerosil" -0.25% (w/w). An aqueous solution (5 mg/ml) of dimethothiazine mesylate was administered to rats.

Methods

All work was carried out in a laboratory screened to exclude light of wavelength up to 470 nm, and, where possible, media containing dimethothiazine or metabolites were handled and stored under an atmosphere of oxygen-free nitrogen.

Animal Experiments

(a) *In vivo studies in rats.* Rats were starved overnight but allowed access to water before oral administration (5 mg/kg) of ¹⁴C-dimethothiazine mesylate. For the duration of the experiment, the animals were housed in a glass metabolism cage (Jencon's Metabowl) with radiocarbon-dioxide collecting facility consisting of two scrubbing towers each containing 5 N ethanolamine (200 ml). The latter was changed after 6, 24, and then each 24 hr. A flow rate of air (300 to 500 ml/min) was maintained through the system. At the end of the experiment, the rats were anesthetized (ether), exsanguinated, and dissected. Urine and feces were collected separately. In the experiments involving neomycin pretreatment, all rats were housed in glass metabolism cages throughout and starved overnight before administration of ^{14}C-dimethothiazine mesylate. Neomycin sulfate was administered orally on three mornings consecutively (100 mg in 1 ml water) and on the third afternoon and fourth morning (50 mg in 0.5 ml water). A control group of rats was given an identical regime of water administrations; 3 hr after the last administration, both groups were given labeled drug (5 mg/kg p.o.). At the end of the experiment, the rats were treated as described above. In all experiments rats were allowed food and water *ad libitum* 3 hr after administration of dimethothiazine. Three rats were used in each experiment; the excreta and tissues were pooled and analyzed immediately or stored at $-20°$ until required.

(b) *In vivo studies in dogs.* Dogs were starved overnight, but allowed access to water, before oral administration (5 mg/kg or 1 mg/kg) of ^{14}C-dimethothiazine mesylate. Each animal was housed in a metal metabolism cage with a radiocarbon-dioxide collecting facility, consisting of two scrubbing towers each containing 5 N ethanolamine (21) which was changed after 6 and 24 hr. A flow rate of air (12 l/min) was maintained through the system. Blood samples were taken from a foreleg vein. Dogs were allowed food and water *ad libitum* 3 hr after administration of dimethothiazine; at the end of the experiment, they were killed by injection of pentobarbital sodium and treated as described for rats.

(c) *In vitro studies with rat liver.* Five male Charles River rats were stunned, exsanguinated, and the liver placed in ice cold 1.15% potassium chloride (3 volumes) and homogenized with ice cooling in a Potter-Elvehjem homogenizer (20 passes) in small batches. The homogenate was centrifuged at 10,000 g for 15 min at 0°C and the supernatant used directly. The incubation medium contained nicotinamide (2 mmoles), magnesium chloride (3 mmoles), glucose-6-phosphate (100 μmoles), NADP (30 μmoles), 0.2 M phosphate buffer, pH 7.4 (20 ml), liver supernatant (40 ml), and unlabeled (27 μmoles) plus ^{14}C-labeled (3 μmoles) dimethothiazine mesylate in a final volume of 100 ml. A similar incubation medium, in which the liver supernatant was boiled for 10 min and cooled before addition, was also prepared. Both media were incubated with shaking at 37°C for 1.5 hr, while a slow flow of air was maintained through the flasks and passed directly to radiocarbon dioxide-collecting towers as used in the *in vivo* rat experiments. At the end of the incubation period, both media were treated as described by Coccia and Westerfeld (7) except that, whereas the volume of the incubation media used in this study was four times greater, the volumes of extracting solvents were increased only twofold. All distillations of solvents following extraction were carried out at 35 to 40°C. The final residue on evaporation of methanol contained 75% of the starting radioactivity in both cases. These residues were dissolved in methanol and subjected to two-dimensional thin-layer chromatography on silica gel G (Merck) in solvent systems—I, (a) cyclohexane–acetone–diethylamine (55:35:10, v/v/v)

(6), (b) methylethylketone–triethylamine (97:3, v/v) and II, (a) as (a) above, and (b) benzene–dioxane–diethylamine–water (70:17.5:7.5:1, v/v/v/v) (8). Spots were visualized under light of 254 nm, scraped off, and the radioactivity determined by liquid scintillation counting.

Determination of Radioactivity

Tissues and feces were homogenized with up to 1 volume of water and an aliquot (100 to 300 mg) of homogenate taken. Small organs, aliquots of bone marrow and spinal cord (both 10 to 30 mg), and blood and plasma (0.1 or 0.2 ml) were treated directly. These samples were either combusted (Packard Tricarb Sample Oxidizer) or digested with 72% (w/w) perchloric acid (0.2 ml) plus 30% (w/v) hydrogen peroxide (0.4 ml) (9) at 70° until dissolved, then cooled and scintillation mixture (15 ml) added. The scintillation mixture metered by the combuster consisted, per vial, of ethanolamine (5 ml), methanol (9 ml), and a scintillator solution (5 ml) comprising 2,5-diphenyloxazole (PPO, 15 g) plus 1,4-*bis*-2-(5-phenyloxazolyl)–benzene (POPOP, 0.5 g) in toluene (11). The scintillation mixture used for the digested samples consisted of PPO (4 g), naphthalene (72 g), toluene (400 ml) and 2-methoxyethanol (500 ml). Ethanolamine solutions containing radiocarbon dioxide and thin-layer chromatography plate scrapings were added directly to this scintillation mixture for counting. Skin (one part by weight) was digested by heating under reflux till dissolved in 2 M potassium hydroxide in 95% ethanol (three parts by volume). When the solution was cool, the pH was adjusted to 7 with 72% (w/w) perchloric acid and the mixture filtered. The supernatant (1 ml) and urine samples (up to 1 ml) were added to Insta-gel (Packard Instrument Co.) (10 ml) for counting. At least two samples from each biological medium were determined. Vials were counted twice in a Packard liquid scintillation spectrometer (model 3003 or 3380) with quench correction by external standard ratio or internal standardization (^{14}C-hexadecane).

Spectrofluorimetric Determinations (3)

(a) *Glassware and reagents.* All glassware was immersed in concentrated nitric acid for 18 hr, then washed thoroughly with water and finally double-distilled water; *n*-heptane was stored over concentrated sulfuric acid for 20 hr with occasional shaking and replacement of the acid after 18 hr. The acid was removed and the organic phase washed with distilled water. Redistilled isoamyl alcohol (2% v/v) was added and the combined organic solvent washed with 2 M sodium hydroxide, distilled water, 0.1 M sulfuric acid and, finally, double-distilled water. 5 M Sodium hydroxide and 0.1 M acetate buffer, pH 8.2, were separately shaken with *n*-heptane–isoamyl alcohol for 10 min, and the organic phase separated and discarded. The pH of the buffer was readjusted to 8.2 with washed sodium hydroxide. Aqueous solutions were prepared in double-distilled water.

(b) *Method.* To the plasma sample (up to 1 ml) were added water (equal volume) and 5 M sodium hydroxide (1 ml), and the mixture shaken thoroughly and left for 5 min before extraction with *n*-heptane–isoamyl alcohol (2 × 5 ml). Centrifugation was used to give complete separation of the phases. The combined organic phase was shaken with 0.1 M acetate buffer, pH 8.2, (5 ml) for 2 min and then with 0.1 M sulfuric acid (1 ml) for 5 min. The acid extract was immediately removed and added to 0.02% potassium permanganate (0.1 ml). After 5 to 10 min, 0.02% hydrogen peroxide (0.1 ml) was added and the fluorescence emission intensity (excitation 350 nm, emission 420 nm) recorded within 10 min (Baird Atomic Model SF 100E Fluorispec spectrofluorimeter). The permanganate-peroxide section of the procedure was adapted from that of Pacha (10).

RESULTS

Plasma Levels

Throughout this chapter, levels of radioactivity are expressed as μgrams of dimethothiazine base per gram of tissue or milliliter of medium to facilitate comparison between experiments. Following oral administration (5 mg/kg) of ^{14}C-dimethothiazine mesylate to two beagle dogs, maximum plasma levels of 1.03 and 1.34 μg/ml were obtained at 2.7 and 3.5 hr, respectively, after administration (Fig. 2), decreasing in one dog to 0.16 μg/ml at 24 hr. At a lower dose (1 mg/kg, p.o.) in another dog, the plasma-decay curve had a similar shape, but the concentration was proportionately higher in relation to the 5 mg/kg dose, with a peak level of 0.36 μg/ml at 2 hr decreasing to 0.06 μg/ml at 25 hr and 0.03 μg/ml at 49 hr. The level in whole blood was generally 70 to 90% of that in plasma. Following oral administration (5 mg/kg), plasma levels in the rat (Table 1) were generally about 30% of those in the dog at the same dose. However in both species plasma levels showed a similar early (8 to 24 hr) decline with a corresponding half-life of 8 to 9 hr.

In a separate study in three beagle dogs at a higher oral dose (8.3 mg/kg), plasma levels of dimethothiazine plus desmethyldimethothiazine were measured by a spectrofluorimetric method (3). This method measures, in addition to dimethothiazine, 70 and 50% of the amounts of desmethyldimethothiazine and desdimethyldimethothiazine respectively present in plasma, extracted sulfoxides having been selectively removed by an acetate buffer wash. Initial examination by thin-layer chromatography has detected little desdimethyldimethothiazine in plasma, and the method may be regarded as measuring mainly dimethothiazine plus part of the desmethyldimethothiazine present. Although the extent of absorption of dimethothia-

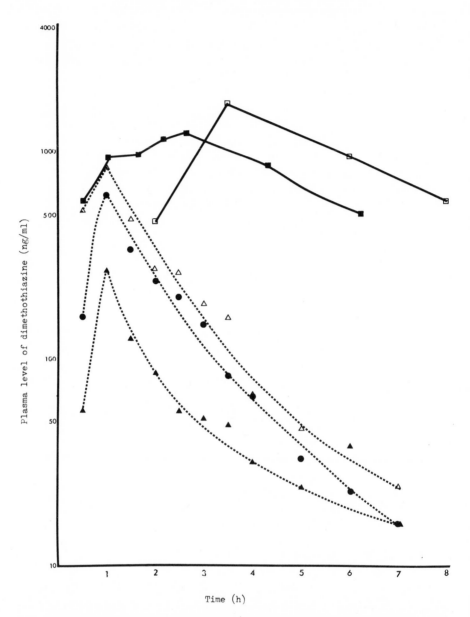

FIG. 2. Plasma levels of radioactivity, expressed as ng of dimethothiazine base per ml, in two dogs (━━━■━━━ and ━━━□━━━) following oral administration (5 mg/kg) of ^{14}C-dimethothiazine mesylate, and of dimethothiazine plus desmethyldimethothiazine determined spectrofluorimetrically in three dogs (▪ ▪ ▪ △ ▪ ▪ ▪ ▪, ▪ ▪ ▪ ● ▪ ▪ ▪, and ▪ ▪ ▪ ▲ ▪ ▪ ▪ ▪ ▪) following oral administration (8.3 mg/kg) of dimethothiazine mesylate.

TABLE 1. Distribution of radioactivity in male Charles River rats[a] following oral administration (5 mg/kg) of ^{14}C-dimethothiazine (DMT) mesylate

Duration of study	1 hr		2 hr		4 hr		24 hr		48 hr		96 hr	
Radioactivity level / Tissue	[14]C as μg DMT base per g of tissue	μg per g tissue/μg per ml plasma	[14]C as μg DMT base per g of tissue	μg per g tissue/μg per ml plasma	[14]C as μg DMT base per g of tissue	μg per g tissue/μg per ml plasma	[14]C as μg DMT base per g of tissue	μg per g tissue/μg per ml plasma	[14]C as μg DMT base per g of tissue	μg per g tissue/μg per ml plasma	[14]C as μg DMT base per g of tissue	μg per g tissue/μg per ml plasma
Whole blood[b]	0.189	1.27	0.122	1.15	0.482	1.35	0.0531	0.844	0.0251	1.08	0.0381	1.10
Plasma[b]	0.149	1.00	0.106	1.00	0.356	1.00	0.0630	1.00	0.0233	1.00	0.0346	1.00
Brain	0.0964	0.648	0.0574	0.541	0.223	0.626	0.0782	1.24	0.0630	2.71	0.0683	1.97
Eye	0.107	0.717	0.0455	0.428	0.317	0.889	0.0595	0.945	0.0410	1.76	0.0354	1.02
Heart	0.314	2.11	0.185	1.74	0.936	2.63	0.0660	1.05	0.0470	2.02	0.0336	0.971
Lung	1.50	10.1	0.930	8.75	5.29	14.8	0.209	3.33	0.116	4.97	0.0580	1.68
Liver	5.00	33.6	3.11	29.3	5.83	16.4	0.681	10.8	0.447	19.2	0.269	7.77
Spleen	0.498	3.35	0.777	7.32	1.94	5.44	0.173	2.75	0.117	5.02	0.0622	1.80
Stomach plus contents	207	1390	317	2980	10.3	28.9	0.302	4.79	0.0461	1.98	0.0510	1.47
Small intestine plus contents	17.8	120	12.8	121	79.8	224	0.841	13.3	0.172	7.41	0.0781	2.26
Large intestine plus contents	0.206	1.38	1.40	13.1	20.5	57.6	4.36	69.3	0.215	9.22	0.122	3.52
Adrenal	0.550	3.70	0.347	3.27	2.31	6.48	0.407	6.46	0.445	19.1	0.210	6.07
Kidney	0.660	4.44	0.528	4.97	4.36	12.2	0.196	3.11	0.172	7.41	0.123	3.56
Testes	0.106	0.711	0.498	4.68	0.460	1.28	0.111	1.76	0.104	4.46	0.0883	2.55
Fat	0.248	1.67	0.358	3.37	1.23	3.45	0.0957	1.52	0.238	10.2	0.0692	2.00
Carcass	0.331	2.22	0.163	1.53	0.701	1.97	0.100	1.59	0.0802	3.44	0.0420	1.21
Bone marrow	n.d.	—	n.d.	—	n.d.	—	0.143	2.26	0.0753	3.23	0.103	2.98
Skin plus fur	0.169	1.13	0.125	1.18	0.463	1.30	0.161	2.55	0.108	4.62	0.0807	2.33

[a] Figures obtained from the pooled media from three rats at each time interval.
[b] Expressed as value per ml of medium in each case.
n.d. – not determined.

zine and the maximum plasma levels obtained varied markedly in the 3 dogs (Fig. 2), the average maximum plasma level of 0.57 μg/ml occurred at 1 hr after administration and declined rapidly to a mean value of 0.019 μg/ml at 7 hr. The latter may be compared to a radioactivity level of 0.73 μg/ml at the same time.

Distribution Data

In the rat, tissue levels of radioactivity (Table 1) were maximal at 4 hr after oral administration (5 mg/kg) and were generally higher than plasma levels, indicating a tendency to concentrate from plasma. However, in most tissues this uptake was readily reversible, the tissue concentration decreasing as the plasma level decreased. From the more limited information available for the dog (Table 2) the same situation appears to hold, although at 48 hr, a greater number of tissues, notably brain and spinal cord, showed a radioactivity level significantly less than that of plasma. In common with the dog, the brain level of radioactivity in the rat was one of the lowest

TABLE 2. *Distribution of radioactivity in beagle dogs following oral administration (5 mg/kg) of* [14]C-*dimethothiazine (DMT) mesylate*

Duration of study sex of dog	6 hr Male beagle		48 hr Female beagle	
Tissue — Radioactivity level	[14]C as μg DMT base per g of tissue	μg per g tissue/μg per ml plasma	[14]C as μg DMT base per g of tissue	μg per g tissue/μg per ml plasma
Whole blood[a]	0.498	1.00	0.125	0.74
Plasma[a]	0.498	1.00	0.171	1.00
Brain	0.561	1.13	0.043	0.254
Spinal cord	0.613	1.23	n.d.	n.d.
Eye	1.21	2.43	0.943	5.52
Heart	1.16	2.33	0.161	0.940
Lung	4.83	9.71	0.608	3.56
Liver	4.94	9.93	1.09	6.35
Spleen	1.38	2.78	0.225	1.32
Stomach plus contents	3.34	6.71	0.175	1.02
Small intestine plus contents	5.49	11.0	0.353	2.07
Large intestine plus contents	48.8	98.0	0.968	5.66
Adrenal	n.d.	n.d.	0.678	3.97
Kidney	1.97	3.95	0.338	1.98
Ovary/Testes	0.987	1.98	n.d.	n.d.
Fat	0.983	1.97	0.155	0.906
Gastrocnemius muscle	0.825	1.66	0.105	0.614
Carcass	0.773	1.55	0.127	0.740
Bone marrow	0.873	1.75	n.d.	n.d.
Skin	0.734	1.47	0.123	0.166

[a] Expressed as value per ml of medium in each case.
n.d. — not determined.

TABLE 3. *Distribution and excretion of radioactivity in male Charles River rats[a] following oral administration (5 mg/kg) of* ^{14}C*-dimethothiazine mesylate*

Medium	Distribution and excretion of radioactivity as a % of the administered dose					
	1 hr	2 hr	4 hr	24 hr	48 hr	96 hr
Liver	4.54	2.60	3.64	0.778	0.471	0.211
Kidney	0.133	0.116	0.837	0.043	0.037	0.022
Stomach plus contents	70.6	73.7	1.50	0.088	0.019	0.013
Small intestine plus contents	18.8	11.6	54.6	0.972	0.211	0.064
Large intestine plus contents	0.185	1.08	7.76	3.84	0.178	0.081
Remaining tissues, carcass, skin, etc.	5.50	3.47	14.5	2.14	1.69	1.02
Total body content	99.8	92.6	82.8	7.86	2.61	1.41
Radiocarbon dioxide	2.18	2.94	11.7	19.4	18.3	18.2
Urine	0.73	0.55	3.85	14.2	12.3	14.2
Cage wash	0.05	0.34	0.81	5.56	1.19	0.28
Feces	0.02	0.01	none	56.2	62.8	62.4
Total excreted	2.98	3.84	16.4	95.4	94.6	95.1
Total recovered	103	96.4	99.2	103	97.2	96.5

[a] Figures obtained from the pooled media from 3 rats at each time interval.

tissue levels, particularly up to 24 hr. Several tissues in this species had a long (48 to 96 hr) half-life of around 50 hr. Generally at 96 hr, tissue levels, excluding those of excretory organs, were low, the maximum being in the adrenal (0.21 $\mu g/g$), which had a tissue/plasma concentration ratio of 6.1.

Excretion Data

Throughout this study, radioactivity following oral administration (5 mg/kg) was concentrated mainly in the gastrointestinal tract plus excreta of both rat (average 92%) and dog (average 82%). After 24 hr, less than 5% of the administered radioactivity remained in the body of either species (Tables 3 and 4) and was concentrated mainly in the carcass, skin, and excretory organs. Fecal excretion predominated in the rat (Table 3) with the level of radioactivity expired as carbon dioxide exceeding that excreted in the urine. A species differences in excretion between rat and dog was evident in that in the latter (Table 4), urinary excretion marginally exceeded fecal excretion, with a considerably lower level of radiocarbon-dioxide expiration. In a separate study of total excretion following oral administration (5 mg/kg) to a male dog, 46% of the dose was excreted in the urine and 21% in the feces in 24 hr, 57% and 30% respectively in 4 days, and 58% and 36% respectively in 8 days. Thus in this dog, the predominance of the urinary

Table 4. *Distribution and excretion of radioactivity in beagle dogs following oral administration (5 mg/kg) of ^{14}C-dimethothiazine mesylate*

Medium	Distribution and excretion of radioactivity as a % of the administered dose	
	6 hr Male beagle	48 hr Female beagle
Liver	4.92	0.951
Kidney	0.366	0.045
Stomach plus contents	5.29	0.063
Small intestine plus contents	8.12	0.419
Large intestine plus contents	28.5	0.510
Remaining tissues, carcass, skin, etc.	16.0	2.58
Total body content	63.2	4.57
Radiocarbon dioxide	n.d.	7.47
Urine	28.7	42.4
Cage wash	2.35	1.07
Feces	0	39.5
Total excreted	31.1	90.4
Total recovered	94.3	95.0

n.d. — not determined

pathway was evident. The minor differences in excretion pattern shown by these two dogs were probably more individual than sex-related. In the rat, the excretion pattern shown by the two sexes was similar. Thus for the female rat at 96 hr after administration (5 mg/kg), urinary excretion was 11.1%, fecal excretion 74.2%, and cage wash 0.21% with expired radiocarbon dioxide amounting to 13.1% and total body content to 1.4% of the administered dose.

Neomycin Pretreatment of Rats

It was observed that during the period of neomycin pretreatment the average weight of both groups of rats decreased from 175 to 160 g, indicating a reduction in the food intake. The level of radiocarbon dioxide expired in 24 hr by the neomycin-treated group was 7.6%; the level expired by the control group was 8.7% of the administered dose.

Studies with Rat Liver In Vitro

For the extracts of both active and deactivated liver incubations, the radioactivity of the dimethothiazine spot was expressed as a proportion of the total radioactivity determined in the silica gel removed from the thin-layer chromatographic plate. From this was obtained the extent of biochemical plus chemical degradation of dimethothiazine occurring in the active liver incubation (82.4% mean of 2 determinations) and of the chemical degradation only occurring in the deactivated liver incubation (25.3%, mean of 2 determinations), thus giving the level (57.1%) of metabolism. The amount of radiocarbon dioxide produced by both incubation media was less than 0.08% of the radioactivity present.

DISCUSSION

Over the 48 hr following oral administration of ^{14}C-dimethothiazine mesylate, plasma levels of radioactivity in the rat (expressed as μg of compound per ml of plasma) were very similar to those observed for ^{35}S-promazine (11), allowing for the difference in dose. In the dog, plasma radioactivity levels were approximately three times those found in the rat after administration of ^{14}C-dimethothiazine mesylate. Also in the dog, the plasma levels of dimethothiazine plus desmethyldimethothiazine determined spectrofluorimetrically in this study were comparable to those determined spectrophotometrically in an earlier study (6), when adjustment was made for the dose. A marked difference was observed however between the plasma levels of dimethothiazine plus desmethyldimethothiazine and radioactivity in the dog. The latter increased from approximately twice the spectrofluorimetrically determined level initially to nearly 40 times at 7 hr

(Fig. 2), thus giving a measure of the level of dimethothiazine metabolites present in plasma over this period. In addition, the plasma radioactivity level was maximal at 2.7 to 3.5 hr, when the spectrofluorimetrically determined level was in steady decline. It is possible that following oral administration this plasma-level difference was due to either absorption — initially of dimethothiazine and subsequently of metabolites formed — in the gastrointestinal tract, or reabsorption of metabolites excreted in the bile, although contributions from both were possible. Support for the latter explanation was obtained from preliminary studies involving intravenous administration (1 mg/kg), where variation in absorption associated with the oral route was eliminated. A similar relationship of plasma levels to that following oral administration was observed (Fig. 3), with the radioactivity level again showing a broad maximum, in this case at 1.25 hr after administration. Also, in the rat, 18% of the intravenous dose was excreted in the bile in the first 2 hr, and of this, less than 1% was present as the parent compound *(unpublished data)*. Thus it is probable that following oral administration, the dimethothiazine absorbed is rapidly metabolized and the metabolites formed are extensively excreted via the bile and then partly reabsorbed. Such enterohepatic circulation was observed with chlorpromazine in the dog (12).

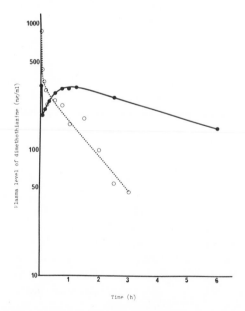

FIG. 3. Plasma levels of radioactivity (━━━━●━━━━), expressed as ng of dimethothiazine base per ml, in a dog following intravenous administration (1 mg/kg) of ¹⁴C-dimethothiazine mesylate, and of dimethothiazine plus desmethyldimethothiazine determed spectrofluorimetrically (■ ■ ■ ✪ ■ ■ ■) in the same dog following dimethothiazine mesylate by the same route and at the same dose, 12 weeks later.

Marked individual variation in the plasma levels of dimethothiazine plus desmethyldimethothiazine was observed in the dog and in preliminary studies in man. This phenomenon has been observed with phenothiazines generally in man (e.g., 13), and makes correlation with pharmacological activity difficult. Thus Crawley et al. (3) found no clear relationship between the plasma levels of dimethothiazine plus desmethyldimethothiazine and the reduction of tonic vibration reflex in man. In the cat and rabbit, we have attempted to correlate the reduction in decerebrate rigidity (2) with plasma levels following both oral and intravenous administration of dimethothiazine mesylate. However, no relationship could be established between these parameters.

The route of excretion of foreign anionic compounds has been shown to be related to the molecular weight of the compound (14) and with phenothiazine derivatives an increase in the size of the N-10 side chain led to an increase in biliary excretion (12) in the dog. Thus, following oral administration of ^{14}C-dimethothiazine (mol. wt. 391) the fecal excretion of radioactivity (62 to 74%) in the rat was greater than that observed (46%) for ^{35}S-chlorpromazine (mol. wt. 319) (15). However, in the dog the fecal excretion of radioactivity (27 to 40%) following ^{14}C-dimethothiazine administration was considerably less than that observed (75 to 89%) following ^{14}C-fluphenazine administration (mol. wt. 437) (16), indicating a low clearance of dimethothiazine and metabolites by this route in the dog and a significant species difference in fecal excretion from the rat.

The expiration of radiocarbon dioxide in both species following oral ^{14}C-dimethothiazine mesylate indicated appreciable metabolism, particularly in the rat, of the N-10 side chain of dimethothiazine, probably resulting in or from its removal from the heterocyclic ring. Degradation of the phenothiazine side chain has been reported in a limited number of instances as a minor route of metabolism, but in few has removal been implied. Thus in one instance (17), promazine and chlorpromazine were metabolized by removal of the side chain in man (0.4%) and dogs (0.8%). There are two probable sites for this route of metabolism of dimethothiazine, namely in the liver or gut microflora and possibly a third, in the gut wall (18).

The first of these routes was examined *in vitro* in the rat using a liver preparation. Although enzymic degradation of dimethothiazine was considerable (57%), no radiocarbon dioxide was liberated, indicating that hepatic enzymes were probably not involved directly in side-chain degradation. Following the treatment of rats with neomycin to suppress gut bacteria, the level of radiocarbon-dioxide production (7.6%) was less than previously found (19.4%). However, the level of radiocarbon-dioxide production by the control group was also low (8.7%). This may be explained by assuming the involvement of gut bacteria in dimethothiazine metabolism, in that during neomycin treatment and before drug administration, the rats were housed in metabolism cages in which their food intake was reduced, resulting in a reduction in gut bacteria. This would lead to a reduction in dimethothiazine side-chain metabolism as observed, apparently to a level at which neomycin treatment had little further effect. It is possible, therefore, that this level (about 8%) of side-chain degradation is carried out by enzyme systems other than those of gut bacteria or liver.

Following oral administration, it is likely that dimethothiazine itself is the substrate for side-chain degradation in the gastrointestinal tract. However, extensive enterohepatic circulation has been shown to occur and preliminary work has indicated that up to 40% of an intravenous dose is expired as radio-carbon dioxide in the rat in 24 hr. Thus, dimethothiazine metabolites can also function as the substrate for the enzyme systems involved.

Following oral administration, it is likely that dimethothiazine itself is the substrate for side-chain degradation in the gastrointestinal tract. However, extensive enterohepatic circulation has been shown to occur and preliminary work has indicated that up to 40% of an intravenous dose is expired as radio-carbon dioxide in the rat in 24 hr. Thus, dimethothiazine metabolites can also function as the substrate for the enzyme systems involved.

SUMMARY

Data on the distribution and excretion of radioactivity following oral administration (5 mg/kg) of [propyl-2-^{14}C] dimethothiazine mesylate to the dog and rat are presented. Plasma levels of radioactivity in the dog were about 3 times those in the rat, but in both species showed a similar early (8 to 24 hr) decline with a half-life of 8 to 9 hr. The plasma level of radioactivity in the dog decreased over the first 7 hr much more slowly than that of dimethothiazine plus desmethyldimethothiazine determined spectrofluorimetrically, indicating the extent of dimethothiazine metabolites present in plasma during this period. Dimethothiazine metabolites underwent extensive enterohepatic circulation. There was little correlation of the plasma levels of dimethothiazine plus desmethyldimethothiazine with the reduction of decerebrate rigidity in the cat and rabbit. Levels of radioactivity in dog brain and spinal cord and rat brain were generally low compared to those in other tissues and plasma. A species difference in the excretion of radioactivity was evident, as in the dog urinary excretion (42 to 52%) marginally exceeded fecal excretion (27 to 40%) whereas in the rat fecal excretion (62 to 74%) predominated over urinary excretion (11 to 14%). Expiration of radiocarbon dioxide in both species indicated metabolism of the N-10 side chain of dimethothiazine. This route of metabolism probably occurs in the intestinal microflora and possibly elsewhere, although it is unlikely that liver is involved, and utilizes dimethothiazine metabolites and probably parent drug as substrates.

ACKNOWLEDGMENT

The authors wish to acknowledge the excellent technical assistance of Miss L. Hiscutt, Miss M. R. Kingdon, Mr. R. Girkin, Mr. K. R. Greenslade, and Mr. R. J. Thomas.

REFERENCES

1. Keary, E. M., and Maxwell, D. R., *Brit. J. Pharmacol. Chemother.,* **30,** 400 (1967).
2. Maxwell, D. R., and Read, M. A., *Neuropharmacology,* **11,** 849 (1972).
3. Crawley, F. E. H., Kennedy, P., and Swash, M., *Brit. J. Pharmacol.,* **47,** 613P (1973).
4. Matthews, W. B., Rushworth, G., and Wakefield, G. S., *Acta Neurol. Scand.,* **48,** 635 (1972).
5. Griffiths, M. I., and Bowie, E. M., *Develop. Med. Child Neurol.,* **15,** 25 (1973).
6. Populaire, P., Decouvelaere, B., Lebreton, G., Pascal, S., and Terlain, B., *Thérapie,* **22,** 1173 (1967).
7. Coccia, P. F., and Westerfeld, W. W., *J. Pharmacol. Exp. Therap.,* **157,** 446 (1967).
8. Beckett, A. H., and Hewick, D. S., *J. Pharm. Pharmacol.,* **19,** 134 (1967).
9. Mahin, D. T., and Lofberg, R. T., *Anal. Biochem.,* **16,** 500 (1966).
10. Pacha, W. L., *Experientia,* **25,** 103 (1969).
11. Walkenstein, S. S., and Seifter, J., *J. Pharmacol. Exp. Therap.,* **125,** 283 (1959).
12. Van Loon, E. J., Flanagen, T. L., Novick, W. J., and Maass, A. R., *J. Pharm. Sci.,* **53,** 1211 (1964).
13. March, J. E., Donato, D., Turano, P., and Turner, W. J., *J. Med. Clin. Exp.,* **3,** 146 (1972).
14. Abdel Aziz, F. T., Hirom, P. C., Millburn, P., Smith, R. L., and Williams, R. T. *Biochem. J.,* **125,** 25P (1971).
15. Emmerson, J. L., and Miya, T. S., *J. Pharmacol. Exp. Therap.,* **137,** 148 (1962).
16. Dreyfuss, J., Ross, J. J., and Schreiber, E. C., *J. Pharm. Sci.,* **60,** 821 (1971).
17. Fishman, V., and Goldenberg, H., *J. Pharmacol. Exp. Therap.,* **150,** 122 (1965).
18. Curry, S. H., D'Mello, A., and Mould, G. P., *Brit. J. Pharmacol.,* **42,** 403 (1971).

The Phenothiazines and Structurally Related Drugs, edited by I. S.
Forrest, C. J. Carr, and E. Usdin. Raven Press, New York © 1974.

Effect of Phenothiazine Drugs on the Stability of Rat Liver Subcellular Particles*

C. S. Popov

Department of Biochemistry, the Georgi Dimitrov Agricultural Academy, Boul. Lenin 73,
Sofia 13, Bulgaria

Phenothiazine drugs cause changes in the stability of biological membranes, which depend on the dose and on some other factors.

The experiments in this field have been performed mainly on the lysosomes using the phenothiazine derivatives promethazine and chlorpromazine (CPZ). These drugs are known to protect the liver against necrosis caused by some toxic agents and to decrease the leakage into plasma of lysosomal acid hydrolases normally associated with such injuries (1–4). Protective effect of CPZ against the labilization of rat liver lysosomes caused by *Escherichia coli* endotoxin and hypervitaminosis A has also been established (5). Phenothiazines prevent mitochondrial swelling and lysis (6–8) as well as the osmotic lysis of erythrocytes (9–11). However, in many investigations phenothiazine drugs have been found to induce damage to biological membranes: labilization of lysosomes (5, 12–22), mitochondria (22, 23, 27), and lysis of erythrocytes (10, 11, 24, 25).

Koenig and Jibril (12) were able to show, by *in vitro* experiments, the activation of the latent lysosomal acid phosphatase and β-glucuronidase in the presence of promazine or CPZ (5 mM). These drugs release more than 50% of the activated enzymes into the solution (nonsedimentable activity) during incubation of large granule fractions for 30 min at 20°C and at pH 7 (barbital buffer).

Our data (26), summarized in Table 1, showed that concentrations of CPZ which activate the latent acid phosphatase ranged from 2.5×10^{-5} to 1.2×10^{-3} M when suspensions of lysosome-rich fractions with protein concentrations of 1.7 to 16.0 mg/ml were used. Therefore, these results indicate the importance of drug concentrations in tissues for demonstrating the membrane-labilizing effect of phenothiazines. Thus it is necessary to specify the drug concentrations and the protein content of the tissues in reporting the results from experiments of this type.

Rat liver mitochondria, lysosomes, and peroxisomes possess different sensitivity to the direct damaging action of phenothiazine drugs. In our *in*

* Paper given by title.

TABLE 1. *Activation of latent acid phosphatase in rat liver large granule fractions by chlorpromazine*

Concentration of chlorpromazine (M)	Concentrations of large granule suspensions (mg protein/ml)					
	1.7	2.5	4.0	7.9	9.0	16.0
None (control)	100	100	100	100	100	100
2.5×10^{-5}	140	100	100	100	100	100
5×10^{-5}	240	124	100	100	100	100
7×10^{-5}	260	170	135	97	100	100
8.3×10^{-5}	280	230	160	100	100	95
10^{-4}	320	330	170	95	105	100
1.7×10^{-4}	–	450	240	91	100	100
3.3×10^{-4}	–	–	–	199	128	102
6.6×10^{-4}	–	–	–	280	250	100
10^{-3}	–	–	–	450	320	113
1.2×10^{-3}	–	–	–	–	390	198

Rat liver large granular fractions, suspended in 0.25 M sucrose solution at pH 7 were preincubated at 18 to 20° for 15 min in the presence of chlorpromazine. The "free" acid phosphatase activity, determined by the method of Gianetto and De Duve (45) is expressed as percent of control.

vitro experiments (27) carried out with rat liver using various concentrations of CPZ, the large granular fractions showed the highest fragility of lysosomes due to this drug. The assessment of stability of subcellular particles was made on the basis of the rate of release into the solution of marker enzymes. Liver peroxisomes are more resistant than other organelles mentioned above, with respect to the adverse effect of the drug used (Table 2). It is interesting that the low concentration of CPZ which caused the release of catalase from peroxisome particles also lowered the nonsedimentable activity of L-α-hydroxy acid oxidase. We assumed that phenothiazines in the concentrations used, would contribute to the binding of the free molecules of this latter enzyme to the granules, and tested this assumption in the experiments on blender-treated large granular fractions in which most of the peroxisomes were disrupted. The results, given in Table 3, indicate that due to the strong inhibition of L-α-hydroxy acid oxidase the proposed enzyme binding induced by CPZ really took place. A low sensitivity of peroxisomes to the harmful effect of CPZ was also seen in *in vivo* studies (22). Rats were treated with CPZ in doses of 20 mg/kg, and the stability of their liver subcellular particles was examined at different time intervals after the application of the drug. Data given in Fig. 1 revealed a decreased release of catalase into the supernatant of granules isolated from liver homogenates of CPZ-treated rats, in comparison with the controls, up to the 48th hr. Hence, peroxisomes of drug-treated rats are more stable than those derived from control animals during the entire experimental period. The results from another series of studies (Nikiforova and Popov, *unpublished data*) showed that CPZ in doses exceeding 40 mg/kg accelerates the redistribution of catalase from the sedimentable to the nonsedimentable

TABLE 2. *Release of acid phosphatase, malate dehydrogenase, catalase, and L-α-hydroxy acid oxidase from rat liver large granular fractions by various concentrations of chlorpromazine*

Concentrations of chlorpromazine (M)	Nonsedimentable enzyme activity (% of total)			
	Acid phosphatase	Malate dehydrogenase	Catalase	L-α-OH acid oxidase
None (control)	6	4	13	9
1×10^{-4}	4	3	11	5
3×10^{-4}	11	3	10	3
5×10^{-4}	22	5	14	2
7×10^{-4}	35	8	12	2
1×10^{-3}	54	19	15	2
2×10^{-3}	61	24	18	6
5×10^{-3}	—	40	50	15

Samples from large granular fractions, suspended in 0.25 M neutral solution of sucrose were preincubated at 18 to 20°. After 20 min, the samples were centrifuged for 20 min at 20,000 × g. The nonsedimentable enzyme activities are expressed in percent of the respective total (sedimentable + nonsedimentable) activities. Triton X-100 in concentration 0.3 % was added to suspensions before determination of sedimentable enzyme activities.

TABLE 3. *Effect of chlorpromazine on the activity and distribution of L-α-hydroxyacid oxidase in fractions, obtained after centrifugation of blender-treated rat liver large granular fractions*

Blender-treated for 1.5 min		Relative enzyme activity (%)
Centrifugation ⟶	supernatant	72
	sediment	28
+CPZ 5×10^{-4} M centrifug. →	supernatant	20
	sediment	48
Centrifugation →	supernat. + CPZ 5×10^{-4} M	38
	sediment + CPZ 5×10^{-4} M	30

15 min after the addition of chlorpromazine (at 18 to 20°C) the samples were separated into sediment and supernatant fractions by the centrifugation for 20 min at 20,000 × g. The enzyme activity of fractions is expressed as % of total activity (sedimentable + nonsedimentable) found in blender-treated and fractionated samples.

form in liver homogenates of rats receiving the drug; this redistribution indicates the extent of damage to peroxisomes.

It was noted that during incubation (as indicated in the legend to Fig. 1), and subsequent centrifugation of the samples, more than half of the peroxisome marker enzyme activity was detected in the supernatant, both in

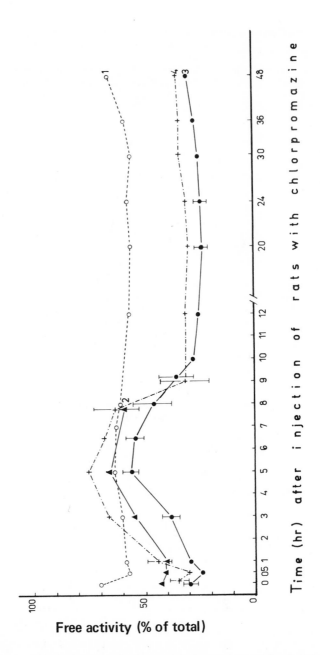

FIG. 1. Release of acid phosphatase, malate dehydrogenase, catalase, and protein from the large granular fractions, isolated from liver homogenates of control rats and rats, killed at different intervals of time after treatment with chlorpromazine.

Two samples of each granular fraction, sedimented between 600 and 20,000 g and washed once, were preincubated in a medium containing 0.25 M sucrose and 0.1 M acetate buffer (pH 5) at 37°. After 30 min, the samples were cooled in an ice water bath and to one of them Triton X-100 was added, to yield a final concentration of 0.2%. After vigorous shaking, the samples were centrifuged at 20,000 g for 20 min.

The nonsedimentable activity of the marker enzymes for the lysosomes, mitochondria, and peroxisomes (determined in supernatants obtained from samples not treated with Triton X-100) was expressed as percent of total enzyme activity, released in the presence of the detergent. The control values are indicated at zero points. 1-catalase; 2-protein; 3-acid phosphatase; 4-malate dehydrogenase.

control fractions and in those from CPZ-treated animals. On the basis of our recent investigations (27), which demonstrated an extremely high sensitivity of peroxisomes to physical factors, it is suggested that the enhanced level of soluble catalase in this case may, to a large extent, be due to disruption of these particles during the preparation of these suspensions. In the experiments mentioned above, the granular sediments were resuspended by means of a Potter-Elvehjem homogenizer consisting of a smooth-walled glass tube fitted with a Teflon pestle at 1,500 rpm.

The release of malate dehydrogenase and acid phosphatase from the large granular fractions isolated from liver homogenates of CPZ-treated rats showed complex dynamics. After the application of the drug a transitory decrease was followed by a gradual elevation, indicating labilization of lysosomes and mitochondria of the nonsedimentable activity of malate dehydrogenase and acid phosphatase. A considerable enhancement of malate dehydrogenase activity in supernatant fractions was detected during the first hour. Such an increase in soluble acid phosphatase activity was observed during the third hour, with a maximum at 5 to 6 hr as in the case of malate dehydrogenase. These changes in the nonsedimentable activity of lysosome and mitochondria marker enzymes indicate that shortly after the treatment of experimental rats with CPZ in doses of 20 mg/kg, their liver mitochondria and lysosomes become more stable than those of the nontreated animals. This stabilizing effect is followed by a gradually increasing labilization with a trend toward earlier damage to the mitochondria. Subsequently, the above-mentioned organelles regain higher stability than that of controls at about 10 hr after the application of CPZ. This condition persists for a long time. Liver mitochondria and lysosomes of treated rats return to their normal level of stability, in some cases within 30 hr and within 48 hr in other instances.

As can be seen from Fig. 1 and Table 2, the results obtained *in vitro* and *in vivo* were not entirely similar. *In vitro,* the mitochondria are less sensitive than the lysosomes to the labilizing effect of CPZ. In living cells, however, these particles undergo earlier changes indicating an increased fragility. It would, however, be premature to conclude that *in vivo* liver mitochondria are more susceptible to the damaging action of phenothiazines than lysosomes, only on the basis of an earlier increase in the nonsedimentable malate dehydrogenase activity, as well as in the rate of release of this enzyme. It is necessary to carry out further investigations with various doses of CPZ in order to elucidate this problem.

EFFECT OF VARIOUS DOSES OF SOME PHENOTHIAZINE DRUGS ON THE STABILITY OF RAT LIVER LYSOSOMES

The *in vivo* effect of the phenothiazine derivatives promazine, promethazine, propionylpromazine, and CPZ, on the stability of rat liver lysosomes was studied comparatively. Considerable differences were found in the doses of various drugs, capable of producing minimal lysosome-labilizing effects. The results given in Fig. 2 showed that CPZ and propionylpromazine in doses of more than 2 mg/kg, promazine in doses more than 17 mg/kg, and promethazine in doses of more than 27 mg/kg, induce accelerated release of acid phosphatase detectable by the methods used, indicating injury to lysosomes (17). However, the doses required for the individual drugs should not be considered inflexible. Under the conditions in which the experiments have been carried out, they show only the potency of various drugs as membrane labilizers, compared to one another. Bearing in mind that a number of factors may affect the potentiation or weakening (in some cases even complete elimination) of the lysosome-labilizing effect of the drugs studied, a considerable variability should be expected for the dose range given in the text to Fig. 2, above which the lysosomes are damaged.

Phenothiazine drugs exert different effects on the biological membranes. Low concentrations induce stabilization, and high ones labilization. The differences between the various representatives of this group found in the studies on their respective lysosome-labilizing effects are quantitative, which is probably due to structural differences. The determination of the concentrations required to produce stabilizing or labilizing effects, is frequently difficult due to the great number of factors determining the phenothiazine effects on the membranes (drug/tissue ratio, a number of antagonists, etc.). The fact that these drugs stabilize the biological membranes both *in vitro* (6–11, 28) and *in vivo* (3–5, 26) and protect them against the damaging effects of direct (vitamin A) and indirect (endotoxins) labilizers indicates that the stabilization effect is probably a direct one. In some cases, phenothiazines protect the biological membranes also indirectly, acting as free radical scavengers and antioxidants (3, 4, 7).

It seems that the mechanism of the membrane-labilizing effect of phenothiazine derivatives both *in vitro* and *in vivo* is different. These drugs induce *in vitro* a direct disruption of the membranes, when they are used in comparatively high concentrations. It is suggested that this is due to their surface-active properties (11, 29). In living cells, however, the damage to biological membranes caused by phenothiazines applied in moderate doses is probably a secondary effect. It is likely that this is due to primary disruption of bioenergetic reactions within the cell, which has been demonstrated in a number of investigations (26, 30–35). It seems that this inhibition of bioenergetic pathways is achieved at concentrations of phenothiazine drugs much lower than those that are able to produce direct injury of the cell organelle membranes; such concentrations in the living cells could be reached during treatment of experimental animals with extremely high doses.

It has been found that phenothiazines act as competitive inhibitors of flavoenzymes (31, 36–38). It is possible that interference with the flavoenzymes functioning in the respiratory chain is of great importance for

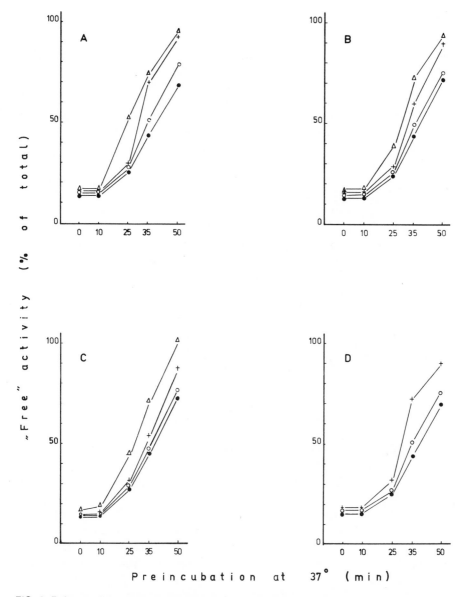

FIG. 2. Release of the acid phosphatase from large granular fractions, isolated from liver homogenates of control and treated rats.

Aliquots of fractions used for determining the enzyme activity were preincubated for 0, 10, 25, 35, and 50 min in a medium containing 0.25 M sucrose and 0.1 M acetate buffer (pH 5) at 37°. The substrate (Na-β-glycerophosphate) yielding a final concentration of 0.05 M was added at the end of the preincubation period and thereafter incubation was continued for 10 min. The "free" activity is expressed as percent of the total activity determined in the presence of Triton X-100 (0.1%) (45).

FIG. 2 (A) ●—● controls; ○—○ rats treated with chlorpromazine (CPZ) in doses of 2 mg/kg; +——+ rats treated with CPZ-5 mg/kg; △——△ rats treated with CPZ, 10 mg/kg; (B) ●—● controls; ○—○ rats treated with propyonylpromazine (PPZ), 2 mg/kg; +——+ rats treated with PPZ, 5 mg/kg; △——△ rats treated with PPZ, 10 mg/kg; (C) ●—● controls; ○——○ rats treated with promethazine (PMZ), 27 mg/kg; +——+ rats treated with PMZ, 30 mg/kg; △——△ rats treated with PMZ, 40 mg/kg; (D) ●—● controls; ○—○ rats treated with promazine (PZ), 17 mg/kg; +——+ rats treated with PZ, 20 mg/kg.

damage to the membrane by these pharmacologically active agents. It is our opinion that membrane damage observed *in vivo* from phenothiazine drugs, correlates with the function of the succinate-oxidizing pathway, which is less sensitive to their inhibitory action than the pathway for the NAD · H_2-oxidation (39). This problem has been discussed in detail elsewhere (26), and supporting data were reported (18, 40). The results in Fig. 1 confirm a concept whereby the function and structure of the mitochondria seem to be affected initially by the treatment of rats with CPZ, with subsequent effects on the structure of the other organelles. The following data also support the hypothesis of indirect labilization of cell organelle membranes *in vivo* by the phenothiazines: (1) Table 1 reveals that rather high concentrations of CPZ per tissue unit are necessary to produce direct damage to liver lysosomes. Considering the fact that after administration of CPZ at the rate of 100 mg/kg, the highest concentration obtained in the liver was 10^{-4} M (41), the damage of liver lysosomes caused by this drug in doses of less than 10 mg/kg is hardly produced by a direct concentration related effect. (2) The slight lysosome-labilizing effect of CPZ observed in animals kept at temperatures of 35 to 37°C after application of the drug also indicates an indirect action rather than a direct one (Fig. 5A). In this case the energy supply of the cells may suffice for the reduced requirement of heat.

FACTORS PRODUCING CHANGES IN THE EFFECT OF PHENOTHIAZINE DRUGS ON BIOLOGICAL MEMBRANES

The results given in this section were obtained mainly from *in vivo* experiments carried out in our laboratory on the lysosome-labilizing effect of CPZ. Conflicting data on the effects of phenothiazine drugs on liver lysosomes have been reported. As stated above, CPZ in doses exceeding 2 mg/kg in rats fed on bread and milk or on a diet of caseine and water acts as a labilizer of liver lysosomes. However, Gaudiano et al. (42) have noted no such effect using much higher doses of drug (20 mg/kg). The differences may be due to the large variety of factors determining phenothiazine effects on the biological membranes.

Diets and Some Dietary Factors

The data from studies by the present author (16, 20, 21) have shown that dietary factors may modify the effect of CPZ on the stability of biological membranes. Most of these factors diminish their damaging action. The results from the investigation on rats fed different diets and treated with CPZ are presented in Fig. 3A. This drug, applied at a rate of 10 mg/kg, caused significant labilization of liver lysosomes of animals fed on bread and milk, oats and milk, and caseine diets. Different results were obtained

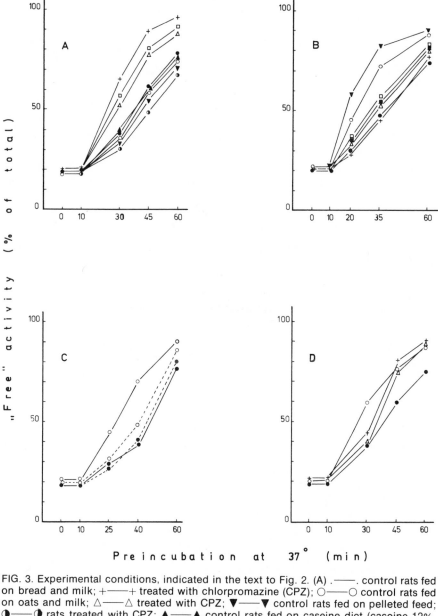

Preincubation at 37° (min)

FIG. 3. Experimental conditions, indicated in the text to Fig. 2. (A) .——. control rats fed on bread and milk; +——+ treated with chlorpromazine (CPZ); ○——○ control rats fed on oats and milk; △——△ treated with CPZ; ▼——▼ control rats fed on pelleted feed; ◗——◗ rats treated with CPZ; ▲——▲ control rats fed on caseine diet (caseine 12%, sucrose 60%, starch 12%, olive oil 6%, dried baker's yeast 4%, and minerals 5%) and milk; □——□ rats treated with CPZ. CPZ was applied in a dose of 10 mg/kg. (B) .——. controls; ○——○ rats treated with chlorpromazine (10 mg/kg CPZ); +——+ rats treated with CPZ + histidine (150 mg/kg and after two hr. 100 mg/kg); △——△ rats treated with CPZ + thiamine hydrochloride (2 × 40 mg/kg); □——□ rats treated with CPZ + arginine (150 and 100 mg/kg); ▼——▼ rats treated with CPZ + lysine hydrochloride (150 and 100 mg/kg); ■——■ CPZ + riboflavin (2 × 10 mg/kg). (C) —— rats fed on caseine diets with 6% dried baker's yeast; – – – rats fed on caseine diet with 20% dried yeast; . . . controls; ○○ treated with chlorpromazine (10 mg/kg). (D) .——. control rats fed on caseine diet (see the text for Fig. 3A); ○——○ rats treated with chlorpromazine (CPZ) in doses of 10 mg/kg; +——+ control rats fed on caseine diet without minerals + milk; △——△ rats treated with CPZ.

for the same CPZ dose in animals fed pellet feed, caseine diet without minerals + milk (21), or caseine diet with 20% dried baker's yeast (20). No labilization of liver lysosomes was seen and even a trend toward their stabilization was noticed (Fig. 3).

Many nutritional factors, as established in our previous studies, may also act as antagonists of phenothiazine drugs with respect to their membrane damaging effects (16, 21, 24). Some vitamins (riboflavin and thiamine) and amino acids (histidine, glutamic acid, and arginine) were found to protect the biological membranes against the harmful effect of CPZ, both *in vitro* and *in vivo*. Thiamine and riboflavin protect rat liver lysosomes from the damage caused by CPZ *in vivo* (Fig. 3). Such an effect was also observed for thiamine *in vitro* (Table 4). Riboflavin protects erythrocytes against CPZ-induced hemolysis *in vitro* (Fig. 4). The influence of some amino acids on the lysosome-labilizing effect of CPZ is shown in Fig. 3B and Table 4. Simultaneous treatment of rats with CPZ and histidine, glutamic acid, or arginine failed to activate the latent acid phosphatase which, in turn, indicates increased permeability of lysosomal membranes observed when the drug alone was administered. *In vitro* histidine and arginine also proved to be strong antagonists of CPZ (Table 4). As indicated in Fig. 3B, lysine applied in combination with CPZ, enhances the lysosome-labilizing action of the latter. A similar effect was obtained when cystine was used (Popov and Tzakov, unpublished data).

TABLE 4. *Activation of latent acid phosphatase activity in rat liver large-granule fractions by chlorpromazine and by chlorpromazine + histidine, arginine, or thiamine*

Compound	"Free" enzyme activity
None (control)	100
Chlorpromazine 6×10^{-4} M	1200
Chlorpromazine + histidine 10 mg/ml	450
Chlorpromazine + histidine 5 mg/ml	270
Chlorpromazine + histidine 2 mg/ml	180
Chlorpromazine + histidine 1 mg/ml	420
Chlorpromazine + arginine 10 mg/ml	600
Chlorpromazine + arginine 5 mg/ml	380
Chlorpromazine + arginine 2 mg/ml	540
Chlorpromazine + arginine 1 mg/ml	950
Chlorpromazine + thiamine 10 mg/ml	320
Chlorpromazine + thiamine 5 mg/ml	460

Chlorpromazine and the other compounds were premixed. Suspensions of isolated lysosomal-mitochomdrial fractions obtained from rat liver homogenates, were added to this mixture after several min. The "free" acid phosphatase activity was determined after preincubation at 37° for 20 min and pH 5 (0.1 M acetate buffer) by the method indicated in the text for Table 1.

The enzyme activity is expressed as percentage of control.

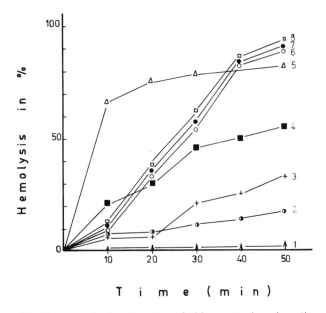

FIG. 4. Lysis of erythrocytes in the presence of chlorpromazine plus other substances. Samples of erythrocytes suspended in isotonic solution of NaCl with various components added to them were incubated at 18 to 20°. Two-ml samples from each suspension were removed after 10, 20, 30, 40 and 50 min and were centrifuged for 2 min at 1,000 g. The hemoglobin measured in the supernatants is expressed as percentage of the maximum amount of pigment released under conditions of complete hemolysis caused by the addition of the nonionic detergent Triton X-100 (0.02%). 1—controls, 3×10^{-4} M ATP and 5×10^{-4} M riboflavin; 2—7×10^{-4} M chlorpromazine (CPZ) $+ 3 \times 10^{-4}$ M ATP mixed before the addition of erythrocytes; 3—7×10^{-4} M CPZ $+ 5 \times 10^{-4}$ M riboflavin; 4—7×10^{-4} M CPZ $+ 3 \times 10^{-4}$ M ATP. CPZ has been added 2 min after mixing erythrocytes with ATP; 5—7×10^{-4} M CPZ $+ 3 \times 10^{-4}$ M ATP. ATP was added 2 min after mixing erythrocytes with CPZ; 6—7×10^{-4} M CPZ $+ 10^{-3}$ M sodium glutamate; 7—7×10^{-4} M CPZ. 8—7×10^{-4} M CPZ $+ 10^{-3}$ M disodium succinate.

Temperature

The effect of environmental temperatures on the lysosome-labilizing action of CPZ was studied previously (19). The data from these experiments are summarized in Fig. 5A. The results from the nontreated rats were included with the three experimental groups since the differences observed did not exceed intersubject variations. There were, however, large differences in the rate of release of the acid phosphatase from the large granular fractions isolated from CPZ-treated rats from the experimental groups: in fractions from animals kept at 14 to 16°C after treatment with the drug, the lysosome-marker enzyme was released very rapidly, whereas in rats kept at 35 to 37°C, the rate was similar to that of controls, and in rats kept at 19 to 20°C, the rate was intermediate. On the basis of the rate of release of acid phosphatase, which was used as criterion for lysosome membrane stability, it can be concluded that in animals treated with CPZ and kept at

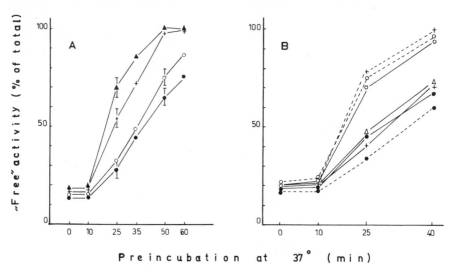

FIG. 5. Experimental conditions as indicated in the legend of Fig. 2. (A) .——. controls; ○——○ treated with CPZ (10 mg/kg) and kept at 35 to 37°; +——+ treated with CPZ and kept at 19 to 20°; ▲——▲ treated with CPZ and kept at 14 to 16°. (B) —— rats kept at temperature 18 to 20° before injection; – – – rats acclimed to cold before injection. . . . . controls; ○○○ treated with CPZ (10 mg/kg); +++ treated with CPZ + ATP (2 × 40 mg/kg); △——△ treated with CPZ + succinate.

temperatures of 35 to 37°C, the damage to liver lysosomes is very slight. When the environmental temperature was decreased, the labilization effect increased although the animals were treated with the same doses of drug.

Rats treated with CPZ and kept at 35 to 37°C do not show the hypothermia normally produced by the drug at lower temperatures. It seems that this fact has no bearing on the damaging action of CPZ on lysosomes, because promethazine at doses which cause hypothermia does not damage the lysosomes. When rats treated with CPZ are kept at 5 to 7°C, or 19 to 20°C, they show practically the same degree of hypothermia, but as can be seen from Fig. 5, liver lysosomes of rats kept at various temperatures after treatment with CPZ have different stability.

Recently we were able to show (43) that liver lysosomes of rats subjected to cold acclimation were resistant to the adverse effects of CPZ administered at a rate of 10 mg/kg (Table 5). It was established that lysosome membranes of rats acclimed three to four times (every day for 1 hr at −5 to −6°C) and treated with the drug used 0.5 hr after the last cooling were more stable than those of the respective controls (acclimed but untreated animals). Their stability was similar to that of the nonacclimed and untreated rats. The effect observed was detected about 16 hr after a single cooling period. It persisted up to 6 days. After 5 to 6 days of acclimation, the animals regained their ability to react as the controls with respect to the labilizing action of CPZ. Forty hr after the last cooling period of three times acclimed rats, the

TABLE 5. *Release of acid phosphatase from large granular fractions, isolated from liver homogenates of control rats, rats subjected to cold acclimation, and rats treated with chlorpromazine*

Number of acclimations	Experimental groups of animals		"Free" activity of the acid phosphatase, determined at different intervals of time after the beginning of preincubation at 37° and pH 5 (0.1 M acetate buffer)			
			0 min	10 min	25 min	40 min
I	Nonacclimed		19	18	44	56
	"	+ chlorpromazine	20	20	73	92
	Acclimed		18	19	38	72
	"	+ chlorpromazine	21	20	67	92
II*	Nonacclimed		18	19	40	59
	"	+ chlorpromazine	20	22	75	89
	Acclimed		21	18	58	75
	"	+ chlorpromazine	22	21	62	87
III	Nonacclimed		16	18	50	58
	"	+ chlorpromazine	18	17	80	98
	Acclimed		17	16	67	72
	"	+ chlorpromazine	16	16	63	67
IV	Nonacclimed		20	20	48	56
	"	+ chlorpromazine	20	21	67	84
	Acclimed		18	20	61	73
	"	+ chlorpromazine	19	18	48	68
VI	Nonacclimed		17	17	40	57
	"	+ chlorpromazine	18	21	68	80
	Acclimed		17	19	37	60
	"	+ chlorpromazine	19	18	38	72
IX	Nonacclimed		21	20	42	50
	"	+ chlorpromazine	19	20	72	93
	Acclimed		19	19	55	65
	"	+ chlorpromazine	20	20	88	95

* Rats were injected with chlorpromazine 16 hr after cooling. In these experiments rats were treated with chlorpromazine at a rate of 10 mg/kg, 0.5 hr after the last cold acclimation. The experimental procedure is the same as indicated in the text to Fig. 2.

membrane damaging effect of phenothiazines was as distinct as in the case of nonacclimed rats. At present, we are unable to explain these observations. Considering similar dynamics of changes in catecholamine levels during cold acclimation (44) and susceptibility of rats to lysosome-labilizing effect of CPZ, we assume that catecholamines may be involved in this case. Preliminary experiments, however, in which CPZ was applied in combination with adrenaline or noradrenaline, did not produce the expected results. The data obtained from these studies with thyroidectomized or adrenalectomized animals as well as with animals treated with thyroxine + CPZ, might be useful for the interpretation of the higher resistance of rats subjected to cold acclimation against the lysosome-labilizing effect of phenothiazine drugs.

Other Factors

ATP protects rat liver lysosomes from the labilizing action of CPZ *in vivo* (Fig. 5) (15) and erythrocytes against the hemolytic effect of this drug *in vitro* (Fig. 4) (24). Protection of lysosome membranes from the CPZ-induced fragility with ATP was found only when the experiments were carried out on rats kept at constant temperature (18 to 20°C) or kept for a long time (more than 8 to 10 days) in rooms with nonconstant temperature (10 to 17°C). In rats subjected three times to cold acclimation and treated 40 hr after the last cooling with CPZ + ATP, the protective effect of the latter was not observed (Fig. 5) (43). The lysosome-labilizing effect of phenothiazines was diminished by succinate *in vivo* (Fig. 5) (18). The protective action of succinate, however, depends to a large extent on various factors (20).

The data above indicate that the dose is not the most important factor in producing the lysosome-labilizing effects of phenothiazine drugs *in vivo*. On the other hand, these results may provide an explanation for the discrepancies between the data obtained by different researchers in their studies of the effect of phenothiazines on the stability of lysosomal membranes.

The protective effects of ATP, thiamine, riboflavin, histidine, and arginine from CPZ-induced injury of biological membranes might be due to complex formation between these agents and phenothiazines, which in turn might render them inactive as membrane labilizers and as enzyme inhibitors. Such complex formation between CPZ and ATP or riboflavin has been reported (29, 31).

SUMMARY

The effects of various phenothiazines on the stability of the membranes of subcellular particles prepared from rat liver were studied. A variety of factors accounting for the effects observed *in vivo* and *in vitro* were considered, among them pretreatment of the animals with phenothiazines, concentrations of phenothiazines, ambient temperatures and prior acclimation of animals, nutritional factors, and interactions with various endogenous substances such as hormones and amino acids.

REFERENCES

1. Rees, K. R., Sinha, K. P., and Spector, W. G., *J. Pathol. Bacteriol.*, **81**, 107 (1961).
2. Bangham, A. D., Rees, K. R., and Shotlander, V. L., *Nature*, **193**, 754 (1962).
3. Slater, T. F., (1966) *Proc. Europ. Soc. for the Study of Drug Toxicity*, Vol. VII, 1966, pp. 30–45.

4. Slater, T. F., in *Lysosomes in Biology and Pathology*, Vol. 1, Norh Holland, Amsterdam, 1969, pp. 469–492.
5. Guth, P. S., Amaro, G., Sellinger, O. Z., and Elmer, L., *Biochem. Pharmacol.*, **14**, 769 (1965).
6. Spirtes, M. A., and Guth, P. S., *Biochem. Pharmacol.*, **12**, 37 (1963).
7. Smith, E. E., Watanabe, C., Louie, J., Jones, W. J., Hoyt, H., and Hunter, E. F., *Biochem. Pharmacol.*, **13**, 643 (1964).
8. Spirtes, M. A., Morgan, E. S., and Cohen, M. S., *Biochem. Pharmacol.*, **14**, 295 (1965).
9. Freeman, A. R., and Spirtes, M. A., *Biochem. Pharmacol.*, **12**, 47 (1963).
10. Van Steveninck, J., Gösund, W. K., and Booij, H. L., *Biochem. Pharmacol.*, **16**, 837 (1967).
11. Seeman, P., and Kwant, O., *Biochim. Biophys. Acta*, 483, 512 (1969).
12. Koenig, H., and Jibril, A., *Biochim. Biophys. Acta*, **65**, 543 (1962).
13. Allison, A. C., and Young, M. R., *Life Sci.*, **3**, 1407 (1963).
14. Baccino, F. M., Rita, G. A., and Dianzani, M. U., *Enzymologia*, **29**, 169 (1965).
15. Popov, Ch. S., *Compt. Rend. Acad. Bulg. Sci.*, **19**, 1071 (1966).
16. Popov, Tsch. S., *Z. Naturforschung*, **22b**, 1157 (1967).
17. Popov, Ch. S., *Compt. Rend. Acad. Bulg. Sci.*, **22**, 1213 (1969).
18. Popov, Ch. S., *Biochem. Pharmacol.*, **18**, 1257 (1969).
19. Popov, Ch. S., *Biochem. Pharmacol.*, **18**, 1778 (1969).
20. Popov, Ch. S., *Experientia*, **27**, 47 (1971).
21. Popov, Ch. S., *Compt. Rend. Acad. Bulg. Sci.*, **25**, 829 (1972).
22. Popov, Ch. S., *Compt. Rend. Acad. Bulg. Sci.*, **25**, 1293 (1972).
23. Haksar, A., and Peron, F. G., *Biochim. Biophys. Acta*, **264**, 548 (1972).
24. Popov, Ch. S., Yordanov, Y. M., and Nikiforova, M., *Compt. Rend. Acad. Bulg. Sci.*, **23**, 221 (1970).
25. Santos-Martinez, J., Aviles, T. A., and Laboy-Torres, J. A., *Arch. Internat. pharmacodyn. et Ther.*, **169**, 83 (1972).
26. Popov, Ch. S., *Dissertation*, VVMI, Sofia, 1971.
27. Popov, Ch. S., Geneva, L. G., Nikiforova, M., and Tzacov, L. *Compt. Rend. Acad. Bulg. Sci.*, **26**, 841 (1973).
28. Weissmann, G., in *Lysosomes in Biology and Pathology*, vol. 1, North Holland, Amsterdam 1969, pp. 276–291.
29. Ira, B., *Arch. Biochem. Biophys.*, **109**, 321 (1965).
30. Dimitrov, O. A., and Kolotilova, A. I., *Biokhimia*, **32**, 156 (1967).
31. Racker, E., (1965) *Mechanisms in Bioenergetics*, Academic, New York, 1965, pp. 161–196.
32. Berger, M. H., Strecker, G., and Waelsch, H., *Nature*, **177**, 1234 (1956).
33. Gey, K. F., Rutishauser, R., and Pletscher, A., *Biochem. Pharmacol.*, **14**, 507 (1965).
34. Løvtrup, S., *J. Neurochem.*, **12**, 743 (1965).
35. Wand, H., *Naturwissenschaften*, **51**, 220 (1964).
36. Gabay, S., and Harris, S. K., *Biochem. Pharmacol.*, **14**, 17 (1965).
37. Gabay, S., and Harris, S. K., *Biochem. Pharmacol.*, **15**, 317 (1966).
38. Gabay, S., and Harris, S. K., *Agressologie*, **9**, 78 (1968).
39. Racker, E., *Mechanisms of Bioenergetics*, Academic, New York, 1965, pp. 122–131.
40. Popov, Ch. S., and Radoutcheva, T., *Compt. Rend. Acad. Bulg. Sci.*, **22**, 799 (1969).
41. Salvador, R. A., and Burton, R. M., *Biochem. Pharmacol.*, **14**, 1185 (1965).
42. Gaudiano, A. G., Petti, A., Polizzi, M., Tartarini, S., and Bartoli, G. M., *Biochem. Pharmacol.*, **18**, 65 (1969).
43. Popov, Ch. S., and Geneva, L. G., *Compt. Rend. Acad. Bulg. Sci.*, **26**, 837 (1973).
44. Stobrovskij, E. M., and Karovin, K. F., *Physiol. J. USSR*, **58**, 414 (1972).
45. Gianetto, R., and De Duve, C., *Biochem. J.*, **59**, 433 (1955).

The Phenothiazines and Structurally Related Drugs, edited by I. S. Forrest, C. J. Carr, and E. Usdin. Raven Press, New York © 1974.

Session II: Discussion

Reporter: L. H. Piette

1. *P. Seeman*

Q. Kaul: It is well established that phenothiazine derivatives which cause parkinsonian symptoms increase the turnover of dopamine and the homovanillic acid concentration in the brain. How do you explain these effects in terms of presynaptic inhibition being the mechanism of action of these drugs in causing extrapyramidal symptoms?

A. Prolonged low dosage chlorpromazine therapy would increase the spontaneous dopamine release, causing bucco-oral tardive dyskinesia, while only minimally affecting impulse-triggered release. Higher dosage of chlorpromazine reduces impulse-triggered release by presynaptic blockade, thus producing parkinsonism, and at the same time reducing the dyskinesia. In other words, dyskinesia may depend on both spontaneous and impulse-triggered release whereas parkinsonism may depend primarily on impulse-triggered release.

2. *A. A. Manian and L. H. Piette*

Q. You interpret the amount of drug lost in your cell-suspending solution as being bound to the RBC membranes. How can you be sure whether this amount of drug is really bound to the membrane or is inside the contents of the cells? Our work has shown that the major portion of the sequestered CPZ metabolites is inside the cells. This may be how the RBC carried CPZ as well, and not merely in the form of drug bound to the membrane.

A. Although we do not know for sure that all of the drug is bound only to the membrane, when we use RBC ghosts instead of intact cells, we get essentially the same results in terms of total drug bound. Also I would expect that with our spin-labeled CPZ derivative that the spectrum we obtained would be quite different, if a portion of drug were bound on the membrane and another protion in the cell itself. We get the same ESR spectrum for spin-labeled ghosts as for intact RBC.

3. *M. A. Bickel*

Q. from floor: Most drug therapy is given orally and as a result of this method of administration we know that over 60 to 70% of the drug is in the gut for as long as 6 hr. Why is it that you did not choose gut tissue for your measurements?

A. These studies are all *in vitro* measurements and not *in vivo,* and therefore the method of administration is not important.

4. *U. Breyer*

Q. from floor: Do you have any idea as to the mechanism of ring cleavage?

A. No, but it possibly occurs after oxidation at the terminal nitrogen.

Q. Is MAO inhibited by these compounds?

A. We don't know.

5. *S. Gabay and C. P. Huang*

Q. Curry: What was the albumin concentration in the difference spectra studied? This is important in relation to the fact that albumin has its own spectrum in the 250 nm region. I am interested to know whether the spectral change is in the CPZ or the albumin molecule, and, if you know the answer, how do you know?

A. The albumin concentration in the difference spectroscopic studies was 1.8×10^{-5} molar. The absorption of albumins in the 250 nm region and that of the phenothiazines also in this region were balanced out by the reference tandem cell containing exactly the same solutions. Only the perturbation absorption was observed. We believe that the spectral changes we see in the 260 nm region were derived mainly from CPZ, the perturbation of tryptophyl- or tyrosinyl-residue should be closer to 300 nm and much weaker.

Q. Wollemann: Does the electrophoretic mobility of your albumin change after treatment with the phenothiazines? We have observed, after incubation of CPZ with sera in equal amounts, that the mobility of several protein bonds, especially the α and β globulins, does change.

A. Our studies showed only the interaction between albumins and phenothiazines at the binding stage, which reaches equilibrium within a fraction of a second. After incubation for a period of time, it is possible that further irreversible change takes place. Also, we are only working with purified serum albumin.

6. *J. W. Gorrod*

Q. Grant: As a point of interest, chlorpromazine may be converted to chlorpromazine sulfoxide in the absence of oxygen, by irradiation of aqueous solutions in the presence of silver, mercuric, ferricyanid, and ferric ions.

Q. Perel: Does remethylation occur in your system?

A. Remethylation has been found by Beckett, but there is no evidence as to the cofactor. One must beware of methodology: once one gets the monodesmethyl derivative, N-hydroxylation can occur. These are very unstable compounds and can lead to breakdown products and artifacts.

7. *J. M. Perel*

Q. Gorrod: We also found remethylation of primary amines to the parent compound in some instances. Did you find N-OH metabolites?

A. We did not distinguish between N-oxides and hydroxides.

Q. Fenner: How specific is your procedure for imipramine metabolites in plasma and tissues?

A. The method, partly developed by Moody in England, was found to be specific by Bickel, using GC/MS.

Session III

Side Effects

Chairmen: Heinz E. Lehmann and Virginia Zaratzian

The Phenothiazines and Structurally Related Drugs, edited by I. S.
Forrest, C. J. Carr, and E. Usdin. Raven Press, New York © 1974.

Sex Differences in Long-Term Adverse Effects of Phenothiazines

Heinz E. Lehmann and Thomas A. Ban

Department of Psychiatry, McGill University, Montreal, Quebec, Canada

INTRODUCTION

There is now sufficient evidence to establish that neuroleptic phenothiazines do not cure schizophrenic patients; regardless of which neuroleptic one prescribes and whatever improvement is obtained, it usually
reaches a plateau in the first 3 to 6 months of treatment. On the other hand,
there is also sufficient clinical evidence to suggest that this initial improvement can be sustained in the majority of patients with maintenance therapy.
In this context, there is a rule of thumb that after the first episode a schizophrenic patient should be maintained on medication for at least 1 yr, after
the second for at least 2 yr, and thereafter for an indefinite period of time.
Early cessation of therapy may lead to relapse within 4 weeks in 25% of
patients, within 8 weeks in 50% and within 12 weeks in 75% (1).

Although maintenance therapy with phenothiazines may prevent relapse
in a considerable percentage of schizophrenic patients, chronic administration of neuroleptics may also lead to skin and eye complications or persistent dyskinesia with or without morphological changes in the substantia
nigra (2). The exact incidence of chronic skin pigmentation is unknown, but
it is estimated to occur in less than 0.1% of all patients treated with chlorpromazine for 2 years or more, and there are indications that in the development of this complication both individual susceptibility and the total amount
of drugs consumed play important roles. Although most patients with skin
pigmentation have ocular complications, a considerably higher percentage
of patients manifest eye rather than skin changes. By slit-lamp examinations, the occurrence of ocular changes in the course of chronic neuroleptic
treatment with chlorpromazine was reported to be as high as 20 to 35%. A
similarly high incidence of persistent dyskinesia in patients on chronic
phenothiazine treatment was reported by Faurbye and his collaborators (3)
and Pryce and Edwards (4), with a slightly higher incidence in females
(44%) than in males (33%) (5). In contradistinction to skin and eye complications, which are dose related, there is no clear correlation between the
dosage and duration of drug administration and the occurrence, time of
onset, duration, or intensity of persistent dyskinesia (1).

In view of these findings, a study was designed to establish the incidence of drug-induced extrapyramidal signs (EPS) in the After-Care Clinic and inpatient population of Douglas Hospital (Verdun, Quebec), as well as the incidence of phenothiazine-induced skin pigmentation in the same hospital, with special reference to sex differences in these long-term adverse effects.

SURVEYS OF DRUG-INDUCED EXTRAPYRAMIDAL MANIFESTATIONS

To establish the incidence of EPS in the After-Care Clinic (ACC) and in the inpatient population of Douglas Hospital, all patients between 15 and 65 yr of age who attended the ACC within a 4-week period and a representative sample of 350 inpatients of the same age group were examined and assessed on a modified version of the extrapyramidal symptom rating scale of Simpson et al. (6) (Table 1). At the same time, the presence or absence of bucco-oral involuntary movements (BOS), a special type of late and often irreversible extrapyramidal manifestation, was noted. Furthermore, tremor was also objectively assessed by recording involuntary finger movements on a graph paper that moved at the rate of 2 cm/sec (employing a Grass SPA-1 transducer) and rigidity by a tapping test, which consisted of pressing two buttons, one after the other consecutively, using the metacarpophalangeal, wrist, or elbow joints (7, 8).

TABLE 1. *EPS rating scale (6)*

Item	Score
1. Tremors	
2. Facial expression	
3. Neck rigidity	0 = absent
4. Gabellar tap	1 = mild
5. Leg pendulousness	2 = moderate
6. Arm drop	3 = severe
7. Shoulder shaking	4 = very severe
8. Elbow movements	
9. Wrist movements	
10. Gait	

A total of 454 patients (199 male, 255 female) with a mean age of 42.3 yr (males 40.9 and females 43.6) attended the ACC and were included in the outpatient survey. Of the 454 patients, 96 (21%) presented extrapyramidal signs. Of them, 43 (44.8%) were men and 53 (55.2%) women. Table 2 shows that BOS alone and associated with parkinsonism was more common among female (20) than male (11) patients, whereas akathisia was slightly more prevalent among male (5) than among female (1) patients.

A total of 350 patients, i.e., 23.7% of the entire hospital population [168

TABLE 2. *Sex distribution of EPS in ACC outpatient study*

EPS	Males	Females	Total
Parkinsonism alone	27	32	59
Parkinsonism with BOS	8	15	23
BOS alone	3	5	8
Akathisia alone	5	1	6
Total	43	53	96

males (48%) and 182 females (52%)], with a mean age of 41.2 yr (males 37.9 and females 43.3) were included in the inpatient survey. Of the 350 patients, 277 (79.1%) presented EPS. Of them, 126 (45.4%) were men and 151 (54.6%) women. Table 3 shows that, as at the ACC, BOS alone and in combination with parkinsonism was more common among female (16) than male (7) patients. Unlike the ACC population, akathisia in inpatients was slightly more prevalent among female (13) than male (6) patients.

TABLE 3. *Sex distribution of EPS in inpatient study*

EPS	Males	Females	Total
Parkinsonism alone	113	122	235
Parkinsonism with BOS	6	14	20
BOS alone	1	2	3
Akathisia	6	13	19
Total	126	151	277

Pooling the data from the ACC and inpatient surveys, a total of 804 patients (367 male, 437 female) with a mean age of 41.75 yr (males 39.40 and females 43.45) were included in the study. Of these 804 patients, 373 (46%) presented EPS. There were 169 (45%) men and 204 (55%) women. Table 4 shows that BOS alone and in combination with parkinsonism was more common among female than male patients, whereas the incidence of parkinsonism alone or akathisia alone was independent of the sex contingent.

TABLE 4. *Sex distribution of EPS (combined population)*

EPS	Males	Females	Total
Parkinsonism alone	140	154	294
Parkinsonism with BOS	14	29	43
BOS alone	4	7	11
Akathisia alone	11	14	25
Total	179	204	373

SURVEY OF PHENOTHIAZINE-INDUCED SKIN PIGMENTATION

The first survey of phenothiazine-induced skin pigmentation was carried out in the Provincial Mental Hospital at Essondale (British Columbia, Canada). It included 6,000 patients and revealed 70 skin-pigmented cases (9). Another survey at approximately the same time, carried out at the Douglas Hospital (then Verdun Protestant Hospital, Verdun, Quebec, Canada) covered 1,500 patients and revealed 15 skin-pigmented cases (10). Although the incidence of phenothiazine-induced skin pigmentation was approximately the same — 1% — in the two psychiatric hospital populations, there was a difference in sex distribution. Phenothiazine-induced skin pigmentation at Essondale was restricted to female patients and was associated in at least 80% of the cases with amenorrhea, whereas at Verdun it affected both sexes — five male and 10 female patients — and the affected female patients were not all amenorrheic.

More recently, a second survey of phenothiazine-induced skin pigmentation was carried out at the Douglas Hospital (11). All 960 adult patients of the hospital (geriatric patients were excluded) were inspected in the daylight by a team, and a total of 28 patients with skin pigmentation were found. Thus the incidence of phenothiazine-induced skin pigmentation increased from 1 to 2.9% during the past 7 yr. When the 143 patients of the acute admission wards were excluded from the total population, there was a further raise in the incidence of skin pigmentation (from 2.9 to 3.4%). As in the first survey, both sexes were affected, with a somewhat higher incidence of skin pigmentation in female (18) than in male (10) patients. It was noted, however, that the age of female patients with skin pigmentation was somewhat higher (range from 20 to 62 yr, mean 44.05 yr, median 32 yr) than of

TABLE 5. *Sex and age distribution*
of skin-pigmented patients

Age (years)	Males (10)	Females (18)	Total (28)
Range	15–58	20–62	15–62
Mean	33.50	44.05	39
Median	32	45	34

TABLE 6. *Relevant information on duration of treatment and*
phenothiazine dosage of skin-pigmented patients

Duration of treatment: range (in years)	3–14
Duration of treatment: mean (in years)	8.6
Dosage range: daily (in CPZ units)	75–9,010
Mean dosage: daily (in CPZ units)	1,228
Dosage range: cumulative (in CPZ units)	550,000–5,570,000
Mean dosage: cumulative (in CPZ units)	2,928,000

the male patients (range from 15 to 58 yr, mean 33.50 yr, median 45 yr). Finally, it was also noted that all of the patients were on phenothiazines (promazine, seven patients; trifluoperazine, 12 patients; prochlorperazine, 12 patients; perphenazine, 12 patients; fluphenazine, two patients), and all except one had received chlorpromazine sometime in the course of treatment. Duration of phenothiazine treatment in the skin-pigmented group ranged from 3 to 14 yr (mean 8.6 yr); the dosage from 75 to 9,010 chlorpromazine units (mean 1,228 units); and the cumulative dose from 550,000 to 5,570,000 chlorpromazine units (mean 2,928,000) (Tables 5 and 6).

DISCUSSION

On the basis of the inpatient and ACC surveys of EPS it was noted that, although there was a higher incidence of EPS in the inpatient (79.1%) than in the outpatient (21%) population, the incidence of BOS was lower in inpatients (6.5%) than in outpatients (14%). The lower incidence of BOS in inpatients is at variance with the contention that in the development of BOS, hospitalization plays an important role. On the other hand, findings in both in- and outpatient populations are in favor of the notion that age and cumulative dose are two important operating factors in the production of BOS. Accordingly, the median age of patients with BOS was found to be somewhat higher (48.4 yr) than the median age of patients with EPS in general (46.65 yr), at least in the ACC population, and the percentage of patients with BOS was higher with large cumulative doses of phenothiazines (inpatients 32.8%; outpatients 24.3%) than with small cumulative doses (inpatients 5.8%; outpatients 3.2%) in both in- and outpatients. Finally, it was noted that in the total population of the in- and outpatient surveys, buccooral dyskinesia occurs more frequently in female (36) than in male (18) patients.

Although surveys of phenothiazine-induced skin pigmentation at the Douglas Hospital could not substantiate the notion that this complication occurs exclusively in females in both surveys, there were indications that in the development of this abnormality the sex contingent does play a role. More female (18) than male (10) patients were affected by this abnormality, and the affected female patients were older (mean 44.05 yr) than the affected male patients (mean 33.5 yr).

SUMMARY

The incidence of phenothiazine-induced extrapyramidal signs (with special reference to bucco-oral dyskinesia) and skin pigmentation was studied in the patient population of a psychiatric hospital. It was noted that the sex factor seems to play a role in the development of both the bucco-oral syndrome and skin pigmentation. Both abnormalities are more frequently encountered in female than in male patients.

ACKNOWLEDGMENT

This study was partially supported by U.S. Public Health Service grant MH–05202–12.

REFERENCES

1. Ayd, F. J., In DiMascio, A., and Shader, R. I. (eds.), *Clinical Handbook of Psychophar-macology*, Science House, New York, 1970.
2. Christiansen, E., Moller, J. E., and Faurbye, A., *Acta Psychiat. Scand.*, **46**, 14 (1970).
3. Faurbye, A., Basch, P., Bender-Petersen, P., Branborg, G., and Pakkenberg, H., *Acta Psychiat. Scand.*, **40**, 10 (1964).
4. Pryce, I. G., and Edwards, H., *Brit. J. Psychiat.*, **114**, 775 (1966).
5. Fann, W. E., Davis, J. M., and Janowsky, F. S., *Dis. Nerv. Syst.*, **33**, 182 (1972).
6. Simpson, G. M., Amnsco, D., Blair, J. H., and Farkas, R., *Arch. Gen. Psychiat.*, **10**, 199 (1964).
7. Guttman, H., Lehmann, H. E., and Ban, T. A., *Laval Medical*, **14**, 449 (1970).
8. Lehmann, H. E., Ban, T. A., and Saxena, B. M., *Laval Medical*, **41**, 909 (1970).
9. Greiner, A. C., and Berry, K., *Canad. Med. Ass. J.*, **9**, 663 (1964).
10. Ban, T. A., and Lehmann, H. E., *Canad. Psychiat. Ass. J.*, **10**, 112 (1965).
11. Ananth, J. V., Ban, T. A., Lehmann, H. E., and Rizvi, F. A., *Indian J. Psychiat.*, **14**, 76 (1972).

The Phenothiazines and Structurally Related Drugs, edited by I. S. Forrest, C. J. Carr, and E. Usdin. Raven Press, New York © 1974.

Evolutionary Origin of Extrapyramidal Disorders in Drug-Treated Mental Patients, Its Significance, and the Role of Neuromelanin

Fred M. Forrest

Veterans Administration Hospital, Palo Alto, California 94304

INTRODUCTION

During the last decades, two developments have dominated neuropsychiatric literature: first, the obvious success of chemotherapy, especially the phenothiazine drugs and related compounds, in emptying the formerly overcrowded mental hospitals, and second, the problems connected with the appearance of late side effects, particularly of the extrapyramidal type. In spite of great progress in the treatment of the parkinsonian syndrome, the overall problem of extrapyramidal side effects is still unresolved. The rate of incidence of the dyskinetic syndrome is variously reported as 3 to 40%, making it obvious that either different patient populations or greatly varying treatment methods or incompatible nosology are being described. The question of reversibility is hotly debated. While some authors advocate discontinuation of the offending drug in tardive dyskinesia (1–3), numerous experienced clinicians report frequent and severe aggravation of the syndrome after reduction of medication. They recommend continuation and even increase of neuroleptic drug doses or appropriate manipulation of antipsychotic drugs in order to eliminate the symptoms (4–6). The regrettable fact of this unsolved treatment problem is reflected in a most recent FDA drug bulletin (7), suggesting "that all antipsychotic agents be discontinued at the first sign of abnormal oral movements or other manifestations of tardive dyskinesia" and that "drug holidays are advisable in patients receiving long-term medication." This unfortunate generalization may induce numerous psychiatrists to withhold optimum dosages from severely ill chronic mental patients on the basis of an exaggerated fear that the side effects might outweigh the therapeutic benefits.

This author has treated, during the last two decades in his hospital practice, over 1500 chronic male mental patients with intensive phenothiazine medication and has seen about 5% of these patients develop tardive dyskinesia (mostly in mild and transitory form) consisting of some involuntary finger movements or tongue twisting or somewhat abnormal gait. Most of these side effects were not severe enough to interfere with the continued use of antipsychotic medication. It was noted that chlorpromazine medication produced less dyskinetic side effects than treatment with the piperazine- and piperidine-linked drugs. The most severe symptoms among our patients were produced by the administration of fluphenazine (Prolixin®), perphenazine (Trilafon®), thioridazine (Mellaril®) and especially trifluoperazine (Stelazine®), most of which could be reversed by substituting chlorpromazine. The danger inherent in "minimal" chemotherapy has been previously described by us and other authors (4, 6, 8). Recent statistics showing a significant increase in homicides committed by prematurely discharged or otherwise undermedicated mental patients should be a warning signal to the present advocates of "minimal" chemotherapy (9). It is, however, not the purpose of this paper to elaborate further on treatment methods and to contribute to a seemingly endless controversy which is partly due to the total lack of understanding of the origin of the syndrome, its complex neuroanatomy, biochemistry, and so far unrecognized phylogenetic aspects. The problem of proper therapy of tardive dyskinesia and especially the use of enzyme inducers such as diphenhydramine (Benadryl®) and barbiturates in combination with chlorpromazine, and the long-term beneficial effect of continuous chlorpromazine treatment will be discussed in a separate paper. The most perplexing treatment problem is the frequently reported observation that tardive dyskinesia in chronically drug-treated hospitalized psychiatric patients tends to be less severe during drug treatment and more severe when the drug is stopped (5, 10–14). Curran (5) recently has pointed out the absurdity of the conclusion "that a drug can produce a syndrome both upon administration and upon withdrawal." Equally perplexing is the bizarreness of most of the dyskinetic movements. They appear useless and have been given such fanciful names as "Rabbit Syndrome" (15) "Flycatcher Tongue" (16) etc., but are strangely coordinated in spite of their awkward appearance. If one introduces the methodology of an ethologist into psychiatry in analyzing the syndrome, one has to ask "What is it good for?" and "Why are these involuntary movements and the parkinsonian tremor performed in a predetermined sequence and rhythmicity?" A logical answer to these questions can only be found in the assumption that there is a genetic component in these muscular movements which otherwise could not be so universally alike. It is a biological axiom that only reflex mechanisms of vital importance during long epochs in the evolution of a species become so engraved in the central nervous system as to be transmitted by heredity.

The next question therefore is "during which period of our evolution might these motoric reflex patterns have had survival value?" Our premammalian ancestors have lived for roughly 400 million years in all sorts of environments, from aquatic and semiaquatic to terrestrial and arboreal surroundings and have developed from fish into amphibians, reptiles, and mammals, all the while preserving the basic structure of our nervous system. By relating extrapyramidal motor manifestations — of the dyskinetic as well as parkinsonian type — to vital reflex mechanisms of the distant past, it will be attempted in the following discussion to gain some insight into the neurodynamics and origin of these symptoms and the pathological conditions capable of reactivating some of the ancestral motor functions buried in our phylogenetically old extrapyramidal nerve centers which comprise the basal ganglia, the subthalamic nucleus, the substantia nigra, the red nucleus, the amygdala as well as parts of the brainstem reticular formation (17).

DESCRIPTION AND EVOLUTIONARY ORIGIN OF EXTRAPYRAMIDAL DISORDERS

Drug-induced dyskinesia is characterized by involuntary, bizarre movements of various body regions including trunk, limbs, mouth, and facial muscles, similar to the motoric disorders caused by organic lesions of the basal ganglia (11, 18, 19).

A. Oral dyskinesia frequently is the only motoric disturbance without involvement of other parts of the body. These involuntary rhythmic mouth movements have been variously described as chewing motions, lip smacking, puffing up of cheeks and protrusion of tongue. Cinefluorographic analysis has shown that this strikingly awkward grimacing is not part of a swallowing cycle. The tongue movement in a normal swallowing act consists of an upward and backward motion in contrast to the consistent forward thrust of the tongue in oral dyskinesia (20). As a matter of fact, the constant innervation of the genioglossus muscle in severe oral dyskinesia interferes with the swallowing of solid food. The dyskinetic rhythmic "lapping" movements of the tongue together with a frequently observable shallow breathing pattern give the impression that these patients suffer from some respiratory distress. Surprisingly they deny this when questioned. These "semibizarre" and "semipurposeful" buccolingual motions resemble most closely the gill breathing motions of fish, especially the labored inhaling of water of an oxygen-starved carp at the bottom of an aquarium. The pursing of the lips and the puffing of the cheeks (evolved from gills) are too similar in sequence, form, and rhythm to be accidental. It seems, therefore, probable that we deal in oral dyskinesia with an ancestral aquatic respiratory reflex, reactivated by pathological stimulation of a phylogenetically old, subcortical, respiratory nerve center. The nerve center involved may be the substantia nigra, which has been described by students of comparative anatomy as the respiratory midbrain center of fish (21). However, other pigmented nuclei of the brainstem may be involved. So far no consistent clinicopathological correlations have been established for specific nuclei and dyskinetic symptoms (11). We will return in later sections of this chapter to the substantia nigra and the significance of its neuromelanin content in the causation of extrapyramidal disorders.

B. Choreoathetotic movements of the upper limbs are seen in many dyskinetic patients. Their arms, hands, and fingers twist and pronate behind their backs and these slow motions are often accompanied by rotation of the shoulders or swivelling of the hips. Again, these movements appear bizarre on terra firma but make sense as swimming movements in an aquatic medium. They are a type of "swim-crawl" similar to the swimming movements of the limbs of some amphibia and some primitive reptiles, e.g., the skinks, whose gyrating locomotion in their present desert environment has been aptly described as "swimming in the sand" (22). This slow athetoid posturing is probably generated by reactivation of subcortical nerve centers in the corpus striatum and possibly putamen (23). These basal ganglia represent our principal premammalian brain centers, are strongly developed in reptiles and have superseded the brainstem nuclei of fish. Their development parallels the evolution of the limbs, but their functions, in turn, were progressively replaced by the evolution of the neocortex, the seat of our conscious mind. The inactivated older centers were thereby forced into some type of quiescence, with slower metabolism and subsequent deposition of neuromelanin. Depigmentation and neuronophagia of the putamen and the substantia nigra have been described in autopsy findings of drug-treated patients (24) and might be correlated to the symptom complex of drug induced choreoathetosis.

C. Akathisia, also described as the symptom of "restless legs," occurs in approximately 10 to 20% of all drug-induced extrapyramidal reactions. It is impossible for the afflicted patients to sit still and they have difficulties in getting complete rest, even when lying down. Some become very distressed over these leg motions and produce considerable secondary anxiety by their futile attempts to suppress this restlessness. These involuntary motions are not subject to our conscious mind. They are not mediated by the pyramidal motor pathways, but by nerve impulses transmitted through the extrapyramidal pathways of the rubrospinal and vestibulospinal tracts which connect the heavily pigmented red nucleus and the vestibular centers to all anterior spinal motor cells. These impulses are transmitted to the reflex arcs of the lumbar and sacral nerve plexus innervating our gluteal, peroneal, and psoas muscles. In turn these muscles, represented by the lowest spinal nerve circuits, are the successors of our original tail. Since the fish tail, as the principal organ of primitive aquatic locomotion, beats the water with alternate strokes, the reactivation of motor nuclei of the sacral plexus produces alternate movements of our gluteal muscles. This rhythmic innervation of gluteal muscles, presently the extensors of our thighs, causes in akathisic patients a repetitive rising from the sitting position and their peculiar dancing steps while standing. Akathisia, therefore, seems to exemplify the transmutation of function of a "fossil" locomotor organ into a motion of involuntary character.

Such automatic movements of an exorgan, insensitive to willful control, frequently produce anxiety. Thereby *exmotion* evolves into *e-motion* and acquires a communicative component, thus becoming a gesture. Any observer will easily interpret this "getting-up" reflex as a symbol of the patient's intention "to go for a walk," even while he is treading on the same spot.

If this phylogenetic interpretation is correct, the neuromelanin content of the globus pallidus or red nucleus could be implicated in the reappearance of the akathisic syndrome (see also the Conclusions section of this chapter).

D. To illustrate the transmutation of "fossil" locomotor function into a gesture, an example familiar also to lay people may be quoted: Everybody recognizes the ubiquitous behavior pattern of dogs wagging their tails when expressing joy. Why doesn't any dog ever flap his ears or use another body part for the expression of friendliness? The phylogenetic origin of this reflex becomes clear only when the question is posed as follows: Why is the tail wagging always done in a *horizontal* plane when joy is expressed and why does the dog reserve a vertical tail movement, namely the pulling in of the tail between his legs, for the expression of fear? It is rather easy to recognize—but to this author's knowledge has never before been explained—that the tail wagging in the horizontal plane is an analogue to the fish tail propelling the fish forward. The fish tail is an organ of approach and the dog tail executes a "fossil" motion to *signalize* approach.

On the other hand, the pulling in of the tail as an expression of fear mirrors the *diving* reflex of fish, amphibium, or primitive reptile in seeking protection in the depths of water. From the standpoint of a useful or purposeful reaction, the tail wagging does not make any sense, since it does not propel the dog forward. Still it is transmitted by heredity and has become the dog's universal greeting gesture. It is understood by his cospecifics and by man as his *intention* of friendly approach. Again exmotion has become a symbol of e-motion. This communicative aspect of the tail wagging had acquired enough survival value to prevent further significant atrophy throughout millions of years of terrestrial evolution.

The tail wagging as the phylogenetically oldest mode of locomotion in vertebrates is probably mediated by the oldest motoric parts of the basal ganglia, the globus pallidus. The nerve impulses leading from the pallidum via efferent extrapyramidal pathways to the tail, however, do not instigate actual approach, which is only done when the cortical pyramidal pathways innervate the limbs.

The globus pallidus has obviously assumed during recent evolution a communicative, emotional, quasipsychic function. (See also the section on Evolution and neurochemistry of the Basal Ganglia.)

A tail wagging dog who actually approaches his master, therefore, innervates simultaneously his extrapyramidal and pyramidal motor systems, the former expressing emotion and motivating the latter into volitional motion. This example of evolution of some animal behavior demonstrates the survival of ancestral aquatic locomotor reflexes in the service of the mental development of mammals.

It also demonstrates that the two mammalian central nervous motor systems can act independently and do not always cooperate harmoniously. Whoever has seen an excited dog greeting his master after prolonged absence, and losing his footing on a polished floor by the violent tail wagging, has witnessed the interference of a conscious motoric action by an unconscious subcortical impulse, a typically schizophrenic-like reaction pattern. Extrapyramidal disorders in man also constitute a type of motoric schizophrenic-like split mind.

That the human species has lost its tail, might be the consequence of the acquisition of language. We no longer need any tail for communication, as we communicate more effectively by wagging our tongues. But we have not completely lost our extrapyramidal impulses with regard to tail motions and can clearly recognize in the wiggling of the hips of a seductive female the communicative component of a long-vanished ancestral tail motion indicating, as in the tail wagging of the dog, a preparedness to approach . . . or to be approached.

E. The parkinsonian syndrome is characterized by a triad of motoric symptoms: general immobility (akinesia), rigidity of trunk and limbs (bradykinesia), and tremor of the hands and fingers (rest tremor). This hand tremor, of a frequency of 3 to 6 per sec, is surprisingly similar, in its rhythm and sequence of muscular action, to the stabilizing movements of the breast fins of many fish. As zoologists know, the breast fins of fish do not primarily serve locomotor function but maintain equilibrium in an unstable aquatic medium.

Consequently, the fins are subject to automatic, rhythmic, vestibular impulses and represent the end organ of a vital reflex arc, holding the fish upright at rest. When the fish moves forward by the motions of its tail and posterior vertebral column, the fins remain immobile. Now, our hands and fingers have evolved from breast fins of fish. The tragic malformations from thalidomide toxicity, in which the ontogenetic development of the long bones of our limbs is inhibited, reminded us painfully of this phylogenetic relationship, accounting for the bizarre appearance of the hands hanging like fins from the trunks of the victims. The similar rhythm and morphological similarity of the parkinsonian rest tremor — misleadingly called "pill rolling," and better characterized as "water flailing" — to the breast fin movements of fish, equally support the hypothesis of an aquatic origin of this common disorder. Parkinsonian rest tremor constitutes probably the reactivation of an equilibrial fin reflex.

On the other hand, when a fish is at rest and does not want to move from its place, be it for resting or lying in wait for prey — it has to keep its body and tail immobile and rigid. Only the eyes, which most fish can not close, are kept open and are directed upwards toward the light to scan for prey or danger from other predators. This combination of general immobility, rigidity of trunk, and stabilizing motion of fins is a vital aquatic motoric reflex mechanism which for the sake of brevity I shall refer to from here on as the "anchoring reflex."

Once more, should it be just coincidence that the motoric triad of the parkinsonian syndrome, namely rigidity, immobility, and rest tremor are identical with the vital muscular reflex phenomena comprising the "anchoring reflex" of a fish at rest or "on the lookout"?

F. Eye muscle spasms, known as oculogyric crises, may occur in connection with the parkinsonian syndrome—the encephalitic type as well as drug induced—with the eyes fixed upwards. Why has no oculogyric crisis with the eyes directed downwards ever occurred? As previously mentioned, observation in an aquatic medium of prey and enemies is obviously facilitated by the pupils directed towards the light. Pathological reactivation of this naturally dominant aquatic oculomotor tonus might well be the cause for the fixed, upwards directed gaze of the oculogyric crises in Parkinson's disease. Therefore, it is proposed to describe the oculogyric crisis as pathological reactivation of an aquatic visual "orienting" reflex. Finally, the entire parkinsonian syndrome may be considered as the pathological reappearance of an aquatic anchoring reflex, used by our remote ancestors trillions of times for most vital aspects of existence and therefore indelibly engraved in our central nervous system.

On the basis of the previous analysis, all extrapyramidal symptoms may be interpreted as reactivations of camouflaged "fossil" functions of our piscine, amphibian, and reptilian ancestors, originally representing vital respiratory, equilibrial, locomotor, anchoring, and orienting reflexes in an aquatic medium.

HISTOPATHOLOGY OF EXTRAPYRAMIDAL DISORDERS

The high incidence of pathological changes in the basal ganglia, especially the substantia nigra and locus coeruleus in Parkinson's disease, has been substantiated in the literature. In these brains, pigmented neurons are decreased in number in the substantia nigra and locus coeruleus. Phase and electronmicroscopic observations of Lewy bodies and melanin granules in these brainstem nuclei showed a decrease in the dense component of melanin before the complete breakdown of the substructure of the neuron itself (25).

It has also been established that similar cell degeneration in the substantia nigra in combination with gliosis in the midbrain and brainstem nuclei takes place in the brains of patients with persistent oral dyskinesia and on long-term neuroleptic therapy. Some autopsies showed diffused cellular gliosis in cerebral cortex, basal ganglia, and midbrain with striking gliosis in the caudate nucleus. Large amounts of pigmented bodies and free pigment were seen in the substantia nigra and to some extent in the globus pallidus and putamen (26–28).

Today it is a recognized fact that the involuntary movement disorders produced by neuroleptic drugs or encephalitic processes have in common the involvement of the pigmented subcortical nerve centers, the neuromelanin of which has been altered within the cells or displaced from them.

EVOLUTION AND NEUROCHEMISTRY OF THE BASAL GANGLIA

The vital nerve centers of the fish brain are located in the brainstem where the neurons of the substantia nigra are already present but not pigmented. The substantia nigra in fish and amphibia is considered to be a motoric respiratory nucleus, the efferent fibers of which probably innervate the gill muscles (21). The pigment of the substantia nigra increases with evolution, and the higher evolved the mammals, the more pigmented are the substantia nigra neurons. Ontogenesis repeats the phylogenetic process. The substantia nigra is not pigmented in human infants until the second year of life. It becomes increasingly pigmented during growth and adolescence (29). The basal ganglia reach their highest motoric development in the reptiles concomitantly with the development of limbs. The globus pallidus, as the oldest and most centrally located motoric basal ganglion of the archipallium, innervates the oldest locomotor organs of our reptilian ancestors, their rump and tail muscles, whereas the caudate nucleus represents the more recent locomotor organs, the limbs. The development of the prefrontal motor cortex during mammalian evolution supersedes the motoric nuclei of the basal ganglia. The human brain can be compared to a multifloored structure in which each floor has retained certain functions, all subordinated to the final decision making top floor, the cortex, from which all conscious action emanates.

The function of neuromelanin in nervous tissue is not clearly understood, but it must have significance since it is preferably deposited in tissues which are phylogenetically old. Marsden seems to have been the first to speculate on the phylogenetic significance of neuromelanin and its relationship to catecholamine synthesis: "In pigmented cells, tyrosine metabolism appears primarily oriented towards neuromelanin synthesis rather than to catecholamine production. Conversely, in nonpigmented neurons, tyrosine metabolism is exclusively directed towards catecholamine synthesis . . . As cerebral evolution progresses, cerebral dominance is transferred from primitive brainstem nuclei to expanding forebrain centers. During this process the demands for catecholamine synthesis diminish in the brainstem nuclei as their functions are taken over by higher centers. Diminished catecholamine synthesis is achieved by diverting L-tyrosine metabolism towards the formation of neuromelanin rather than catecholamine. Thus, as evolution of the brain takes place, primitive brainstem nuclei associated with the central autonomic and extrapyramidal systems become increasingly pigmented. Neuromelanin is thus a recent phylogenetic development and it appears that the intensity of pigmentation is related to the degree of evolution" (30, 31).

If Marsden's hypothesis is correct, neuromelanin must have some inhibitive action on the bioelectric activity of the nerve cell and produce some decrease in the cell's discharge frequency. It is interesting that neuromelanin is usually deposited most intensively around the axon hillock of the cell (29) which may mean that it serves as a barrier to the electron flow from the cytoplasm into the original axon cylinder of the nerve cell. Actually this is in agreement with the physical qualities of melanin as an electron acceptor or electron trap. If therefore dopamine as an electron donor (e.g., in a pigmented neuron of the substantia nigra) is inactivated by neuromelanin as an electron acceptor, the cell would become bioelectrically inactive and lead a "quasihibernating" existence. According to biological principles such an inactive cell should have eventually atrophied. This, however, was not the case. The substantia nigra continued to exist, and as a group of Swedish researchers have recently shown by use of histofluorescence methods, (32–35), the neurons of the substantia nigra contain dopamine as well as neuromelanin. Dopamine was found to be transported via the nigrostriatal pathway centripetally to the nucleus caudatus. When these fibers are cut, the caudate nucleus becomes deficient in dopamine and a parkinsonian syndrome is produced (36–38).

At a remote point in evolution at which no caudate nucleus had as yet developed in our aquatic ancestors, the substantia nigra obviously had a purely motoric function, mediated through centrifugal fibers. Its present centripetal connections and the transmission of dopamine to higher nerve centers of more recent development permit the conclusion that the substantia nigra has undergone a fundamental change from a motoric to a secretory function. As long as part of the cell metabolism is directed towards neuromelanin formation, the neuron does not act as a motoric but as a secretory unit. Logically therefore, if the axonal impulse inhibition of neuromelanin can be eliminated, the cell should revert from its secretory or endocrine function to its original motoric function. Since this original function served aquatic reflex mechanisms, the result is the reappearance of involuntary, bizarre motions of the dyskinetic syndrome or of parkinsonian character.

Apparently phenothiazines, especially chlorpromazine, are able to inactivate neuromelanin in basal ganglia and thereby interfere with the phylogenetically more recent secretory activity of the pigmented neurons. This, in turn, causes the cell metabolism to revert to its original, more primitive aquatic metabolic patterns, as elaborated below (see Table 1).

TABLE 1. *Phylogenetic origin of extrapyramidal disorders*

Vital functions and reflex mechanisms in vertebrates	Evolutional adaptation of vital functions from aquatic to terrestrial life			Phenothiazine side effects by inactivation of melanin and reactivation of aquatic reflex mechanisms in man and primates
	Fish Coelacanth	Amphibia Reptilia	Mammals Man	
1. Blood pressure	Low		Higher	Lower (orthostatic hypotension)
2. Heat regulation	Temp. 40–80°		Higher (98°)	Lowering of temperature
3. Equilibrium	Unstable in water		Stable on land	Unstable – vestibular stimulus: reactivation of fin rhythm 3–6 p. sec.: parkinsonian tremor
4. Respiration and metabolism	Gill action Pentose cycle		Lung action Krebs cycle	Reactivation of gill movements (oral dyskinesia) reactivation of pentose cycle-glia (48)
5. Locomotion	Body twist Tail mvts.	Body twist Limb mvts. Crawl Tail mvts.	— Quadrupedal Gait Bipedal gait Assoc. mvts.	Body twist (Torsion spasm) Swim–Crawl (Athetotic mvts.) Sacral plexus refl. (glut. plantar) (akathisia)
6. Resting activity	Anchoring reflex: Immobility Rigidity Fin rhythm	Immobility Rigidity	Immobility	Reactivation of anchoring reflex: Immobility (akinesia) Rigidity (bradykinesia) Fin rhythm (rest tremor) Parkinsonian syndrome
7. Orienting refl. ocular mvts.	Eyes fixed upward	Eyes mobile	Eyes forward	Reactivation of orienting reflex: eyes fixed upward (spasm) (oculogyric crisis)

INTERACTION BETWEEN NEUROMELANIN AND CHLORPROMAZINE

The interaction between chlorpromazine and melanin has been extensively studied and reported. Potts was the first to hypothesize on this subject (39). Van Woert found that the oxidating activity of melanin is inhibited by pharmacologic compounds such as phenothiazine and chloroquine (40). Forrest et al. have elucidated the interaction of chlorpromazine with melanoprotein *in vivo* and *in vitro* (41). It was conclusively shown by the work of Forrest and Gutmann, and Bolt and Forrest that the phenothiazines act as electron donors and the melanin as electron acceptor (41, 42). This results in tight *in vivo* binding of these drugs to any melanin bearing tissues, such as retina, hair, melanoma etc. (39, 43, 44). It was furthermore found that the paramagnetic signal of melanoprotein was reduced upon addition of chlorpromazine (41) which means that the two opposite charges neutralize one another, leaving a bioelectrically more or less inert compound. Applying the same concept to the neuromelanin of the pigmented neurons of the basal ganglia, the following interpretation of the cause of drug induced extrapyramidal manifestations may be advanced: Phenothiazines — and probably many other electron-donating neuroletpic drugs — attach themselves to the neuromelanin inside the pigmented neuron and thereby produce an inert compound which loses its function as an electron trap. It seems, therefore, justified to add yet another quality to the many other well established biological effects of chlorpromazine and call it "melanostatic."

To the same degree as neuromelanin is inactivated by chlorpromazine in the substantia nigra, the synthesis of dopamine will increase since the tyrosine — as the precursor of either — will be fully available for dopamine synthesis. The excess of available dopamine pushes into the formerly blocked axon cylinder, bypassing the now inert neuromelanin barrier. This bioelectric impulse may stimulate the remyelinization of the original motoric axon cylinder whose Swan cell sheath had atrophied due to inactivity. The regeneration of an axon cylinder sheath is a slow process requiring weeks or months for full regrowth, depending on the length of the axon. This slow regeneration might explain the tardive appearance of dyskinetic symptoms.

Clinical experience of this and other authors has shown that continued chlorpromazine therapy will eventually be accompanied in most cases by the disappearance of the symptoms of tardive dyskinesia (4–6, 10). A possible explanation for this curious fact could be the finding that long-term chlorpromazine therapy leads eventually to the destruction of pigmented neurons and to neuronophagia. Forrest et al. reported depigmentation of neurons of the substantia nigra in a patient on long-term chlorpromazine therapy who had not shown any dyskinetic symptoms at the time of his death (caused by heart attack) (24). Total loss of substantia nigra cells has apparently no deleterious effect on vital neural functions since other dopamine producing ganglia in the corpus striatum seem to be able to compensate for the partial loss of dopamine. The capacity of the brain to compensate functionally for the loss of the destroyed elements is enormous (45). When this stage of neuronophagia is reached, the afflicted cells cease to exist and the dyskinetic syndrome comes to an end. This could be compared to the surgical removal of an appendix, troublesome while it was malfunctioning, however without pathological sequelae, after removal.

On the other hand, interruption of therapy with chlorpromazine or other neuroleptics leads frequently to paradoxical aggravation of the dyskinetic syndrome, probably due to sudden availability of excess dopamine: While the bond between chlorpromazine and melanin is very stable and persisting (44, 46), the presumable bond between chlorpromazine and dopamine would be much weaker and readily broken after discontinuation of the drug (46, 47). Thus, dopamine liberated from a loose complex with chlorpromazine would become abundantly available, producing dyskinetic and/or hyperkinetic manifestations.

Research literature on extrapyramidal disorders is confusing and difficult to evaluate. Considering the many neural structures which are involved in the regulation of our motor activity, representing hundreds of millions of years of evolution in diverse environments, this is not astonishing. In the absence of any existing plausible explanation of extrapyramidal symptomatology, the foregoing theory of reactivation of ancestral reflex mechanisms by inactivation of neuromelanin through the melanostatic action of chlorpromazine and other neuroleptic drugs might contribute to a better understanding of these phenomena. Admittedly many aspects are speculative and will need correction as new knowledge and factual data become available.

CONCLUSIONS

1. Extrapyramidal drug-induced disorders, including all forms of dyskinesia, hyperkinesia, and bradykinesia have a common phylogenetic origin and represent ancestral aquatic or semiaquatic reflex mechanisms, reactivated by the melanostatic effect of chlorpromazine or other neuroleptic drugs within the pigmented neurons of the brainstem or the basal ganglia.

2. Neuromelanin within the nerve cells of the pigmented nuclei, e.g., substantia nigra, red nucleus, locus coeruleus, globus pallidus, etc. has a dual function: By blocking the axonal outflow and its original motoric function it causes the neuron to go into "motoric" hibernation. The subsequent accumulation of the primary neurotransmitter transforms the cell into a secretory unit, a "quasiendocrine" gland.

3. Neuromelanin can therefore be considered an impulse inhibitor and its inactivation will cause the reappearance of various types of ancestral reflex activity specific for each pigmented nucleus.

4. Neuroleptic drugs, and especially chlorpromazine among the pheno-

thiazines, have a special affinity and attach themselves to the neuromelanin of the extrapyramidal neurons producing charge-transfer complexes. The resulting addition compounds are bioelectrically inert and lose the electron trapping function of melanin. Once this impulse barrier is eliminated, the original transmitter substance attempts to restore axonal flow leading to slow regeneration of the atrophied original axon cylinder. Such regeneration may require many months before contact with the muscular end organs is restored. This is probably the reason for the delayed onset of the syndrome of tardive dyskinesia.

5. Dyskinetic symptoms appear in various forms or intensity during the melanostatic stage of chlorpromazine therapy, but frequently regress or disappear when the treatment is continued. That stage may amount to chemosurgery, eliminating the extrapyramidal symptomatology.

6. Histopathological autopsy findings on dyskinetic and drug-treated patients seem to confirm the causative relationship between drug induced extrapyramidal disorders and the neuromelanin of the pigmented subcortical nuclei. Inert melanin-chlorpromazine compounds are eventually expelled as foreign bodies from the neuron, which itself may disintegrate in the process.

SUMMARY

To date no plausible theory has been advanced for the origin and prevention of drug-induced extrapyramidal disorders. In view of the paradoxical and totally unexplained phenomenon of aggravation of symptoms after discontinuation of the offending drug, a new theory based on the evolution of our central nervous system and its neuromelanin content is proposed. It has been formerly established that due to electron donation of phenothiazines, charge-transfer complexes are formed with melanin *in vivo* and *in vitro*. It has been furthermore demonstrated that extrapyramidal disorders have their pathological correlates in many of the pigmented subcortical motoric basal ganglia. It is now proposed that the functional balance between dopamine and neuromelanin within the substantia nigra and other pigmented nuclei, as well as the balance between other neurotransmitters and neuromelanin, e.g., in locus coeruleus, red nucleus, globus pallidus, etc. is disturbed by the "melanostatic" action of phenothiazines and certain other neuroleptic drugs. Consequently, these phylogenetically old, subcortical nerve centers resume a bioelectric activity consistent with their original vital functions in our ancestral aquatic and semiaquatic environment. The similarity of the various dyskinetic and parkinsonian manifestations with old aquatic reflex mechanisms is pointed out. This theory offers an adequate interpretation for the seemingly bizarre extrapyramidal manifestations, the delayed onset of the symptoms as well as the paradoxical fact of aggravation of the symptoms upon withdrawal of the drug.

REFERENCES

1. Crane, G. E., *Agressologie*, **9**, 209 (1968).
2. Crane, G. E., et al., *Activitas Nerv. Superior*, **11**, 1 (1969).
3. Ayd, F. J., Jr., *Medical Science*, **18**:32 (1967).
4. Kline, N. S., *Amer. J. Psychiat.*, **124** (Supp.), 48 (1968).
5. Curran, J. P., *Am. J. Psychiat.*, **130**, 4 (1973).
6. Freedman, D. X., *Arch. of Gen. Psychiat.*, **28**, 463 (1973).
7. FDA Bulletin, Mailing to Psychiatrists, May 1973.
8. Forrest, F. M., et al., *Amer. J. Psychiat.*, **121**, 33 (1964).
9. San Francisco Examiner and Palo Alto Times, Relative to Recent Discharge Practices from California Mental Hospitals, June 1973.
10. Hollister, L. E., *Psychiatric Annals*, **3**, 7 (1973).
11. Faurbye, A., *Acta Psychiat. Scand.*, **40**, 10 (1964).
12. Turck, I., et al., *Brit. J. Psychiat.*, **121** (565), 605, (1972).
13. Degkwitz, R., et al., *Arzneimittelforsch.*, **16**, 276 (1966).
14. Degkwitz, R., *Activitas Nerv. Superior*, **9**, 389 (1967).
15. Jus, K., et al., *Dis. Nerv. System*, **34**, 27 (1973).
16. Lambert, P., et al., *Psychotropic Drugs and Dysfunctions of the Basal Ganglia, A Multidiscip. Workshop*, Public Health Serv. Publ. No. 1938, 1969, p. 10.
17. Hornykiewicz, O., *Brit. Med. Bull.*, **29**, 172 (1973).
18. Uhrbrand, L., and Faurbye, A., *Psychopharmacologia*, **1**, 408 (1960).
19. Barbeau, A., et al., *Rev. Can. Biol.*, **22**, Nos. 3–4 (1963).
20. Massengill, R., Jr., and Nashold, B., *Acta-oto-laryng*, **68**, 457 (1969).
21. Jacob, Chr., *Das Menschenhirn*, Lehmann's Verlag, München, 1911.
22. International Wild Life Encyclopedia, Marshall Cavendish, New York, 1970, vol. 16, p. 2156.
23. DeLong, M. R., *Science*, **179**, 1240 (1973).
24. Forrest, F. M., et al., *Agressologie*, **4**, 259 (1963).
25. Tennyson, V., et al., *Brain Res.*, **53**, 307 (1973).
26. Christensen, E., et al., *Acta Psychiat. Scand.*, **46**, 14 (1970).
27. Cammermeyer, J., *Psychotropic Drugs and Dysfunctions of the Basal Ganglia, A Multidiscip. Workshop*, Public Health Serv. Publ. No. 1938, 1969, p. 19.
28. Gross, H., and Kaltenbäck, E., in *The Present Status of Psychotropic Drugs. Pharmacological and Clinical Aspects*, Cerletti, A., and Bove, F. J. (Eds.), Excerpta Medica, Amsterdam, 1969, pp. 474–476.
29. Fenichel, G. M., and Bazelon, M., *Neurology*, **18**, 817 (1968).
30. Marsden, C. D., *Lancet*, **2**, 475 (1965).
31. Marsden, C. D., *Lancet*, **2**, 1244 (1965).
32. Andén, N. E., et al., *Life Sciences*, **3**, 523 (1964).
33. Andén, N. E., et al., *Acta Physiol. Scand.*, **67**, 306 (1966).
34. Fuxe, K., and Andén, N. E., in *Biochem. and Pharmacol. of the Basal Ganglia, Proceed. of the 2nd. Symp. of the Parkinson's Dis. Inf. and Res. Ctr.*, Coll. of Physicians and Surgeons of Columbia University, New York, Nov. 29–30, 1965, p. 123.
35. Dahlstrom, A., and Fuxe, K., *Acta Physiol. Scand.*, **62**, (Supp.), 232 (1964).
36. Andén, N. E., et al., *Am. J. Anatomy*, **116**, 329 (1965).
37. Poirier, L. J., and Sourkes, T. L., *Brain*, **88**, 181 (1965).
38. Faull, R. L. M., and Laverty, R., *Expt'l. Neurol.*, **23**, 332 (1969).
39. Potts, A. M., *Trans. Am. Ophthal. Soc.*, **60**, 517 (1962).
40. Van Woert, M. H., *Proceed. Soc. for Exptl. Med.*, **129**, 165 (1968).
41. Forrest, I. S., et al., *Agressologie*, **7**, 147 (1966).
42. Bolt, A. G., and Forrest, I. S., *Recent Adv. in Biol. Psych.*, **10**, 29 (1968).
43. Rutschmann, J., et al., *Psychopharm. Serv. Ctr. Bull.*, **2**, (5), 73 (1962).
44. Blois, M. S., Jr., *J. Invest. Dermatology*, **45**, 475 (1965).
45. Thoenen, H., and Tranzer, J. P., *Ann. Rev. of Pharmacol.*, **13**, 169 (1973).
46. Lindquist, N. G., *Acta Radiologica*, (Supp.) 325, 77 (1973).
47. Gutmann, F. (*Personal communication, this symposium*, 1973).
48. Laborit, H., *Neurophysiologie. Aspects metaboliques et pharmacologiques*, Masson et Cie., Paris, 1969.

The Phenothiazines and Structurally Related Drugs, edited by I. S.
Forrest, C. J. Carr, and E. Usdin. Raven Press, New York © 1974.

Factors Predisposing to Drug-Induced Neurologic Effects

George E. Crane

Spring Grove State Hospital, Catonsville, Maryland 21228

INTRODUCTION

Several attempts have been made to relate age, sex, dose levels, and other variables to the neurologic side effects of psychoactive drugs. It is fairly well established that children and young adults are more susceptible to acute dystonia, whereas older subjects are more likely to develop pseudoparkinsonism. It has also been claimed that parkinsonian symptoms are more frequent in females than in males. Publications on the factors contributing to tardive dyskinesia are numerous and have been reviewed in a recent paper (1); hence, it will suffice here to summarize the most significant findings.

The prevalence of tardive dyskinesia ranges from a minimum of 0.5 to a maximum of over 40%. This discrepancy is attributable to a number of factors, such as age, chronicity of patients, and size of the samples. The lack of standardization of the methods used for the assessment of symptoms also plays a major role. With two exceptions, most investigators agree that the frequency of tardive dyskinesia increases with age. On the other hand, in only seven of 11 studies are females more likely to be so affected. With one notable exception, clinicians have not been able to demonstrate a clear-cut relationship between brain damage and tardive dyskinesia. Duration of treatment plays an important role, as most authors have described dyskinetic manifestations only after 2 yr of drug therapy. Clinical observations and theoretical considerations (2) suggest that antiparkinsonian drugs uncover latent dyskinesias.

Little is known about the effects of dosage and types of neuroleptics. Inaccurate treatment records, the use of many neuroleptics alone or in combinations, continuous adjustments of dose levels, and the addition of ancillary drugs permit only an approximate estimate of the intensity of drug exposure. Furthermore, dosage, duration of treatment, and the use of antiparkinsonian drugs are highly interrelated, as will be shown in this chapter, whereas the effects of certain variables tend to neutralize each other. For instance, older subjects tend to develop tardive dyskinesia to a significant degree, but receive smaller doses of neuroleptics. Similarly, the administration of high doses of neuroleptics tends to suppress overt manifestations of this disorder but, at the same time, creates a condition favoring the development of long-term, persistent motor disorders (3, 4). At the 1971 meeting of the American Psychiatric Association, I reported data obtained from a sample of 398 chronic hospitalized patients (5). Of the seven variables studied, only age and exposure to drugs were significantly related to tardive dyskinesia or parkinsonism.

The material to be presented here is based on a larger sample of patients and on more sensitive statistical analyses of data.

METHODS

Definitions and Measures

The characteristics of the patients' sample are detailed in Table 1. Doses of the several drugs prescribed to patients are expressed in milligrams of chlorpromazine equivalents per day. Maximum dose is based on the highest dose prescribed for a period of at least six months at any one time in the course of treatment. (In the event the highest dose is administered for less than six months, it is averaged with the next highest dose.) Duration of treatment is the number of years on drug therapy. (Patients with frequent or prolonged absences from the hospital or with inadequate records from this and other institutions are excluded from the study.) Continuity of treatment is measured in percentages of drug exposure from the initiation of treatment to 1970, when the survey was conducted. The use of antiparkinsonian agents refers to their administration at the time of the survey. Central nervous system (CNS) disorder includes organic brain diseases so diagnosed at the time of admission or in the course of hospitalization. Convulsive disorder, postlobotomy status, active or inactive CNS lues are also included in this category. Patients with well-documented extrapyramidal disorders (Huntington's disease, viral encephalitis, idiopathic, or senile parkinsonism) antedating drug therapy are not included. Some patients may have developed one of these conditions while receiving neuroleptic therapy but, except for

TABLE 1. *Characteristics of 669 chronic patients*

1. Median age	53 years
2. Sex	Male 287, female 382
3. Median maximum dose	430 mg
4. Median duration treatment	6.5 years
5. Continuous treatment	>90%, 217; <90%, 452
6. Median current dose	240 mg
7. Antiparkinsonian	Yes 165, no 504
8. CNS disorder	Yes 112, no 557

1–8: See text.

mild senile tremor and an occasional idiopathic case of parkinsonism, the number must have been negligible. Symptoms of tardive dyskinesia and parkinsonism were recorded separately and rated from a minimum of 0 to a maximum of 6 for each category.[1] All examinations were carried out blindly with regard to treatment.

Patient Population

In 1970, a survey for neurologic side effects was made of the total patient population in the chronic areas of Spring Grove State Hospital (except for geriatric services which have the main function of treating newly admitted patients over 65). The sample studied, however, includes a sizeable proportion of subjects who became geriatric cases during their prolonged stay in the hospital. Of the 900 patients housed in the various services, 669 were included in this investigation; the other 231 were excluded because of poor cooperation or the inadequacy of available medical records. Average total and average continuous hospitalization were 16 and 13 years, respectively. The correlation matrix in Table 2 shows the following. (a) Females are older than males, reflecting a general trend in this direction reported in most mental institutions. (b) Maximum dose, duration of treatment, continuity of drug administration, current dose levels, and the use of antiparkinsonian drugs are all interrelated (physicians tend to treat the same patients with high doses of medication plus antiparkinsonian drugs continuously and for long periods of time). (c) Maximum and current doses are inversely related to age, which also correlates with current medical practices. (d) The prevalence of CNS damage shows only a slight tendency to be greater in the older persons, mainly because the sample includes a fairly large number of patients with convulsive disorder and only a few with chronic brain syndromes due to age.

FINDINGS

Data on the prevalence of tardive dyskinesia and parkinsonism are summarized in Table 3. The frequency of tardive dyskinesia in this sample is comparable to that of studies reporting a high percentage of this disorder.[2] On the other hand, the frequency of the most severe cases approaches that of studies at the other extreme. Parkinsonism is less prevalent than tardive dyskinesia and may include extrapyramidal disorder due to age.

Tardive dyskinesia seems to be positively related to age, duration of treatment, and the use of antiparkinsonians, whereas there is no significant relationship between this disorder and the other five variables (zero correlation

---

[1] For classification and rating of neurologic effects, reference is made to Crane, G. E., and Naranjo, E. S., *Arch. Gen. Psychiat.*, **24**, 179 (1971).

[2] According to a study now in progress, signs consistent with minimal dyskinesia may not be drug related in patients over 65.

TABLE 2. *Correlation matrix*

Variable	Age	Sex	Mx dose	Duration	Continuous	Current	Antipark	CNS
1. Age								
2. Sex (Male)	$-0.1844^{a,b}$							
3. Maximum dose	-0.3909^a	-0.0158						
4. Duration treatment	0.013	0.0493	0.5062^a					
5. Continuous treatment	-0.0696	-0.0232	0.3046^a	0.4260^a				
6. Current dose	-0.309^*	-0.0640	0.6780^a	0.3442^a	0.2878^a			
7. Antiparkinsonian	-0.0811	0.0492	0.1993^a	0.1262^a	0.1438^a	0.2002^a		
8. CNS disorder	0.0910	-0.0128	-0.1445^a	-0.1441^a	-0.0720	-0.0720	-0.0509	

[a] Significant at <0.01 level.
[b] Males are significantly younger than females at <0.01 level, 1–8: see text.

TABLE 3. *Prevalence of tardive dyskinesia and parkinsonism*

Rating	Tardive dyskinesia		Parkinsonism	
	N	(%)	N	(%)
Minimal (1, 2)	213	(32)	159	(24)
Moderate (3, 4)	71	(11)	65	(10)
Severe (5, 6)	16	(2.4)	17	(2.5)

of Table 4). When the effects of age and the level of current dosage are averaged, the relation between tardive dyskinesia and maximum dose becomes significant. When maximum dose or duration is held constant, current dose levels become inversely related to tardive dyskinesia. On the other hand, duration of treatment is no longer a significant factor when continuity of treatment is controlled. The use of antiparkinsonian drugs, with its high correlation with the intensity of treatment, ceases to be positively related to tardive dyskinesia at the 0.01 level, when most factors related to drug administrations are averaged.

Parkinsonism is positively related to age and duration of treatment irrespective of the role played by the other variables. Female sex loses its significance as a contributing factor to parkinsonism when age is averaged out. Maximum dose is inversely related to parkinsonism if duration of treatment is held constant. The use of antiparkinsonian drugs becomes a significant factor when age is controlled.

Data on the effects of length of hospitalization on tardive dyskinesia or parkinsonism were not reported in Table 4, because the correlation between duration of hospitalization and of treatment was so high that the separation of the effects of the two variables on neurological effects was impossible. Consequently, a study was made of 287 patients admitted to the hospital prior to 1955, the year when the large-scale use of neuroleptics began in this hospital. In this subsample, there was no significant relationship between hospitalization and duration of treatment. The coefficient of correlation between tardive dyskinesia and hospitalization was 0.05, between parkinsonism and hospitalization 0.09 (both insignificant), suggesting that institutionalization *per se* does not produce neurologic side effects, at least in a very chronic population.

In view of the importance of age as a contributor to neurologic side effects, maximum dose and duration of treatment were analyzed separately in a sample of 311 patients aged 55 or over (Figs. 1, 2). The prevalence of tardive dyskinesia increased sharply in subjects receiving doses in excess of 200 mg of chlorpromazine equivalent a day for 6 months or longer. Similarly, the number of patients with moderate or severe dyskinesia became substantial when the duration of treatment was longer than 2 yr. (In this

TABLE 4. Coefficient of correlation (r) between tardive dyskinesia, parkinsonism, and eight variables

	Zero order correlation	Partial correlation controlling for							
	Tard. dysk.	Age	Sex	Mx dose	Dur. tr.	Cont. tr	curr. ds	Antpk.	CNS dis.
1. Age	0.2496	–	0.2297	0.2636	0.2515	0.2746	0.2441	0.2609	0.2521
2. Sex (male)	-0.0467	NS	–	NS	NS	NS	NS	NS	NS
3. Max dose	0.0720	0.1902	NS	–	NS	NS	0.1561	NS	NS
4. Dur. treat.	0.1409	0.1423	0.1435	0.1214	–	NS	0.1734	0.1277	0.1402
5. Cont treat.	0.0500	NS	NS	NS	NS	–	NS	NS	NS
6. Curr. dose	-0.0627	NS	NS	-0.1521	-0.1200	NS	–	NS	NS
7. Antipark.	0.1200	0.1453	NS	NS	NS	NS	0.1356	–	0.1200
8. CNS dis.	-0.0155	NS	NS	NS	NS	NS	NS	NS	–
Parkinsonism									
1. Age	0.2808	–	0.2618	0.2975	0.2834	0.3070	0.3011	0.2924	0.2835
2. Sex (male)	-0.1415	NS	–	-0.1418	-0.1534	-0.1518	-0.1418	-0.1480	-0.1417
3. Max dose	-0.0180	NS	NS	–	-0.1309	NS	NS	NS	NS
4. Dur. treat.	0.1838	0.1880	0.1930	0.2237	–	0.1401	0.1957	0.1724	0.1834
5. Cont. treat.	0.0830	NS	NS	NS	NS	–	NS	NS	NS
6. Curr. dose	0.0002	NS	NS	NS	NS	NS	–	NS	NS
7. Antipark.	0.1096	0.1384	NS	NS	NS	NS	NS	–	NS
8. CNS dis.	-0.0161	NS	NS	NS	NS	NS	NS	NS	–

r with abolute value >0.12 significant at <0.01 level, 1–8: see text.

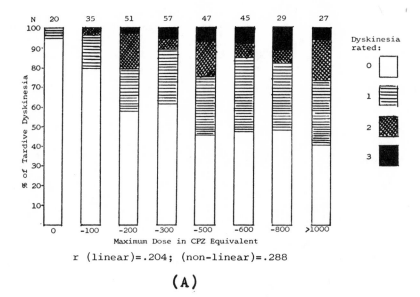

r (linear)=.204; (non-linear)=.288

(A)

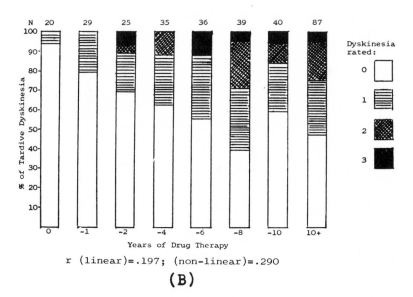

r (linear)=.197; (non-linear)=.290

(B)

FIG. 1. Percentage of tardive dyskinesia (A) by maximum dose and (B) by duration of drug treatment.

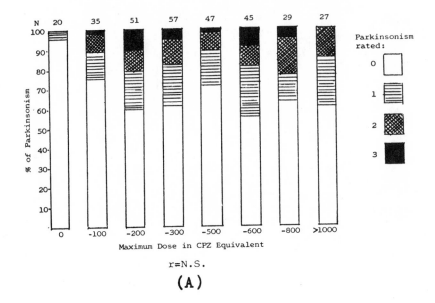

r=N.S.

(A)

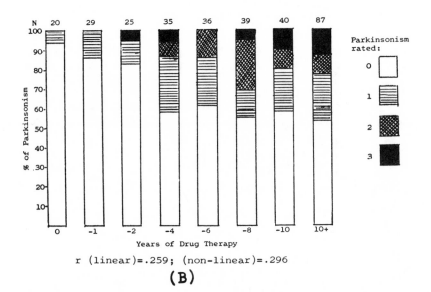

r (linear)=.259; (non-linear)=.296

(B)

FIG. 2. Percentage of parkinsonism (A) by maximum dose and (B) by duration of drug treatment.

sample, patients who were treated for short periods of time also received rather small doses of neuroleptics.) As for parkinsonism, the pattern was similar to that of tardive dyskinesia with regard to duration, but not with regard to maximum dose. In patients under 55, data were inconclusive. Dyskinesia was only marginally more prevalent in subjects treated with maximum doses exceeding 1,000 mg of chlorpromazine equivalent a day.

DISCUSSION

Data obtained from a study of this type must be interpreted with great caution because the administration of drugs, choice of dosage, and the use of antiparkinsonian agents were not random procedures. The patients' mental status as well as untoward drug effects may have influenced the physicians in their selection of types of neuroleptics, doses, and antidotes. For instance, the use of antiparkinsonian agents is positively related to symptoms of parkinsonism, at least in older patients. A simplistic interpretation of this finding may suggest that these compounds contribute to parkinsonism, when the truth of the matter is that patients exhibiting this syndrome are more likely to be treated with a substance designed to correct it, albeit ineffectively. The data presented here do not permit a rational interpretation unless one makes the following three assumptions: (a) physicians are generally more concerned about the control of psychotic manifestations than about discomfort of side effects or long-lasting neurologic effects; (b) in 1970, when the survey was conducted, the average physician had little awareness of tardive dyskinesia, and therefore, the presence of this disorder was not likely to affect his decision regarding treatment; and (c) parkinsonism, on the other hand, was usually diagnosed, particularly when it was severe. Doses were reduced and antiparkinsonian agents prescribed, but the administration of neuroleptics was seldom discontinued except for short periods of time.

It is legitimate to conclude that tardive dyskinesia increases with age, regardless of sex or duration of hospitalization. Organic brain disorder (based on diagnosis rather than on the degree of intellectual impairment) is not a significant factor. The use of high doses of neuroleptics in the course of chemotherapy contributes to tardive dyskinesia in older subjects only; a finding which is in agreement with the results of a previous study (4). The data on duration of treatment do not provide satisfactory information as to the length of drug exposure necessary for the development of tardive dyskinesia, because the symptoms detected at the time of this survey may have been present for some time. The syndrome of tardive dyskinesia, however, increases sharply only after the second year of therapy, as pointed out by several authors. In certain conditions, higher doses tend to reduce the severity of symptoms, thus indirectly confirming the observation that the reinstitution of drug therapy following withdrawal of medication tends to suppress the overt manifestations of dyskinesia. Antiparkinsonian drugs may uncover tardive dyskinesia in older subjects under certain circumstances.

The interpretation of data on parkinsonism is more difficult for reasons stated earlier. Age unquestionably is an important factor, but sex does not appear to play a significant role. Contrary to traditional belief (6), females are not more susceptible to this disorder than males, at least not after prolonged exposure to drugs. Parkinsonism, on the other hand, tends to increase with the duration of treatment, since length of therapy is positively related to parkinsonism, irrespective of the other variables. Hence, the contention that parkinsonism often tends to subside in the course of treatment (or with the use of antiparkinsonian agents) may be applicable only to the early stages of treatment.

In conclusion, age and exposure to drugs are contributing factors to neurologic side effects, but the individual's vulnerability to the neurotoxicity of phenothiazines and related drugs must play a major role, too. Otherwise, it would be difficult to explain why certain subjects in their thirties or forties develop rather severe dyskinesia after an intake of medication which is not excessive, while a certain percentage of elderly subjects remain neurologically intact despite intensive exposure to drugs. Inasmuch as these individual factors are not known, the administration of neuroleptics must be kept at a minimum, particularly for older patients. The amount of neuroleptic medication received by these Spring Grove State Hospital patients is fairly representative of a population of this type (7). Thus, the high proportion of persons exhibiting tardive dyskinesia and/or parkinsonism clearly indicates that the current practices of prescribing these drugs are in need of revision.

SUMMARY

An attempt was made to relate nine variables to tardive dyskinesia and parkinsonism in a chronic hospital population. The data indicate that tardive dyskinesia is positively related to age, regardless of the effects of other variables. In patients over 55, exposure to drugs is also positively related to this disorder, while high current doses seem to suppress it. Parkinsonism increases with age and the duration of treatment. Thus, duration of treatment and/or high dosage contribute to both tardive dyskinesia and parkinsonism, particularly in patients older than 55. The fact that a large number of patients are affected by neurologic side effects in a sample which is fairly representative of long-term hospitalized populations suggests that current practices of drug administration should be revised.

REFERENCES

1. Crane, G. E., *Brit. J. Psychiat.,* **122,** 395 (1973).
2. Rubovitz, R., and Klawans, H. L., *Arch. Gen. Psychiat.,* **27,** 502 (1972).

3. Crane, G. E., *Aggressol.,* **9,** 209 (1968).
4. Crane, G. E., *Arch. Neurol.,* **22,** 176 (1970).
5. Crane, G. E., *Scientific Proceedings (Abstracts) 124th Annual Meeting, American Psychiatric Association,* 112, 1971, Washington, D.C.
6. Duvoisin, R. E., In *Psychopharmacology,* Efron, D. H., (ed.), Public Health Service Publication 1836, U.S. Government Printing Office, Washington, D.C., 1968, pp. 561–573.
7. Prien, R. F., and Klett, C. J., *Schizophrenia Bulletin,* **5,** 64 (1972).

The Phenothiazines and Structurally Related Drugs, edited by I. S. Forrest, C. J. Carr, and E. Usdin. Raven Press, New York © 1974.

Effects of Promazine and Chlorpromazine Metabolites on the Cornea

H. Richard Adams, Albert A. Manian, Marie L. Steenberg, and Joseph P. Buckley

Department of Pharmacology, University of Texas Southwestern Medical School at Dallas, Dallas, Texas 75235, Psychopharmacology Research Branch, NIMH, Rockville, Maryland 20852, and Department of Pharmacology, University of Pittsburgh School of Pharmacy, Pittsburgh, Pennsylvania 15213.

INTRODUCTION

Ophthalmopathies have been observed in man and in experimental animals after administration of the phenothiazine-derivative tranquilizers, and at least three entities have been described. Corneal-lenticular opacities have been observed concomitantly with pigmentation and discoloration of exposed portions of the skin during chronic chlorpromazine administration (1–7), and this syndrome is thought to be related to the photosensitizing qualities of the phenothiazine-like compounds. Pigmentary degenerative changes of the retina have also been associated with certain phenothiazine derivatives (3, 5, 8–10), and are believed to be due to concentration of these agents in the melanin-rich uveal tract. Corneal and lenticular opacities, which may not be related to melanin interaction and which have been present without concurrent skin disorders, have also been observed following the prolonged administration of chlorpromazine (5–7).

Although several investigations have attempted to define the pathophysiologic processes involved in chlorpromazine-related corneal disorders, the etiologic origin(s) has not been determined. It has been suggested that biotransformation products, rather than the parent molecule, may be responsible for ocular disorders observed following the administration of phenothiazine-derivative tranquilizers (3, 4, 7). The present studies were conducted to determine the effects of promazine, chlorpromazine, and certain of their metabolites on the cornea when injected directly into the anterior chamber of eyes of laboratory animals.

MATERIALS AND METHODS

One hundred and eighty-eight rabbits, weighing between 2 and 4 kg, of both sexes, were utilized in the present study; 48 of these were pigmented (black and white or brown and white) and the remainder were albino (New Zealand).

Three domestic short-haired cats, two beagle dogs, one rhesus monkey *(Macaca mulatta),* and two cynomolgus monkeys *(M. iris)* were also utilized.

All animals were clinically healthy as determined by physical examination, had been laboratory maintained for a period of at least one week (rabbits) or several months, and had not knowingly been exposed to any chemical agent for at least the interval during which they were housed in the laboratory (rabbits) or for several weeks prior to an experiment.

The intracameral injection technique utilized in the present study necessitated anesthetization. Methohexital or pentobarbital was administered intravenously to rabbits until a surgical level of anesthesia was reached. Pentobarbital was similarly used in the dogs. Ketamine was given intramuscularly to the cats, and phencyclidine was used in the subhuman primates.

Following anesthetization, the anterior chamber was entered through the superior aspect of the cornea in approximately the "12:00 o'clock" position, anterior to the limbus 2 to 4 mm, with a 26.5-gauge hypodermic needle connected to a 1-ml syringe. Location of the needle in the anterior chamber was ascertained by visual observation (Fig. 1), and the drug was then injected. The needle was withdrawn after injection of the agent, and no attempt was made to stop leakage of the aqueous humor through the puncture site. A modification of this procedure was utilized in some cases in which the superficial portion of the cornea was first incised using an ophthalmic "needle-knife," and the anterior chamber was then entered by insertion of a needle through the incision. The globe was immobilized by digital pressure or by scleral fixation.

Eyes were examined at 6, 12, 18, and 24 hr, and periodically thereafter, following the injection of the test compounds. Histopathologic and slit-lamp microscopic examination of affected corneas were conducted in certain instances.

One of the following phenothiazine derivatives was injected directly into the anterior chamber during general anesthesia: promazine hydrochloride (PZ); chlorpromazine hydrochloride (CPZ); chlorpromazine sulfoxide hydrochloride (CPZ-SO); 7-hydroxychlorpromazine (7-OH-CPZ); 8-hydroxychlorpromazine (8-OH-CPZ); 7-methoxychlorpromazine (7-MO-CPZ); 2-hydroxypromazine (2-OH-PZ); 3-hydroxypromazine (3-OH-PZ); 2,3-dihydroxypromazine (2,3-Di-OH-PZ); 7,8-dihydroxychlorpromazine (7,8-Di-OH-CPZ); 0.9% NaCl; and 0.1 N HCl. Initially, 100 to 200 μg of each compound in 0.1 ml diluent (0.9% NaCl solution, and in some cases a few drops of HCl) was injected into eight to 28 different eyes, which were then observed periodically for 2 weeks. If a compound did not induce corneal changes within that period, additional experiments with that agent were excluded from the study.

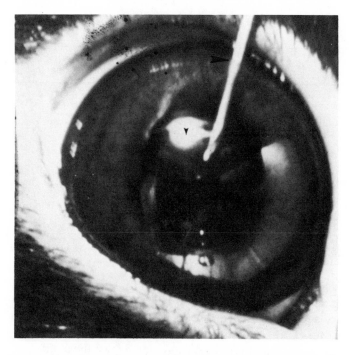

FIG. 1. Intracameral injection technique: large horizontal arrow points to the entry of the needle through the cornea, small perpendicular arrow is imprinted on a "highlight" (reflection of flash bulb). Note the complete transparency of the cornea (pigmented rabbit).

RESULTS

The results obtained with pigmented and albino rabbits during the present investigation are summarized in Table 1. Since initial studies utilizing 48 pigmented and 24 albino rabbits indicated no essential differences in the responsiveness of albino rabbit eyes when compared with the eyes of pigmented rabbits, subsequent studies utilized albino rabbits due to their greater commercial availability.

Controls

It is readily apparent that the trauma and related disruption of ocular homeostasis resulting from intracameral injections have no readily discernible effect on corneal transparency at the time intervals studied. Sterile isotonic saline in a volume of 0.1 ml was injected into the anterior chamber of 44 different eyes of 62 rabbits; in no instance was corneal opacity observed (Table 1). A small (< 0.25 mm) white scar was often observed at the corneal puncture site in control as well as in treated eyes. Fibrin clots were also occasionally observed in the anterior chamber of treated and control eyes, but usually disappeared within a 24- to 48-hr period. Similarly,

TABLE 1. *Effect of intracameral injection of PZ, CPZ, and certain metabolites of these agents on the cornea of rabbits*

Compound	Dose injected	Number of eyes injected	Incidence (number) of corneal opacity	% Incidence
0.9% NaCl	0.1 ml	44	0	0
0.1 N HCl	0.1 ml	14	0	0
PZ	100 μg	16	0	0
CPZ	100 μg	28	0	0
	200 μg	4	0	0
CPZ-SO	100 μg	4	0	0
	200 μg	4	0	0
2-OH-PZ	100 μg	10	0	0
3-OH-PZ	100 μg	10	0	0
7-MO-CPZ	100 μg	10	0	0
7-OH-CPZ	100 μg	26	7	27
8-OH-CPZ	100 μg	40	21	50
2,3-Di-OH-PZ	100 μg	37	26	70
7,8-Di-OH-CPZ	100 μg	69	61	88

transient vascular congestion was periodically seen in treated and control eyes in the superior aspect of the episcleral tissue. In three control and one treated eye, hemorrhage occurred following inadvertent tearing of the iris, and these eyes were deleted from the study. Apparent purulent infection occurred in one eye and this animal was deleted from the study.

Additional "control" eyes were injected with 0.1 ml of 0.1 N HCl since several of the compounds presently studied are acidic. However, the injection of 0.1 N HCl (pH < 4) into 14 eyes of nine rabbits elicited no visible changes in corneal transparency (Table 1). During each separate experiment conducted throughout the study, saline or HCl was always administered in several eyes as a continuous control measure.

PZ, CPZ, CPZ-SO, 7-MO-CPZ, 2-OH-PZ, and 3-OH-PZ

These compounds were injected individually in doses of 100 or 200 μg (see Table 1) into eight to 28 separate eyes. Corneal opacity was not induced by these agents.

7-Hydroxychlorpromazine

Twenty-six eyes were injected with 7-OH-CPZ (100 μg) and corneal opacity occurred in seven eyes, an incidence of approximately 27% (Table 1). Corneal opacity was seen within 18 to 24 hr after injection, was usually present for 3 or 4 days, and rarely lasted longer than 5 days.

8-Hydroxychlorpromazine

Forty eyes were injected with the 8-hydroxy derivative of chlorpromazine and corneal opacity occurred in 21 eyes, an incidence of approximately

50% (Table 1). Corneal changes were seen within 18 to 24 hr and they were usually absent by the 4th or 5th day after injection.

2,3-Dihydroxypromazine

The 2,3-dihydroxy derivative of promazine was injected into 37 eyes and corneal opacity was induced in 26 eyes, an incidence of approximately 70% (Table 1). Opacity developed within 24 hr after injection and was usually present for 7 to 8 days.

7,8-Dihydroxychlorpromazine

The 7,8-dihydroxy derivative of chlorpromazine induced corneal opacity in 61 of the 69 eyes in which it was injected, an incidence of approximately 88% (Table 1). Corneal changes were present within 24 hr after injection and they were usually visible for 11 to 16 days. The quantity of 7,8-Di-OH-CPZ utilized throughout the study was usually 100 μg due to the highly reproducible corneal lesions seen at this dose level; however, corneal opacity occurred following the similar injection of 50 μg of the metabolite and occasionally with 25 μg.

The topical application of these metabolites onto the epithelial surface of the cornea had no visible effect on corneal transparency.

Corneal changes induced by the intracameral injection of 7-OH-CPZ, 8-OH-CPZ, 2,3-Di-OH-PZ, and 7,8-Di-OH-CPZ appeared similar, with the exception of the stated differences in incidence and in the length of time that changes were visible. Gross observation of affected eyes revealed a diffuse cloudy "milky" opacification of the cornea (Fig. 2). Coloration of corneal opacity varied from "milky white" to "milky gray-white" and occasionally "milky blue." Characteristically, the entire cornea was affected, but less severe involvement was usually observed when lower doses of the compounds were tested. A clear dose-response relationship was not consistently obtainable; however, this could be attributed to the inability to control the amount of compound and aqueous humor which leaked through the corneal puncture following withdrawal of the injection needle. Affected corneas appeared markedly thickened; however, gross observation indicated no apparent increase in globe size. In addition, these corneal changes did not seem to elicit pain since rabbits with affected corneas did not physically react to ophthalmic examination to any greater extent than nontreated rabbits. In fact, treated and control rabbits were quite immobile during rather prolonged slit-lamp examinations when grasped by the scruff of the neck with one hand and held around the pelvic region with the other hand.

It was extremely difficult to assess visual acuity in the rabbits. It seemed, however, that vision was impaired during the duration of severe corneal opacity as evidenced by decreased avoidance of approaching objects. How-

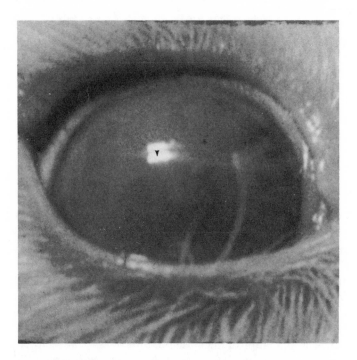

FIG. 2. Corneal opacity induced by 100 µg of 7,8-Di-OH-CPZ injected into the anterior chamber 24 hr prior to photograph. Note lack of corneal transparency: the iris and pupil are not visible. Compare with corneas in Figs. 1 and 4. Small arrow is imprinted on a reflection of the flash bulb (pigmented rabbit).

ever, as corneal transparency recurred, vision apparently returned to normal. In addition, the lenses were not visible due to the severity of corneal involvement and resulting lack of transparency. Following resolution of corneal changes, however, the lens appeared grossly normal.

Since 7,8-Di-OH-CPZ consistently induced corneal opacity, additional studied were conducted with this compound. In order to determine if light had an effect on the corneal changes, 12 albino rabbits were used. Saline (0.1 ml) was injected into one eye and 7,8-Di-OH-CPZ (100 µg in 0.1 ml) into the other eye of each rabbit. Six of the rabbits were maintained in a darkened room and the other six were placed in an animal room maintained on a 12-hr light-dark cycle. In this experiment, corneal opacity developed in all eyes injected with 7,8-Di-OH-CPZ whether the rabbits were maintained in the dark or lighted room (Table 2). Again, the similar injection of NaCl had no apparent effect on corneal transparency.

Slit-lamp biomicroscopic examination conducted 24 hr after injection of the compounds indicated that corneas exposed to 7,8-Di-OH-CPZ were markedly thickened and the stroma appeared diffusely edematous (Fig. 3). In addition, diffuse yellowish-gray discoloration was observed in the

TABLE 2. *Effect of dark or light-dark environment on incidence of corneal opacity induced by intracameral injection of 7,8-Di-OH-CPZ in rabbits*

Compound	Dose injected	Light condition	Eyes injected	Incidence of corneal opacity
0.9% NaCl	0.1 ml	Dark	6	0
		Light-Dark	6	0
7,8-Di-OH-CPZ	100 μg	Dark	6	6
		Light-Dark	6	6

posterior portion of the cornea. However, CPZ had no apparent effect on the cornea (Fig. 4).

In order to examine histological characteristics of affected corneas, the 7,8-Di-OH derivative of CPZ (100 μg) was injected into an additional four eyes of eight rabbits, and CPZ (100 μg) was injected into the remaining

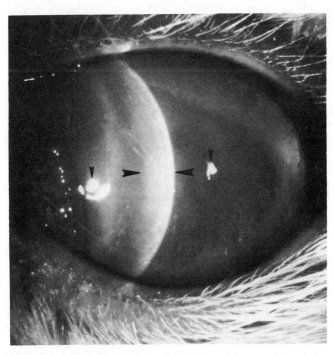

FIG. 3. Slit-lamp appearance of corneal opacity induced by 100 μg of 7,8-Di-OH-CPZ injected into the anterior chamber 24 hr prior to photograph. Note lack of corneal transparency: the iris and pupil are not visible. The distance between the large horizontal arrows indicates the thickness of the slit-lamp reflection and represents the thickness of the cornea. Compare the lack of corneal transparency and the markedly thickened cornea with the normal cornea in Fig. 4. Small perpendicular arrows are pointing toward reflections of the flash bulb (albino rabbit).

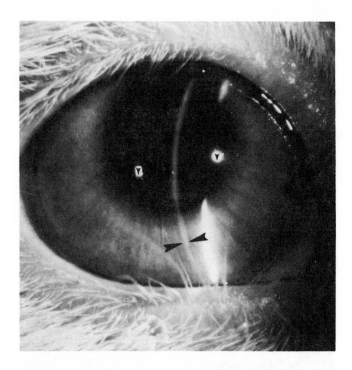

FIG. 4. Lack of effect of CPZ on the cornea, 100 μg injected into the anterior chamber 24 hr prior to photograph. Note transparency of cornea: the iris and pupil are visible. The distance between the large semihorizontal arrows indicates the thickness of the slit-lamp reflection and represents the thickness of the cornea. Small perpendicular arrows are imprinted on reflections of the flash bulb (albino rabbit).

four eyes. The rabbits were euthanatized by acute pentobarbital overdosage 24 to 30 hr after injection of the agents. Both eyeballs were removed and placed in 10% potassium phosphate-buffered formalin. After formalin fixation, the eyeballs were imbedded in paraffin, sectioned, and stained with hematoxylin and eosin. Histopathologic examination of eyes treated with 7,8-Di-OH-CPZ indicated diffuse stromal edema of affected corneas. CPZ had no apparent effect on the cornea.

Additional studies with 7,8-Di-OH-CPZ indicate that this compound induces similar corneal opacity in cats, dogs, and monkeys *(M. mulatta* and *M. iris)*. An example of typical corneal opacity induced by this agent in a monkey is seen in Fig. 5.

DISCUSSION

Phenothiazine-derivative tranquilizers have been widely utilized in the chronic pharmacotherapeutic management of psychiatric patients. Within the past decade, several investigators have associated long-term high-dose

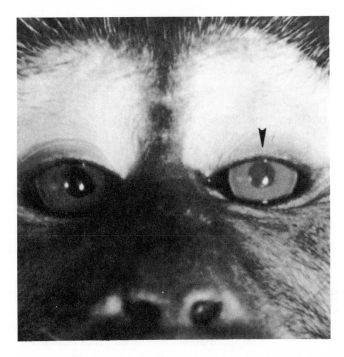

FIG. 5. Corneal opacity induced in a monkey (*M. iris*) by 100 μg of 7,8-Di-OH-CPZ injected into the anterior chamber 24 hr prior to the photograph. Arrow indicates eye injected with 7,8-Di-OH-CPZ: the other eye was injected with saline 24 hr prior to photograph. Note diffuse haze of affected cornea.

administration of several of these agents, particularly chlorpromazine, with different types of ocular disorders. Despite the repeated incidence of chlorpromazine-induced ophthalmopathies, little is known regarding the etiologic origin of these conditions. Several investigators have suggested that breakdown products rather than the parent chlorpromazine molecule may be responsible for ocular changes observed following prolonged administration (3, 4, 7). In the present study, evidence is presented which suggests that specific hydroxylated metabolites of chlorpromazine, but not the parent drug, may be causally related to the induction of corneal opacity observed in man following chronic chlorpromazine administration.

Previous reports have indicated that at least three different pathologic ocular entities may result following exposure of patients to phenothiazine-related tranquilizers. These are (a) corneal-lenticular opacities observed concomitantly with photosensitivity-related skin pigmentation (1–7), (b) pigmentary retinopathy associated with concentration of phenothiazine-compounds in the melanin-rich uveal tract (5, 8–10), and (c) lenticular and corneal opacities observed without the concurrent presence of skin changes (5–7).

Greiner and Berry (1) first reported the occurrence of skin pigmentation and corneal and lenticular opacities in amenorrheic women following long-term high-dose administration of chlorpromazine for control of various mental illnesses. Skin pigmentation and corneal-sclera changes were observed only on those areas normally exposed to light. Subsequent reports by several investigators have substantiated the occurrence of oculocutaneous pigmentation in chronically treated patients of both sexes (2–7). Due to the presence of discoloration only in those areas exposed to light, it is believed that these changes are related to the photosensitizing characteristics of phenothiazine-like compounds. In the present investigation, corneal opacification occurred in rabbits maintained in darkness as well as in rabbits housed in a light-dark environment. It therefore seems untenable to associate these corneal changes directly with photosensitization. However, present data should not be interpreted to exclude the possibility that these metabolite-induced corneal abnormalities may predispose the eye in some way to photosensitivity-related disorders.

Interaction of chlorpromazine with melanin has also been suggested as a potential contributing factor to oculocutaneous pigmentation changes since melanin apparently forms a charge-transfer complex *in vitro* and *in vivo* with chlorpromazine compounds (11). In addition, phenothiazine-derivatives concentrate in the melanin-rich uveal tract of pigmented animals (12), but such localization is not observed in albino animals. This interaction with melanin has been postulated as a potential mediating factor in chorio-retinal damage observed following treatment with related tranquilizers (12, 13). In the present study, corneal opacity was observed in albino rabbits as well as in pigmented rabbits. The interaction of injected metabolites with melanin may, therefore, be excluded as a contributing factor.

Ocular changes that may not be directly related to either photosensitivity or melanin interaction have been observed in man following repeated administration of chlorpromazine. Barsa et al. (14) observed anterior lenticular and posterior corneal opacities in 175 of 658 mentally ill patients receiving phenothiazine tranquilizers. Of these 175 patients, 67 were reported as showing no evidence of skin photosensitivity. Tredici et al. (7) and Margolis and Goble (15) have also reported the occurrence of ocular disorders without the concomitant presence of skin photosensitivity changes.

In the present study, diffuse corneal opacity was observed in rabbits following the intracameral injection of certain metabolites of promazine and of chlorpromazine. It is unlikely that these changes are directly related either to photosensitization or to melanin interaction, as previously discussed. Therefore, the present observations suggest that at least certain types of corneal changes observed following chronic administration of chlorpromazine may be related to specific ophthalmic toxicity of hydroxylated metabolites of that compound. That metabolites may play a role in ocular toxicity of the phenothiazines in man has been previously suggested (3, 4, 7). In addition, the corneal lesions produced in rabbits in the present study were similar to certain changes seen in man. Corneal opacities have been repeatedly observed in psychiatric patients receiving chronic chlorpromazine therapy (1–7), and discoloration (white, whitish-brown, yellowish-brown), primarily of the posterior cornea, are routine. In the present study, opacity of the cornea and diffuse yellowish discoloration located primarily in the posterior cornea were observed. Unlike lesions seen in man after chronic chlorpromazine treatment, however, marked diffuse edema of the stroma was observed in rabbit corneas following a single injection of hydroxylated metabolites. It would be interesting to observe the effects of repeated injections of subminimal doses of the metabolites into the anterior chamber over a period of time. This procedure not only would provide additional information concerning the manner of formation and nature of the corneal opacity but might also demonstrate anterior lenticular-lesion development.

The mechanism of corneal opacification induced by promazine and chlorpromazine metabolites in rabbits has not been determined. Corneal damage could theoretically result from such nonspecific causes as precipitation of the involved compounds in the anterior chamber. Such chemical changes, although not visually observed, cannot be completely discounted. It seems unlikely, though, that only certain metabolites would be affected in this manner. The dihydroxylated derivatives are the more polar compounds and it would be expected that their relatively greater water solubility would actually decrease the likelihood of their precipitation in the aqueous humor. Yet, these metabolites consistently induced corneal changes.

The acute onset of corneal edema suggests rather pronounced effects on membrane permeability of the corneal endothelial cells. The corneal endothelium, composed of a mono layer of endothelial cells, is the innermost layer of the cornea, and it functions to maintain the cornea relatively free of aqueous humor. This is accomplished either by providing a simple barrier to aqueous flow or by pumping the aqueous back into the anterior chamber. Thus, the rapid onset of corneal edema induced by presently studied metabolites suggests rather marked interference with endothelial function. Alternatively, membrane permeability of corneal stromal cells or their ultra structures may be adversely affected by these metabolites so that the water-electrolyte fluxes essential to normal cell function are altered. Previous studies have clearly indicated, in fact, that at least certain types of mammalian cells are affected by phenothiazine derivatives with resulting alterations in membrane permeability (16–18).

Although the mechanism remains unclear, the fact remains that under present experimental conditions, only specific metabolites of chlorpromazine and promazine induce corneal changes when injected directly into the ocular anterior chamber. 7-OH-CPZ, 8-OH-CPZ, 2,3-Di-OH-PZ, and

7,8-Di-OH-CPZ induce reproducible diffuse corneal opacity, whereas the parent compounds PZ and CPZ and several other metabolites of these drugs have no discernible effect on corneal transparency.

SUMMARY

Promazine (PZ), chlorpromazine (CPZ), and several metabolites of these phenothiazine-derivative tranquilizers were injected individually into the anterior chamber of rabbit eyes. The 2,3-dihydroxy (Di-OH) derivative of PZ and the 7,8-Di-OH derivative of CPZ consistently (> 70 and 88%, respectively) induced diffuse corneal opacity in both pigmented and albino rabbits. Corneal opacity occurred in rabbits maintained in a darkened room as well as in those rabbits housed in a light-dark environment. The 7-hydroxy (OH)-CPZ and 8-OH-CPZ derivatives variably induced corneal opacity (27 and 50% incidence, respectively); whereas PZ, CPZ, CPZ-sulfoxide, 7-methoxy-CPZ, 2-OH-PZ, 3-OH-PZ, 0.9% NaCl solution, and 0.1 N HCl had no apparent effects on corneal transparency. Corneal opacity was evident within 18 to 24 hr after injection of the compounds. Corneal opacity induced by either the 7 or 8 monohydroxy CPZ derivative or 2,3-Di-OH-PZ lasted 5 to 8 days, whereas 11 to 16 days was usually required for resolution of corneal changes produced by 7,8-Di-OH-CPZ. Histopathologic examinations of rabbit eyes treated with 7,8-Di-OH-CPZ revealed extensive stromal edema in affected corneas. A markedly thickened and diffusely edematous cornea with yellowish-gray discoloration in the posterior portion of the cornea was observed upon slit-lamp biomicroscopy. Present findings indicate that only specific hydroxylated metabolites of PZ and CPZ, but not the parent molecules PZ and CPZ, induce corneal opacity when injected into the ocular anterior chamber.

ACKNOWLEDGMENTS

This work was supported in part by U.S. Public Health Service contract FDA 72-312 from the Food and Drug Administration, and contract HSM-42-71-72 from the National Institute of Mental Health.

The authors gratefully acknowledge the contributions of Dr. J. Lynn and Mr. W. Stenstrom of the Ophthalmology Department, University of Texas Southwestern Medical School at Dallas, and of Dr. P. Marineau, Department of Pathology, McKeesport Hospital, Pittsburgh.

REFERENCES

1. Greiner, A. C., and Berry, K., *Canad. Med. Ass. J.*, **90**, 663 (1964).
2. Feldman, P. E., and Frierson, B. D., *Am. J. Psychiat.*, **121**, 187 (1964).
3. Siddall, J. R., *Arch. Ophth.*, **74**, 460 (1965).
4. Sandvig, K., *Acta Ophthalmol.*, **43**, 730 (1965).

5. Mathalon, M. B. R., *Lancet, 2,* 111 (1965).
6. McClanahan, W. S., Harris, J. E., Knobloch, W. H., Tredici, L. M., and Udasco, R. L., *Arch. Ophth., 75,* 319 (1966).
7. Tredici, L. M., Schiele, B. C., and McClanahan, W. S., *Minn. Med., 48,* 569 (1965).
8. Weekley, R. D., Potts, A. M., Reboton, J., and May, R. H., *Arch. Ophth., 64,* 65 (1960).
9. May, R. H., Selymes, P., Weekley, R. D., and Potts, A. M., *J. Nerv. and Ment. Dis., 130,* 230 (1960).
10. Siddall, J. R., *Canad. J. Ophthal., 1,* 190 (1966).
11. Bolt, A. G., and Forrest, I. S., *Rec. Adv. Biol. Psychiatr., 10,* 20 (1968).
12. Potts, A. M., *Invest. Ophth., 1,* 522 (1962).
13. Potts, A. M., *Invest. Ophth., 1,* 290 (1962).
14. Barsa, J. A., Newton, J. C., and Saunders, J. C., *J. A. M. A., 193,* 98 (1965).
15. Margolis, L. H., and Goble, J. L., *J. A. M. A., 193,* 95 (1965).
16. Freeman, A. R., and Spirtes, M. A., *Biochem. Pharmacol., 11,* 161 (1962).
17. Freeman, A. R., and Spirtes, M. A., *Biochem. Pharmacol., 12,* 47 (1963).
18. Holmes, D. E., and Piette, L. H., *J. Pharmacol. Exp. Therap., 173,* 78 (1970).

The Phenothiazines and Structurally Related Drugs, edited by I. S.
Forrest, C. J. Carr, and E. Usdin. Raven Press, New York © 1974.

Pigmented Hyperkeratosis Among Schizophrenic Patients Treated with Nicotinic Acid

J. R. Wittenborn, Robert Nenno, Harvey Rothberg, and Walter B. Shelley

Interdisciplinary Research Center, Rutgers University, The State University of New Jersey, New Brunswick, New Jersey 08903, New Jersey College of Medicine and Dentistry, Newark, New Jersey, New Jersey College of Medicine and Dentistry, New Brunswick, New Jersey, and Department of Dermatology, University of Pennsylvania School of Medicine, Philadelphia, Pennsylvania

INTRODUCTION

The present report describes acanthosis nigricans-like lesions among patients receiving high levels of both nicotinic acid (3,000 mg per day) and phenothiazines over an extended period of time (1). Although for some years this particular dermatosis has been known to be associated with nicotinic acid, relatively few instances are described in the literature.

Acanthosis nigricans was described in the latter part of the nineteenth century (2, 3). The condition appears as a darkened, slightly raised epidermis which is generally smooth in its appearance and may become conspicuous on those portions of the body which are relatively moist and ordinarily covered by clothing, particularly the axillary, antecubital, pubic, and popliteal regions, and the waist. Furthermore, continuing pressure from other surfaces appears to be a factor. The condition has been associated with internal malignancy, endrocrinopathies, liver disorders, and nicotinic acid.

After describing the appearance of acanthosis nigricans-like lesions in a hypercholesteremic patient who had received 4,000 mg nicotinic acid per day for a period of 4 months, Tromovitch et al. (4) offered a threefold classification for acanthosis nigricans: (a) benign acanthosis nigricans, a genodermatosis inherited through regular or irregular dominance not associated with internal malignancy; (b) malignant acanthosis nigricans, which is always associated with internal malignancy; and (c) pseudoacanthosis nigricans associated with obesity on a nutritional, constitutional, or endocrine basis.

In a 1968 review of 90 cases of acanthosis nigricans seen at the Mayo Clinic between 1935 and 1966, Brown and Winkelmann (5) proposed that the disease be divided into two types: malignant and benign, with the benign cases further classified in terms of etiologic subtypes.

Three cases associated with drugs as a subgroup of the benign type included two cases associated with nicotinic acid. Two such cases had been described also by Parsons and Flinn in an earlier report (6) of the treatment of hypercholesteremia with nicotinic acid.

FINDINGS FROM THE PRESENT SAMPLE

In the course of an investigation designed to test the hypothesis that nicotinic acid at a high dosage level (3,000 mg per day) is an effective supplement in the treatment of schizophrenia, 47 patients were maintained on nicotinic acid for a period of 24 months. The patients were all schizophrenic males recently admitted to the New Jersey State Hospital at Marlboro. As suitable patients came to the Male Admission Ward, they were assigned to the treatment regimen.

Nicotinic acid was administered daily as a supplement to the patient's usual treatment regimen, which almost invariably began with a phenothiazine, and for most patients the continuing medication included phenothiazines. For some individuals, however, the phenothiazine dosage level was reduced in correspondence with amelioration of the symptoms. In keeping with current practices, most of the patients left the hospital after 4 or 5 months of inpatient care and were maintained according to their needs on an outpatient basis.

Regardless of their outpatient status, however, all patients were closely monitored throughout their treatment period with regard to actual ingestion of prescribed nicotinic acid.

In May 1969, one of the outpatients appeared with a pattern of marked pigmentation which was sufficiently well developed to be a cause for alarm in both the patient and the treatment staff. Physical examination revealed a pattern of pigmented hyperkeratosis distributed over the trunk, upper thighs, and upper arms. The pigmentation was most marked about the axillae, pubic area, and small of the back. There was no evidence of dermatosis of the hands, face, or feet. In other respects, the physical examination was unremarkable. Were it not for the freedom from pigmentation in areas exposed to the sun, the condition would have been suggestive of a pellagra-type dermatosis.[1] The biopsy material revealed a prominent hyperkeratosis, papillomatosis, and moderate irregular acanthosis. The malphigian layer was thin with a flattening of the basal layer and an effacement of the rete ridges. No evidence of malignancy was indicated, and the histologic features were considered to be nonspecific.[2]

As a result of the development of this dermatosis, all patients were examined for evidence of pigmentation, and thereafter the regularly scheduled

---

[1] Internist's report.
[2] Biopsy report.

physical examination included scrutiny of all body surfaces. Twenty-three of the 47 patients who continued on nicotinic acid for the full 24 months developed the characteristic pattern of pigmentation to an unmistakable and cosmetically undesirable degree. There were no significant variations in biopsy reports. The superficial resemblance to acanthosis nigricans was noted, but the papillamatosis was considered to be too minimal and the papillary edema too slight to support this diagnosis.[3] Some of the patients reported that this hyperkeratotic epidermis could be removed by vigorous abrasive scrubbing. Discussion of this condition with numerous dermatologists at the AMA meeting in New York was not fruitful.[4]

Because of the prevalence of this condition and the uniformity with which the various cases were described by several consulting dermatologists, the possible extrinsic sources of this dermatosis were explored. The nicotinic acid was supplied through the courtesy of Squibb; the manufacturer was Cobb-Warner. The processing and packaging of this particular lot of nicotinic acid was carefully reviewed, and several samples of the medication distributed to patients were examined for foreign chemicals. No possible source of contamination was revealed, and no foreign substance could be found in the samples tested. Since some of the patients were in the hospital for a very short period of time and developed the pigmentation months later while on an outpatient status, it could not be associated with the hospital. The appearance of the pigmentation was also unrelated to the season.

For various reasons characteristic of clinical research, all of the patients who entered the study did not continue through the full 24 month schedule of treatment. Among the 47 patients completing the nicotinic acid series, 23 developed the characteristic pattern of pigmentation. In no instance did this pigmentation occur prior to the fourth month of treatment, and in one patient its appearance was delayed until the 17th month. Analysis of the data revealed that all of the patients developing this pattern of pigmentation had been receiving phenothiazine medication concurrently with the nicotinic acid. Of the patients receiving both phenothiazines and niacin treatment, about 60% developed the characteristic pigmentation. Of those who failed to develop pigmentation, 10 (about 40%) had been maintained on a reduced phenothiazine regimen or treatment by some other psychotropic drugs.

Very few of the patients developing the pigmentation were over 35 years of age: only two (22%) of those over 35 were pigmented, whereas 21 (58%) of the patients 35 or under were pigmented. Thus in the present sample it appears that the emergence of this characteristic pigmentation in response to nicotinic acid therapy not only involved the substantial use of pheno-

---

[3] Dermatologist's report.
[4] Dermatologist's report.

thiazines, but occurred almost exclusively in patients 35 years of age or under.

DISCUSSION

Presumably, all reports describing the occurrence of acanthosis nigricans-like dermatoses in patients treated with nicotinic acid have not come to our attention, but the reports cited here suggest that this development is relatively rare. In the Parson's sample of 44 cholesteremic patients who were receiving nicotinic acid (6), two developed the characteristic pattern of pigmentation. Brown and Winkelmann (5) reviewed 90 patients with a diagnosis of acanthosis nigricans, and in this group two patients had developed the characteristic pigmentation in association with nicotinic acid treatment. In the Tromovitch et al. description of one patient who developed the acanthosis nigricans-like pigmentation in association with nicotinic acid (4), no indication of the size of the sample treated with nicotinic acid is provided. In a review of 28 hypercholesteremic patients who received nicotinic acid for at least 1 year, Christensen et al. (7) do not refer to an acanthosis nigricans-like reaction. Such patterns of pigmentation have appeared among patients in an ongoing cardiac study which involves continued treatment with nicotinic acid, but data indicating the relative incidence of this development are not available at this time. In that sample, the incidence appears to be much less frequent than the incidence in the present sample of schizophrenic patients.[5]

On the basis of the Parson's (6) data, it may be estimated that the incidence of acanthosis nigricans-like dermatosis might be between 4 and 5% for the cholesteremic patients treated with nicotinic acid. In the present sample of schizophrenic patients, however, the incidence is approximately 49% for those who remained in treatment for the full 24 months. There are several important and presumably relevant differences between the cholesteremic and the schizophrenic patients. Specifically, the schizophrenic patients were much younger than the cholesteremic patients. In addition, very few, if any, of the cholesteremic patients were receiving phenothiazines, and all the schizophrenic patients had had a recent if not current hospitalization in a state mental hospital.

Reports of this pattern of pigmentation among psychiatric patients receiving nicotinic acid are limited to a few observations by Hoffer, who stated that flexor surfaces of the body became dark like a severe sun tan. He considers this to be a result from an increased deposition of adrenochrome pigment in the skin, nails, and hair—and not a sign of toxicity. He further notes that this pigmentation tends to disappear within a year or two, and that it

---

[5] Personal communication.

may be removed by vigorous scrubbing after a bath.[6] Lehmann, Ban, and their associates (8–11), who have conducted several studies in Canada, have seen no indication of the pigmented dermatosis. According to their published reports, very few of the patients were maintained on high-dosage nicotinic acid for a lengthy period of time (more than 6 months). Thus it is possible that in the Canadian samples, the acanthosis nigricans-like pigmentation did not have a sufficient opportunity to develop. It is also possible that their patients are different in other ways from those involved in the Marlboro study, e.g., maybe older or receiving less phenothiazine treatment. Other clinicians using nicotinic acid in private psychiatric practice have reported the characteristic dermatosis.[7] The fact that such a development has been less commonly observed by other investigators may, in part, reflect the possibility that their patients did not continue with the daily ingestion of large quantities of nicotinic acid over a sufficiently long period of time. It is also possible that other investigators did not require their patients to remove all clothing on the occasion of physical examinations subsequent to the fourth month of treatment.

In conclusion, it is hypothesized that a concurrent regimen of phenothiazine treatment enhances the apparent potential of continued high dosage of nicotinic acid to bring about an acanthosis nigricans-like pattern of pigmented dermatosis, and the susceptibility to this particular reaction to nicotinic acid treatment in the presence of phenothiazine medication is greatest in patients 35 years of age or younger.

ACKNOWLEDGMENTS

The writers gratefully acknowledge the contribution of numerous professionals who, at some time, were employed in the work of the project. Among them specific mention is made of Ann Adams, Mary Brown, R.N., Antonio DeLiz, M.D., Sarah Fallon, M.SW., Jennifer Gerrish, M.SW., Nafi Kiremitci, M.D., Helen Maurer, M.SW., Donald McDonald, Ph.D., and E. S. P. Weber, M.D.

The inquiry described in this report was conducted under U.S. Public Health Service Grant MH 13731.

REFERENCES

1. Wittenborn, J. R., Weber, E. S. P., and Brown, M., *Arch. Gen. Psychiat.*, **28**, 308, (1973).
2. Pollitzer, S., in *International Atlas of Rare Skin Diseases*, Unna, P. G., Morris, M., Besnier, E., and Duhring, L. A., (eds.), Pt. IV, No. 10, H. K. Lewis, London, 1890, p. 6.
3. Janovsky, V., in *International Atlas of Rare Skin Diseases*, Unna, P. G., Morris, M., Besnier, E., and Duhring, L. A., (eds.), Pt. IV, No. XI, H. K. Lewis, London, 1890, p. 1.

---

[6] Personal communication.

[7] Personal communication.

4. Tromovitch, T. A., Jacobs, Ph. H., and Kern, S., *Arch. Dermatol.,* **89,** 222 (1964).
5. Brown, J., and Winkelmann, R. K., *Medicine,* **47,** 33 (1968).
6. Parsons, W. B., and Flinn, J. H., *AMA Arch. Int. Med.,* **103,** 783 (1959).
7. Christensen, N. A., Achor, R. W. P., Berge, K. G., and Mason, H. L., *J.A.M.A.,* **177,** 76 (1961).
8. Ananth, J. V., Ban, T. A., Lehmann, H. E., and Bennett, J., *Canad. Psychiat. Ass. J.,* **15,** 15 (1970).
9. Ban, T. A., and Lehmann, H. E., *Nicotinic Acid in the Treatment of Schizophrenias,* Canadian Mental Health Association, Toronto, Canada, 1970.
10. Ramsay, R. A., Ban, T. A., Lehmann, H. E., Sazena, B. M., and Bennett, J., *Canad. Med. Ass. J.,* **102,** 939 (1970).
11. Ban, T. A., *Nicotinic Acid in the Treatment of Schizophrenias,* Canadian Mental Health Association, Toronto, Canada (1971).

The Phenothiazines and Structurally Related Drugs, edited by I. S.
Forrest, C. J. Carr, and E. Usdin. Raven Press, New York © 1974.

Side Effects of Depot Fluphenazines

Frank J. Ayd, Jr.

International Drug Therapy Newsletter, 917 West Lake Avenue, Baltimore, Maryland 21210

INTRODUCTION

Fluphenazine is considered the most potent of the piperazine phenothiazine neuroleptics. More than 17 yr of clinical experience with this compound, in vast numbers of patients of all ages with almost every known
psychiatric and physical disorder, have proven it to be a very safe neuroleptic (1). This same extensive clinical experience, especially some well-
designed, well-controlled, and well-executed studies, has verified the
therapeutic efficacy of this compound.

Since oral fluphenazine is so safe and effective, it is not surprising that the
long-acting injectable forms, fluphenazine enanthate and fluphenazine decanoate, which are even more potent on a milligram-per-milligram basis
than the oral form, have proven to be as safe and as effective as the oral
form. This review of the side effects that have occurred in patients treated
with the enanthate and the decanoate provides the data that substantiate
their safety.

PHARMACOLOGIC EFFECTS

Fluphenazine enanthate and fluphenazine decanoate have been given to
enough patients (over 125,000) to permit evaluation of their safety for short-
term and long-term therapy. An analysis of the published reports on these
drugs verifies conclusively that they are remarkably safe compounds. They
are capable of causing minor autonomic side effects, infrequent hypotensive
responses, and sporadic dermatologic disorders. Generally, these have
been mild and not severe enough to discontinue treatment. Usually they
subside spontaneously as treatment with the same dosage is continued or
after dosage is reduced.

Depending on the dosage and individual susceptibility, some patients
experience varying degrees of drowsiness and lethargy after an injection of
the enanthate or the decanoate. As a rule, these reactions occur after the
initial injection. Generally they are mild, do not require counteracting medication, and abate spontaneously within a week. Should these pharmacologic
effects be pronounced, they usually can be mitigated or abolished by 10

or 20 mg of methylphenidate once or twice daily for a few days postinjection. Sometimes, several cups of coffee is a sufficient stimulant to overcome these reactions.

EXTRAPYRAMIDAL REACTIONS

Although it is widely believed that fluphenazine enanthate and decanoate have a greater tendency to cause extrapyramidal reactions than other potent neuroleptics, this has not been proven by well-designed, rigidly controlled, and well-executed comparative studies. Actually, the published studies comparing the depot fluphenazines with oral antipsychotic drugs, when analyzed *in toto,* indicate that these drugs are no more liable to evoke striopallidal symptoms than other potent neuroleptics. There is evidence that suggests that the incidence of neurologic reactions due to the decanoate is somewhat less than that of the enanthate. Only the time of onset of each of the extrapyramidal reactions induced by fluphenazine enanthate and decanoate differs significantly from the time of onset of these same reactions elicited by the potent oral neuroleptics. Whereas, as shown in Fig. 1, 90% of dyskinesias and 90% of cases of parkinsonism and 90% of the akathisias caused by oral neuroleptics develop in the first 4.5 days, 72 days, and 73 days, respectively, 90% of each of these reactions due to fluphenazine enanthate or decanoate appear as follows: dyskinesia 12 to 24 hr postinjec-

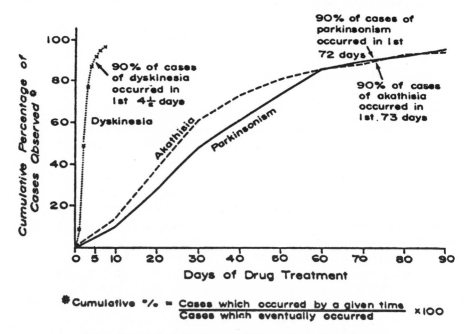

FIG. 1. Drug-induced extrapyramidal reactions: time of onset.

tion; akathisia 1 to 4 days postinjection; and parkinsonism 2 to 5 days post-injection. Because of the dramatic onset of depot neuroleptic-induced striopallidal reactions, especially the dyskinesias, some clinicians think these are more severe than those caused by the oral neuroleptics. Whether this is factual or a mirage is uncertain at this time. I am unaware of any study that provides data which permit a definitive conclusion about this.

When treatment with fluphenazine enanthate or decanoate is started, some patients develop mild to moderate degrees of the extrapyramidal reaction, akinesia. This can mimic the drug-induced lethargy and drowsiness discussed above. This neurologic reaction is not relieved by methylphenidate but it is very responsive to antiparkinsonian medication. Should the latter be indicated, it usually has to be prescribed for a few days, since even untreated akinesia tends to wane progressively in the first postinjection week.

Other patients develop mild akathisia immediately after an injection. This manifests itself by muscle cramps and some insomnia. Since this is a striopallidal reaction, it can be managed easily by an antiparkinsonian drug. It also can be eased by the bedtime administration of an antihistamine, such as diphenhydramine hydrochloride, which has both antiparkinsonian and hypnotic effects. It is seldom necessary to prescribe such counteracting agents for more than a week postinjection.

Akathisia is often described by the patient as the "jitters." Moderate to severe forms of this neurologic reaction cause the patient to feel compelled to walk or pace the floor. When sitting he constantly shifts his legs or taps his feet and complains of feeling jittery or anxious. When standing the patient may continuously rock his body forward, backward, and side to side, or constantly shift his weight from one foot to the other. Simultaneously, there may be chewing movements of the jaw, a rolling or smacking of the tongue, and a twisting of the fingers.

Most patients are annoyed by akathisia and will not tolerate it long. Relief can be achieved by an antiparkinsonian drug taken orally twice daily, often without any need to lower the dose of subsequent injections. Sometimes only partial relief can be obtained with moderate doses of an antiparkinsonian drug. Larger doses are inadvisable, since these drugs exert psychotropic effects of their own and their coadministration in large doses with depot fluphenazines may precipitate a toxic psychosis. Safer control of severe akathisia can be secured by the simultaneous prescription of moderate doses of an antiparkinsonian agent and small doses of a barbiturate, a sedative phenothiazine such as chlorpromazine, or an antihistamine.

Dyskinesia or dystonic reactions are characterized by the abrupt onset of retrocollis, torticollis, facial grimacing and distortions, dysarthria, labored breathing, and involuntary muscle movements. These may be accompanied by scoliosis, lordosis, opisthotonos, tortipelvis, and the characteristic gait of dystonia.

Another form of dyskinesia is oculogyric crisis. The attack begins with a fixed stare for a few moments. Then the eyes are rotated upwards and laterally and fixed in that position. The patient is barely able to move his eyes. At the same time, the head is tilted backwards and laterally, the mouth is opened wide, the tongue is protruded, and the facial expression suggests pain.

Dystonic reactions can be relieved promptly by the intravenous administration of diazepam or by the intravenous or intramuscular injection of 1 to 2 mg benztropine mesylate or 1 to 2 mg biperiden, which may be repeated in a half hour if necessary. Thereafter, oral antiparkinsonian medication should be prescribed every 4 to 6 hr for three or four doses. As alternate therapy, the patient could be given a quick-acting barbiturate (e.g., chlorpromazine 25 or 50 mg) or an antihistamine. Recovery also can be expedited by having the patient lie down in a quiet, darkened room. After recovery, depot fluphenazine can be continued in lower doses or concomitantly with an antiparkinsonian drug, since dystonic reactions are not a contraindication to further therapy with these drugs.

Depot fluphenazine-induced parkinsonism is manifested by varying degrees of intensity and combinations of loss of associated movements, rigidity of limbs, cogwheel phenomenon, tremors, facial rigidity, poverty of movement, gait and posture disturbances, drooling, and skin changes. These usually are relieved by adequate doses of an antiparkinsonian agent.

It is now well established that any neuroleptic, especially when administered in high doses or for months or years continuously, may cause a neurological syndrome called persistent or tardive dyskinesia. In contrast to acute dyskinesia, which comes on abruptly in the first few days of treatment and often is preceded by or accompanied by subjective anxiety and which usually responds to antiparkinson drug therapy, persistent dyskinesia evolves as imperceptibly as the unfolding of a flower after months of therapy, seldom causes any subjective distress, and is resistant to all chemotherapeutic remedies for striopallidal reactions. In fact, antiparkinson drugs may make the symptoms worse.

A comprehensive description of the manifestations of persistent dyskinesia has been written by Ayd and also by Crane (2, 3). When this disorder develops, it continues unmodified or worsens as long as the patient receives the same dose of the causal drug. When medication is discontinued or the dosage is reduced substantially, there may be some modification of symptoms, but, as a rule, symptoms persist for months or years and in most cases appear to be irreversible.

Persistent dyskinesia has been detected in patients being treated with depot fluphenazines. However, each patient had a history of previous treatment for varying lengths of time (usually several years) with different doses of one or more oral neuroleptics (more often the latter). *To date no verified case of persistent dyskinesia has been reported in patients treated exclusively with a depot fluphenazine.*

That treatment with a depot fluphenazine may cause persistent dyskinesia is a possibility. The probability of this happening may be quite low, since depot fluphenazines exert antipsychotic effect with a fraction of the dose of oral neuroleptics. Nevertheless, therapists using depot fluphenazines should carefully monitor their patients to avoid this neurologic complication or to lessen the risk of its occurrence. The art of pharmacotherapy with depot fluphenazines includes the administration of the lowest effective dose as infrequently as possible. This means that patients should *not* routinely receive the same dose at fixed intervals, but progressively lower doses at widening intervals.

DEPRESSIVE REACTIONS

In 1969, Alarcon and Carney called attention to severe depressive mood changes in 16 patients, initially diagnosed schizophrenic, who were being treated with fluphenazine enanthate or decanoate (4). These severe melancholias appeared usually within a few days postinjection. Generally, they did not last long. In five patients the depression was thought to have been responsible for suicide. In eight out of 10 patients, the depression remitted after electroconvulsive therapy.

Subsequent to Alarcon and Carney's report, a few other clinicians also reported severe depressive reactions during treatment with depot fluphenazines (5). These melancholias were responsive to either ECT or antidepressant drug therapy. Such citations naturally raise the question: "Are fluphenazine enanthate and decanoate depressogenic pharmaceuticals?"

Alarcon and Carney, and other clinicians, seem convinced that the depressive mood changes they observed were due to fluphenazine enanthate or decanoate. Yet, Alarcon and Carney acknowledged that in several of their patients, the original diagnosis of schizophrenia was changed to schizoaffective reaction, manic depressive reaction, or depression with hysterical features. Furthermore, they retreated seven of ten patients with either the enanthate or the decanoate after the depression cleared for up to nine months without a recurrence of melancholia.

An analysis of their five patients who committed suicide reveals that: (1) all were over age 30, (2) more men than women (2:1) did suicide, (3) three of the five patients had depressive episodes prior to depot fluphenazine therapy, and (4) 50% had a history of one or more suicidal attempts before depot fluphenazine therapy. In addition, three of the ten who did not suicide were found on reassessment to have an affective disorder.

In evaluating the significance of this data of Alarcon and Carney, it must be remembered that the gravest risk of mental illness, especially depression, is suicide. Although anyone may commit suicide, the rate increases with advancing age, with 70% of suicides happening after age 40. Suicide attempts in older patients are made three times more often by men. Suicide is a masculine type of reaction. Significantly more men than women suicide after age 30, a fact that has been constant the world over ever since data on this subject have been assembled. Finally, the risk of suicide is greater in those with a history of prior suicidal attempts (6).

Although Alarcon and Carney believe that fluphenazine may convert schizophrenia into an acute depression, it must be stressed that: (1) acute melancholia occurs very frequently in the course of untreated schizophrenia, (2) schizophrenia itself carries some risk of suicide, and (3) depressive reactions can happen during the administration of any neuroleptic. Imlah has aptly commented that we do not conclude that electroconvulsive therapy or antidepressants are depressant because of the suicidal incidence following their use (7).

Alarcon and Carney also have stated that: "Lesser changes of affect that may occur are being observed as part of a more extensive and detailed assessment of fluphenazine." This may be an affective manifestation of an extrapyramidal reaction. All effective antipsychotic drugs—phenothiazines, reserpine, butyrophenones, thioxanthenes—may produce a syndrome that closely resembles an endogenous depression (early waking, morning retardation, self-reproachfulness, and a depressed mood). To determine whether or not the symptoms are drug-induced, give an antiparkinson drug orally or intravenously. If the symptoms are drug-induced, they subside promptly, often within one-half hour after administration of the antiparkinson medication (8).

CONVULSIONS

Convulsions may be sparked by any neuroleptic, especially in epileptics, and in nonepileptics if large doses are given, particularly to patients with organic brain damage or who have had many ECTs. However, seizures are a rare side effect of oral and depot fluphenazines (9). In fact, these drugs have been administered to many seizure-free epileptics without provoking convulsions, as well as to many partially controlled epileptics without affecting the frequency or severity of their fits (10). Examples of long-acting injectable neuroleptic-induced seizures in nonepileptics have been cited by Capstick and by Neal and Imlah (11). The former had a postlobotomy patient who had a grand mal seizure 5 months after the first injection of fluphenazine enanthate. The latter had a patient who had a seizure 2 days after the first injection of 25 mg fluphenazine decanoate following which the patient became overactive and physically aggressive. Eleven days later, this patient was given a second injection of 25 mg fluphenazine decanoate without adverse consequences.

On the basis of personal experience as well as information from colleagues with extensive experience with potent neuroleptics, it appears that the precipitation of a convulsion by any of these drugs (oral or long-acting injectable) is not an absolute contraindication to further treatment with the same neuroleptics. In most instances, continued neuroleptic therapy does not cause a recurrence of convulsions.

JAUNDICE

Only very rarely have the oral piperazine phenothiazines been judged responsible for hepatic dysfunction. These drugs have been administered to patients with a history of jaundice due to the less potent phenothiazines without causing any signs or symptoms of ill-effects on the liver. These same drugs have been given to thousands of patients with liver damage due to diverse etiologies, chiefly alcohol, also without apparent or readily detectable adverse hepatic effects. Finally, although piperazines, like fluphenazine, have been prescribed continuously for many years for a large number of patients, clinical or laboratory evidence of liver toxicity is very scant indeed.

Of all the piperazine phenothiazines, fluphenazine apparently has caused the lowest incidence of jaundice. Mild, transient jaundice during oral fluphenazine therapy has been reported three times (12–14). In each case the reporting clinicians expressed uncertainty about the role of fluphenazine in causing the jaundice. If these were definitely fluphenazine-induced icterus, the incidence is still less than 1 in 4 million patients treated. In view of this fact, it is not surprising, therefore, that neither fluphenazine enanthate nor decanoate has been responsible for a single case of jaundice, even though each has been administered to enough patients at all dose levels and for a sufficient period of time to reasonably assume that any hepatotoxic effects would have appeared. Furthermore, like oral fluphenazine, the enanthate and decanoate have been given to many patients with varying degrees and types of liver pathology without adverse consequences. Also the continuous administration of each of these depot neuroleptics, even in very high doses, for months and years, has not resulted in clinical or laboratory evidence of hepatotoxicity. Thus, it appears that neither fluphenazine enanthate nor decanoate, even when administered for prolonged periods, is likely to have any deleterious effects on the liver.

AGRANULOCYTOSIS

There are rare reports of agranulocytosis due to piperazine phenothiazines, none of which was attributed to oral fluphenazine. Thus, it can be affirmed that, in view of the many thousands of patients treated with this drug, the risk of fluphenazine causing this blood dyscrasia is very low indeed.

So far, agranulocytosis has not been attributed to fluphenazine enanthate or decanoate, despite their administration in low and high doses to an estimated 125,000 patients in the past 9 yr. Nevertheless, the occurrence of agranulocytosis and other adverse hematological reactions in patients treated with oral neuroleptics has generated concern about the possible toxic effects on the bone marrow of long-acting injectable neuroleptics. Fluctuations in the leucocyte count have occurred in patients receiving fluphenazine enanthate and decanoate, just as they happen in patients treated with oral neuroleptics. These are independent of the drug. Thus, it can be said that even the prolonged administration of depot fluphenazines is not likely to have adverse effects on the hematopoietic system.

SKIN AND EYE CHANGES

Because ocular and dermatologic changes have occurred in some patients receiving phenothiazines (chlorpromazine, levomepromazine, and thioridazine) over a long period or in very high doses, it should be noted that there has not been a report in the medical literature of any form of fluphenazine causing skin or eye changes (15–24). In fact, these drugs have been administered to patients with lens and corneal opacities and/or skin pigmentation due to other phenothiazines without worsening either condition.

INTERACTION WITH OTHER DRUGS

The fear that adverse interactions might occur between fluphenazine enanthate or decanoate and any other drug(s) a patient may require after either drug had been injected has proven to be groundless. Almost 9 yr of experience with the enanthate and 7 yr with the decanoate in thousands of patients have shown that almost any drug can be coprescribed with them with little or no risk of harmful potentiation or of other forms of adverse interaction. Even the potentiation of barbiturates, sedatives, and alcohol by a neuroleptic declines rapidly, so that after a few weeks most people being treated with a neuroleptic can take a barbiturate, a sedative, or drink alcohol with miniscule risk of any serious potentiation.

The extensive clinical experience to date with fluphenazine enanthate and decanoate indicates that there is little reason to fear adverse interaction with these drugs. Many patients being treated with depot fluphenazines have taken regularly or intermittently one or more other medicines—psychoactive compounds, including lithium, sedatives, barbiturate and nonbarbiturate hypnotics, analgesics, antiarthritics, antibiotics, anticoagulants, anticonvulsants, antispasmodics, antituberculosis agents, cardiovascular preparations, CNS stimulants, anorexics, oral contraceptives and other hormones, diuretics, hypoglycemics, muscle relaxants, and innumerable over-the-counter remedies. Over 100 different drugs have been taken along with fluphenazine enanthate or decanoate without untoward interactions occurring. It appears that depot fluphenazines can be combined safely with the majority of drugs physicians commonly prescribe.

COMMENT AND CONCLUSION

One prevalent concern about depot neuroleptics is based on the fact that once the substance is injected, it cannot be removed from the body when this would seem desirable. This is true not only for long-acting injectable neuroleptics but also for oral neuroleptics after a few doses. Once the body is impregnated with an oral neuroleptic, it cannot be removed any more quickly than if the same substance in equivalent dosage has been injected. Clinical experience has shown that serious adverse reactions to depot fluphenazines are no more frequent and usually less so, than similar reactions to other potent oral neuroleptics. When these have happened with oral neuroleptics, they were usually seen after multiple doses have been absorbed into the body, have acted on receptor sites and have resulted in the drug and/or its metabolites being bound to proteins, so that rapid excretion is most unlikely, if not impossible. Pragmatically, this does not differ from what happens when a depot neuroleptic has been injected. Consequently, clinicians have no more reason to be concerned about the possible consequences of injecting a depot neuroleptic than they have for the consequences of administering oral neuroleptics.

The data on the safety of fluphenazine enanthate and decanoate are convincing and consoling. These drugs are as safe, if not more so, than any potent oral neuroleptic.

REFERENCES

1. Ayd, F. J., Jr., *Dis. Nerv. Syst.*, **29**, 744 (1968).
2. Ayd, F. J., Jr., *Med. Sci.*, **18**, 32 (1967).
3. Crane, G. E., *Arch. Gen. Psychiat.*, **24**, 179 (1971).
4. Alarcon, R., and Carney, M. W. P., *Brit. Med. J.*, **3**, 564 (1969).
5. Segal, M., and Ropschitz, D. H., *Brit. Med. J.*, **4**, 169 (1969).
6. Ayd, F. J., Jr., *Recognizing The Depressed Patient*, Grune and Stratton, Inc., New York, 1961.
7. Imlah, N. W., *Brit. Med. J.*, **4**, 49 (1969).
8. Ayd, F. J., Jr., *Int. Drug Ther. Newsletter*, **1**, 3 (1966).
9. Ayd, F. J., Jr., *Med. Clin. North Amer.*, **45**, 1027 (1961).
10. Capstick, N., *Dis. Nerv. Syst. (Supp)*, **31**, 15 (1970).
11. Neal, C. D., and Imlah, N. W., *Dis. Nerv. Syst. (Supp)*, **31**, 24 (1970).
12. N.I.M.H.-PSC Collaborative Study Group, *Arch. Gen. Psychiat.*, **10**, 246 (1964).
13. Fogel, E. J., and Matheu, H. M., *Cur. Ther. Res.*, **4**, 213 (1962).
14. Walters, G. M., Terrence, C., and Steckel, R., *Amer. J. Psychiat.*, **120**, 81 (1963).
15. Ayd, F. J., Jr., *Int. Drug Ther. Newsletter*, **1**, 1 (1966).
16. Ayd, F. J., Jr., *Int. Drug Ther. Newsletter*, **1**, 5 (1966).
17. Ayd, F. J., Jr., *Int. Drug Ther. Newsletter*, **1**, 20 (1966).
18. Ayd, F. J., Jr., *Int. Drug Ther. Newsletter*, **1**, 33 (1966).
19. Ayd, F. J., Jr., *Int. Drug Ther. Newsletter*, **2**, 2 (1967).
20. Ayd, F. J., Jr., *Int. Drug Ther. Newsletter*, **2**, 11 (1967).
21. Ayd, F. J., Jr., *Int. Drug Ther. Newsletter*, **3**, 1 (1968).
22. Ayd, F. J., Jr., *Int. Drug Ther. Newsletter*, **3**, 6 (1968).
23. Ayd, F. J., Jr., *Int. Drug Ther. Newsletter*, **3**, 11 (1968).
24. Ayd, F. J., Jr., *Int. Drug Ther. Newsletter*, **6**, 7 (1971).

The Phenothiazines and Structurally Related Drugs, edited by I. S. Forrest, C. J. Carr, and E. Usdin. Raven Press, New York © 1974.

Session III: Discussion

Reporter: J. R. Wittenborn

1. *H. Lehmann*

Q. Crane: Were the same investigators examining both the inpatients and the outpatients?

A. Yes, the same team and at the same time.

F. Forrest: I have an explanation for more extrapyramidal symptoms in outpatients. Outpatients are less likely to continue drug treatment.

Q. Vinars: Did you look at sex differences in treatment intake?

A. Yes, they were almost identical. Female patients did not take higher dosages.

2. *G. E. Crane*

Winsberg: I would like to ask Dr. Crane to elaborate on his observations regarding tardive dyskinesia to encompass a cautionary note to the pediatric psychopharmacologist. At least two investigators (McAndrews and Engelhardt) have reported on the prevalence of tardive dyskinesia in the pediatric age range among children on long-term high-dose neuroleptic pharmacotherapy. Since the reversibility of this syndrome is unknown in adults and most certainly unknown in children, precautionary measures and careful observations in the pediatric age range seem obligatory.

A. The parkinsonism in children is more or less reversible, but the stereotype of the older female patient with parkinsonism should no longer exist. It can be seen in younger females.

Q. Winsberg: Was there no correlation with organicity?

A. No, but my evaluation was based on the clinic diagnosis only. Edwards, to whom you refer, had a different basis for his classification.

Denber: Dr. Crane's serious concern for the rational use of antipsychotic drugs should be heeded. But the data that he presents raise several questions. Although tardive dyskinesia generally seems to be more prevalent in older females than males, on treatment for relatively long periods of time and at high dosages, leading to a suspicion that antedating organic factors may have a role, he states that there was no evidence of such findings. Yet his data contain no reference to EEG studies, psychodiagnostic tests, neurologic examinations, or lumbar punctures. His statement that on the basis of his finding of frequent tardive dyskinesia, prescription practices may have to be revised, may give rise to alarm in medical circles, not to mention among patients, and in the press and elsewhere. It is clear that tardive dyskinesia exists, for the French authors described the syndrome already in 1958 to 1959. I have seen it in a patient 17 years of age, but a review of published cases shows that it is most prevalent after 50 years, and Crane's data bear that out. Unless the future evidence is clear-cut, which it is not here, one must be very cautious and prudent before making sweeping generalizations which can only have a very negative effect on the treatment of the mentally ill.

A. I did the best I could. I suggest the physicians be more careful in the use of drugs.

Glassman: I don't think it is incumbent on Dr. Crane to prove his point beyond doubt. It is incumbent on the psychiatrists to show that Dr. Crane's claim is not true.

Lehmann: It is more common among the elderly. Each clinician must make his own judgment.

3. *F. Forrest*

From floor: One must distinguish between electron acceptors and electron donors. I feel it is a question of electron affinity.

Turner: About 100 years ago Hughlings Jackson differentiated between the positive and the negative aspects of damage to the nervous system. The negative aspect dealt with the loss of function; the positive, with the appearance of functions of the remaining intact nervous system, essentially a release phenomenon when "higher" controls were withdrawn.

As I recall, it was perhaps 35 years ago that Foster Kennedy showed that an epileptic in a grand-mal seizure, turned face downward or placed face down in water, made swimming motions. This example is but one of a large number which show that the upright or face-up posture of man obscures the real significance of many neurologic disorders. We must thank Dr. Forrest for his efforts in drawing our attention to other examples.

4. *H. R. Adams*

Q. I. Forrest: Is this a suitable model for opacities in man? I think that the corneal swelling after direct injection of phenolic CPZ metabolites is not a valid model for CPZ-induced ocular opacities, which may be due to accumulation of insoluble aglycones of CPZ-glucuronides, hydrolized by β-glucuronidase in ocular chamber fluid.

A. It may take years for the corneal opacity to form in man.

Unknown: Quinones may polymerize and form the opacities.

5. *F. J. Ayd, Jr.*

Q. Simpson: I believe we will get tardive dyskinesia from this form of medication, just as we have from other types of drug administration.

A. Yes, perhaps, but the risk is greatly reduced, and it is easier to separate the treatments by suitable intervals.

Crane: Dr. Ayd is the inventor of the "Drug Holidays." I think this is a nice principle, and it may explain why the drug in this form is well tolerated.

A. It has been assumed that there is a slow increase in blood drug level, but that the level may be possibly too low for assay in the plasma. Nevertheless, no efficacy is lost.

6. *J. R. Wittenborn*

Q. F. Forrest: Perhaps the pigmentation may be associated with the detergent.

A. Since most of the patients were out of the hospital at the time of pigmentation, it is probable that all of the usual detergents were involved. We also have the problem of explaining the absence of pigmentation in the controls and the relatively older patients and patients not getting phenothiazines.

Unknown: Perhaps it was air pollution.

A. Marlboro is in a rural area and there is no industry nearby. A clinician near Princeton tells me that he has seen several cases of this pigmentation among his recent patients.

Session IV

Chlorpromazine Metabolism, Distribution and Excretion: Assay Procedures

Chairmen: Ursula Breyer and Liisa Ahtee

The *Phenothiazines and Structurally Related Drugs,* edited by I. S. Forrest, C. J. Carr, and E. Usdin. Raven Press, New York © 1974.

Further Studies of Chlorpromazine Metabolism in Schizophrenic Men

Patricia Turano, W. J. Turner, and Donald Donato

Research Division, Central Islip State Hospital, Central Islip, New York 11722

Chlorpromazine (CPZ) [1] and 35 of its derivatives have been identified by comparison with synthetic standards using two-dimensional thin-layer chromatography (TLC) of extracts from the urine, feces, and blood of schizophrenic men on long-term CPZ therapy (1–3). A number of still unidentified compounds have also been detected.

Variations of Curry's method for preparing plasma for gas chromatography of CPZ (4) and methods using ether or dichloromethane (DCM), followed by gas chromatography (GC) and TLC, respectively, revealed that TLC permitted identification and quantitation of more compounds than did GC (5, 6). As many as 16 compounds could be measured by TLC in plasma extracts either 2 hr after the first morning medication or 12 to 15 hr after the last evening medication. From washed erythrocyte hemolysates also, there were as many as 16 compounds identified and quantitated; no more than trace amounts of these were conjugated (5). Only two of the spots, yielding a pink color with the Forrest spray, are still unidentified.

CPZ, as well as its mono- and nonhydroxylated derivatives, remains unchanged for many months when dissolved in absolute ethanol and stored at $-10°C$. The dihydroxylated and hydroxymethoxy derivatives are much less stable and yield multiple spots even when freshly prepared and protected from light and heat (3).

CPZ and its metabolites are known to undergo extensive changes in light and in the presence of Fe^{2+}, both in aerobic and anaerobic conditions (1, 7–10). Experiments in our laboratory, however, demonstrated that

---

[1] Abbreviations used in this text for chlorpromazine and its metabolites are: CPZ, chlorpromazine; CPZ-SO, chlorpromazine sulfoxide; Nor_1CPZ, monodesmethylchlorpromazine; Nor_1CPZ-SO, monodesmethylchlorpromazine sulfoxide; Nor_2CPZ, didesmethylchlorpromazine; Nor_2CPZ-SO, didesmethylchlorpromazine sulfoxide; CPZ-NO, chlorpromazine N-oxide; CPZ-NO-SO, chlorpromazine N-oxide sulfoxide; 7-OH-CPZ, 7-hydroxychlorpromazine; 7-OH-CPZ-SO, 7-hydroxychlorpromazine sulfoxide; 7-OH-Nor_1CPZ, 7-hydroxy monodesmethyl chlorpromazine; 7-OH-Nor_1CPZ-SO, 7-hydroxy monodesmethylchlorpromazine sulfoxide; 7-OH-Nor_2CPZ, 7-hydroxy didesmethylchlorpromazine; 7-OH-Nor_2CPZ-SO, 7-hydroxy didesmethylchlorpromazine sulfoxide; 8-OH-CPZ, 8-hydroxychlorpromazine; $3,7-(OCH_3)_2$-CPZ, 3,7 dimethoxychlorpromazine.

photodecomposition was not required to account for the number and variety of CPZ derivatives we have encountered, nor did work-up of CPZ urines in the dark result in fewer or a smaller quantity of derivatives. A closer inquiry has revealed that many of these may occur on prolonged contact at room or elevated temperatures with sundry solvents, including distilled, deionized water. Whether, or to what extent, these derivatives may also be truly of metabolic origin we cannot now say.

METHODS AND MATERIALS

Our routine methods for the extraction of CPZ from biological materials have been reported previously (3, 5, 6). In an attempt to identify sources of artifacts, we examined each step of our procedures leading up to and including TLC of metabolites in biological material (Fig. 1).

No CPZ derivatives arise during TLC by our methods, and no confusing spots appear on extraction and TLC of control urines. None arise from the solvents themselves. Therefore, any artifacts must arise from CPZ during processes of extraction, of incubation, or of evaporation of solvents. Indeed, it appears that at each step such artifacts may appear. It is not possible in this short space to provide all details of the evidence, but a number of experiments may be cited. These, performed with pure standards, simulate each step in preparation of CPZ-containing urine for final TLC and quantification.

Representative of solvents studied were distilled, deionized water, aqueous solutions buffered at pH 4.5 (acetate) or 9.5 (phosphate), redistilled DCM, freshly redistilled isoamyl alcohol (which, 5% v/v in DCM, is

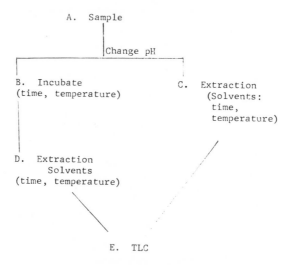

FIG. 1. Schematic diagram of procedure.

designated as DCMI), and absolute and 95% ethanol and ethyl ether, freshly distilled from ferrous sulfate. Fresh control urines used had pH values above 5.6. Representative volumes of solvents were 1, 5, or 100 ml. Solvents were evaporated under nitrogen, on a steam bath, at room temperature, or in a heating block at 60°C.

Although nine standards have been examined in detail, we report here chiefly on CPZ and 7-OH-CPZ as representative of nonhydroxylated and monohydroxylated derivatives, respectively.

(A) CPZ and 7-OH-CPZ were added to distilled water and aliquots were at once brought to dryness under nitrogen with or without heat. These were taken up in a few microliters of absolute ethanol and chromatographed immediately. Other aliquots were allowed to stand at 10, 20, or 37°C for 1 and 2 hr to note any changes over time.

(B) CPZ or 7-OH-CPZ in distilled water and in CPZ-free urine was brought to pH 4.5. Aliquots were immediately removed. The remainder was placed in a 37°C incubator for 1 and 2 hr. At zero time, 1- and 2-hr samples were immediately adjusted to pH 9.5 and extracted into DCMI, evaporated under nitrogen over a steam bath, and chromatographed at once.

(C) Standards were each added to various volumes of solvents, brought to dryness under nitrogen with or without heat and chromatographed.

Each TLC plate was spotted with mixtures of synthetic standards as well as with the preparations under investigation. Although most TLC has been done in two dimensions, in order to conserve space, the figures in this paper are in only one dimension. On occasion, TLC was supplemented by GC as described by us previously (3).

RESULTS

CPZ and 7-OH-CPZ, added to 0.5 ml distilled water and evaporated immediately under a stream of nitrogen at room temperature or alternatively in a heating block at 60°C, then chromatographed from absolute alcohol, yielded six to eight spots, as seen in Fig. 2. Figure 2 shows a TLC plate presenting the effect of incubation of CPZ, CPZ-SO, and 7-OH-CPZ in water and in a CPZ-free erythrocyte suspension in the dark at 37°C for 18 hr. 7-OH-CPZ suffered a more extensive degradation in water than in red blood cell suspensions. This was true also in the water–urine comparisons. Such effects, then, may arise during standing of urine in the laboratory or during β-glucuronidase incubation. The major spots from CPZ were due to CPZ, CPZ-SO, Nor_1CPZ; minor spots were due to Nor_1CPZ-SO, CPZ-NO, and CPZ-NO-SO. These could arise when urine stands in the laboratory or during extraction. The major derivatives of 7-OH-CPZ were its sulfoxide, 7-OH-Nor_1CPZ, 7-OH-Nor_1CPZ-SO, and a compound tentatively identified as 3,7-dihydroxy-CPZ. This was always present in considerable amount from water, but had hitherto been found by us only in extracts of urine and

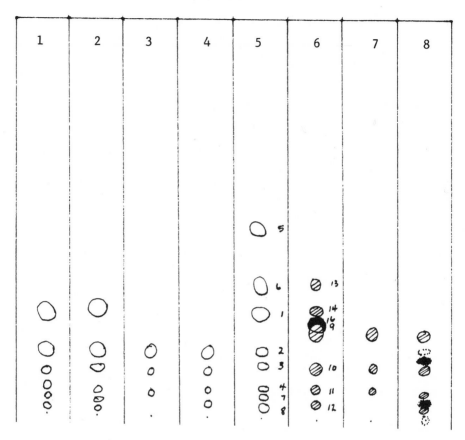

FIG. 2. Three standards after incubation in RBC and distilled water (Solvent system II). Column 1 is CPZ in rbc; 2, CPZ in H_2O; 3, CPZSO in rbc; 4, CPZSO in H_2O; 5, N P Mix; 6, OH mix; 7, 7-OHCPZ in rbc; 8, 7-OHCPZ in H_2O. Open spots, pink; lined spots, purple; solid spots, blue.

feces. In the figures the numbers adjacent to the spots correspond to the standards (3).

Figure 3 represents the consequences of addition of CPZ and 7-OH-CPZ to 100 ml of several commonly used organic solvents evaporated immediately on a steam bath under nitrogen and chromatographed from absolute alcohol. In this instance, the final solution of CPZ was subjected to TLC and GC; there was excellent agreement between the two. The derivatives found here depend to a great extent upon the solvent used. DCM yielded only the parent compound and its sulfoxide, whereas DCMI gave the parent compound, its sulfoxide, and the corresponding Nor_1 derivative. Ether yielded the parent compound, its sulfoxide, the corresponding Nor_1 derivative, and its sulfoxide. In addition, 7-OH-CPZ with ether gave two unknowns, one of which may be the 3,7-dihydroxy derivative.

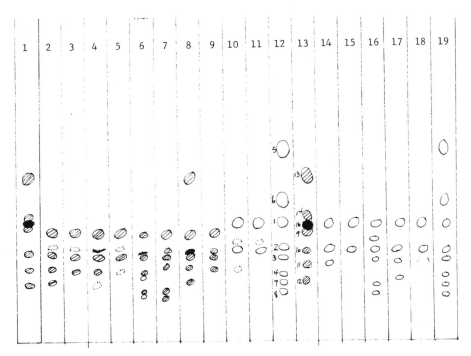

FIG. 3. CPZ and 7-OH-CPZ standard in various organic solvents (Solvent system II). Column 1 is OH mix; 2, 95% ethanol; 3, absolute ethanol; 4, spectroanalyzed DCMI; 5, spectroanalyzed DCM; 6, iso amyl alcohol; 7, distilled ether; 8, distilled DCM; 9, freeze dried DCM; 10, 95% ethanol; 11, absolute ethanol; 12, N P mix; 13, OH mix; 14, spectroanalyzed DCMI; 15, spectroanalyzed DCM; 16, iso amyl alcohol; 17, distilled ether; 18, distilled DCM; N P mix in column 19. (See Fig. 2 for color key.)

Chromatography in two dimensions with the many standards available to us has led to no further identifications.

Solutions of CPZ or of 7-OH-CPZ in DCM or in DCMI, respectively, as commonly occurs with urine extractions, were evaporated with N_2 at room temperature or alternatively on a steam bath. At room temperature, the time required was, of course, much longer than on the steam bath. TLC of these preparations is shown in Fig. 4. Here we found more extensive breakdown at room temperature than with heat. At room temperature, there were recovered the unchanged compound, its sulfoxide, and its corresponding Nor_1 derivative and its sulfoxide, the N-oxide and its sulfoxide, and a large pink spot with R_f 0.75 (solvent system II[2]). This last appears to be a mixture of two of the pink unknowns previously reported by us (3), possibly the propionic or acetic acid derivatives. These two pink spots occur in all biological material we have examined.

---

[2]Solvent system II: acetone-methanol-ammonia (100:40:1).

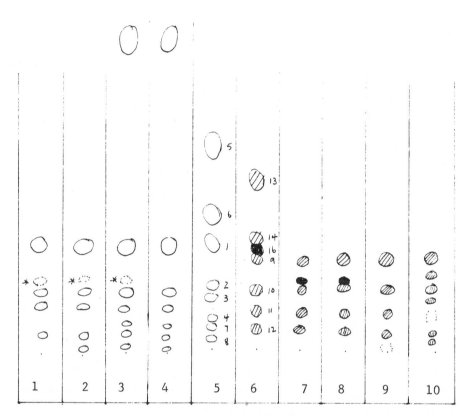

FIG. 4. CPZ and 7-OH-CPZ in DCM and DCMI, on steam bath and at room temperature (Solvent system II). Column 1, CPZ plus distilled DCM plus heat; column 2, CPZ plus distilled DCMI plus heat; 3, CPZ plus distilled DCM and no heat; 4, CPZ plus distilled DCMI and no heat; column 5 is the non polar mixture; column 6, OH mixture; 7, 7-OH plus distilled DCM plus heat; 8, 7-OH plus distilled DCMI plus heat; 9, 7-OH plus distilled DCM, no heat; 10, 7-OH plus distilled DCMI, no heat. (See Fig. 2 for color key.)

When CPZ was added to 5 ml ether and evaporated at 60°C under N_2, only the CPZ spot appeared in TLC and the CPZ peak in GC.

DISCUSSION

Coccia and Westerfeld (10), in their extensive work on metabolism of CPZ and its derivatives by liver microsomes, reported that no nonenzymatic alteration occurred, except in the presence of ferrous ion, even under conditions of extraction and with large volumes of solvents, evidently requiring hours to work up. They used essentially the same conditions of TLC as we do, both in one and two dimensions. They also used radiolabeled CPZ to confirm completeness of recovery of metabolites. In the presence of ferrous ion, particularly with added ascorbic acid, extensive mono- and didesmethylation and ring hydroxylation occurred. These phenomena have largely been confirmed by others (11, 12).

We believe that our results cannot be due to the presence of trace amounts of Fe^{2+} for the following reasons: (a) failure to detect Fe^{2+} and Fe^{3+} on evaporation of 500 ml of our water to 1 ml and addition of o-phenanthroline, (b) occurrence of alterations in redistilled organic solvents, and (c) simple monodesmethylation and sulfoxide formation in the absence of ascorbic acid and of sulfoxide formation alone in its presence.

We will not attempt to explain the discrepancies but will rather point out that of the large number of compounds which have been revealed in extracts of biological material very few could have arisen merely as artifacts. Quantitatively, the monodesmethylated derivatives and their corresponding sulfoxides, N-oxides, and N-sulfoxides may well, in part, arise nonenzymatically, so this must be considered in analytic studies. Similarly 3,7-dihydroxy CPZ and its sulfoxide may well be completely artifactual.

However, the following alterations in the molecule appear clearly to be totally of metabolic origin: didesmethylation, 7-hydroxylation, 7,8-dihydroxylation, and O-methylation. The occurrence of 8-OH-CPZ presents some problems and may be the result of dihydrodiol formation from the 7-hydroxy-CPZ followed by dehydration and dismutation. The occurrence of 3,7-$(OCH_3)_2$-CPZ in urine extracts is not yet certain, although it seems highly probable; it could arise by nonenzymatic formation of the corresponding dihydroxy-CPZ and enzymatic O-methylation, but in either case would not arise as an *in vitro* artifact.

The occurrence of two pink spots with R_f near 0.9 in our preparations (apparently acetic or propionic acid derivatives) and their occurrence in extracts from urine leaves open the question of a possible metabolic origin. Coccia and Westerfeld (10) did not find these in their microsomal preparations, yet Rodriguez and Johnson (13) found the propionic acid derivative in urine, and Hammar, Holmstedt, and Ryhage (14) found it in plasma, as we do also. The compounds we find occur, surprisingly, in extracts from alkaline solutions; they must therefore arise by oxidation of a precursor. Inasmuch as the corresponding aldehyde has been found in microsomal preparations, we may suppose that the aldehyde is of metabolic origin; oxidation would produce the acid, but also possibly dismutation could produce both the acid and the alcohol. However, this latter has not been detected in our work.

SUMMARY

Nonenzymatic oxidation of CPZ and 7-OH-CPZ was shown to occur at each of the steps in preparation of biological materials for quantitation by

TLC or GC. The oxidations, in absence of Fe^{2+}, in light or in dark, in water or in organic solvents, led to monodesmethylation, sulfoxidation, and formation of N-S dioxides. In water, CPZ also gave rise probably to acidic derivatives. In water or diethyl ether, 3,7-dihydroxy-CPZ arose from 7-OH-CPZ. Ascorbic acid increased sulfoxide formation but restricted further oxidation.

ACKNOWLEDGMENT

We wish to acknowledge the excellent technical assistance of John T. Brady, Robert T. Leyra, and David Danielson. This study was supported in part by Grant MH 05096 (from the National Institute of Mental Health).

REFERENCES

1. Usdin, E., *CRC Crit. Rev. Clin. Lab. Sci.,* **2,** 347 (1971).
2. Turano, P., Canton, C., Turner, W. J., and Merlis, S., *Aggressol.,* **9,** 193 (1968).
3. Turano, P., Turner, W. J., and Manian, A., *J. Chromatog.,* **75,** 277 (1973).
4. Curry, S. H., *Anal. Chem.,* **40,** 1251 (1968).
5. Turano, P., March, J., Turner, W. J., and Merlis, S., *J. Med. Exp. Clin.,* **3,** 109 (1972).
6. Turano, P., and Turner, W. J., *J. Chromatog.,* **64,** 347 (1972).
7. Huang, C. L., and Sands, F. L., *J. Chromatog.,* **13,** 246 (1964).
8. Huang, C. L., and Sands, F. L., *J. Pharm. Sci.,* **56,** 259 (1967).
9. Grant, F. W., and Greene, J., *Appl. Pharmacol.,* **23,** 71 (1972).
10. Coccia, P. F., and Westerfeld, W. W., *J. Pharmacol. Exp. Ther.* **157,** 446 (1967).
11. Brookes, L. G., and Forrest, I., *Exp. Med. Surg.,* **29,** 61 (1971).
12. Daly, J. W., and Manian, A. A., *Biochem. Pharmacol.,* **16,** 2131 (1967).
13. Rodriguez, C. F., and Johnson, D., *Life Sci.,* **5,** 1283 (1966).
14. Hammar, C. G., Holmstedt, B., and Ryhage, R., *Anal. Biochem.,* **25,** 532 (1968).

The Phenothiazines and Structurally Related Drugs, edited by I. S.
Forrest, C. J. Carr, and E. Usdin. Raven Press, New York © 1974.

Quantitation of Chlorpromazine and Its Metabolites in Human Plasma and Urine by Direct Spectrodensitometry of Thin-Layer Chromatograms

T. L. Chan, G. Sakalis, and S. Gershon

Neuropsychopharmacology Research Unit, Department of Psychiatry, New York
University Medical Center, New York, New York 10016

INTRODUCTION

The development of assay procedures for chlorpromazine (CPZ) and its metabolites has been quite difficult, not only because of low plasma levels, but also because of the unusual complexity of CPZ metabolism in humans. After comparison of all possible quantitation methods, we have chosen and developed a direct-scan technique for the simultaneous quantitation of CPZ and of its 17 metabolites in human plasma and urine. This quantitative thin-layer chromatography (TLC) method is coupled with a selective extraction procedure. Details of this method have been published elsewhere (1, 2). Preliminary results on plasma levels of CPZ and its metabolites by this assay procedure have also been reported (3, 4).

This chapter describes: (a) new data on methodology, (b) plasma and urine levels of CPZ and its metabolites from two schizophrenic patients on CPZ medication over a period of 4 weeks, and (c) some other aspects of chlorpromazine metabolism in humans.

EXPERIMENTAL PROCEDURE

Materials and methods not herein described were the same as previously reported (1, 2). Recently, our technique of extraction and quantitative TLC has been standardized and will be presented in detail elsewhere (5).

CPZ in liquid form was administered orally, three times daily. Blood was drawn 3 hr after the first dose. After centrifugation, plasma was extracted as soon as possible within 1 hr without freezing. Twenty-four hr urine samples were collected, and urine creatinine was assayed according to Folin and Wu (6).

RESULTS AND DISCUSSION

Qualitative and Quantitative Analyses of CPZ and Its Metabolites from Human Plasma and Urine

Typical scans of plasma extracts from a patient and a healthy subject are shown in Fig. 1. Unknown metabolites are identified and quantitated by comparing with reference compounds developed alongside on the same plate. It is seen that there is no measurable absorption in the control plasma samples. Nonphenolics (absorption at 525 nm) and phenolics (absorption at 560 nm) are selectively separated into two groups. The nonphenolics are identified as CPZ, Nor_1CPZ, Nor_2CPZ, CPZ-SO, Nor_1CPZ-SO, Nor_2CPZ-SO, and CPZ-NO. The phenolics are 7-OH CPZ, 7-OH Nor_1CPZ, 7-OH Nor_2CPZ, 7-OH CPZ-SO, 7-OH Nor_1CPZ-SO, and 7-OH Nor_2CPZ-SO. All metabolites could be easily quantitated according to the integral numbers shown below. Scans of urine extracts from a patient are shown in Fig. 2. Nonphenolics and phenolics (free and conjugated) are separated into two groups. A wide spectrum of CPZ metabolites are found in this sample.

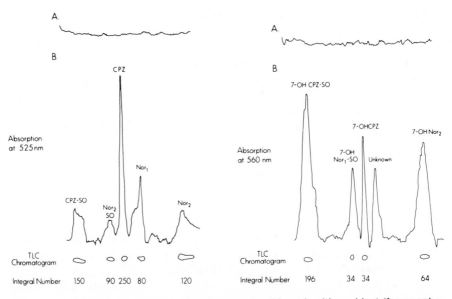

FIG. 1. (A, left): trace of scanning of a plasma extract from healthy subject (for nonphenolics); (B, left): trace of scanning of the plasma extract from patient S.H. receiving 600 mg CPZ t.i.d. (for nonphenolics); (A, right): trace of scanning of a plasma extract from a healthy subject (for 7-hydroxylates); (B, right): trace of scanning of a plasma extract from patient S.H. receiving 600 mg CPZ t.i.d. (for 7-hydroxylates).

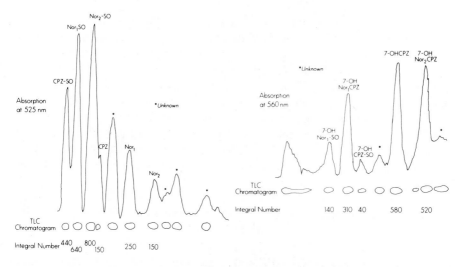

FIG. 2. (Left, absorption at 525 nm): trace of scanning of urine extract from patient H.G. receiving 900 mg CPZ/day (for nonphenolics); (right, absorption at 560 nm): trace of scanning of a urine extract from patient H.G. receiving 900 mg of CPZ/day (for total 7-OH CPZ's and glucuronides).

Reproducibility for Quantitation

In order to evaluate the accuracy and reliability of this standardized direct-scan technique, mixtures of phenolic and nonphenolic CPZ metabolites, at different concentrations, were separated by TLC; after color de-

TABLE 1. Average values of absorption for standard CPZ metabolites after color development

Metabolite	λ max (nm)	N^a	Concn. (nmole)	Absorption[b] Mean	±S.E.
CPZ	525	43	5	286.2	2.9
Nor_1CPZ	525	18	5	268.9	11.7
Nor_2CPZ	525	25	5	297.8	8.6
CPZ-SO	525	41	5	179.9	2.0
Nor_1CPZ-SO	525	30	5	193.1	2.3
Nor_2CPZ-SO	525	25	5	211.8	3.4
CPZ-NO	525	26	5	256.9	5.0
7-OH CPZ	560	49	5	333.1	4.4
7-OH Nor_1CPZ	560	40	5	298.2	5.4
7-OH Nor_2CPZ	560	44	5	323.8	4.7
7-OH CPZ-SO	560	44	5	307.5	4.4
7-OH Nor_1CPZ-SO	560	28	5	257.7	6.7
7-OH Nor_2CPZ-SO	560	32	5	317.8	4.6

[a] Number of experiments.
[b] Absorption expressed as total counts of peak area × sensitivity factor.

velopment, total absorption for each CPZ metabolite was measured. These results (Table 1) are somewhat different from those reported previously (1, 2). First, the total absorption for each component is generally higher. Second, the reproducibility is approximately ± 10% (an improvement over our earlier procedures). Thus, the standardized technique (5) further enhances the accuracy and reliability of this assay procedure. It is interesting to point out that spotting and spraying may be the two critical steps in obtaining better results. Results on duplicate assays of the same plasma and urine samples are summarized in Tables 2 and 3, respectively. The reproducibility of the overall method is once again in the range of ± 10% or better.

Simultaneous Measurement of Plasma and Urine Levels of CPZ and Its Metabolites

Plasma and urine levels of CPZ and its metabolites from two schizophrenic patients on CPZ medication over a period of 4 weeks are summarized in Figs. 3 and 4. In general, results were about the same for both patients. More metabolites were detected in urine than in plasma. With regard to the nonphenolic urinary metabolites, including CPZ, steady-state excretion rates were achieved after the first week. The metabolic patterns of the phenolic metabolites varied very significantly. While the sulfoxides achieved a low steady-state early, the nonsulfoxides (7-OH CPZ, 7-OH Nor_1CPZ, and 7-OH Nor_2CPZ) rose to levels several-fold greater than those of the sulfoxides, suggesting that one or more enzymes (hydroxylating and/or conjugating enzymes) have been induced during treatment. Sakalis et al. (7) have discussed this possibility. Despite the fact that aryl-hydroxylase activity was induced by CPZ in animals (8, 9), discrepancies were recently reported (10).

With regard to plasma levels, one of the patients (A.J., Fig. 3) showed a dramatic rise in CPZ, CPZ-SO, and CPZ-NO over the first 2 weeks, followed by a sharp decline. Patient M.D. (Fig. 4) did not exhibit this pattern. After 28 days, the main metabolites in plasma and urine were the same and were present in the same relative concentrations. Since this effect would be expected, it indicates that our analytical procedure is reliable.

In conclusion, the unusual complexity of CPZ metabolism in humans is fully demonstrated by the metabolite profiles of plasma and urine samples.

Time Course of CPZ and Its Metabolites in Plasma

A time course curve of CPZ and its metabolites in plasma of patient L.A., who received a single dose of 600 mg CPZ, is presented in Fig. 5. It is shown that the time peak of CPZ in plasma occurs at 3 hr. However, the kinetics of other metabolites are quite different. CPZ-SO has a plasma peak beyond 3 hr, but the 7-OH Nor_2CPZ has a much shorter half-life than the parent

TABLE 2. *Reproducibility of plasma assays (nmole/ml plasma)*

Patient	S.M. 2/22				M.D. 3/1				A.J. 3/14				E.S. 4/2			
Duplicate / Metabolite	A	B	Mean	S.D.	A	B	Mean	S.D.	A	B	Mean	S.D.	A	B	Mean	S.D.
Nonconjugate																
CPZ	0.14	0.17	0.155	±0.015	0.35	0.33	0.340	±0.010	1.03	1.03	1.03	±0.0	0.22	0.24	0.23	±0.010
Nor$_1$	0.00	0.00	0.00	—	0.00	0.00	0.00	—	0.08	0.10	0.09	±0.010	0.00	0.00	0.00	—
Nor$_2$	0.00	0.00	0.00	—	0.00	0.00	0.00	—	0.00	0.00	0.00	—	0.00	0.00	0.00	—
CPZ-SO	0.31	0.31	0.310	±0.0	0.13	0.16	0.145	±0.015	1.11	1.11	1.110	±0.0	0.5	0.45	0.475	±0.025
Nor$_1$-SO	0.00	0.00	0.00	—	0.00	0.00	0.00	—	0.14	0.17	0.155	±0.015	0.00	0.00	0.00	—
Nor$_2$-SO	0.00	0.00	0.00	—	0.00	0.00	0.00	—	0.00	0.00	0.00	—	0.00	0.00	0.00	—
CPZ-NO	0.21	0.23	0.220	±0.010	0.00	0.00	0.00	—	0.52	0.48	0.50	±0.020	0.00	0.00	0.00	—
7-OH-CPZ	0.37	0.38	0.375	±0.005	0.24	0.26	0.25	±0.010	0.00	0.00	0.00	—	0.22	0.20	0.21	±0.010
7-OH-Nor$_1$	0.00	0.00	0.00	—	0.00	0.00	0.00	—	0.00	0.00	0.00	—	0.00	0.00	0.00	—
7-OH-Nor$_2$	0.21	0.25	0.230	±0.020	0.066	0.053	0.0595	±0.065	0.00	0.00	0.00	—	0.00	0.00	0.00	—
7-OH CPZ-SO	0.22	0.19	0.205	±0.015	0.00	0.00	0.00	—	0.00	0.00	0.00	—	0.25	0.23	0.24	±0.010
7-OH-Nor$_1$-SO	0.00	0.00	0.00	—	0.00	0.00	0.00	—	0.00	0.00	0.00	—	0.00	0.00	0.00	—
7-OH-Nor$_2$-SO	0.00	0.00	0.00	—	0.00	0.00	0.00	—	0.00	0.00	0.00	—	0.00	0.00	0.00	—
Conjugate																
7-OH-CPZ	0.77	0.72	0.745	±0.025	0.47	0.49	0.48	±0.010	0.24	0.22	0.23	±0.010	0.09	0.08	0.085	±0.005
7-OH-Nor$_1$	0.62	0.53	0.575	±0.045	0.31	0.25	0.28	±0.030	0.29	0.31	0.30	±0.010	0.30	0.33	0.315	±0.015
7-OH-Nor$_2$	0.56	0.49	0.525	±0.035	0.41	0.54	0.475	±0.065	0.24	0.29	0.265	±0.025	0.00	0.00	0.00	—
7-OH-CPZ-SO	0.54	0.51	0.525	±0.015	0.14	0.15	0.145	±0.005	0.27	0.27	0.270	±0.0	0.17	0.21	0.19	±0.020
7-OH-Nor$_1$-SO	0.59	0.66	0.625	±0.035	0.14	0.125	0.1325	±0.0075	0.39	0.33	0.36	±0.030	0.00	0.00	0.00	—
7-OH-Nor$_2$-SO	0.00	0.00	0.00	—	0.23	0.21	0.22	±0.010	0.12	0.10	0.11	±0.010	0.18	0.21	0.195	±0.015

TABLE 3. Reproducibility of urine assays (nmole/ml urine)

Patient	A.J. 3/7				M.D. 3/9				A.J. 3/27				S.S. 4/16			
Duplicate Metabolite	A	B	Mean	S.D.	A	B	Mean	S.D.	A	B	Mean	S.D.	A	B	Mean	S.D.
CPZ	1.23	1.16	1.195	±0.035	2.64	2.64	2.64	±0.0	3.75	3.91	3.83	±0.080	0.34	0.34	0.34	±0.0
Nor$_1$	0.00	0.00	0.00	—	0.00	0.00	0.00	—	5.00	5.00	5.00	±0.0	1.98	1.89	1.935	±0.045
Nor$_2$	1.59	1.36	1.475	±0.115	2.50	3.07	2.785	±0.285	7.16	7.39	7.275	±0.115	2.17	2.02	2.095	±0.075
CPZ-SO	2.34	2.22	2.28	±0.060	4.16	4.13	4.145	±0.015	6.41	6.41	6.41	±0.0	2.61	2.61	2.61	±0.0
Nor$_1$-SO	8.49	7.55	8.02	±0.470	10.38	10.61	10.50	±0.115	22.50	24.17	23.34	±0.835	6.25	6.91	6.58	±0.330
Nor$_2$-SO	17.95	16.59	17.27	±0.680	16.82	16.36	16.59	±0.230	35.14	37.84	36.49	±1.35	10.4	10.6	10.5	±0.10
CPZ-NO	11.67	11.31	11.49	±0.180	20.83	20.60	20.72	±0.12	14.04	13.83	13.94	±0.105	3.33	3.16	3.25	±0.085
7-OH CPZ	17.65	17.65	17.65	±0.0	47.65	47.65	47.65	±0.0	77.78	85.19	81.49	±3.635	18.5	18.0	18.0	±0.25
7-OH Nor$_1$	24.44	23.70	24.07	±0.370	55.56	54.81	55.19	±0.375	123.3	130.0	126.7	±3.335	24.1	26.0	25.5	±0.95
7-OH Nor$_2$	43.93	47.21	45.57	±1.64	62.95	68.20	65.58	±2.625	152.4	158.7	155.6	±2.825	65.8	64.1	64.5	±0.85
7-OH CPZ-SO	5.22	4.06	4.64	±0.58	6.96	7.30	7.13	±0.170	14.71	14.71	14.71	±0.0	5.08	5.08	5.08	±0.0
7-OH Nor$_1$-SO	0.00	0.00	0.00	—	0.00	0.00	0.00	—	17.39	17.39	17.39	±0.0	9.78	9.78	9.78	±0.0
7-OH Nor$_2$-SO	11.43	9.52	10.48	±0.955	10.16	11.43	10.80	±0.635	36.36	39.39	37.88	±1.515	16.2	16.8	16.5	±0.25

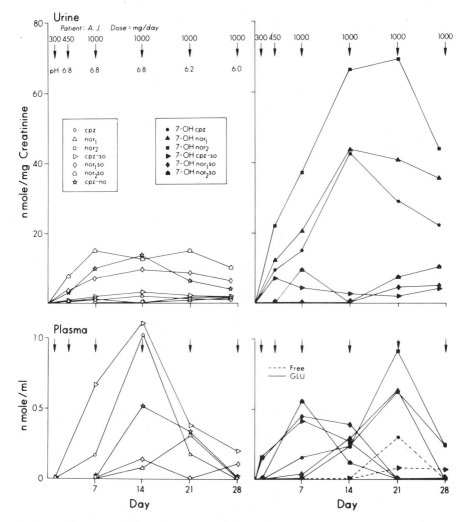

FIG. 3. Plasma and urine levels of CPZ and its metabolites from patient A.J. on CPZ medication over a period of 4 weeks. The open symbols are for nonphenolics; the closed symbols are for 7-OH CPZ's.

drug. Therefore, any interpretation of data or conclusions based on plasma levels will be misleading unless the complete picture of the complex pharmacokinetics and interactions of different components is considered.

Percentage Recovery of CPZ and Its Metabolites in a Urine Sample

Since free 7-OH CPZ and its Nor_1, Nor_2, and SO metabolites were not separated from their glucuronides in our urine routine assay, it would be helpful to include some data on the percentage recovery of CPZ and dif-

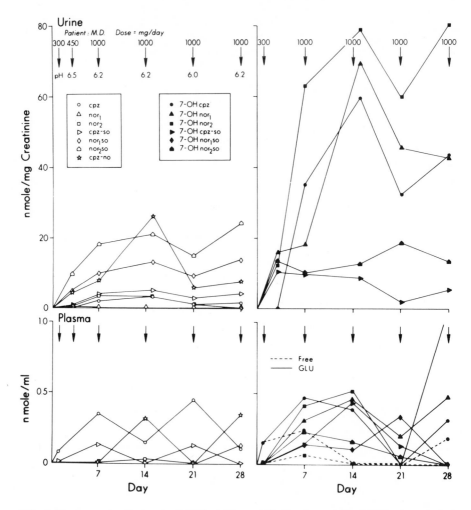

FIG. 4. Plasma and urine levels of CPZ and its metabolites from patient M.D. over a period of 4 weeks. The open symbols are for nonphenolics; the closed symbols are for 7-OH CPZ's.

ferent groups of metabolites in a urine sample. Results are summarized in Table 4. It can be seen that the percentage distribution of nonphenolics, free 7-OH CPZ, and 7-glucuronides in urine is 24.8, 8.9, and 66.3%, respectively. The ratio of nonconjugates to conjugates is in agreement with that reported by others (11, 12). However, these ratios may change dramatically from sample to sample, as shown in Figs. 3 and 4. Moreover, the high content of 7-glucuronides excreted in the urine is also compatible with the considerable concentration of glucuronides found in plasma.

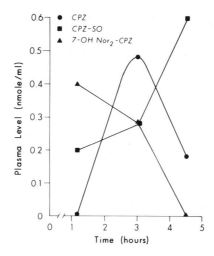

FIG. 5. Time course of CPZ and its metabolites in plasma of patient L.A. receiving a single dose of 600 mg CPZ.

TABLE 4. *Distribution of CPZ and its metabolites in a 24-hours urine sample of patient J.G. receiving 900 mgs CPZ/day*

Metabolite	Urine level (nmole/ml)	% of total
Nonconjugate		
CPZ	0.14	
Nor_1	1.26	
Nor_2	1.36	24.8%
CPZ-SO	2.09	(Nonphenolics)
Nor_1CPZ-SO	6.35	
Nor_2CPZ-SO	13.40	
7-OH CPZ	2.62	
7-OH-Nor_1CPZ	0.49	
7-OH-Nor_2CPZ	2.08	8.9%
7-OH CPZ-SO	0.46	(Free 7-OH CPZs)
7-OH-Nor_1CPZ-SO	0.93	
7-OH-Nor_2CPZ-SO	2.35	
Glucuronide		
7-OH CPZ	2.94	
7-OH-Nor_1CPZ	13.95	
7-OH-Nor_2CPZ	12.00	66.3%
7-OH CPZ-SO	1.51	(Glucuronides)
7-OH-Nor_1CPZ-SO	6.00	
7-OH-Nor_2CPZ-SO	29.45	

Erythrocyte Levels of CPZ and Its Metabolites

A comparison of plasma and erythrocyte levels of CPZ and its metabolites is summarized in Table 5. It is demonstrated that the erythrocytes contain as much as 50% of the total CPZ and its metabolites in the whole blood sample. Only certain metabolites, however, are taken up by red blood cells.

TABLE 5. *Comparison of plasma and erythrocyte levels of CPZ and its metabolites from a blood sample of patient J.G. receiving 900 mg CPZ/day*

Metabolite	Plasma level (nmole/ml) (A)	RBC level (nmole/ml) (B)	Whole blood level (nmole/ml) (A) + (B)[a]
CPZ	0.64	0.36	1.00
Nor_1	0.00	0.00	0.00
Nor_2	0.00	0.32	0.32
CPZ-SO	0.00	0.11	0.11
Nor_1CPZ-SO	0.00	0.23	0.23
Nor_2CPZ-SO	0.00	0.72	0.72
7-OH CPZ	0.17	0.00	0.17
7-OH-Nor_1CPZ	0.37	0.00	0.37
7-OH-Nor_2CPZ	0.00	0.00	0.00
7-OH CPZ-SO	0.27	0.00	0.27
7-OH-Nor_1CPZ-SO	0.00	0.00	0.00
7-OH-Nor_2CPZ-SO	0.37	0.00	0.37
Total	1.72	1.74	3.46
%	~ 50%	~ 50%	100%

[a] Assuming equal volume of both fractions.

SUMMARY

A direct-scan technique employing quantitative TLC for visible absorption of color complexes of CPZ and its metabolites by spectrophotometric method with the use of Schoeffel double-beam spectrodensitometer Model SD 3000 and density computer SDC 300 is described. CPZ and 17 metabolites have been analyzed qualitatively and quantitatively. This method has been applied for routine assays of CPZ and its metabolites in both human plasma and urine. The reproducibility of this method is in the range of ± 10%

ACKNOWLEDGMENTS

This work is in collaboration with Drs. N. Schooler and J. Levine of N.I.M.H.-PRB. We would like to thank Drs. E. Usdin and A. Manian for their helpful suggestions and supplies of metabolites. We also wish to thank

Dr. J. W. Schweitzer for reading the manuscript, and Miss Fong Y. Moy, Mrs. Sheila Olewitz, Mrs. Mei Y. Lu, and Mr. J. Romero for expert technical assistance.

This work was supported by N.I.M.H. Grant MH 17968.

REFERENCES

1. Chan, T. L., and Gershon, S., *Mikrochim. Acta*, **3**, 435 (1973).
2. Chan, T. L., and Gershon, S., in *Quantitative Thin-Layer Chromatography*, Touchstone, J. (Ed.), Wiley, New York, 1973, Chapter 14.
3. Chan, T. L., Sakalis, G., and Gershon, S., *Clin. Pharmacol. Ther.*, **14**, 133 (1973).
4. Sakalis, G., Chan, T. L., and Gershon, S., *Psychopharmacologia* (*in press*, 1973).
5. Chan, T. L., and Gershon, S., *Psychopharmacol. Bull.*, N.I.M.H., U.S.A., (*in press*, 1973).
6. Folin, O., and Wu, H., in *Practical Physiological Chemistry*, Hawk, Oser, and Summerson (Eds.), The Blakiston Co., 1952, p. 506, p. 839.
7. Sakalis, G., Curry, S. H., Mould, G. P., and Lader, M. H., *Clin. Pharmacol. Ther.*, **13**, 931 (1972).
8. Wattenberg, L. W., (*This proceedings*, 1973).
9. Breyer, U., (*Personal communication*).
10. Stevenson, I. H., O'Malley, K., Turnbull, M. J., and Ballinger, B. R., *J. Pharm. Pharmac.*, **24**, 577 (1972).
11. Bolt, A. G., and Forrest, I. S., *J. Pharm. Sci.*, **56**, 1533 (1967).
12. Hollister, L. E., and Curry, S. H., *Res. Comm. in Chem. Path. and Pharmacol.*, **2**, 330 (1971).

The Phenothiazines and Structurally Related Drugs, edited by I. S.
Forrest, C. J. Carr, and E. Usdin. Raven Press, New York © 1974.

Chlorpromazine Analysis by Gas Chromatography with an Electron-Capture Detector

Stephen H. Curry

*Department of Pharmacology and Therapeutics, The London Hospital Medical College,
Turner Street, London, E. 1., England*

INTRODUCTION

The development of a gas-chromatographic method for the analysis of chlorpromazine in clinical samples was announced at the second symposium in this series in 1967 (1, 2). The method was published in full in 1968 (3). It has since been used in studies of chlorpromazine concentrations in human plasma (4), of the disposition of the drug in animals (5), of chlorpromazine absorption *in vivo* and *in vitro* (6), and of the relation between concentrations and effects in man (7, 8). It appears to have been the technique of choice over the last 6 years for the determination of, particularly, unmetabolized chlorpromazine. However, it is not without its difficulties, and it has been described as "difficult to replicate" (9). A number of constructive suggestions for modification of the method have been made, both in published reports and in private discussions (10, 11).

Extensive experience at the London Hospital has revealed occasional but important difficulties in applying the method. For example, (a) the benzodiazepine series of drugs have been found to have retention times and extraction characteristics similar to those of chlorpromazine, and these compounds are sometimes found in the plasma of chlorpromazine-treated patients; (b) certain electron-capture detectors are insensitive to chlorpromazine, particularly when the drug is contaminated with biological material; (c) recovery varies with different anticoagulants, and between individuals, and this can be complicated by variable degrees of adsorption of chlorpromazine onto glass and onto protein plugs; (d) certain experimental samples, when assayed in duplicate as two supposedly identical aliquots, give rise to a pair of widely divergent figures; and (e) occasional batches of the column packing fail to separate the demethylated metabolites from unmetabolized chlorpromazine.

In view of the above difficulties, it seemed appropriate to reassess the

335

method in regard to chromatographic separation, contamination, detector sensitivity, recovery with and without internal standards, and variation in results. This chapter describes a series of relevant experiments, and this symposium seems an appropriate place for this report, after 6 years of experience of chlorpromazine analysis.

EXPERIMENTAL

Reagents and Materials

Columns of 3% OV-17 on Chromosorb W HP (80–100 mesh) were manufactured in the laboratory. Chromatography materials were purchased from Perkin Elmer, Limited (Beaconsfield, London). Solvents and inorganic chemicals were reagent grade and were obtained from Hopkin and Williams, Limited (London). Reference samples of chlorpromazine were donated by May and Baker, Limited (Dagenham, England), and by Smith, Kline, and French Laboratories (Philadelphia, Pa.). Reference samples of benzodiazepine drugs were donated by Roche Products, Limited (Welwyn Garden City, England) and Boehringer Ingelheim, Limited (London). ^{35}S-Chlorpromazine was purchased from The Radiochemical Centre (Amersham, England), with a specific activity at the time of purchase of 27.6 mCi/mmole. Polycarbonate centrifuge tubes were obtained from Measuring and Scientific Equipment, Limited (London), and tapered glass centrifuge tubes (15 ml) from Quickfit, Limited (Staffordshire, England).

Standard solutions of chlorpromazine were prepared by dissolving the hydrochloride in water. Treatment of 1-ml samples of these solutions with 1 ml of ammonia solution (N) and total extraction into 1 ml of toluene containing 15% isoamyl alcohol gave solutions suitable as chromatographic standards. Standard solutions of benzodiazepines were prepared in ethanol. Heparinized and oxalated blood samples were obtained from healthy volunteers and from patients receiving chlorpromazine.

Apparatus

Gas chromatography was performed with a Pye Model 104 instrument equipped with a 15 mCi ^{63}Ni ionization detector operated at 49 V d.c., with a pulse space of 150 μsec. Coiled 9-foot glass columns, 3.5 mm, internal diameter, were operated at 265°. Dry nitrogen was the carrier gas at an initial pressure of 40 psi, giving a flow rate of 80 ml/min. The inlet and detector temperatures were 275°C.

Extraction

The extraction technique was the "nonselective" method of the earlier report (3). To 1 to 5 ml of plasma in a 25-ml stoppered polycarbonate centrifuge tube were added 1 ml of N NaOH and 10 ml of *n*-heptane containing 1.5% isoamyl alcohol. The tube was shaken mechanically for 30 min and centrifuged. A 9-ml aliquot of the organic layer was transferred to a 15-ml, glass-stoppered centrifuge tube containing 2 ml of 0.05 N HCl. The tube was shaken mechanically for 10 min and centrifuged. A 1.8-ml aliquot of the aqueous layer was transferred to a 15-ml, tapered, glass-stoppered centrifuge tube. The solution was made alkaline with 0.2 ml of ammonia solution (N) in water and extracted with 100 μl of toluene containing 15% isoamyl alcohol. The tube was shaken mechanically for 15 min and centrifuged. The aqueous layer was removed by aspiration, and the organic layer was collected in the tapered portion of the tube. Samples of the organic layer (1 to 10 μl) were examined by gas chromatography and by liquid scintillation spectrometry when radioactive chlorpromazine was used.

pH-Partition

Five-ml samples of 10-ml heptane extracts from solutions containing chlorpromazine, "apparent chlorpromazine," or diazepam (100 ng/ml) were added to 5 ml samples of various buffer solutions (pH 2.4 to 6.8) or of 0.1 N HCl. After mechanical shaking for 30 min and centrifugation, aliquots of the buffer solutions were removed, made alkaline with ammonia, and extracted as in the previous section into 100 μl of toluene containing 15% isoamyl alcohol. Samples of the toluene layer were examined by gas chromatography.

RESULTS AND DISCUSSION

Contamination with Benzodiazepine Drugs

Contamination with benzodiazepines was first noticed when it was found that a number of plasma samples from subjects involved in single-dose (25 mg) chlorpromazine studies appeared at first sight to contain unusually high concentrations of the drug. However, detailed retention time measurements indicated that the gas-chromatographic peak had a retention time approximately 10% longer than the time expected. The presence of an important impurity was therefore proved. Concentrations of the impurity, estimated in five subjects and calculated as "apparent chlorpromazine," were much higher than the concentrations of chlorpromazine in subjects when the authenticity of the chlorpromazine peak was undoubted, and the material was also detected in supposedly blank samples (time 0), and its concentration changed less over the 24-hr period than was the case with authentic chlorpromazine.

The characteristics of the impurity were assessed by pH-partition studies and chromatographic analysis. The influence of pH on the heptane/water partition characteristics of the "apparent chlorpromazine" was different from the influence of pH on the heptane/water partition characteristics of pure chlorpromazine and of authentic, recovered chlorpromazine (Fig. 1). Investigations with diazepam showed that this compound had the same partition characteristics as the "apparent chlorpromazine," and this led to the recording of a gas-chromatographic trace for chlorpromazine and diazepam, together with the related benzodiazepines medazepam, nordiazepam, and oxazepam (Fig. 2). It is of great importance that the electron-capture detector used was extremely sensitive to the benzodiazepines whereas its sensitivity to chlorpromazine was an order of magnitude lower. The concentrations of diazepam in the experimental samples mentioned earlier were those which might have persisted as long as 3 months after a single dose of the drug, so that neither subject nor investigator would necessarily have suspected that diazepam had been consumed at a relevant time.

Contaminating signals have plagued chlorpromazine analysis, and identification of the unwanted materials has not proved easy. Diazepam is obviously one of the potential contaminants, and Fig. 2 indicates that oxazepam is another. Even mass spectra have not fully clarified the problem. In one study, an apparent contaminant appeared to have the mass spectrum of chlorpromazine (11). It obviously was chlorpromazine in that case, clinging to tubes and other glassware in the laboratory in question. However, it should be noted that, on the basis of Fig. 2, a mixture of nine parts chlorpromazine and one part diazepam will give a chromatographic signal which predominantly indicates diazepam, whereas the highest mass number in the mass spectrum will be that of chlorpromazine, which has the higher molecular weight.

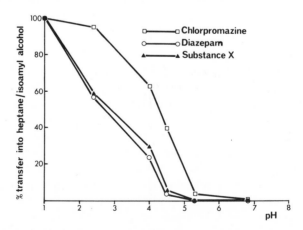

FIG. 1. pH-Dependent distribution of chlorpromazine, diazepam, and a contaminant of experimental plasma (substance X) between heptane containing 1.5% isoamyl alcohol and water.

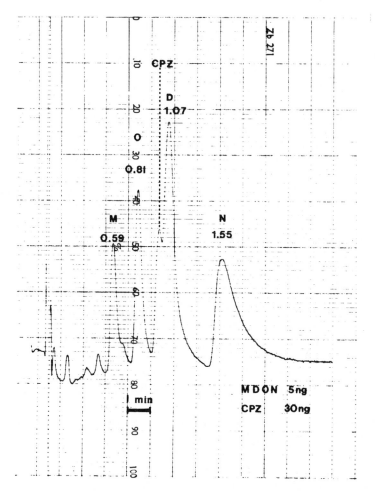

FIG. 2. Gas-chromatographic trace of chlorpromazine (CPZ) in the presence of medazepam (M), diazepam (D), nordiazepam (N), and oxazepam (O).

Detector Sensitivity

A number of individual detectors have been examined. In general, the
presence of biological material has been found not to interfere with the
response of electron-capture detectors to chlorpromazine. However, problems occasionally arise from this source, and the results of one relevant
experiment are shown in Fig. 3. The detector in question gave a linear
response to chlorpromazine in standard solutions in toluene. The response
was also linear to varied quantities of chlorpromazine in an extract prepared
as in the Experimental Section of this chapter, but when chlorpromazine
in a solution of the pure compound was added to a biological extract, the

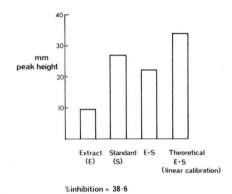

%inhibition = 38·6

FIG. 3. Inhibition of GLC response. Chromatographic signal to various chlorpromazine samples, recorded with a detector subject to contamination-induced inhibition of the chlorpromazine signal.

chlorpromazine signal was reduced by approximately 40%. The reason for this reduction is unknown. It occurs with different detectors of apparently identical design. In any application of gas chromatography in chlorpromazine analysis, it is obviously essential to know the characteristics of the detector, although it is not necessary to eliminate from use a detector which gives a reproducible, but reduced, signal.

Recovery with and without Radioactive Internal Standard

Extracts were made from water, individual heparinized blank plasma samples, and pooled batches made from individual heparinized and oxalated blank plasma samples. Recovery of chlorpromazine was measured by gas chromatography and from radioactivity, as a percentage of the material originally in the water or plasma, found in the final toluene solution, and corrected for the aliquot volumes. Both methods indicated better than 95% recovery from water (Fig. 4). This confirmed the original observation (3).

Mean recovery from seven individual heparinized plasma samples was 62% (radioactivity) and 58% (gas chromatography). Mean recovery from nine aliquots from a pooled batch made from quantities of the seven individual samples was comparable at 69% (radioactivity) and 68% (gas chromatography). It was not identical to the 62% and 58% recorded earlier because of unequal contributions from the various samples. The mean recoveries (radioactivity) in four sets of six serial samples, each set from a different subject were 60, 72, 74, and 75%, showing that recovery varied between subjects. This last set of determinations could only be made with radioactivity measurements, as trace quantities of radioactive chlorpromazine were added to the chlorpromazine already present following the dose.

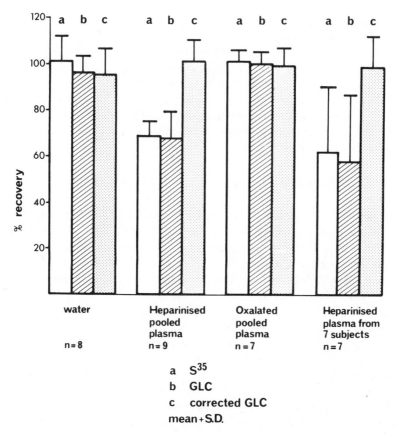

FIG. 4. Recovery (mean + S.D.) of chlorpromazine from various aqueous solutions by radioactivity (a), gas chromatography (b), and corrected gas-chromatographic measurements. See text for details.

Variation in recovery figures within the groups was of interest. The standard deviation on gas-chromatography data from water confirmed the original observations (3). The variation in determinations in pooled experimental plasma from a group of subjects was comparable, but the variation in determinations in a series of individual experimental plasma samples from different subjects was much greater (Fig. 4). This confirmed that recovery varied between subjects. The variation within each batch of six samples collected at time points after chlorpromazine administration was similar to, or less than, the variation in pooled plasma. This indicated that recovery was a feature more of the individual subject than of the individual plasma sample.

With oxalated plasma, all mean recoveries were greater than with heparinized plasma, at 100%. Variations were comparable with those with heparinized plasma when pooled plasma was used. They were less than those recorded when a series of individual plasma samples from several subjects were considered.

In the experiments in which chlorpromazine was assayed by both GLC and ^{35}S, correction of the GLC data by multiplying by factors ($100/^{35}$S data) always gave mean recoveries in the range 95 to 101%. High recoveries were found by ^{35}S measurements in solutions in which high recoveries were found by chromatographic measurements, and low recoveries were found by ^{35}S measurements in solutions in which low recoveries were found by chromatographic measurements.

Duplicate Assays of Experimental Samples

Duplicate assays with samples from patients treated with chlorpromazine sometimes failed to provide pairs of numbers with differences in agreement with the degree of variation expected on the basis of the data presented in the previous section of this paper (8, 12). In about 50% of cases, the paired figures were within three standard deviations of their own mean (based on the figure of 6% of the mean for the standard deviation determined with pooled control plasma), whereas with a normally distributed phenomenon, more than 95% of pairs should have fallen into this category. Study of large numbers of control chlorpromazine assay results has shown that the analysis is a normally distributed phenomenon.

The discrepancy is shown in Fig. 5. Forty-four experimental plasma samples were assayed in duplicate. The mean of each pair of figures was calculated. The deviation of the individual numbers in each case was calculated from the mean of the pair in each case and expressed as a percentage of the mean. This percentage was divided by 6, to give an estimate of the mean in terms of the number of the predetermined value for the standard deviation. The whole procedure was also carried out with 44 pairs of control samples.

The distribution of the pairs is shown in Fig. 5. Quite clearly, the pairs were normally distributed when control samples were studied, but bimodally distributed with experimental samples. Control experiments have so far failed to reveal a reason for this bimodal distribution. Experiments with all possible variations of technique for the preparation of plasma from whole blood have been tried, involving variations in centrifugation conditions and in the proportion of the plasma removed from the centrifuged blood, and involving measurement of recovery of radioactive chlorpromazine as described previously. The only possibility remaining is that the difference is real, indicating that plasma is not always homogenous with respect to chlorpromazine. Perhaps this is not as impossible as it sounds at first hearing, especially for a drug that is 99% bound to plasma protein by a process much influenced by extraneous factors. Although this apparent variation is obviously of extreme importance in the interpretation of measurements of chlorpromazine concentrations in plasma, it should be noted that the

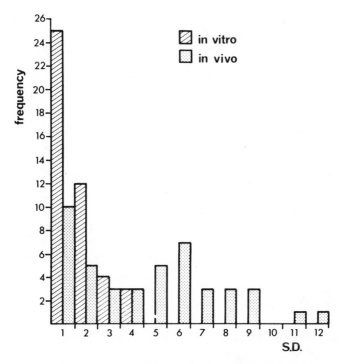

FIG. 5. Frequency distribution diagram for chlorpromazine analysis in solutions from laboratory *(in vitro)* and human *(in vivo)* sources. The S.D. axis indicates the number of standard deviations from the mean (see text for details).

greatest deviation ever recorded is approximately 70% from the mean of a pair, which is in line with the accuracy of many of the analyses performed in clinical laboratories.

General Considerations

These observations are obviously of importance to those using gas chromatography for the analysis of chlorpromazine. First, the use of a radio-active internal standard apparently failed to reduce appreciably the variation in results obtained by multiple analysis of standard solutions in water and pooled plasma, but it did confirm the validity of the gas-chromatographic analyses. The routine use of a radioactive internal standard would provide the means for a simple recovery correction in the calculation of the drug content of individual samples when heparinized plasma is studied. However, since recovery appears to be a characteristic of the subject rather than of the individual sample, the same result would probably be achieved by the determination of a "recovery constant" for each subject, to be used in all calculations for that subject. This constant could be determined in a blank sample with gas chromatography or radioactivity measurements, with both combined, or in an experimental sample by radioactivity measurements alone. This approach should overcome all problems resulting from variations in recovery, whether caused by differences in anticoagulants, individual variation, adsorption onto glass and protein plugs, or unknown factors. Careful use of radioactive internal standards will also permit allowance to be made for relatively unsatisfactory electron-capture detectors, when the use of such detectors cannot be avoided. This particular problem would obviously be reduced in significance by the use of a gas-chromatographic internal standard, as recommended by other workers (10).

It would seem prudent to assay samples in duplicate in the future, since, using the method as originally described, without internal standards, a single determination will in 94% of cases be within 12% of the mean result that would have been obtained from multiple determinations. The mean of two will be correspondingly more accurate. However, this does not allow for the apparently uncontrollable, and still unexplained, variation within some experimental—as opposed to control—plasma samples.

Interfering contaminants, such as diazepam, will continue to present a problem to those using the method, but the careful use of retention-time measurements, serial assays, and partition-coefficient measurements will ensure detection of contaminants of this type. It would seem prudent to omit subjects with such impurities from further chlorpromazine experiments, although the partition-coefficient differences may well be such as to allow exploitation of counter-current principles in the separation of the materials by solvent extraction. Related problems will arise from rare failures of particular column batches to separate efficiently demethylated chlorpromazine metabolites from the unchanged drug, but relevant to this problem is the fact that adequate methods for nonchromatographic separation, by acetylation of the metabolites, or by extraction with buffer solutions, have already been described (3, 13).

CONCLUSION

It is considered that the analytical problems discussed in this chapter, and others that may arise in the future, can be overcome by the careful application of the chemical, analytical, and statistical principles described. One real problem concerning duplicate experimental samples, remains unsolved, but this is a biological rather than an analytical problem.

REFERENCES

1. Curry, S. H., *Agressologie,* **9,** 115 (1968).
2. Curry, S. H., and Brodie, B. B., *Fed. Proc.,* **26,** 761 (1967).
3. Curry, S. H., *Anal. Chem.,* **40,** 1251 (1968).
4. Curry, S. H., Davis, J. M., Janowsky, D. S., and Marshall, J. H. L., *Arch. Gen. Psychiat.,* **22,** 209 (1970).

5. Curry, S. H., Derr, J. E., and Maling, H. M., *Proc. Soc. Exp. Biol. Med.*, **134,** 314 (1970).
6. Curry, S. H., D'Mello, A., and Mould, G. P., *Brit. J. Pharmacol.*, **42,** 403 (1971).
7. Curry, S. H., Marshall, J. H. L., Davis, J. M., and Janowsky, D. S., *Arch. Gen. Psychiat.*, **22,** 289 (1970).
8. Sakalis, G., Lader, M. H., Curry, S. H., and Mould, G. P., *Clin. Pharmac. Ther.*, **13,** 1931 (1972).
9. Usdin, E., *Critical Reviews in Clinical Laboratory Sciences*, **2,** 347 (1971).
10. Flint, D. R., Ferullo, C. R., Levandoski, P., and Hwang, B., *Clin. Chem.*, **17,** 830 (1971).
11. Spirtes, M. A., *Clin. Chem.*, **18** (1972).
12. Hollister, L. E., Kanter, S. L., Curry, S. H., and Derr, J. E., *Clin. Pharmac. Ther.*, **11,** 49 (1970).
13. Curry, S. H., and Marshall, J. H. L., *Life Sciences*, **7,** 9 (1968).

The Phenothiazines and Structurally Related Drugs, edited by I. S. Forrest, C. J. Carr, and E. Usdin. Raven Press, New York © 1974.

Total Excretion of ^{3}H-Chlorpromazine and ^{3}H-Prochlorperazine in Chronically Dosed Animals: Balance Sheet

I. S. Forrest, J. Fox*, D. E. Green, A. P. Melikian, and M. T. Serra

Biochemical Research Laboratory, Veterans Administration Hospital, Palo Alto, California 94304

INTRODUCTION

Chlorpromazine has been universally and successfully used in the therapy of mental illness and in general medicine for 20 yr and has been investigated clinically and chemically at an unprecedented level of intensity. It therefore seems hard to believe that major problems of drug metabolism still persist, and that whole areas remain in which our knowledge is deficient.

Far fewer data have been obtained for the piperazine-linked phenothiazines. Prochlorperazine was selected for study of this subgroup because it has the same chlorine substituent at position 2 of the phenothiazine nucleus, so differences in metabolism and excretion can be entirely attributed to the differences in the side chains of the two drugs, i.e., the dimethylaminopropyl aliphatic tail of chlorpromazine versus the 3-(4-methyl-1-piperazinyl)propyl side chain of prochlorperazine.

Even in the case of chlorpromazine, the literature is vague on rates of total excretion via the urine and feces and the period of time required for total excretion. We attempted to ascertain these data for the two phenothiazine drugs in various mammals, primarily by radioquantitation, and disregarded minor and finer points, such as excretion into the saliva, or irreversible losses from transpiration, tears, nasal secretion, or incorporation of drug metabolites into hair and nails.

Fecal excretion in man has not been extensively investigated. Curry et al. (1), who determined unchanged chlorpromazine only, found less than 1% of the dose in several days' collections from three patients on various doses of chlorpromazine. Turner and Turano reported approximately 5%

---

* Formerly at the Department of Animal Laboratory Medicine, Stanford University School of Medicine, Stanford, California. Current address: Animal Care Facility, Colorado University Medical Center, Denver, Colorado 80220.

total chlorpromazine plus metabolites during workshops on assay procedures of chlorpromazine at N.I.M.H., held in 1971 and 1972.

Total urinary excretion rates of unlabeled, chronically administered chlorpromazine were previously reported by us (2). Obviously, radio-quantitation is the most convenient method for determining total drug excretion. Since there are difficulties in obtaining permission in California to administer isotopically labeled drugs to man for other than diagnostic or therapeutic purposes, we selected rhesus monkey as the most suitable animal model. Of 13 species of mammals studied with regard to *in vitro* chlorpromazine metabolism (3), seven of which were also studied *in vivo* (4), rhesus emerged as the animal model most closely resembling man with regard to type of metabolites formed, as well as routes and rates of excretion (5). The data obtained for rhesus monkeys were compared to those for rabbits and guinea pigs, for which information had previously been obtained in our laboratory.

MATERIALS AND METHODS

Dutch Belt rabbits, short-haired, pigmented guinea pigs, and rhesus monkeys were used in the studies of total chlorpromazine and prochlorperazine excretion via the urine and feces. Male and female animals were studied, and the data for both sexes were quite similar. "Chronic drug administration" as referred to below, specifies animals at steady state, who have received the drug for more than 4 weeks, and for several months in most instances. Acute single-dose administrations were given to animals without any drug level.

The drugs employed, chlorpromazine hydrochloride and prochlorperazine dihydrochloride or dimaleate, both unlabeled and tritium-labeled at position 9 of the nucleus, were gifts of Smith Kline and French Laboratories, for which we thank Dr. Harry Green. All reference metabolites used in chromatographic identification of excreted metabolites were obtained from the Psychopharmacology Research Branch, N.I.M.H., for which we thank Dr. Albert A. Manian in particular.

Oral drug administration was somewhat unconventional. Since we had observed that rabbits and guinea pigs struggle increasingly against the introduction of a stomach tube during prolonged periods of chronic drug administration by gavage and sometimes bite off the rubber tubing so as to choke on the inserted end, this procedure was abandoned. Instead, the restraining boxes, holding the animals with only the heads protruding from the box, were tilted upward by 90°, a wooden dowel with an appropriate hole was inserted to hold the jaws apart, and the drug dose in form of liquid concentrate was delivered by means of a short rubber-tipped pipette through the hole in the dowel.

In the more precious rhesus monkeys, we wanted to avoid all stressful procedures and experimented with various forms of oral drug doses to be voluntarily ingested by the animals. The maximum chlorpromazine dose acceptable to the animals was 20 mg/kg/day embedded in various foods such as slices of apple or orange, marshmallows, or their standard monkey chow biscuits. In all instances, chlorpromazine hydrochloride was converted into the free base which is apparently less soluble in saliva and hence perceived as less objectionably bitter. The animals were observed for approximately 30 min until all of the drug-containing food was swallowed. This was always offered as the first food of the day, regardless of the food vehicle selected.

In the case of prochlorperazine, which was given in smaller daily doses, no conversion of the salt to the free-base form of the drug was required.

The tracer doses of the labeled drugs were administered in the same way, at the rate of approximately 20 μCi/kg of body weight.

Collection of urine and feces from all animals was made in metabolic cages equipped with stainless steel pans retaining the feces quantitatively, and a stainless steel wire screen covering the hole in the pan through which the urine was funneled into ice-cooled polypropylene bottles for the 24-hr collection period. Excreta were stored at $-20°C$ until they were worked up. All animals had *ad libitum* access to water and stock diet.

Radioquantitation was performed by direct scintillation counting of a maximum of 500 μl of urine in a Packard Tri-Carb Spectrometer, Model 2002, using a scintillation cocktail containing 100 g of naphthalene, 5 g of PPO, 0.3 g of dimethyl-POPOP, 730 ml of dioxane, 135 ml of toluene, and 45 ml of methanol.

All 24-hr feces samples were totally homogenized in three to five volumes of tetrahydrofuran. One-hundred- to 500-μl aliquots of the homogenate were oxidized in the Packard Sample Oxidizer, Model 305. The resulting tritiated water was collected in the same dioxane-based cocktail described above for scintillation counting.

Reagents used were ACS or scintillation grades.

Modifications of the previously reported methods (2, 6–9) were improvements suggested by Kaul (10, 11), i.e., addition of 15% propanol to dichloromethane for extraction of unconjugated chlorpromazine metabolites, and the use of alkaline hydrolysis instead of the slower enzymatic hydrolysis of conjugated chlorpromazine metabolites.

RESULTS AND DISCUSSION

Total excretion of tritiated chlorpromazine and prochlorperazine administered to rabbits, guinea pigs, and rhesus monkeys was studied by radioquantitation, under various conditions of prior treatment of these animals, as illustrated in Tables 1 and 2. Steady-state conditions under chronic drug administration of unlabeled drug prior to administration of the labeled dose were always verified by the reproducibility of chemical assays of the urinary drug-excretion rate on several consecutive 24-hr collections.

TABLE 1. *Total excretion of ³H-chlorpromazine (CP)*

Animal	Medication CP, mg/kg/day, p.o.	% ³H in urine (averaged)	% ³H in feces (averaged)	Total %[a] ³H excreted (averaged)
Rabbit				
chronic (2)	30, cold dose continued after ³H-CP	48.1	35.9	84.0
acute (2), single dose	~ 1 mg/kg	28.2	13.1	41.3
Guinea pig				
chronic (2)	30, cold dose continued after ³H-CP	62.7	33.9	96.6
acute (6), single dose	~ 1 mg/kg	20.5	31.0	51.5
Rhesus monkey				
chronic (2)	20, cold dose continued after ³H-CP	83.5	13.3	96.8
chronic (2)	20, cold dose stopped after ³H-CP	51.9	31.1	83.0

[a] ³H-CP was administered at approximately 20 μC/kg of animal weight. Collection of excreta was continued until DPM counts became insignificant, i.e., for periods of 10 to 20 days.
Number in parentheses indicates number of animals.

In the case of chlorpromazine (Table 1), the excretion of the label was nearly quantitative in all chronically dosed animals in whom the dose of cold chlorpromazine was maintained after administration of the label. It was 84% in rabbit and 97% in guinea pig and rhesus monkey, with the urinary excretion accounting for the majority of the label in all species. The highest ratio of urinary versus fecal excretion was seen in rhesus monkey and equalled 6.3.

Acute drug administration in form of a single dose containing tracer material was studied in rabbit and guinea pigs only. The excretion of label under these conditions amounted to approximately one-half that observed under chronic drug administration.

In rhesus monkey another aspect was studied: after the tracer dose was administered to chronically pretreated animals, the maintenance dose of unlabeled chlorpromazine was abruptly discontinued. This not only lowered the total excretion rate of the label by 14%, but also caused a very significant decrease in the ratio of urinary versus fecal excretion, from 6.3 to 1.7. A ratio as low as 1.7 is uncharacteristic of the primates rhesus monkey and man, and has not previously been seen during acute or chronic drug administration. This aspect should be studied further in man, since it might yield significant information on desirable practices of drug administration and discontinuation.

Figure 1 illustrates the day-to-day excretion of the tritium label over a 7-day period in two chronically dosed rhesus monkeys in whom the unlabeled chronic daily dosage was maintained after administration of the label. It shows the relatively rapid excretion of the label in these animals within the first week, whereas the following week's collection accounted for less than 10% of the total recoverable radioactivity.

Figure 2 illustrates the excretion of the label over a 10-day period as the average from two rhesus monkeys, chronically dosed as described before, but in whom all drug was abruptly withdrawn after the last dose containing the label. From the second day on, a shift toward increased fecal excretion and decreased urinary excretion was noted, which persisted through the sixth day. Thereafter, total excretion became very small, so the ratio of urinary to fecal excretion was not a significant parameter.

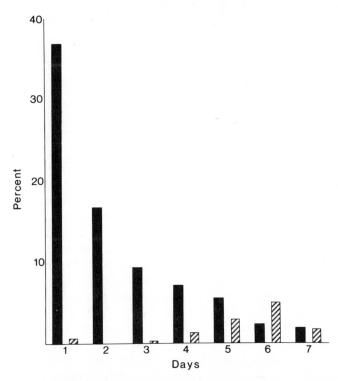

FIG. 1. ³H-Chlorpromazine excretion: average of 2 rhesus monkeys chronically dosed with 20 mg/kg/day, p.o. Drug dosage maintained throughout collection period: urinary excretion = solid black bars, fecal excretion = crosshatched bars, days (abscissa) = days after administration of label, % (ordinate) = % of applied radioactivity excreted per day.

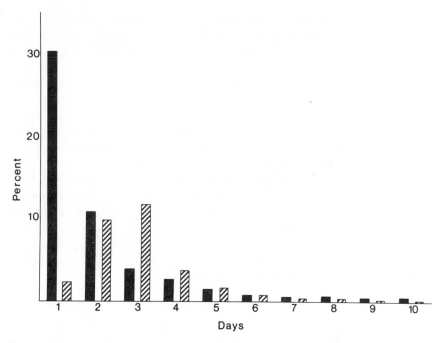

FIG. 2. ³H-Chlorpromazine excretion: average of 2 rhesus monkeys chronically dosed with 20 mg/kg/day, p.o. Drug dosage discontinued at administration of label. Urinary excretion = solid black bars, fecal excretion = crosshatched bars, days (abscissa) = days after administration of label, % (ordinate) = % of applied radioactivity excreted per day.

The analogous data for prochlorperazine are shown in Table 2 for the same three species of mammals. Rabbits and guinea pigs were studied with regard to total prochlorperazine excretion on two different chronic dosage levels, i.e., 5 and 25 mg/day/kg, p.o., respectively. Compared to chlorpromazine, the overall excretion rates were slightly lower, whereas the total period of measurable excretion of radioactivity was the same. In addition to three rhesus monkeys chronically dosed with 2 mg/kg/day, one animal was studied after a single, labeled, i.m. dose of 1 mg/kg. The fact that total urinary and fecal excretion after the single i.m. dose was greater than in the three orally and chronically dosed monkeys is somewhat suspect. The labels of single drug doses—regardless of the route of administration—are normally recovered to a lesser extent than those at chronic drug dosage, in which tissue saturation has been achieved. In this instance the lesser recovery of label after chronic drug dosage suggests that the monkeys did not actually ingest all of the food containing the labeled dose, but may have removed morsels from their cheek pouches after the usual 30-min observation period. In future trials at least the important tracer dose will be delivered by i.m. injection.

Figure 3 illustrates the day-to-day urinary and fecal excretion of pro-

TABLE 2. *Total excretion of ³H-prochlorperazine (PCP)*

Animal	Medication	% ³H in urine (averaged)	% ³H in feces (averaged)	Total %* ³H excreted (averaged)
Rabbit				
chronic (3)	5 mg/kg/day, p.o.	17.4	73.6	91.0
chronic (2)	25 mg/kg/day, p.o.	24.5	62.8	87.3
Guinea pig				
chronic (3)	5 mg/kg/day, p.o.	9.5	67.3	76.8
chronic (2)	25 mg/kg/day, p.o.	12.7	55.5	68.2
Rhesus monkey				
chronic (3)	2 mg/kg/day, p.o.	18.6	48.9	67.5
acute (1)	1 mg/kg, i.m.	24.0	57.0	81.0

* ³H-Prochlorperazine was administered at approximately 20 µC/kg of animal weight. Collection of excreta was continued until DPM counts became insignificant, i.e., for periods of 8 to 20 days.

Number in parentheses indicates number of animals.

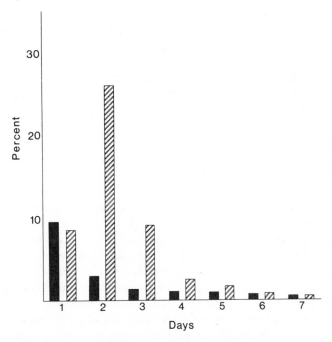

FIG. 3. ³H-Prochlorperazine excretion: average of 3 rhesus monkeys chronically dosed with 2 mg/kg/day, p.o. Drug dosage maintained throughout collection period. Urinary excretion = solid black bars, fecal excretion = crosshatched bars, days (abscissa) = days after administration of label, % (ordinate) = % of applied radioactivity excreted per day.

chlorperazine as the average from three chronically dosed animals. The chronic dose of 2 mg/kg/day of unlabeled prochlorperazine was maintained after administration of the label. Compared to the analogous conditions using chlorpromazine (see Fig. 1), the great majority of the label is excreted within the first 4 days in both instances. With chlorpromazine, however, the overwhelming majority is excreted via the urine; in the case of pro-chlorperazine, the urinary and fecal excretion rates are almost equal on the first day, and fecal excretion predominates from day 2 on. This may well be characteristic of all piperazine-linked phenothiazines, but all available data on record by Symchowicz et al. for perphenazine (12) and by Phillips and Miya for prochlorperazine (13, 14) supporting this observation have been obtained for the rat, which is known to eliminate most drugs via the feces. In the present study, the predominance of fecal over urinary excretion was seen in rabbit, guinea pig, and rhesus monkey—and would presumably apply to man. It therefore appears that all phenothiazine drugs cannot be assumed to be equivalent in therapeutic application, if one assumes that drug metabolism, distribution, and excretion are significant parameters.

Radioquantitation, using tritiated chlorpromazine and prochlorperazine and three species of mammals, thus appeared to be a reasonably satisfactory procedure which indicated that urinary and fecal excretion was essentially complete within 10 to 20 days.

When we tried to correlate these data with chemical assays of the urinary and fecal drug content, we found that all currently used procedures, based on solvent extraction of the drug content, or on column chromatography (6, 9), with subsequent spectrophotometric assays of groups of metabolites (2, 6) or thin-layer chromatography (7), yielded lower recoveries than radioquantitation. The discrepancies varied for the individual mammals, whereby the differences seen in guinea pigs were smaller than in the other species. Less than 10% discrepancy was considered tolerable in view of the various steps involved in solvent extraction and the subsequent assay procedures used. However, 30% discrepancy as observed primarily in conjugated drug fractions appeared excessive and is currently being studied. Tritium exchange, which would yield excessive excretion values, cannot be ruled out at this time and will have to be proved or disproved by the use of ¹⁴C-ring-labeled chlorpromazine as the tracer material. In view of the metabolically inactive position 9 of the nucleus (the site of the tritium label used), however, tritium exchange does not appear probable. Another theoretically possible explanation might be the breakdown of the phenothiazine nucleus, resulting in fragments not determinable by the usual methodology. Again, this appears highly improbable, and no such incidence has been reported for biotransformations. This leaves the uncomfortable probability that all methodology in current use is not adequate to determine the numerous metabolites of the phenothiazine drugs, known and unknown, or that methods thought to separate conjugated from unconjugated drug metabolites are not as satisfactory as assumed.

We plan to pursue these studies further in view of their implications for clinical therapeutics as well as for toxicology, since most phenothiazine drugs are administered for long periods of time and in high daily doses.

SUMMARY

Phenothiazine drugs are administered to large numbers of patients, frequently for indefinite periods of time and in high daily doses. It therefore seems important to study their biotransformation, distribution, and excretion in man and appropriate animal models as parameters which eventually will help elucidate their mode of action. After 20 years of intensive study of the phenothiazines, even as simple an aspect as a balance sheet — input versus output under chronic or acute conditions of drug administration — is a controversial subject. Using three species of mammals and two phenothiazine drugs tritiated at the metabolically insensitive position 9 of the nucleus, it was found that under chronic drug dosage, recovery of the label was essentially complete within 10 to 20 days. Lesser recoveries prevailed under acute conditions. Correlated chemical assays (spectrophotometric or chromatographic) proved less satisfactory and from 10 to 30% of the daily dose excreted in urine and feces according to radioquantitation remained unaccounted for. This discrepancy is tentatively attributed to inadequate methodology for determination of all known and unknown metabolites of the phenothiazine drugs.

ACKNOWLEDGMENTS

This study was supported in part by U.S. Public Health Service grants MH 18190 and MH 20094 as well as by research support from the Veterans Administration.

REFERENCES

1. Curry, S. H., Davis, J. M., Janowsky, D. S., and Marshall, J. H. L., *Arch. Gen. Psychiat.*, **22**, 209 (1970).
2. Bolt, A. G., Forrest, I. S., and Serra, M. T., *J. Pharm. Sci.*, **55**, 1205 (1966).
3. Brookes, L. G., and Forrest, I. S., *Exp. Med. Surg.*, **29**, 61 (1971).
4. Forrest, I. S., and Brookes, L. G., in *Proc. Seventh Congress of Collegium Internationale Neuro-Psychopharmacologicum*, Prague, August 1970.
5. Forrest, I. S., Brookes, L. G., Deneau, G. A., and Mellett, L. B., *The Pharmacologist*, **12** (2), 273 (1970).
6. Bolt, A. G., and Forrest, I. S., *J. Pharm. Sci.*, **56**, 1533 (1967).
7. Forrest, I. S., Bolt, A. G., and Serra, M. T., *Biochem. Pharmacol.*, **17**, 2061 (1968).
8. Forrest, I. S., Rose, S. D., Brookes, L. G., Halpern, B., Bacon, V. A., and Silberg, I. A., *Agressologie*, **11**, 127 (1970).

9. Forrest, I. S., Green, D. E., and Serra, M. T., *Psychopharmacology Bulletin,* **9 (2),** 20 (1973).
10. Kaul, P. N., Conway, M. W., Ticku, M. K., and Clark, M. L., *J. Pharm. Sci.,* **61,** 581 (1972).
11. Kaul, P. N., Conway, M. W., Ticku, M. K., and Clark, M. L., *J. Lab. Clin. Med.,* **81,** 467 (1973).
12. Symchowicz, S., Peckham, W. D., Eisler, M., and Perlman, P. L., *Biochem. Pharmacol.,* **11,** 417 (1962).
13. Phillips, B. M., and Miya, T. S., *Proc. Soc. Exp. Biol. Med.,* **112,** 706 (1963).
14. Phillips, B. M., and Miya, T. S., *J. Pharm. Sci.,* **53,** 1098 (1964).

The Phenothiazines and Structurally Related Drugs, edited by I. S. Forrest, C. J. Carr, and E. Usdin. Raven Press, New York © 1974.

High-Pressure Chromatographic Analysis of Phenothiazine-Related Compounds

William C. Landgraf

Applications Research Department, Quality Control Division, Syntex Laboratories, Inc., Palo Alto, California 94304

INTRODUCTION

In the past few years, a single technique has emerged strongly to support the needs of biological, analytical, and pharmaceutical chemists in their analysis of complex mixtures. This method of analysis, high-pressure liquid chromatography (HPLC), is unusual in that it has been applied to a wide variety of compounds such as steroids (1, 2), amino acids, proteins, sulfa drugs (3), antioxidants, and other pharmaceuticals (4). The technique can be applied at relatively low concentrations when the appropriate detector is used. Important considerations are that HPLC techniques generally do not require derivatives, and they operate at or near room temperature, thereby avoiding thermal stressing of compounds. Our earlier efforts have been directed to the analytical application of HPLC techniques to steroid-related separations where it is highly successful. In the current work we have attempted to determine phenothiazine-related drugs and some metabolites by HPLC methods. Its principal focus was on the attempt to achieve separation and identification of these products.

THE HPLC TECHNIQUE

To illustrate this method in detail we will begin by relating to developments in our own HPLC system, which consists of a mechanical pump, columns, injection port, and detector system.

For a particular separation attempt, one selects a solvent system, polar, nonpolar or some intermediate combination which is appropriate to the task.

The separation of components on the column depends on the principle of partitioning between the mobile phase and the permanently bound polar phase on the surface of the substrate. This latter consists of spherical particles that have been chemically treated to yield surfaces with distinct levels of polarity. $P = x_1/W/(x_0 = x_1)/L$ (5, 6) is an expression which can be

357

used to relate such partitioning on the columns where $(x_0 - x_1)/L$ equals the concentration of solute in extracting phase and x_1/W equals concentration remaining in original solution. Collander might express this distribution as $\log P_2 = a \log P_1 + b$, where P_2 and P_1 represent the two phases and coefficient a represents a goodness of fit parameter in linear equation, when the data is compared to some reference system.

For optimum sample introduction, one employs loop injection which maintains constant operating conditions on the column. Errors relating to operational variables are significantly decreased by using the loop injectors. Many HPLC systems employ a single meter column while we use three meters and an ultraviolet (UV) detector, operating at 254 nm, for strongly UV absorbing steroids. Other detectors sensing other physical parameters have been employed. During the course of this present work, as with our earlier efforts, we have noticed that substantial care is required in the selection and subsequent treatment of these particles in order to achieve good partitioning characteristics for our columns (5, 7). For example, several levels of chemical treatment have been employed and these result in distinct activity levels for the columns employed. The higher levels result in very polar columns, which have very high loading capacities, longer retention times, and also can tolerate milligram quantities of materials. However, more frequently, moderate levels of chemical treatment yield more reasonable retention times.

In order to assure flexibility in the composition of the mobile phase, a ternary system is employed. This consists of trimethyl pentane, isopropanol, and acetonitrile, the combination of which is partially variable. This variation permits some control of the polarity of the mobile-phase system, which affects the retention time in our columns. In addition to these rather polar columns, an octadecyl silane (ODS) column for reverse phase partitioning has been employed with excellent results. Here again, the composition of the mobile phase is multicomponent. For example, trimethyl pentane, isopropanol, a secondary amine, and water are used in varying quantities depending on the resolution requirements of the compounds. The usual operating conditions are typical and variable from 1,500 to 2,800 psi with flow velocities of 0.5 to 2.0 cc/min.

APPLICATION OF TECHNIQUE TO SPECIFIC PROBLEMS

The utility of the HPLC method has been extended by us to a number of pharmaceutical areas. In particular, it is used for the analysis of disodium cromoglycate (8), an antiasthmatic compound, many steroids, sulfa drugs, phenolics, and prostaglandins. For the steroids, it has been demonstrated that this method is capable of differentiating many steroids which have similar substituents. Tables 1 and 2 list the relative retention times of these compounds and in some cases the difference in retention times.

TABLE 1. *Retention times of various steroids*

No.	Compound	Retention time (min)
(1)	Norethindrone (17-Hydroxy-19-Nor-17α-pregn-4-ene-20-yn-3-one)	15.7
(2)	Progesterone (4-Pregnene-3,20-dione)	15.8
(3)	Fluocinonide (6α,9α-Difluoro-11β,16α,17-trihydroxy-21-acetate-pregna-1,4-diene-3,20-dione cyclic 16,17-acetal with acetone)	18.5
(4)	Deoxycorticosterone (21-Hydroxy-pregn-4-ene-3,20-dione)	20.4
(5)	Flurandrenolide (6α-Fluoro-11β,21-dihydroxy-pregn-4-ene-3,20-dione)	22.0
(6)	Paramethasone Acetate (6α-Fluoro-11β,17α-dihydroxy-21-acetate-16α-methyl-1,4-pregnadiene-3,20-dione)	22.0
(7)	11-Deoxycortisol (17α,21-Dihydroxy-4-pregnene-3,20-dione)	23.2
(8)	Corticosterone (11β,21-Dihydroxy-pregn-4-ene-3,20-dione)	26.0
(9)	Cortisone acetate (17α,21-Acetate-hydroxy-pregn-4-ene-3,11,20-trione)	28.2
(10)	Fluocinolone Acetonide (6α,9α-Difluoro-11β,16α,17,21-tetrahydroxypregna-1,4-diene-3,20-dione cyclic 16,17-acetal with acetone)	27.6
(11)	Lactone from (10) (6α,9α-Difluoro-11β,16ξ,20ξ-trihydroxypregna-1,4-diene-3-one-21-oic-16-lactone)	64.0
(12)	21-Aldehyde from (10) (6α,9α-Difluoro-11β,16α,17α-trihydroxypregna-1,4-diene-3,20-dione-21-AL-16,17-acetonide)	66.0
(13)	21-Acid from (10) (6α,9α-Difluoro-11β,16α,17α 20 tetrahydroxypregna-1,4-diene-3-one-21 carboxy-16,17-acetonide)	> 60.0

TABLE 2. *Retention time increments*

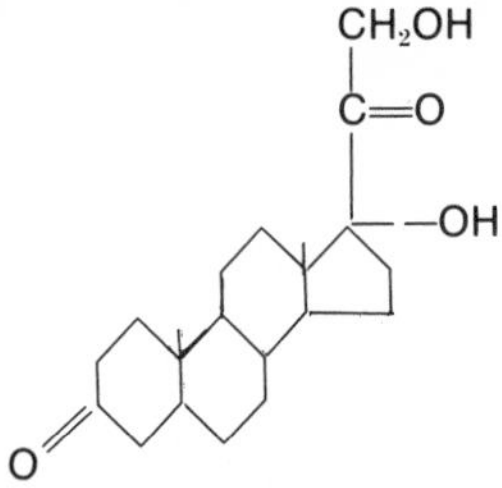

CH$_2$OH

C=O

—OH

O

11-Deoxycortisol
23.2

	Substitution	R.T. increment	
Cortisone	11-ONE	+17.8	
Cortisone acetate	11-ONE, 21 AC	+ 5.6 $\big\rbrace$ 12.2	
Hydrocortisone acetate	11-OH, 21 AC	+ 4.5 $\big\rbrace$ 1.1	2.0
Hydrocortisone	11-OH	+19.8	
Paramethasone acetate	5 F1, 11-OH, 21 AC 16 Me = 5.7	—	
Desoxy	-17 (OH)	− 2.8	
Chloromadinone acetate	5 CL, 17 AC, 5–6 ENE	− 3.4	
Prednisone	H-ONE, 1Δ-ENE	+17.8, +4.4	

The most interesting aspect may be that the partitioning of compounds is effected on columns, the overall plate efficiency (HETP), which is calculated to be no greater than 400/m of column. This observation is in contrast to the relatively high values of plate efficiency stated by numerous commercial houses (9–11). We have prepared such plate number columns in our laboratory, but they do not, in our estimation, yield as good a resolution for the compounds we have examined.

The urine samples we examined for chlorpromazine metabolites were supplied to us by a local hospital laboratory. In the analyses of the urine extracts, much use was made of the reference compounds supplied to us by Dr. Manian of N.I.M.H., whose help is gratefully acknowledged.

The urine sample of a specific individual treated with 1,200 mg/day chlorpromazine was extracted using a combination of techniques, ion exchange and partitioning into a solvent system. This concentrate was used for injection onto the HPLC columns. As previously described, the samples were partitioned on our HPLC system using the ternary system of trimethylene pentane, ethanol, and acetonitrile as the mobile phase. The separated compounds were detected with a 254 nm UV detector (12). Each of these retention times was compared to values of retention times of reference compounds (Tables 3 and 4).

TABLE 3. *Retention times*

Compound	Retention time (min)
7 MeO-Promazine	14.6
6 (OH) Cl Promazine	29.9
7,8 (MEO)$_2$ CP	18.1
7 (OH) CP	27.8
Chlorpromazine sulfone	25.6
Nor$_1$-CP · HCl	33.0
Estrone	24.4
Equilin	29.3
2 Cl-Phenothiazine	11.8
Nor$_1$ CP · HCl	22.0
7 OH-8 MeO CP	23.6
Nor$_1$ CP SO	40.9
CPN-Oxide	81.5
7 OH Nor$_1$ CP	48 (Broad)
7 OH-Nor$_2$ CP-SO	
CP Sulfoxide SKF (CP 5-Oxide)	19.3

CP = Chlorpromazine.

TABLE 4. *Component of urine sample*

Compound		Based on 254 nm ABS Approximate concentration
1	2 Cl Phenothiazine	20%
2	Nor$_1$-CP	35%
3	7,8 (MeO)$_2$ CP -or- CP 5-oxide	35%
4	7 OH CP	3%
5	Nor$_1$ CP-SO	3%
6	CP N-oxide	5%

DISCUSSION

Examination of the data for retention times of the reference compounds (Table 3) with the data from the HPLC analysis of the urine (Table 4) establishes several points. First, compounds 4, 5, and 6 do appear to be consistent with previously reported data. Second, compound 3 CP 5-oxide correlates well with prior reports and permits us to reject the other alternative 7,8 (MeO)$_2$ CP from consideration. However, with 2-chlorophenothiazine (compound 1) and the Nor$_1$ CP (compound 2), the current data are significantly in excess of prior reports: 1 to 2% versus 20 to 35%. Therefore, a more reasonable interpretation of these data might be to suggest that the compounds in question are indeed the Nor$_1$ CP and 2-chlorophenothiazine, but that they are incompletely resolved from other components, which for the present cannot be uniquely identified. It is most reasonable to expect that these compounds will be identified by reference to other compounds soon to be examined by us.

The results reported here tend to support the GLC determinations made by Johnson et al. (13); however, they do differ in actual concentration of metabolites found. Furthermore, the results differ from those observed by Forrest (14) in a recent study on rhesus monkeys.

SUMMARY

The use of HPLC as an analytical technique to separate urinary metabolites of chlorpromazine has been explored. For comparison, HPLC data for various steroids are given, as the data and techniques for these compounds are considerably further advanced. Furthermore, steroids — both exogenous and endogenous — are subject to biotransformation, which are quite similar to phenothiazines, e.g., hydroxylation and formation of glucuronides. The effect of substituents on the basic structure will be similar (for retention times) for the various phenothiazine compounds.

Tentative quantitation of some phenothiazine metabolites has been made by a comparison of the retention times of the compounds isolated from urine with those of reference compounds. The technique has not yet been developed to the extent that qualitative and quantitative results by HPLC can be compared with the analytical results from other assay techniques.

REFERENCES

1. Landgraf, W. C., and Jennings, E. C., *J. Pharm. Sci.,* **62**, 278 (1972).
2. Krol, G. J., Masserano, R., Carrey, J., and Khan, T., *J. Pharm. Sci.,* **10**, 1483 (1970).
3. Poet, R. B., and Pu, H. H., *J. Pharm. Sci.,* **62**, 809 (1973).
4. Roos, R. W., *J. Pharm. Sci.,* **61**, 1979 (1972).
   Rabel, F. M., *Anal. Chem.,* **45**, 957 (1973).
5. Leo, A., Hansch, C., and Elkins, D., *Chem. Rev.,* **71**, 525 (1971).
6. Hoy, K. B. L., *J. Paint. Tech.,* **42**, 76 (1970).
7. Bossant, C. J., *ISA-Transact.,* **7**, 283 (1968).
8. Cox, J. S. C., Woodard, G. D., and McCrone, W. C., *J. Pharm. Sci.,* **60**, 1458 (1971).
9. Kirkland, J. J., *Anal. Chem.,* **41**, 218 (1969).
10. Kirkland, J. J., and DeStefano, J., *J. Chrom. Sci.,* **8**, 309 (1970).
11. Kirkland, J. J., *J. Chrom. Sci.,* **7**, 7 (1969).
12. Veenings, H., *J. Chem. Ed.,* **11**, A749 (1970).
13. Johnson, D. E., Rodriguez, C. F., and Burchfield, H. P., *Biochem. Pharm.,* **14**, 1453 (1969).
14. Forrest, I. S. *(unpublished data).*

The Phenothiazines and Structurally Related Drugs, edited by I. S. Forrest, C. J. Carr, and E. Usdin. Raven Press, New York © 1974.

Development of Antibodies to Chlorpromazine

Sydney Spector

Roche Institute of Molecular Biology, Nutley, New Jersey 07110

Radioimmunoassays, when introduced by Yalow and Berson (1), were used for the measurement of protein hormones; it soon became apparent that this method had applicability for compounds other than protein hormones. Thus, polypeptide hormones, nonpeptide hormones, and drugs are all presently being measured by radioimmunoassay. Radioimmunoassay offers many advantages in the determination of physiologically and pharmacologically active substances in biologic fluids or tissues. The procedure is relatively easy to carry out. It is based on the principle of competition between a labeled and unlabeled antigen for a specific antibody.

Antigen* + Antibody $\rightleftarrows$ Antigen* − Antibody,
Antigen* + Antigen + Antibody $\rightleftarrows$ Antigen* − Antibody + Antigen
$$− Antibody.$$

The critical factor in establishing a satisfactory radioimmunoassay is the development of a satisfactory antiserum; for the antiserum to meet that criterium, it should possess high avidity and a great specificity for the antigen.

Immunogenicity of a compound is related to a number of factors; molecular weight is of prime importance. The minimal molecular weight necessary to stimulate antibody production has been markedly reduced; it has been reported that some small peptides such as angiotensin II (2) and oxytocin (3) can elicit antibody formation. However, most drugs require conjugation to a carrier as they are not immunogenic by themselves. We coupled the haptenic group, chlorpromazine, to bovine serum albumin by complexing the diazotized *p*-amino benzoic acid to chlorpromazine and then conjugated the diazotized complex to the protein using a water soluble carbodiimide reagent. Figure 1 indicates the postulated conjugated protein used for immunization.

Rabbits were immunized in the foot pads with an emulsion containing the immunogen in Freund's complete adjuvant. The injections were repeated at weekly intervals for 4 weeks; a fifth injection containing the immunogen alone was administered intradermally into multiple sites along the flank of

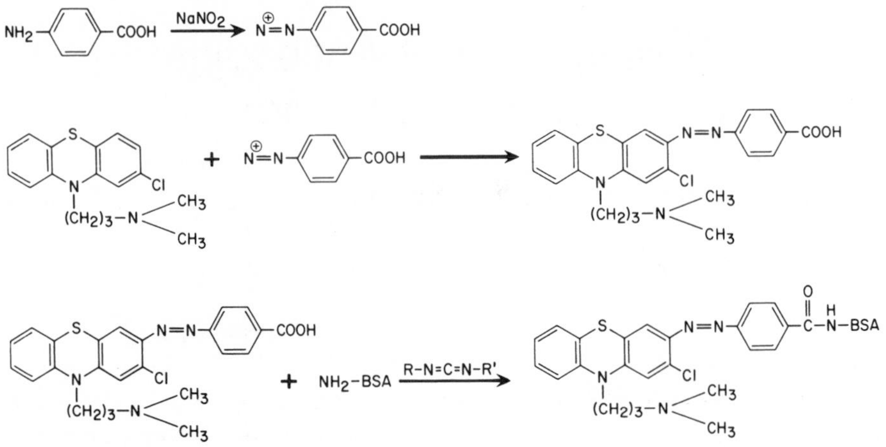

FIG. 1. Conjugation of CPZ to protein carrier.

the animal a month later. Rabbits were bled 10 days later. The sera of the immunized animals were then tested for the presence of antibodies by incubating varying dilutions of the antiserum with a constant amount of labeled antigen. The antibody-antigen* complex was separated from the antigen*-free fraction by the Farr procedure.

Although we have been able to generate antibodies which are specific for chlorpromazine and fail to bind chlorpromazine sulfoxide, we have not determined the full specificity of the antibodies. Problems have arisen in the development of a radioimmunoassay for chlorpromazine: we have had great difficulty in obtaining antibodies possessing a high titer or high avidity for the haptenic group, and sensitivity of the assay will be determined by the affinity of the antibody.

Another problem to be resolved before we have a good radioimmunoassay for chlorpromazine is its protein-binding capacity. Since the assay is dependent on the binding of the haptenic group to a limited number of sites on the antibody, anything that binds the hapten nonspecifically will affect the assay adversely.

There are many techniques to measure chlorpromazine. Most are time consuming and complex. Although to date a satisfactory radioimmunoassay for chlorpromazine has not been developed, the method offers the inherent advantages of specificity and simplicity.

REFERENCES

1. Yalow, R. S., and Berson, S. A., *J. Clin. Invest.*, **39**, 1157 (1960).
2. Boyd, G. W., Landon, J., and Peart, W. S., *Lancet*, **II**, 1002 (1967).
3. Chard, T., Kitan, M. J., and Landon, J., *J. Endocr.*, **46**, 269 (1970).

The Phenothiazines and Structurally Related Drugs, edited by I. S. Forrest, C. J. Carr, and E. Usdin. Raven Press, New York © 1974.

Immunological Properties of Some Phenothiazines

M. Shostak

New York State Psychiatric Institute, 722 West 168th Street, New York, New York 10032

INTRODUCTION

The measurement of drug levels in tissues and biological fluids has proved to be a valuable technique both by furthering our theoretical understanding of drug action and by providing a rational basis for clinical use. In the case of phenothiazines, efforts have been hampered by the minute amounts of drug involved and by the multiplicity of metabolites simultaneously present. Numerous techniques have been developed for measuring these substances: spectrophotometry (1, 2), radioactive derivative formation (3), fluorescent derivative formation (4, 5), gas-liquid chromatography (6), and thin-layer chromatography (7). The limitations and pitfalls of these and other techniques have been critically reviewed by Usdin (8). All of the methods currently in use are complex and require so much time, labor, and meticulous attention that studies have, of necessity, been limited in size, with correspondingly limited data. Small sample size is a particularly severe constraint in psychiatric studies since response to a neuroleptic drug is not a simple one-dimensional variable which can be readily and accurately measured. Furthermore, psychiatric diagnostic categories are themselves somewhat ambiguous. This combination of technical, methodological, and conceptual factors may explain the conflicting results obtained by various laboratories and the poor correlation between drug levels and clinical response.

This paper describes the results of a study of the immunogenicity of phenothiazines in animals.[1] It was initiated in an attempt to develop a simpler, more readily applied method of measuring drug levels using radioimmunoassay.

The major part of this study was focused on chlorpromazine (CPZ), since it is the most widely used neuroleptic and since many of its metabolites have been identified and characterized. Because it is difficult to couple to CPZ, two compounds with similar structures but reactive functional groups were

---

[1] The phenothiazines used in this study, together with their structures and nomenclature, are listed in Table 1.

TABLE 1. *Phenothiazine structure and nomenclature*

Compound/Abbreviation	R_2	R_5	R_7	R_{10}
Chlorpromazine/CPZ 2-Chloro-10-(3-dimethylaminopropyl)phenothiazine	Cl	—	H	$-CH_2CH_2CH_2N(CH_3)_2$
Promazine/PRZ 10-(3-dimethylaminopropyl)phenothiazine	H	—	H	$-CH_2CH_2CH_2N(CH_3)_2$
Trifluopromazine/TFP 10-[3-(dimethylamino)propyl]-2-trifluoromethylphenothiazine	CF_3	—	H	$-CH_2CH_2CH_2N(CH_3)_2$
Chlorpromazine sulfoxide/CPZ-SO 2-Chloro-10-[3-(dimethylamino)propyl]phenothiazine 5-oxide	Cl	O	H	$-CH_2CH_2CH_2N(CH_3)_2$
7-Hydroxychlorpromazine/7-OH-CPZ 2-Chloro-7hydroxy-10-[3-(dimethylamino)propyl]phenothiazine	Cl	—	OH	$-CH_2CH_2CH_2N(CH_3)_2$
Desdimethylchlorpromazine/Nor$_2$CPZ 2-Chloro-10-(3-aminopropyl)phenothiazine	Cl	—	H	$-CH_2CH_2CH_2NH_2$
Quaternary Chlorpromazine/CPZ-QA 2-Chloro-10-[3-(trimethylamino)propyl]phenothiazine Iodide	Cl	—	H	$-CH_2CH_2CH_2\overset{+}{N}(CH_3)_3I^-$
Desdimethylchlorpromazine Mono Amide/Nor$_2$CPZ-MA 2-Chloro-10-[3-(acetamino)propyl]phenothiazine	Cl	—	H	$-CH_2CH_2CH_2NHCOCH_3$
Perphenazine/PER 2-Chloro-10-{3-[1-(2-hydroxyethyl)-4-piperazynl]propyl}phenothiazine	Cl	—	H	$-CH_2CH_2CH_2-$ $N(CH_2)_2(CH_2)_2NCH_2CH_2OH$
Perphenazine Hemisuccinate/PHS 2-Chloro-10-{3-[1-(2-succinoylethyl)-4-piperazynl]propyl}phenothiazine	Cl	—	H	$-CH_2CH_2CH_2-$ $N(CH_2)_2(CH_2)_2N-$ $CH_2CH_2OCOCH_2CH_2COOH$

used: perphenazine and desdimethylchlorpromazine. It was assumed that, because of the structural similarity, antibodies to either or both of these drugs would cross-react sufficiently well with CPZ to be usable in an assay for CPZ.

MATERIALS AND METHODS

Animals

New Zealand white female rabbits, weight 6 to 8 lbs, were obtained from Marland Farms (Wayne, N.J.). Pirbright guinea pigs, weight 500 to 800 g, were obtained from a colony maintained by Dr. J. R. Battisto at the Albert Einstein College of Medicine.

Materials

CPZ hydrochloride, desdimethylated CPZ hydrochloride, and CPZ sulfoxide hydrochloride were obtained from Smith, Kline, and French Laboratories (Philadelphia, Pa.). Perphenazine base was obtained from the Schering Corporation (Bloomfield, N.J.). Dr. Albert Manian of N.I.M.H. supplied 7-hydroxychlorpromazine hydrochloride. Promazine hydrochloride was obtained from Wyeth Laboratories (Philadelphia, Pa.) and triflupromazine hydrochloride from E. R. Squibb and Sons (Princeton, N.J.). Ring-labeled ^{14}C-CPZ (30 mCi/mM) was obtained from Applied Science Laboratories (State College, Pa.). Bovine serum albumin powder, fraction V, was obtained from Metrix (Chicago, Ill.), crystalline rabbit serum albumin from Sigma (St. Louis, Mo.), and dextran T-70 from Pharmacia (Uppsala, Sweden). 1-Ethyl-3-(dimethyl aminopropyl) carbodiimide HCl was obtained from Ott Chemical Co. (Muskegan, Mich.); succinic anhydride and iso-butylchlorocarbonate were supplied by Eastman. Other chemicals and solvents were reagent grade unless otherwise stated. Disposable plastic ware was used throughout except where organic solvents were present. Radioimmunoassay was carried out in disposable Falcon 12 × 75 mm polypropylene or polystyrene tubes.

Procedures

Perphenazine hemisuccinate · 2HCl (PHS · 2HCl). The perphenazine ester was prepared by a modification of the method of Erlanger et al. (9). Perphenazine base (2 g) was refluxed with 2.4 g of succinic anhydride in 20 ml of dry pyridine. After 4 hr of reflux, a 10-ml aliquot was dried *in vacuo* at 60°C and the residue dissolved in 100 ml chloroform. After 10 washes with 25-ml portions of water, the chloroform was dried over sodium sulfate with 100 mg Norit-A. The product was dried *in vacuo* at 40°C and the residue dissolved in hot ethanol containing 6 ml of 1 N HCl. Ethanol was added to turbidity and the product allowed to crystallize. Yield after three crystallizations was 50%. Low actinic glassware was used throughout.

Quaternary chlorpromazine (CPZ-QA). CPZ HCl (100 mg) was mixed into 0.3 ml 1 N NaOH solution and extracted twice with 2 ml of benzene. Methyl iodide (25 μl) was added and the mixture placed in a water bath at 50°C for 2 hr. The bath was allowed to cool to 20°C over 24 hr and the crystals of CPZ-QA washed three times with cold benzene. Yield after drying was 100%.

Desdimethylchlorpromazine monoamide (Nor$_2$CPZ-MA). Nor$_2$CPZ HCl 100 mg was mixed into 0.3 ml 1 N NaOH solution and extracted twice with 2 ml of benzene. Acetic anhydride 0.2 ml and pyridine 0.05 ml were added and the mixture allowed to react 72 hr at 37°C in a low actinic flask. The contents were evaporated *in vacuo* at 60°C, and the residue dissolved in 5 ml benzene. After three washes with 2 ml of 0.1 N HCl, the volume was reduced by evaporation to about 0.5 ml and ethanol added to turbidity. The yield was 30%.

Calculated: C 61.35, H 5.15, Cl 10.65, N 8.42, S 9.63, O 4.81.
Found: C 61.61, H 5.39, Cl 10.70, N 8.35, S 9.33, O 5.01.

Hapten-protein conjugates. Bovine serum albumin (BSA) 75 mg was dissolved in 2 ml of water and 1 ml of dioxane. pH was adjusted to 8.0 at which point the solution was clear. Approximately 250 mg of 1-ethyl-3-(dimethylaminopropyl) carbodiimide HCl (ECDI) in 0.5 ml of water was added. Nor$_2$CPZ · HCl 25 mg was dissolved in 0.25 ml dioxane plus 0.25 ml water. The solution was added to the protein with stirring and the reaction allowed to proceed for 1 hr at room temperature. The conjugate was dialyzed exhaustively, lyophilized, and washed in cold ether. Approximately 11 moles of hapten coupled to each mole of protein as measured by ultraviolet (UV) absorption. The same procedure was used to couple Nor$_2$CPZ to rabbit serum albumin (RSA).

PHS was coupled to BSA using the mixed anhydride method (9). A mixture of dioxane (2.5 ml), tributylamine (0.4 ml), and dimethyl sulfoxide (2.5 ml) was used to dissolve 290 mg of perphenazine hemisuccinate dihydrochloride (PHS · 2HCl). The mixture was chilled to 5°C, 0.07 ml isobutylchlorocarbonate added, and the reaction allowed to proceed 45 min. BSA (0.62 g) was dissolved in 16 ml water. The pH was adjusted to 9.5, and 16 ml dioxane was added. The solution was chilled to 5°C and the first solution added dropwise with stirring. Reaction was allowed to proceed 4 hr with addition of NaOH to maintain pH at 9. The conjugate was then dialyzed exhaustively. Cold acetone (200 ml) was added and the pH adjusted to maximum precipitation (about 6.5). After centrifugation, the wash with acetone-water was repeated once and the precipitate dissolved in saline and lyophilized. Approximately 15 moles of hapten were coupled to each mole of protein, as determined by UV absorption. The same procedure was used to couple PHS to RSA.

Immunization. Twenty mg of Nor_2CPZ-BSA conjugate was dissolved in 4 ml of phosphate-buffered saline, pH 8.3, and emulsified with 4 ml of complete Freund's Adjuvant (FA). Rabbits were inoculated with 0.25 ml of emulsion in each foot pad. Thirty days later, a second inoculation of 2.5 mg of conjugate in incomplete FA was made, and the rabbits were bled 10 days after that. Sera were stored at $-10°C$. PHS-BSA conjugate was used to immunize a second group of rabbits. Each animal received 2.5 mg in complete FA. One group of control animals received 40 mg of CPZ in complete FA, as described by Ueki (10). Another group of controls received 40 mg of perphenazine in complete FA. Both control groups received boosters at 30 days and were bled 10 days later. A 5-ml sample of blood was taken from each animal used in this study *before* immunization.

Passive cutaneous anaphylaxis (PCA). Sera from immunized animals were assayed in guinea pigs using PCA as described by Ovary (11). Intradermal injections of 0.1 ml were made with appropriate dilutions of serum and the animals challenged 24 hr later with 10 mg of hapten-rabbit albumin conjugate and 12 mg of Evans Blue given intravenously. Reactions were scored for size and intensity 1 hr later. Controls included hapten alone, carrier alone, and a mixture of the two.

^{14}C-*CPZ binding.* All sera, pre- and postimmunization, were assayed for CPZ* binding. A 0.9-ml aliquot of serum, diluted 1:100, was placed in a plastic 12×75 mm test tube, and 0.1 ml of CPZ* containing 5,000 cpm was added. After 24 hr incubation at 4°C, 1 ml of charcoal dextran solution in 2% normal rabbit serum was added, and the tubes centrifuged 1 hr at 2,000 rpm. A 1-ml aliquot from each tube was then counted in a Nuclear Chicago Mark 1 Scintillation Spectrometer. The charcoal dextran solution was made up in phosphate-buffered saline, pH 7.2, and contained 2 mg of Norit A and 2 mg of dextran T-70 per ml. The time interval between the first addition of charcoal and centrifugation was variable but generally between 5 to 10 min.

Binding inhibition curves. Competitive inhibition of CPZ* binding by various metabolites of CPZ and by related drugs was measured for concentrations ranging from 10 to 1,000 ng/ml for each drug. Eight to 12 concentrations were used per compound, and each concentration was done in duplicate. A suitable aliquot of compound, diluted in PBS, pH 7.2, was first pipetted into each tube, followed by 0.1 ml of CPZ* and sufficient buffer to bring the volume to 0.5 ml. Antiserum to Nor_2CPZ-BSA was diluted 1:75 and 0.5 ml added to each tube, resulting in a final concentration of 1:150. After incubation for 24 hr at 4°C, free CPZ* was separated by adding 1 ml of charcoal dextran solution followed by centrifugation at 2,000 rpm for 1 hr. A 1-ml aliquot of each supernatant was counted. Each set of tubes also included a pair with normal serum, a pair to which buffer but no charcoal was added, and a pair at the end to which no drug was added.

RESULTS

Both conjugates proved highly immunogenic in rabbits. Heterocytotrophic antiserum was produced by five out of five animals immunized with Nor_2-CPZ-BSA and by six of six immunized with PHS-BSA. Table 2 summarizes the data obtained using PCA in guinea pigs. Anti PHS-BSA serum reacted only with PHS-RSA. Hapten alone (0.1 mg), RSA alone (10 mg), and a mixture of the two were ineffective. Antiserum titers, defined as the maximum dilution causing a 10-mm blue reaction, were in the range of 1:500. Sera from animals immunized with drug not coupled to a carrier were uniformly negative, despite the use of FA.

TABLE 2. *Rabbit antiphenothiazine antibody detection using PCA in the guinea pig*

Immunizing antigen	Challenge antigen[b]	No. pos./ No. tested	Titer[a]
PHS-BSA	PHS-RSA	6/6	1:600
	Nor$_2$CPZ-RSA	0/6	—
	RSA	0/6	—
	PHS	0/6	—
	RSA + PHS[c]	0/6	—
Nor$_2$CPZ-BSA	Nor$_2$CPZ-RSA	5/5	1:400
	PHS-RSA	5/5	1:400
	RSA	0/5	—
	CPZ	0/5	—
	CPZ + RSA[c]	0/5	—
PHS	PHS	0/3	—
CPZ	CPZ	0/3	—

[a] Antiserum titer is the greatest dilution causing a 10-mm blue reaction.
[b] Challenge antigen given intravenously 20–24 hr after intradermal injections of antiserum.
[c] Mixture of hapten and carrier (not covalently bound).

Table 3 summarizes CPZ* binding by various types of sera. Preimmunization sera (i.e., normal sera) bound 50 to 110 cpm, with a mean of 70. Sera from animals immunized with drug alone did not differ significantly from normal sera. Sera from animals immunized with Nor$_2$CPZ-BSA bound 830 to 3,000 cpm, with a mean of 980. Anti-PHS-BSA serum bound 200 to 1,700 cpm, with a mean of 600.

The radioactivity bound by an anti-Nor$_2$CPZ-BSA serum as a function of dilution is shown in Fig. 1. At low dilutions, 1:10 or less, essentially all of the added label is bound, approximately 20 ng of CPZ*. The amount bound decreases as the antiserum is diluted, reaching 50% at 1:150 and 0%

TABLE 3. ^{14}C-CPZ binding by pre- and postimmunization sera—all sera diluted 1:100. Total radioactivity added 5,000 cpm—25 ng CPZ*

Immunizing antigen	No. of rabbits	Range	Mean CPM bound
Preimmunization	30	50–100	70
PHS-BSA	6	200–1700	600
Nor₂CPZ-BSA	5	830–3000	980
PHS	3	60–70	68
CPZ	3	68–108	88

at 1:2,000. For comparison, a curve using ammonium sulfate to separate free from bound CPZ* is also shown. The two methods yield very similar results, indicating that dextran-coated charcoal does not cause significant dissociation of hapten-antibody complex. The problem of dissociation is a critical one in using dextran-coated charcoal. Figure 2 illustrates dissociation as a function of time elapsed between addition of charcoal and centrifugation. Normal serum equilibrates almost instantly, reaching a constant level of 1 to 2% in less than 1 min. Antiserum equilibrates in two steps: a rapid phase from 0 to 2 min and then a slow phase from 55% at 3 min to 45% at 30 min. When a series of tubes was processed, the time between pipetting into the first tube and start of centrifugation was always less than 12 min in order to minimize error due to dissociation.

The effect of several ring-altered metabolites and of unlabeled CPZ on CPZ* binding is shown in Fig. 3. In the absence of any compound except CPZ*, about 60% or 2,500 cpm of the radioactive tracer is bound. As in-

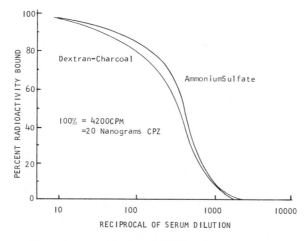

FIG. 1. Percent radioactivity bound by Nor₂CPZ-BSA antiserum as a function of dilution. Bound and free hapten were separated by dextran-charcoal (lower curve) and by precipitation with ammonium sulfate (upper curve).

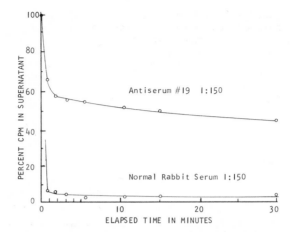

FIG. 2. Dissociation of Nor₂CPZ-BSA antiserum complexed with CPZ*, by dextran-coated charcoal. Time between addition of charcoal and initiation of centrifugation is shown on the abscissa. About 20 ng of CPZ*, 4,200 cpm, was added to the antiserum and the mixture incubated 24 hr at 4°C before separation.

creasing amounts of another, unlabeled drug are added, binding decreases. This effect is most pronounced in the case of unlabeled CPZ, where 50% inhibition is observed with 70 ng of drug. At 1,000 ng, binding has decreased to less than 10%. PHS, indicated by discrete points, behaves in a manner identical to CPZ. Inhibition curves for two ring-altered metabolites, 7-OH-CPZ and CPZ-SO, are also shown. The 50% inhibition values for these

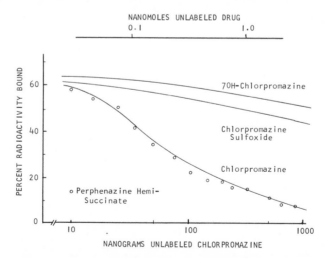

FIG. 3. Competitive inhibition curves for perphenazine, CPZ, and ring-altered metabolites of CPZ. The ordinate represents radioactivity bound by a fixed amount of Nor₂CPZ-BSA antiserum in the presence of variable amounts of other unlabeled drugs. The upper abscissa (nm) applies to all curves; The lower abscissa (ng) applies only to CPZ. Antiserum diluted 1:150.

compounds are over 10,000 ng. Mass of other compounds may be obtained by multiplying the lower abscissa values (Fig. 3) by the ratio MW/319.

Inhibition curves for promazine and triflupromazine are shown in Fig. 4. These drugs are identical to CPZ except for the substituent at position 2 (see Table 1). Promazine, which is not substituted at position 2, is weakly bound and has a 50% inhibition mass of about 1,500 ng. Triflupromazine, which has a trifluoromethyl group, is intermediate between promazine and CPZ, with a 50% inhibition mass of 350 ng.

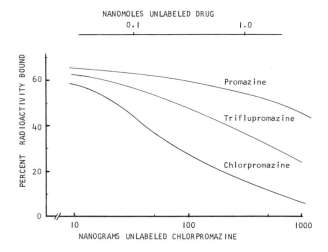

FIG. 4. Competitive inhibition curves for CPZ, promazine, and triflupromazine. Ordinate and abscissa as in Fig. 3.

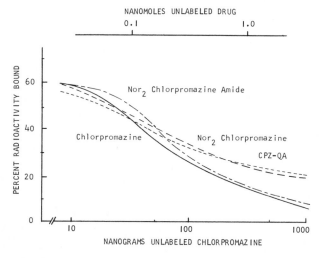

FIG. 5. Competitive inhibition curves for CPZ and side-chain altered compounds. Ordinate and abscissa as in Fig. 3.

Figure 5 illustrates the inhibition curves for a number of side-chain altered compounds. Nor_2CPZ amide (monoamide) is almost as effective as CPZ in competing for binding sites on the antibody; 50% inhibition occurs with about 90 ng. Nor_2CPZ is about as effective as CPZ-QA, and both are inferior to CPZ; 50% inhibition for these compounds occurs at about 130 ng.

DISCUSSION

Perphenazine and Nor_2CPZ, when individually covalently coupled to carrier proteins, elicited synthesis of hapten-specific antibody in rabbits, whereas the drugs alone did not. Because of the structural similarity of these compounds to CPZ, both types of antisera exhibited a high degree of reactivity with CPZ. Antiserum to Nor_2CPZ-BSA conjugate, diluted 1:150, bound 60% of a tracer dose of 20 ng (4,200 cpm) of CPZ*. Addition of unlabeled drug resulted in a decrease in bound radioactivity; 50% inhibition required 70 ng of unlabeled CPZ. A high degree of specificity for the heterocyclic ring structure of CPZ was observed. While only 70 ng of CPZ was required for 50% inhibition, more than 10,000 ng of CPZ-SO or 7-OH-CPZ was needed to achieve the same result. This type of specificity would thus permit determination of CPZ levels in the presence of large amounts of ring-altered metabolites.

When this study was initiated, it was assumed that plasma from CPZ-treated patients would contain moderate to large amounts of unchanged CPZ, moderate amounts of CPZ-SO and 7-OH-CPZ, and relatively small amounts (10 to 15%) of mono- or didesmethylated compounds (Curry: 6, 12, 13). As long as this assumption holds, the use of a serum which is insensitive to side-chain alterations does not introduce excessive error. The antisera described in this study (see especially Fig. 5) are relatively insensitive to perturbations in side-chain structure. This is a direct consequence of using the side-chain terminal nitrogen as a coupling site. Any desmethylated compounds present (unless they are ring altered as well) will simply increase the measured value of CPZ.

Some recently published studies have reported the predominance of desmethylated compounds, with only small amounts of unchanged CPZ present (14, 15). Under these conditions, an antiserum insensitive to side-chain variations would cause serious errors. Several approaches to this kind of difficulty are possible.

One solution is to measure an aliquot of serum before and after reaction with a sterically bulky reagent such as biphenyl sulfonic acid. This reagent, which reacts with primary and secondary amines, would alter the side chain sufficiently to prevent binding with antibody. After reaction with such a reagent, only free CPZ would be measured. The difference between initial and final values would represent total desmethylated metabolites.

Another possibility is to form the hapten-protein conjugate by coupling to one of the rings of CPZ. The side-chain nitrogen atom, together with its methyl groups, should then form an integral part of the structure to which antibody is directed. Because of the rotational freedom of the side chain, it is not obvious *a priori* how much specificity to this part of the molecule could be achieved. This is a question which can only be answered empirically, and we are presently investigating the properties of an antiserum against CPZ-BSA coupled via the 2 (chlorine) position.

The metabolism of CPZ is extremely complicated, and only a few dozen of the many theoretically possible metabolites have been isolated and characterized. The problem is compounded because it is unclear if the therapeutic benefit derived from CPZ is due to the unchanged drug, to one or more metabolites, or to some combination. In view of these difficulties, it would be unrealistic to expect radioimmunoassay, or any other single technique, to provide a definitive solution to so complex a problem. Perhaps the situation is best conceived of in terms of the state of the art prevailing in endocrinology, a field where radioimmunoassay has been developed to a high degree of perfection. The endocrinologist, faced with the task of measuring a hormone in a sample containing dozens, has developed many types of antisera. These sera, together with a variety of extraction and separation techniques, provide a reasonably satisfactory solution, without the use of extremely complicated and expensive equipment. The same type of approach could be applied to the problem of CPZ and its metabolites.

We have described the results of an investigation of the immunogenicity of phenothiazines. The data indicate that antisera are readily elicitable when the drugs are covalently coupled to a carrier protein. These antisera have been tested with a variety of compounds and shown to have properties which are very useful for radioimmunoassay. The sensitivity using a tracer of specific activity 30 mCi/mM is approximately 25 ng, but clearly increasing the specific activity would increase the sensitivity correspondingly.

SUMMARY

A study of the immunogenicity of phenothiazines in animals is described. Perphenazine and Nor_2CPZ, when individually covalently coupled to carrier proteins, elicited synthesis of hapten-specific antibody in rabbits, whereas either drug alone did not.

Antisera were assayed by two methods: *in vivo* by PCA, and *in vitro* by measurement of binding of the radioactive parent compound (CPZ*). Using dextran-coated charcoal to adsorb free drug, antisera to Nor_2CPZ-protein conjugate bound 8 to 36 times as much CPZ* as normal serum, while antisera to perphenazine-protein conjugate bound 2 to 17 times as much. Suitability for radioimmunoassay was tested by competitive inhibition of CPZ* binding by unlabeled CPZ and a number of metabolites and related compounds. All of the compounds tested caused some inhibition. CPZ was the most effective, 50% inhibition occurring at 70 ng. CPZ-SO and 7-OH-CPZ were only slightly bound; over 10,000 ng were required for 50% inhibition. The 50% values for promazine and triflupromazine were 1,500 and 350 ng, respectively. A number of side-chain-altered compounds were tested in a similar manner. Nor_2CPZ, Nor_2CPZ monoamide, and CPZ-QA were all significantly bound; the 50% inhibitory values were 140, 90, and 130 nanograms respectively. Perphenazine and unlabeled CPZ were equally effective in displacing CPZ*, indicating that a Nor_2CPZ antiserum can be used to measure either drug.

The results obtained in this study indicate that it is readily possible to make antisera to phenothiazines when they are coupled to a carrier, and suggest that these sera will be useful in the assay of phenothiazines as they are encountered in clinical practice.

ACKNOWLEDGMENTS

This work was supported in part by Grant MH 21297–01. The author wishes to thank Dr. Paul Newman (Department of Chemistry, Manhattan College, New York) who provided many helpful suggestions concerning organic syntheses; Dr. Robert Rosenfeld (Steroid Institute, Montefiore Hospital, New York) who suggested the use of perphenazine and made the first sample of hemisuccinate; and Dr. James Perel (New York State Psychiatric Institute, New York) who made many helpful suggestions concerning the measurement of phenothiazine compounds.

The author is especially indebted to Dr. J. R. Battisto, (Department of Microbiology and Immunology, Albert Einstein College of Medicine) for the use of his laboratory facilities, for his inexhaustible patience and enthusiasm, and for many valuable suggestions concerning immunological problems which arose during this study.

Dr. Tobias Yellin, Smith Kline and French Laboratories, Philadelphia Pa., made available generous amounts of Nor_2CPZ; and Dr. Albert Manian, N.I.M.H., supplied ultrapure samples of 7-OH-CPZ and CPZ-SO.

REFERENCES

1. Bolt, A. G., Forrest, I. S., and Serra, M. T., *J. Pharm. Sci.*, **55**, 1205 (1966).
2. Bolt, A. G. and Forrest, I. S., *J. Pharm. Sci.*, **56**, 1208 (1967).
3. Efron, D. H., Gaudette, L. E., and Harris, S. R., *Agressologie*, **9**, 103 (1968).
4. Kaul, P. N., Conway, M. W., Clark, M. L., and Huffine, J., *J. Pharm. Sci.*, **59**, 1745 (1970).
5. Forrest, I. S., Rose, S. D., Brookes, L. G., Halpern, B., Bacon, V. A., and Silberg, I. A., *Agressologie*, **11**, 127 (1970).
6. Curry, S. H., *Agressologie*, **9**, 115 (1968).
7. Turano, P., and Turner, W. J., *J. Chromatogr.*, **75**, 277 (1973).
8. Usdin, E., *CRC Crit. Rev. in Clin. Lab. Sci.*, Sept., 347 (1971).
9. Erlanger, B., Borek, F., Beiser, S., and Lieberman, S., *J. Biol. Chem.*, **234**, 1090 (1959).
10. Ueki, A., Tadi, H., and Seno, S., *Acta Medicina Okayama*, **24**, 323 (1970).

11. Ovary, Z., in *Immunological Methods,* Ackroyd, J. F. (ed.), Blackwell Scientific Publications, Oxford, 1964, pp. 259–283.
12. Curry, S. H., *Anal. Chem.,* **40,** 1251 (1968).
13. Curry, S. H., Davis, M., Janowsky, D. S., and Marshall, J., *Arch. Gen. Psychiat.,* **22,** 209 (1970).
14. March, J. E., Donato, D., Turano, P., and Turner, W., *J. Med.,* **3,** 146 (1972).
15. Turano, P., and Turner, W., *J. Chromatogr.,* **75,** 277 (1973).

The Phenothiazines and Structurally Related Drugs, edited by I. S.
Forrest, C. J. Carr, and E. Usdin. Raven Press, New York © 1974.

The Inhibition of the Uptake of Monoamines by Blood Platelets by Phenothiazines and Other Drugs

Liisa Ahtee, David J. Boullin, Laila Saarnivaara,
and Matti K. Paasonen

*Department of Pharmacology, University of Helsinki, Siltavuorenpenger 10, SF-00170,
Helsinki 17, Finland*

INTRODUCTION

A characteristic of monoamine-storing cells is that they accumulate the monoamines against a considerable concentration gradient. In addition to transporting the monoamine stored by the cell concerned, catecholamine-containing cells accumulate indolylamines such as 5-hydroxytryptamine (5HT) and vice versa. The accumulation of monoamines can be inhibited by various drugs among which the most potent are the tricyclic compounds such as phenothiazines and tricyclic antidepressants.

The blood platelets are a commonly used model for studying the effects of drugs on the uptake of 5HT (1–3). This amine is accumulated by the platelets so that the platelet:amine ratio exceeds 1000:1 (4, 5). The blood platelets have also been proposed as useful pharmacological models for adrenergic neurons, although they take up norepinephrine and epinephrine only slightly (6–8). However, the norepinephrine analogue metaraminol is taken up by human and rabbit platelets with an accumulation ratio of 40:1 to 50:1 (9, 10). Metaraminol, which is not deaminated by monoamine oxidase, has a high affinity for the storage sites of norepinephrine and can be used for studying the neuronal uptake of norepinephrine (11–14). Unlike epinephrine and norepinephrine, the catecholamine dopamine is accumulated by blood platelets to about a similar degree as metaraminol (15, 16).

The purpose of the present work was (a) to characterize the monoamine-uptake systems in the platelets by using drugs which are known to inhibit the monoamine uptake and (b) to study how the monoamine-uptake inhibiting activity is related to the chemical structure of the drugs. The drugs studied were the phenothiazine derivatives chlorpromazine, trifluoperazine, and thioridazine; the tricyclic antidepressants chlorimipramine, imipramine, desipramine, amitriptyline, nortriptyline, and protriptyline; as well as methadone, morphine, cocaine, and atropine.

PREPARATION AND INCUBATION OF PLATELETS

Blood from anesthetized rabbits was collected through a carotid cannula and mixed with one-ninth volume of 1.5% disodium edetate. The platelets were separated by centrifugation as described earlier (10) and resuspended in Ca-free Krebs solution. One-ml samples were incubated with gentle shaking at 37°C in air. Drugs dissolved in 0.9% NaCl solution were added to the platelet suspension 10 min before adding ^{14}C-5HT (Radiochemical Centre, Amersham), ^{14}C-dopamine (Radiochemical Centre, Amersham), or ^{3}H-(±)-metaraminol (New England Nuclear Corp.). Thereafter the incubation was continued for a further 10 min. The platelets were immediately separated from the incubation medium by centrifugation. The platelet pellets were homogenized by ultrasonification, and their radioactivity was counted in a liquid scintillation counter Decem NTL 314.

RESULTS AND DISCUSSION

The Accumulation of 5HT, Dopamine, and Metaraminol by Blood Platelets

Table 1 shows that the platelet/medium concentration ratio for 1 μm 5HT after 10-min incubation of rabbit platelets suspended in Ca-free Krebs solution was 133. Under similar conditions, dopamine and metaraminol were concentrated to a ratio of 18:1 to 20:1. These experiments agree with the well-established fact that the platelet monoamine transport system most efficiently accumulates 5HT.

TABLE 1. *Platelet/medium concentration ratio* (C_i/C_o)
after 10 min incubation with 1 μM monoamine

Monoamine	C_i/C_o (mean ± S.E.; n)
5HT	133 ± 27 (3)
Dopamine	18 ± 4 (6)
Metaraminol	20 ± 7 (4)

Rabbit platelets suspended in Ca-free Krebs solution were incubated at 37°C in air for 10 min with 1 μM 5HT, dopamine, or (±)-metaraminol.

The monoamine transport system functions in two steps at least; first, the amine is transferred through the cell membrane, and second, it is taken up by the storage granule. Both 5HT and dopamine are concentrated by the 5HT storage granules of the platelets (17). Figure 1 gives evidence that metaraminol is also taken up by the 5HT storage granules because metaraminol releases 5HT stoichiometrically from the platelets. From both human and rabbit platelets, the accumulated metaraminol can be released by throm-

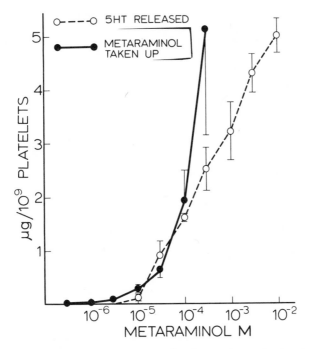

FIG. 1. Uptake of metaraminol by and release of 5HT from rabbit platelets incubated with various concentrations of metaraminol. Two ml samples of platelet suspension were incubated with 0.3 μM to 10 mM (−)-metaraminol for 1 hr. Data were taken from Ref. 10.

bin (Ahtee and Mills, *unpublished results*). Since thrombin selectively releases the platelet particles, this observation also suggests that the accumulated metaraminol is not localized in the cytoplasm but is in a bound form, most probably in the storage granules.

Inhibition of 5HT Uptake by Drugs

Table 2 gives the concentrations of the drugs which caused 50% inhibition (IC_{50}) of 5HT uptake by platelets. The most potent drug was chlorimipramine, which caused 50% inhibition of 5HT uptake at 1.6×10^{-8} M concentration. Chlorimipramine was over 200 times more active than the corresponding phenothiazine derivative chlorpromazine and nearly 4,000 times more active than morphine, the least potent of the drugs studied. All the tricyclic antidepressants studied (chlorimipramine > amitriptyline > nortriptyline > imipramine > protriptyline > desipramine) were more potent inhibitors of 5HT uptake than the phenothiazines studied (trifluoperazine > chlorpromazine > thioridazine).

Contrary to morphine, methadone, another narcotic analgesic, was a relatively potent inhibitor of 5HT uptake. In our earlier study (10) methadone

TABLE 2. *Inhibition of the uptake of 5HT by rabbit platelets by phenothiazines, tricyclic antidepressants, and other drugs*

Drugs in decreasing order of potency	IC_{50} (μM)	Relative inhibitory concentrations
Chlorimipramine	0.016	1
Amitriptyline	0.046	2.9
Nortriptyline	0.062	3.9
Methadone	0.42	26.3
Imipramine	0.47	29.4
Protriptyline	0.94	58.8
Desipramine	1.1	69
Trifluoperazine	1.8	113
Chlorpromazine	3.4	213
Cocaine	4.3	270
Thioridazine	4.8	300
Atropine	28	1,750
Morphine	63	3,940

Rabbit platelets suspended in Ca-free Krebs solution were incubated at 37°C in air, under gentle shaking. (IC_{50}) values were determined by calculating regression lines for the percentage inhibition of 5HT uptake against drug concentration (10 nM to 1 mM). Drugs were added 10 min before 5HT (1 μM), and the incubation was continued thereafter for 10 min.

was also the most potent inhibitor of 5HT uptake of 10 narcotic analgesics studied. Naloxone did not antagonize this effect of methadone, and the effects of narcotic analgesics on 5HT uptake did not correlate with their pain-relieving properties. Cocaine, a potent inhibitor of norepinephrine uptake, was about as potent an inhibitor of 5HT uptake as the least-active phenothiazine derivative studied, thioridazine.

Table 3 shows that phenothiazines and tricyclic antidepressants cause 5HT release from rabbit platelets only in concentrations 100 to 10,000 times higher than those in which they inhibit the uptake of 5HT. This discrepancy in concentrations needed was also shown for several other phenothiazines and tricyclic antidepressants (19), as well as for narcotic analgesics (10). Moreover, the order of potency of these drugs in releasing 5HT is different from their order of potency in inhibiting the uptake of 5HT. The phenothiazines and tricyclic antidepressants with the tertiary amine group in the alkylamino side chain are the most potent inhibitors of 5HT uptake by both neurons and platelets (19–21). On the other hand, the compounds with a secondary amine in the side chain are the most potent 5HT releasers (18, 22), as shown in Fig. 2. Furthermore, piminodine, which also possesses a secondary amine group, is the most potent 5HT releaser of the narcotic analgesics, whereas methadone, the most potent 5HT uptake inhibitor, has a tertiary amine in the molecule (10).

The phenothiazines and tricyclic antidepressants release 5HT from platelets at about the same concentrations at which they cause hemolysis and decrease surface tension (Fig. 2; Refs. 18 and 23). Therefore it is most probable that the 5HT release from platelets induced by these drugs is at

TABLE 3. *Release of 5HT from rabbit platelets by phenothiazines and tricyclic antidepressants*

Drugs in decreasing order of potency	Mean (±S.E.) release at different drug concentrations (% of original content)	
	100 μM	300 μM
Nortriptyline	26 ± 5	75 ± 8
Desipramine	16 ± 5	63 ± 9
Thioridazine	18 ± 6	56 ± 10
Amitriptyline	12 ± 4	50 ± 8
Trifluoperazine	5 ± 2	50 ± 3
Chlorpromazine	10 ± 1	49 ± 3
Imipramine	7 ± 1	39 ± 3

Rabbit platelet-rich plasma was incubated with or without drugs for 1 hr at 37°C, in air. Values from (18).

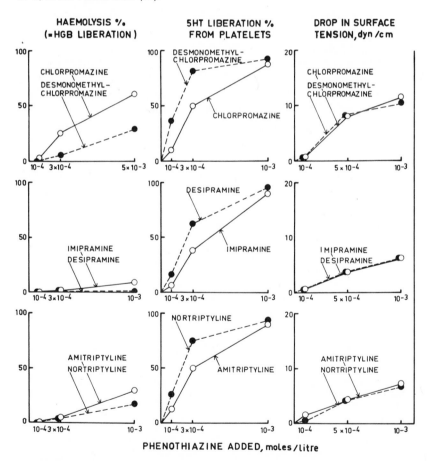

FIG. 2. Effect of desmonomethylation of the terminal dimethylamine group in chlorpromazine, imipramine, and amitriptyline on their haemolytic, platelet-5HT releasing, and surface activities (from Ref. 18; courtesy of *Ann. Med. Exp. Fenn.*).

least partially due to their effects on membrane permeability. The effects of these drugs on 5HT uptake by platelets may also partially result from their effects on membrane permeability. However, distinctly lower concentrations of phenothiazines and tricyclic antidepressants inhibit the uptake of 5HT than release 5HT or decrease the surface tension, and the concentration range of drugs for uptake inhibition is wider than for 5HT release. The very low concentrations of drugs needed to inhibit 5HT uptake, as well as the different order of potency of the drugs in releasing 5HT and in inhibiting 5HT uptake, suggest that the drugs studied, especially the tricyclic antidepressants, inhibit the uptake of 5HT by platelets by acting on a specific transport system and not by having a general effect on membranes.

Inhibition of Dopamine Uptake

Table 4 gives the IC_{50} values for the drugs that inhibited dopamine uptake into platelets. The IC_{50}'s of phenothiazines and tricyclic antidepressants ranged from 3.1 to 7.9 μM. Thioridazine was the most potent inhibitor of dopamine uptake followed by chlorimipramine > amitriptyline = chlorpromazine > trifluoperazine > desipramine > protriptyline = nortriptyline > imipramine. Methadone and especially atropine, morphine, and cocaine were clearly less active than the tricyclic compounds.

The amine structure of the side chain does not seem to influence the ability of the drugs to inhibit dopamine uptake by platelets. Neither does the structure of the central ring of the tricyclic compounds seem to affect the dopamine uptake-inhibiting ability of these drugs. This result is in accordance with that obtained by Horn, Coyle, and Snyder (24) who found that the

TABLE 4. *Inhibition of the uptake of dopamine by rabbit platelets by phenothiazines, tricyclic antidepressants, and other drugs*

Drugs in decreasing order of potency	IC_{50} (μM)	Relative inhibitory concentrations
Thioridazine	3.1	1
Chlorimipramine	3.8	1.2
Amitriptyline	4.9	1.6
Chlorpromazine	4.9	1.6
Trifluoperazine	5.3	1.7
Desipramine	5.9	1.9
Protriptyline	6.1	2.0
Nortriptyline	6.2	2.0
Imipramine	7.9	2.5
Methadone	26	8.2
Atropine	124	40
Morphine	264	85
Cocaine	320	103

Dopamine was added in the final concentration of 1 μM; otherwise the experiments were carried out as described in Table 2.

phenothiazines and tricyclic antidepressants were about as active as inhibitors of dopamine uptake by rat striatal synaptosomes.

Inhibition of Metaraminol Uptake

Table 5 shows that the phenothiazines and tricyclic antidepressants inhibited 50% of metaraminol uptake by platelets in concentrations ranging from 7.2 to 45 μM. The most active compound — thioridazine — inhibited the metaraminol uptake at one-sixth of the concentration needed of imipramine, the least active tricyclic compound. Methadone, atropine, cocaine, and morphine were clearly less active than the tricyclic compounds. As shown before (9), the compounds with a secondary amine structure in the side chain (desipramine, nortriptyline) were more active than the corresponding tertiary amines in inhibiting the metaraminol uptake by platelets. A similar superiority of the desmethyl series of antidepressive drugs in inhibiting the uptake of norepinephrine or metaraminol by peripheral or central neurons has been demonstrated several times (25–27).

TABLE 5. *Inhibition of the uptake of metaraminol by rabbit platelets by phenothiazines, tricyclic antidepressants, and other drugs*

Drugs in decreasing order of potency	IC_{50} (μM)	Relative inhibitory concentrations
Thioridazine	7.2	1
Nortriptyline	13	1.8
Chlorimipramine	21	2.9
Chlorpromazine	22	3.0
Amitriptyline	22	3.1
Protriptyline	24	3.3
Trifluoperazine	24	3.4
Desipramine	30	4.2
Imipramine	45	6.3
Methadone	59	8.2
Atropine	296	41
Cocaine	332	46
Morphine	421	59

($\pm$)-Metaraminol was added in the final concentration of 1 μM; otherwise the experiments were carried out as described in Table 2.

Comparison of the Drugs as Inhibitors of 5HT, Dopamine, and Metaraminol Uptake into Platelets

Figure 3 and Table 6 give information about the relative potencies of the drugs studied as inhibitors of the uptake of 5HT, dopamine, and metaraminol into platelets. First, the relative inhibitory potency of a certain drug could vary up to 1,300-fold (chlorimipramine) in inhibiting the uptake of different

TABLE 6. *Comparison of IC_{50}'s for 5HT, dopamine (DA), and metaraminol (MA) uptake*

Drug	$\dfrac{IC_{50}\ DA}{IC_{50}\ 5HT}$	$\dfrac{IC_{50}\ MA}{IC_{50}\ 5HT}$	$\dfrac{IC_{50}\ MA}{IC_{50}\ DA}$
Chlorpromazine	1.4	6.4	4.5
Trifluoperazine	2.9	13	4.6
Thioridazine	0.6	1.5	2.3
Chlorimipramine	238	1300	5.5
Imipramine	17	96	5.7
Desipramine	5.4	27	5.6
Amitriptyline	107	478	4.5
Nortriptyline	100	205	2.1
Protriptyline	6.5	25	3.9
Methadone	61	141	2.3
Morphine	4.2	6.7	1.6
Atropine	4.4	11	2.4
Cocaine	74	77	1.0

monoamines. Second, the orders of potency of the drugs in inhibiting the uptake of 5HT, dopamine, and metaraminol were dissimilar.

The uptake of 5HT into platelets was especially sensitive to tricyclic antidepressants and methadone. These drugs inhibited the 5HT accumulation in 1/5 to 1/1,300 of the concentrations needed to inhibit the uptake of dopamine or metaraminol. The phenothiazines were clearly less active than the tricyclic compounds in inhibiting the uptake of 5HT. By contrast, the phenothiazines and tricyclic antidepressants inhibited the uptake of dopamine and metaraminol in about similar concentrations. For instance, chlorpromazine and chlorimipramine, which differ only in the central ring structure, were about equipotent in inhibiting the accumulation of dopamine or metaraminol into platelets, whereas the IC_{50}'s of these drugs in 5HT uptake differ by a factor of 200. The phenothiazines inhibited the uptake of 5HT and dopamine in about similar concentrations. The uptake of metaraminol into platelets was slightly more resistant to phenothiazines and tricyclic antidepressants than that of dopamine.

Cocaine inhibited the 5HT uptake first in a relatively high concentration. However, it seems to possess a certain affinity for the 5HT transport system because about 75-times higher cocaine concentration was needed to inhibit the accumulation of dopamine or metaraminol than that of 5HT. Morphine and atropine were very weak inhibitors of uptake of all three monoamines. The uptake of 5HT was slightly more sensitive to even these drugs than to the uptake of dopamine or metaraminol; this is probably an unspecific effect which is associated with the accumulation rate of 5HT, being 6 to 7 times faster than that of dopamine or metaraminol.

These results again emphasize the suitability of blood platelets as a

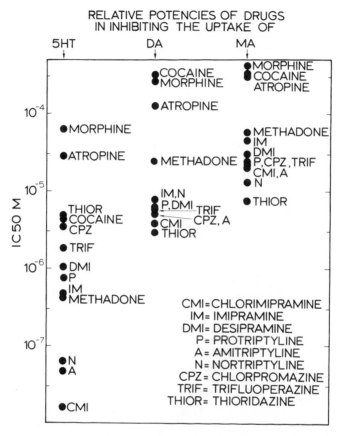

FIG. 3. Relative potencies of phenothiazines, tricyclic antidepressants, and other drugs in inhibiting the uptake of 5HT, dopamine (DA), and metaraminol (MA) into rabbit platelets. The IC_{50}'s are taken from Tables 2, 4, and 5.

pharmacological model for testing 5HT transport. The differences in the order of potency of drugs in inhibiting the uptake of different monoamines suggest that the monoamine transport system of the platelets can also give clues about the effects of drugs on the uptake of other monoamines.

SUMMARY

The effects of phenothiazines, tricyclic antidepressants, and some other drugs affecting the central nervous system on the accumulation of 5HT, dopamine, and metaraminol into blood platelets were studied. During 10-min incubation with 1 μM monoamine, the platelets concentrated six to seven times more 5HT than dopamine or metaraminol. Differences were found both in the relative inhibitory potencies of drugs and in the order of potency of drugs in inhibiting the uptake of different monoamines. The tricyclic antidepressants were clearly more potent inhibitors of 5HT uptake than the phenothiazines, but the two groups of drugs were about equipotent inhibitors of dopamine and metaraminol uptake. Methadone and cocaine had an affinity for the 5HT transport system, whereas morphine and atropine inhibited only slightly the uptake of any of the monoamines studied.

ACKNOWLEDGMENT

This work was supported by grants from the Sigrid Jusélius Foundation and the National Research Council for Medical Sciences, Finland.

REFERENCES

1. Paasonen, M. K., *Ann. Med. Exp. Fenn.*, **46**, 416 (1968).
2. Paasonen, M. K., Ahtee, L., and Solatunturi, E., *Progr. Brain Res.*, **34**, 269 (1971).
3. Sneddon, J. M., in *Progress in Neurobiology*, Vol. 1, Part 2, Kerkut, G. A., and Phillis, J. W., (eds.), Pergamon Press, New York, 1973, pp. 151–198.
4. Born, G. V. R., and Gillson, R. E., *J. Physiol. (Lond.)*, **146**, 472 (1959).
5. Stacey, R. S., *Brit. J. Pharmacol.*, **16**, 284 (1961).
6. Abrams, W. B., and Solomon, H. N., *Clin. Pharmacol. Ther.*, **10**, 702 (1969).
7. Born, G. V. R., and Smith, J. B., *Brit. J. Pharmacol.*, **39**, 765 (1970).
8. McLean, J. R., and Potoczak, D., *Arch. Biochem. Biophys.*, **132**, 416 (1969).
9. Ahtee, L., and Saarnivaara, L., *J. Pharm. Pharmacol.*, **23**, 495 (1971).
10. Ahtee, L., and Saarnivaara, L., *Brit. J. Pharmacol.*, **47**, 808 (1973).
11. Andén, N.-E., *Acta Pharmacol. (Kbh.)*, **21**, 260 (1964).
12. Shore, P. A., Busfield, D., and Alpers, H. S., *J. Pharmacol. Exp. Ther.*, **146**, 194 (1964).
13. Carlsson, A., and Waldeck, B., *Acta Pharmacol. (Kbh.)*, **22**, 293 (1965).
14. Iversen, L. L., in *The Uptake and Storage of Noradrenaline in Sympathetic Nerves*, University Press, Cambridge, 1967, p. 155.
15. Boullin, D. J., and O'Brien, R. A., *Brit. J. Pharmacol.*, **39**, 779 (1970).
16. Solomon, H. M., Spirt, N. M., and Abrams, W. B., *Clin. Pharmacol. Ther.*, **11**, 838 (1970).
17. Da Prada, M., and Pletscher, A., *Life Sci.*, **8**, 65 (1969).
18. Ahtee, L., *Ann. Med. Exp. Fenn.*, **44**, 431 (1966).
19. Ahtee, L., Tuomisto, J., Solatunturi, E., and Paasonen, M. K., *Ann. Med. Exp. Fenn.*, **46**, 429 (1968).
20. Carlsson, A., Corrodi, H., Fuxe, K., and Hökfelt, T., *Eur. J. Pharmacol.*, **5**, 357 (1969).
21. Todrick, A., and Tait, A. C., *J. Pharm. Pharmacol.*, **21**, 751 (1969).
22. Ahtee, L., and Paasonen, M. K., *Acta Pharmacol. (Kbh.)*, **26**, 213 (1968).
23. Ahtee, L., *Ann. Med. Exp. Fenn.*, **44**, 453 (1966).
24. Horn, A. S., Coyle, J. T., and Snyder, S. H., *Mol. Pharmacol.*, **7**, 66 (1971).
25. Callingham, R. A., in *Proceedings of the First International Symposium on Antidepressant Drugs*, Garattini, S., and Dukes, M. V. G. (eds.), International Congress Series No. 122, Excerpta Medica Foundation, Amsterdam, 1966, pp. 35–43.
26. Waldeck, B., *J. Pharm. Pharmacol.*, **20**, 111 (1968).
27. Carlsson, A., Corrodi, H., Fuxe, K., and Hökfelt, T., *Eur. J. Pharmacol.*, **5**, 367 (1969).

The *Phenothiazines and Structurally Related Drugs,* edited by I. S. Forrest, C. J. Carr, and E. Usdin. Raven Press, New York © 1974.

Session IV: Discussion

Reporter: S. Hess

1. *P. Turano*

Gorrod: I can only say that in our system, i.e., *n*-butanol extraction and concentration under vacuum followed by TLC, all under N_2, we do not see any nonmetabolic artifacts except some S-oxidation.

Grant: You indicated that 2-chlorophenothiazine was a metabolite of chlorpromazine and was never observed as an artifact of the work-up procedure. However, we have observed 2-chlorophenothiazine as a product of the solar irradiation of chlorpromazine in nonpolar solvents and it is, therefore, a potential artifact.

3. *S. H. Curry*

Turner: 2,4-Dichlorpromazine, supplied by Smith, Kline and French, is an excellent internal standard. We have added CPZ and four metabolites to control plasma at several concentrations and have found excellent recoveries at all levels.

4. *I. S. Forrest*

Q. Gorrod: Rabbits and guinea pigs have alkaline urine. What is the pH of monkey urine?
A. About 7.5.

Curry: We found that variations in urinary pH in patients over the range 5 to 8 caused pH-dependent changes in urinary excretion of unmetabolized CPZ, amounting to less than 1%.

Q. Grant: Do you have any evidence that stress has an influence on the excretion of drugs in your animals?
A. No — it would be difficult to measure and control.

7. *M. Shostak*

Grant: In reference to your comment that promazine has never been found as a metabolite of chlorpromazine, we have consistently found Nor_2- and Nor_1-promazine sulfoxide in the urines of patients on chlorpromazine, but we have also found that promazine is invariably found in SKF chlorpromazine medication presumably arising by a photoreduction during manufacture or compounding.

8. *L. Ahtee*

Q. Breyer: Can you comment on the difference in the potency of amitriptyline and imipramine to inhibit 5-HT uptake? Are there comparable
studies with brain synaptosomal preparations?

A. Imipramine is a more potent inhibitor of 5-HT uptake by human
platelets than amitriptyline [Ahtee et al., *Ann. Med. Exp. Fenn.*, **46,** 429
(1968)] as well as of the 5-HT uptake in slices of mouse brain [Ross and
Renyi, *Eur. J. Pharmacol.*, **7,** 270 (1969)]. I cannot explain the fact that
amitriptyline was more potent in rabbit platelets.

Session V

Metabolism

Chairmen: James Perel and George J. Wright

The Phenothiazines and Structurally Related Drugs, edited by I. S.
Forrest, C. J. Carr, and E. Usdin. Raven Press, New York © 1974.

Pharmacokinetics of Chlorpromazine Metabolites — A Colossal Problem

Pushkar N. Kaul, Michael W. Conway, and Mervin L. Clark

University of Oklahoma and Central State Griffin Memorial Hospital, Norman, Oklahoma
73069

The determination of circulating blood levels of drugs by means of suitable assay procedures possessing adequate sensitivity and precision is essential if valid data are sought relative to the pharmacokinetics, bioavailability, and dose-response relationships of the drugs. Most assay methodologies generally entail two major aspects: (a) the isolation of the compound(s) from biologic material and (b) subsequent quantitation by an appropriate analytical method. In the case of chlorpromazine (CPZ) and its metabolites, several analytical methods have been proposed and partially developed during the past 22 years, but there are still no unequivocal data on the blood levels of these compounds. This failure in itself reflects the magnitude of the difficulties in the precise quantitation of CPZ and its metabolites.

The major problems seem to arise from at least two facts. First, CPZ and many of its metabolites are not stable when subjected to the usual laboratory procedures used in isolating the compounds from biologic materials prior to analysis. Second, the apparent blood levels obtained following the usual therapeutic doses of CPZ are in the nanogram per milliliter range which limits the use of analytical methods to only fluorometric (1), gas-chromatographic (2), radioquantitative (3), chemical vapor analyses (CVA) (4) and the yet to be developed mass spectrometry of deuterated CPZ discussed by Dr. Jenden at this conference. Of these, CVA has not yet been explored to any significant extent, but the other methods, though available for 3 to 6 years, have yielded conflicting and at best unconfirmed data.

We have concerned ourselves with the development of assay methodology for CPZ and its major metabolites by using fluorescent tagging and subsequent fluorometric determinations, bearing in mind a methodology possibly adaptable to clinical laboratory use. In essence, the assay for metabolites (1, 5) involves the extraction of a 3-ml sonicated blood sample at basic pH with an appropriate organic solvent, evaporation of the extract, and subsequent reaction with dansyl chloride. In a preliminary application of the dansylation assay, we were able to determine blood levels of several metabolites in schizophrenic patients receiving variable doses of CPZ (6). The data, however, appeared to correlate poorly with the dose of CPZ and also lacked precision, which confirms the criticism of other investigators employing other assay methods in their laboratories.

During the past year, we have addressed ourselves to the very basic issue of why an analytical method such as gas chromatography or fluorometry, which are otherwise fairly precise techniques, should show poor precision when applied to measuring CPZ metabolites. This, in our opinion, is the key question relative to the CPZ assay story at this time.

Reliability and Precision of Dansylation Assay

Since quantitation in most of this work was carried out with the help of a dansylation assay which has not yet been widely adopted, we felt it necessary to validate the method by employing at least two approaches: (a) application of the method to a relatively stable dansylable amine, and for this we chose desipramine, and (b) comparison of the method with another standard analytical method, for which we selected gas chromatography (GC).

Application to Desipramine

Lack of day-to-day precision in the dansylation assay when applied to CPZ metabolites necessitated the verification of the precision on desipramine. This compound reacted with dansyl chloride (DNS-Cl) in a stoichiometric fashion and yielded fairly good day-to-day precision (Table 1). However, when the dansylation assay procedure, restandardized on desipramine, was again applied to CPZ metabolites, we continued to observe

TABLE 1. *Reproducibility of dansylation reaction in dioxane*

Compound (conc.)	Assay value (% Day I) ($N = 6$)	Significance
Desipramine (10 μg/reaction)		
DAY: I	100 ± 3.2	—
II	93 ± 1.1	N.S.
III	98 ± 1.1	N.S.
Monodesmethyl CPZ (20 μg/reaction)		
DAY: I	100 ± 1.0	—
II	125 ± 7.3	$p < 0.05$
III	93 ± 3.9	N.S.
IV	75 ± 8.1	$p < 0.05$
V	132 ± 2.5	$p < 0.05$

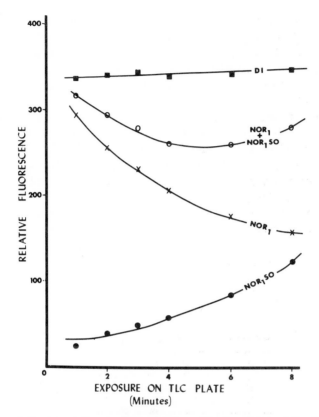

FIG. 1. Effect of dioxane as the reaction solvent on the dansylation of Nor₁CPZ. The loss of Nor₁ and the appearance of its sulfoxide seem to occur when the reaction mixture is spotted on silica-gel plates for TLC separation prior to fluorometry. No such detrimental effect is seen on desipramine (DI).

poor day-to-day precision. At least part of the loss in the case of mono-desmethyl CPZ (Nor₁CPZ) could be accounted for by its conversion to sulfoxide (Fig. 1). After a critical study of the dansylation reaction, it was possible to ascribe this oxidation and loss of the metabolite to the presence of dioxane in the dansylation-reaction mixture. When acetone was substituted for dioxane, there was no conversion of the metabolite to its sulfoxide, nor was there any significant loss following the dansylation reaction in acetone.

Dansylation Compared to GC

Gas chromatography is a fairly standard analytical method used by several laboratories involved in CPZ assay methodology. To compare the reliability of dansylation to that of GC, parallel assays were run on a set of four solutions of different concentrations of Nor₁CPZ employing both the

GC and the dansyl-fluorometric methods of analyses. A Hewlett-Packard model 5750 fitted with a flame ionization detector and a 3% OV-17 on Chromsorb W-HP (80 to 100 mesh) glass column (6 ft long, $1/8^{th}$ in i.d.) was used for GC determinations, with the injection-port temperature at 290°C, the column at 240°C and the detector at 325°C. Cholesterol was used as an internal standard.

The dansylation assay, in essence, involved reacting the metabolite (up to 50 nmoles) in 0.1-ml acetone containing 0.4 μmoles of DNS-Cl, 2μmoles of pH 12 phosphate buffer, and 20% water for a period of 10 min at room temperature. Aliquots of the reacted mixture were spotted on 100-μ silica-gel thin-layer chromatography (TLC) plates and developed in suitable solvents to separate the dansyl derivatives for fluorometric determination (1). Table 2 shows the comparative data obtained by the two methods, and they appear to be reasonably comparable.

TABLE 2. *Comparison of dansylation assay with GC*

	Relative strength % A	
Solution	Dansylation ($N = 6$)	GC ($N = 3$)
A	100.0 ± 2.2	100.0 ± 3.5
B	47.0 ± 1.5	59.9 ± 0.6
C	92.2 ± 2.9	95.6 ± 6.2
D	101.8 ± 3.7	91.1 ± 3.6

INSTABILITY OF METABOLITES

Even after standardization of the dansylation reaction on desipramine and obtaining fairly reproducible data on Nor₁CPZ, it was difficult to obtain acceptable precision (within $\pm$ 10%) when the dansylation assay was applied to blood samples containing known amounts of this and other metabolites. This suggested the necessity of studying the stability of all metabolites individually with respect to their behavior during the prequantitation phase of the assay procedure.

Table 3 includes some of the data pertaining to the effect of various organic solvents on a few metabolites of CPZ during evaporation under nitrogen. The data indicate that different metabolites exhibit different degrees of stability, a part of which, at least, appears to be solvent dependent.

Of the solvents investigated, ethylacetate and dichloromethane appeared to be quite detrimental, whereas hexane appeared less destructive in this respect. Decomposition of the metabolites in ethylacetate was particularly revealing, for this solvent is widely used in extracting many compounds

TABLE 3. *Instability of CPZ metabolites on evaporation in organic solvents*

Metabolite	Vol. evap. (ml)	Rel. fluoresc.		% Loss
		Control	Test	
		Hexane		
7-OH[b]	5	846 ± 16	815 ± 39	4
Nor$_2$[c]	5	6,780 ± 94	4,363 ± 65	36
Nor$_1$[e]	10	1,582 ± 35	1,770 ± 64	0
CPZ (GC)[a]	10	68.5 ± 1.6	68.8 ± 1.01	0
		Benzene		
7-OH	2.5	93 ± 2	92 ± 2	1
Nor$_2$	2.5	1,530 ± 40	1,390 ± 14	9
Nor$_1$	2.5	1,760 ± 18	1,710 ± 24	3
Nor$_2$SO[d]	2.5	1,242 ± 7	735 ± 66	41
		Ethylacetate		
7-OH	2.5	231 ± 5	132 ± 7	43
Nor$_2$	5	6,780 ± 94	2,020 ± 117	70
Nor$_1$	2.5	1,690 ± 27	770 ± 20	54
Nor$_2$SO	2.5	969 ± 8	420 ± 14	58
CPZ (GC)[a]	10	68.5 ± 1.6	39.2 ± 0.9	43
		Dichloromethane		
7-OH	5	923 ± 25	1,040 ± 13	0
Nor$_2$	5	6,780 ± 94	5,040 ± 51	26
Nor$_1$	5	7,150 ± 34	6,428 ± 66	10
CPZ (GC)[a]	10	68.5 ± 1.6	0	100

[a]CPZ was determined by GC and the values represent areas under the GC curves ($N = 3$).
[b]7-Hydroxy CPZ ($N = 6$).
[c]Didesmethyl CPZ ($N = 6$).
[d]Didesmethyl CPZ sulfoxide ($N = 6$).
[e]Monodesmethyl CPZ ($N = 6$).
All solvents used were of commercial Nanograde® (Mallinckrodt) purity (prepared in glass-lined vessels).

TABLE 4. *Effect of ethylacetate on the evaporation of monodesmethyl CPZ*

Metabolite in solvent (2.36 × 10^{-8} M)	Dansylation assay		GC assay	
	Rel. fluor. ($\bar{X}$ ± S.E.)	% control	Rel. curve area ($\bar{X}$ ± S.E.)	% Control
Ethyl acetate				
standing	1,740 ± 39	100	71.6 ± 2.5	100
evaporated	817 ± 26	47	42.8 ± 0.5	60
n-Hexane				
standing	1,588 ± 35	100	68.6 ± 4.5	100
evaporated	1,770 ± 64	111	65.3 ± 2.6	95

Dansylation assay: $N = 6$.
GC assay: $N = 3$.

other than phenothiazines and has recently been adopted by some laboratories for CPZ and its metabolites. That the loss of metabolite in this solvent is real was further confirmed by subjecting ethylacetate solutions of Nor_1-CPZ to both the dansylation and GC assays before and after evaporation under nitrogen (Table 4).

Of the five metabolites investigated Nor_2CPZ and its sulfoxide appeared most vulnerable to destruction during evaporation under nitrogen regardless of the solvent.

KINETIC STUDY

Following validation of dansylation with desipramine and GC and by paying particular attention to the various factors affecting stability of the metabolites, it was possible to develop methodology that gives reasonable precision ($\pm$ 10%) for two metabolites, namely Nor_1CPZ and 7-OH CPZ, to the extent that preliminary kinetic data in sheep could be obtained. Figures 2 and 3 show the time-based disappearance curves of intravenously administered Nor_1CPZ and 7-OH CPZ, each point representing at least six chromatographic determinations from a single blood sample split into three tubes at the beginning of the assay. However, considerably more data from experiments presently under way are required before we are able to describe pharmacokinetic profiles in a meaningful way.

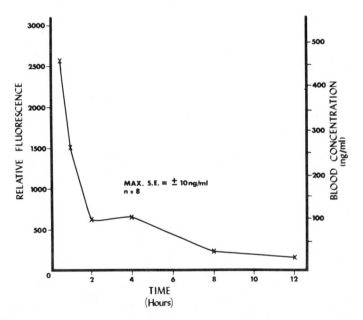

FIG. 2. Disappearance with time of intravenously given Nor_1CPZ (5 mg/kg) in the blood of sheep.

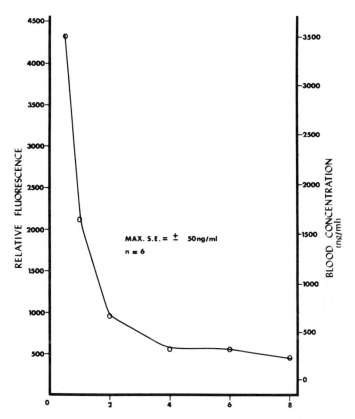

FIG. 3. Disappearance with time of intravenously given 7-OH CPZ (10 mg/kg) in the blood of sheep.

DISCUSSION

It is evident that the accurate quantitation of CPZ and its metabolites in blood and other body fluids for pharmacokinetic computations, bioavailability comparisons of generic products, dose-response studies, etc., warrant the development of a reliable assay methodology. It is all too apparent, however, that a precise and dependable assay methodology depends upon the determination of precise solvent and experimental conditions, particularly in the prequantitation phase. In view of the data presented here, which suggest that the isolation of each individual metabolite may require its own specific solvent and experimental conditions, and considering the number of potential metabolites, it is not difficult to appreciate the enormity of the problem still ahead relative to the pharmacokinetics of CPZ.

Furthermore, the fate of more than 80% of a given dose of this drug in terms of actual metabolites is not unequivocally known. Perhaps a major contribution in this regard is the recent discovery by Beckett and Essien

(7) of the existence of a new metabolite, a hydroxylamine derivative of Nor₁CPZ. Even if this finding is well corroborated, it still accounts for only some 10% of the given dose of CPZ (7). The major metabolites of this drug are, therefore, yet to be discovered. Alternatively, the lack of a precise prequantitation assay methodology may well account for the general failure of investigators in producing unequivocal data on both the qualitative and quantitative aspects of CPZ metabolism.

SUMMARY

Quantitation by fluorescence analysis following dansylation was further validated by its application to desipramine and by its comparison with gas chromatography. Further investigation of the prequantitative aspects of the dansylation assay methodology applicable to CPZ metabolites has revealed the possibility of decomposition during evaporation under nitrogen of organic extracts of the blood, depending on the solvent and the metabolite. Employing an appropriate solvent and rigidly controlled conditions of assay procedure, it was possible to obtain reproducible data on at least mono-desmethyl and 7-hydroxy derivatives of CPZ. The kinetics of disappearance of these metabolites in the blood of sheep following intravenous administration has been presented.

ACKNOWLEDGMENT

These studies were carried out with the support of Grant MH 21408 (from the National Institute of Mental Health). We are indebted to Drs. P. R. Pabrai and Roland Lehr, Ms. Olivia Crane, Mr. Lloyd Whitfield, and Mr. Luke San for their valuable scientific comment and technical assistance. The authors also wish to thank Dr. A. Manian, Psychopharmacology Research Branch, National Institute of Mental Health, for providing a generous supply of CPZ metabolites, and Drs. Irene Forrest and Earl Usdin for stimulating discussion and comment.

REFERENCES

1. Kaul, P. N., Conway, M. W., Ticku, M. K., Clark, M. L., and Huffine, J., *J. Pharm. Sci.,* **59**, 1745 (1970).
2. Curry, S. H., *Anal. Chem.,* **40**, 1251 (1968).
3. Efron, D. H., Hanis, S. R., Manian, A. A., and Gaudette, L. E., *Psychopharmacologia,* **19**, 207 (1971).
4. Green, D. E., and Forrest, I. S., in *Proceedings of the Fifth International Congress on Pharmacology,* San Francisco, California, July 23–28, 1972.
5. Kaul, P. N., Conway, M. W., Ticku, M. K., and Clark, M. L., *J. Pharm. Sci.,* **61**, 581 (1972).
6. Kaul, P. N., Ticku, M. K., and Clark, M. L., *J. Pharm. Sci.,* **61**, 1753 (1972).
7. Beckett, A. H., and Essien, E. E., *J. Pharm. Pharmac.,* **25**, 188 (1973).

The Phenothiazines and Structurally Related Drugs, edited by I. S. Forrest, C. J. Carr, and E. Usdin. Raven Press, New York © 1974.

Two Types of Metabolically Produced Trifluoperazine N-Oxides

M. A. Spirtes

Veterans Administration Hospital, New Orleans, Louisiana 70140, and Tulane University, School of Medicine, Department of Pharmacology, New Orleans, Louisiana 70112

INTRODUCTION

Trifluoperazine (Stelazine®) is one of the most potent phenothiazines commonly in use as a psychotherapeutic agent. In schizophrenia, the average daily dose is about a tenth that for chlorpromazine (CPZ). In contrast to the latter, trifluoperazine metabolism has been relatively little studied. A sulfoxide had been described (1) as well as a demethylation of the N-CH$_3$ grouping in the piperazine ring of the drug structure (2). Finally Gaertner and Breyer (3) and Breyer (4) reported on a trifluoperazine metabolite in which degradation of the piperazine ring structure occurred as well as an N-oxide of perazine. It is not clear from Breyer's N-oxide work where the oxygen is attached on the piperazine ring. Extensions of this work are discussed by Breyer elsewhere in this volume. A perusal of the propyl side-chain of trifluoperazine indicates the possibility of N-oxide formation at the two N-atoms shown in Fig. 1, whereas only one N-oxide is possible at the end of the propyl side chain of CPZ. When CPZ-NO is subjected to gas chromatography (GC) at temperatures over 200°C, a CPZ-metabolite in which the propyl side chain changes to an allyl grouping appears (4). This allyl metabolite, which has a smaller molecular weight and therefore a lower boiling point as well as less polarity, emerges from the gas-chromatographic column before the parent compound. Preliminary experiments in 1970 using a rabbit-liver microsomal-enzyme preparation indicated that, as a result of trifluoperazine metabolism, a similar metabolite also emerges from the column before the parent compound. Occasionally, in addition to this, another unknown peak appeared after the parent. Using Ziegler's amine oxidase, partially purified, to remove a large part of the cyt P-450 of the liver microsomes (5), I was able to increase the size of this peak fivefold and to have it analyzed by gas chromatography/mass spectrometry (GC/MS). Results indicated that the peak existing before the parent was a trifluoperazine N-O with the oxygen bound on the nitrogen located at the end of the propyl side chain, whereas the second unknown peak turned out to be an N-oxide with the oxygen on the *para*-positioned N on the piperazine ring.

399

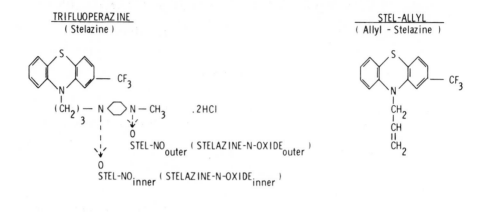

FIG. 1. Stelazine® and CPZ N-oxides and allyl-Stelazine® structures.

METHODS

Liver microsomes from female rabbits fed on Purina Rabbit Chow were prepared as previously described (6) or according to Ziegler (5). The latter's amine-oxidizing complex was also purified according to his procedure (5). The enzyme reaction mixtures used to metabolize trifluoperazine contained the following components: 0.3 mmoles glycine buffer, pH 8.2; 6.0 μmoles neutralized semicarbazide; 6.6 μmoles NADPH; 1.5 μmoles trifluoperazine; and 0.14 mmoles $MgCl_2$ when added; 12 mg of microsomal protein. Final volume of the mixture was 10 ml, and temperature of the reaction 37°C. At 0, 10 and 20 min after the reaction began, aliquots were removed for analyses of trifluoperazine and metabolites and extracted for GC runs as previously reported (6), using a Varian 2100 gas chromatograph. Before such analyses, the metabolic mixtures were deproteinized by the addition of trichloracetic acid to a final concentration of 5%, homogenized after a 10-min pause, and centrifuged for 10 min at 3,000 × *g* at 5°C. When necessary, the metabolites were sent to the University of Pittsburgh, School of Public Health, Department of Biochemistry, for analysis with their gas chromatograph-mass spectrometer.

RESULTS AND DISCUSSION

Figure 2 indicates the metabolites of CPZ produced by a rabbit microsomal mixture similar to the one described under Methods, and extracted in a similar manner. To be noted is the peak emerging at 3 min after injection of the extract and before the 4.5-min peak is seen. These represented CPZ-NO and CPZ, respectively, as determined by pure samples of these compounds obtained from Drs. Efron and Manian, N.I.M.H. Following these are peaks representing, first, monodemethyl-CPZ, then didemethyl-CPZ, CPZ-sulfoxide (CPZ-SO), and finally monodemethyl CPZ-SO (MD-CPZ-SO). Peak heights do not indicate the relative amounts of the metabolites in the extract because of attenuation changes during the course of the run.

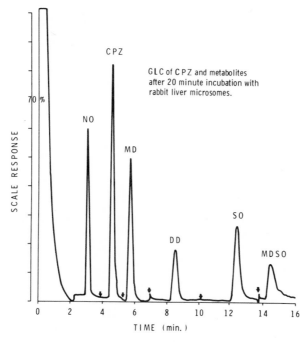

FIG. 2. GC peaks of extracts of metabolites of CPZ obtained from experiments using rabbit-liver microsomes.

Figure 3 shows the trifluoperazine metabolites produced by the rabbit liver microsomal mixture recorded under Methods. It can be seen that there is an emerging peak marked Stel-NO$_{inner}$ at about 3 min, whereas the parent compound peak emerges from the column at about 11 min. This was followed by the emergence of a demethyl-Stelazine® (DM-Stel) peak and, immediately afterward, a small peak marked Stel-NO$_{outer}$.

No attenuation change was made between these two or the last peak at 16 min marked Stel-NO. The identity of the Stel-NO$_{inner}$, Stel, and DM-Stel, as well as Stel-SO peaks, was assured by chromatographing true samples of these metabolites again obtained from N.I.M.H. The Stel-NO$_{outer}$ peak was only infrequently seen, when a crude microsomal mixture was used in the metabolic experiment. When a partially purified microsomal preparation made according to Ziegler (5) was substituted and the metabolites were extracted and chromatographed in the same manner, both the Stel-NO$_{inner-outer}$ peaks increased in height (Fig. 4). The Stel-NO$_{outer}$ was now about five times greater in height and area, and was about the same height and area as the somewhat smaller DM-Stel peak. Also, it appeared in every experiment in which the purified microsomal preparation was used. Because of the possibility of two trifluoperazine-N-oxides as noted in Fig. 1, each of the trifluoperazine metabolite peaks as well as the parent peak itself was subjected to GC/MS analysis. Figure 5 portrays the mass spectra of the 3-min and 12.5-min emerging GC peaks. The former represents the Stel-NO$_{inner}$ (actually the Stel-allyl peak), and the latter represents Stel-NO$_{outer}$. Since the mass spectrum of the GC 3-min peak represents the Stel-allyl

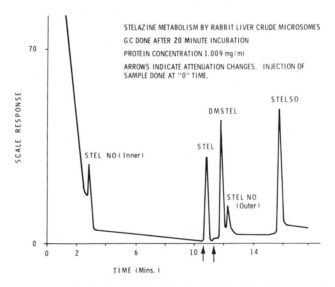

FIG. 3. GC peaks of extracts of metabolites of Stelazine® obtained from experiments using crude rabbit-liver microsomes.

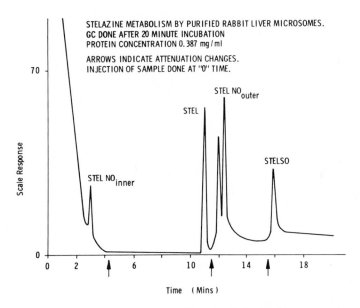

FIG. 4. GC peaks of extracts of metabolites of Stelazine® obtained from experiments using a partially purified rabbit-liver microsomal preparation made according to Ziegler and Mitchell (5).

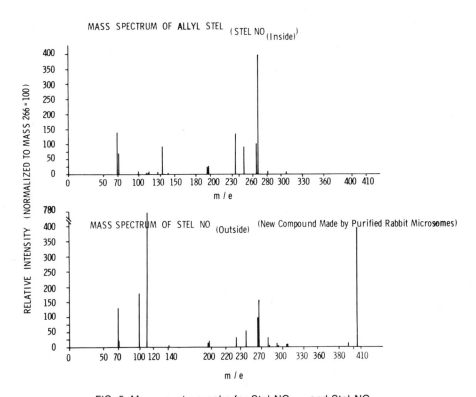

FIG. 5. Mass spectrographs for Stel-NO$_{inner}$ and Stel-NO$_{outer}$.

fragment, no piperazine-containing masses would be expected to be seen, and this is indeed the case. In addition no m/e ions of 423 or 405 would be expected since the piperazine ring is not present and this is also true. The 12.5-min GC peak, when passed through the MS, allows a peak to emerge of m/e of 405. Were 18 added for the stripping of a molecule of H_2O from this ion, an m/e of 423 would result which equals the molecular weight of Stel-NO. Some major piperazine fragments are also seen, indicating that the electron stream does break off a considerable number of different piperazine fragments. The mass spectra for trifluoperazine, Stel-NO, and DE-Stel were also obtained and will be published shortly.

CONCLUSION

The presence of two different trifluoperazine N-oxides has been ascertained among the trifluoperazine metabolites produced by a rabbit liver microsomal metabolic system as described above.

REFERENCES

1. Huang, C. L., and Bhansali, K. G., *J. Pharmaceut. Sci.,* **57,** 1511 (1968).
2. Bickel, M. H., Flückiger, M., and Baggiolini, M., *Naunyn-Schmiedeberg's Arch. Pharmak. u. Exp. Path.,* **256,** 360 (1967).
3. Gaertner, H. J., and Breyer, U., *Arzneim-Forschung,* **22,** 1084 (1972).
4. Breyer, U., *Biochem. Pharmacol.,* **18,** 777 (1969).
5. Ziegler, D. M., and Mitchell, C. H., *Arch. Biochem. Biophys.,* **150,** 116 (1972).
6. Berman, H. M. and Spirtes, M. A., *Biochem. Pharmacol.,* **20,** 2275 (1971).

The Phenothiazines and Structurally Related Drugs, edited by I. S. Forrest, C. J. Carr, and E. Usdin. Raven Press, New York © 1974.

The Use of Combined Gas Chromatography–Mass Spectrometry Techniques for the Identification of Hydroxylated and Dihydroxylated Metabolites of Phenothiazine Drugs

J. Cymerman Craig, W. A. Garland, L. D. Gruenke, L. R. Kray, and K. A. M. Walker

Department of Pharmaceutical Chemistry, School of Pharmacy, University of California, San Francisco, California 94143

The possible relationship between the clinical responsiveness to chlorpromazine (CPZ) and the blood levels of the drug or of its metabolites has given rise to an extensive series of investigations of the metabolic fate of CPZ. In addition to demethylation, S-oxidation, N-oxidation, and more extensive dealkylation resulting in the complete loss of the 10 side chain (1–6), hydroxylation in the aromatic rings has been reported at the 3, 7, and 8 positions (7–10). Moreover, there is now reliable evidence for the existence of dihydroxylated products (10–16) and their monomethylated derivatives (15, 16).

The role of the hydroxylated and dihydroxylated phenothiazine metabolites in the psychotropic activity of CPZ is still unknown. Although many derivatives of CPZ are available from N.I.M.H. (17), few biological evaluation studies on the activity of the hydroxylated metabolites have as yet been carried out. Recent investigations (6, 11, 18–22) report marked pharmacological activity in 7-hydroxychlorpromazine and 3,7-dihydroxychlorpromazine, with lesser, but definite effects in several other dioxygenated products.

The separation and identification of CPZ metabolites is almost entirely carried out (17) by thin-layer chromatography (TLC), and the most recent and thorough study by Turano and Turner (23) employs both two-dimensional TLC and two-dimensional direct-scanning microdensitometry. Their extremely careful and painstaking work (16) has shown that not only does the presence of one metabolite alter the mobility of the others, but that many of the standards changed character more or less rapidly both in solution and on gas chromatography (GC).

Although good results have been reported for GC separation of many

CPZ metabolites, particularly the demethylated products and their sulf-oxides (3, 24, 25) and N-oxides (26), only one reference exists to the use of GC for any hydroxylated metabolite of CPZ: Johnson et al. (3) report the retention time of the O-acetate of 7-hydroxy CPZ, using a polar column packing (cyanosilicone XE-60 and polyethylene glycol carbowax-20000) and temperature programming.

Our investigations (26, 27) showed that the use of a nonpolar column (methylsilicone SE-30) with a low percentage of packing (3%) permitted the separation and identification of all hydroxychlorpromazines at quite moderate temperatures (200°C). The results (Table 1) reveal that while the 1- and 9-hydroxy and the 7- and 8-hydroxy derivatives have very close retention times within each pair, the separation between pairs, as well as between the 3- and 6-hydroxy compounds, was satisfactory. In order to permit unequivocal identification of isomers, the trimethylsiloxy ethers were prepared using N,O-*bis*(trimethylsilyl) acetamide (BSA) (28), and showed excellent separation (Table 1). All times are given relative to CPZ.

A further derivative of general utility was the acetoxy compound, which was best prepared using the N-acetylimidazole reagent (28). Here again good separation was achieved, and it is clear that the use of *two* derivatives will unequivocally identify any hydroxylated CPZ from its isomers.

The method used was to treat the compound (about 1 μg), as a 1% solution in benzene-pyridine (1:1), with an approximately 10-fold excess of the derivatizing agent, shake for 2 min, and inject 1 μl of this solution into an all-glass GC system. It was advantageous to check that the derivative had indeed formed, and this could be done readily by low-resolution mass spectrometry (MS), employing the direct insertion probe, which required about 10 ng of material only. All derivatives were identified by determining their accurate mass using chemical-ionization mass spectrometry (CI-MS) at high resolution. In view of the slight variations found in the retention time of CPZ even on successive determinations, it was essential to have CPZ present in each GC run, and this was done routinely by adding approximately 1 μg of CPZ to each solution to be injected. Under these conditions, triplicate determinations agreed to within 1 to 2%.

A particularly difficult problem was presented by the differentiation between 7- and 8-hydroxychlorpromazine. In view of the close similarity between the GC retention times and also between the mass spectra, both using electron-impact (EI) (29, 30) and CI-MS (31) of these isomers, the trifluoroacetoxy esters prepared in the same way using trifluoroacetylimi-dazole (28) were made and proved to give excellent separation (Table 2). This permitted identification of the 8-hydroxy metabolite (8), using a non-polar packing (methylsilicone, OV-1) with a low percentage (1.5%) packing.

The same methods were successful in the identification and separation of the dioxygenated CPZ metabolites shown in Table 3. Here, the use of diazomethane as an additional derivatizing agent was useful. However,

TABLE 1. GC of hydroxylated CPZs[a]

Substituent R at position	Relative retention time (CPZ = 1.00)[b]		
	R = OH	R = OSi(CH$_3$)$_3$	R = OCOCH$_3$
1	1.25	1.04	1.31
3	2.90	1.73	3.70
6	2.10	2.28	2.60
7	3.63	2.65	3.30
8	3.60	1.98	2.80
9	1.26	0.75	1.47

[a] Column, 2 m × 3 mm, 3% SE-30, column temperature 200°C.
[b] CPZ retention time about 10 min.

TABLE 2. GC of hydroxylated CPZs[a]

Substituent R at position	Relative retention time (CPZ = 1.00)[b]			
	R = OH	R = OSi(CH$_3$)$_3$	R = OCOCH$_3$	R = OCOCF$_3$
7	2.94	2.63	3.39	1.38
8	2.92	2.41	2.82	1.12

[a] Column, 2 m × 3 mm, 1.5% OV-1, Column temperature 210°C.
[b] CPZ retention time about 13 min.

TABLE 3. GC of dioxygenated CPZs[a]

	Relative retention time (CPZ = 1.00)[b]				
Dioxygenated CPZ	Free hydroxy compound	Trimethylsilyl ether	Acetate ester	Trifluoro acetate ester	Methyl ether
7,8-dihydroxy		4.25	7.07		3.46
7-hydroxy-8-methoxy	3.70	3.94	4.96	2.14	3.46
8-hydroxy-7-methoxy	3.58	3.83	4.57	1.99	3.46
3,7-dihydroxy		6.08	9.22		4.46

[a] Column, 2 m × 3 mm, 1.5% OV-1, column temperature 210°C.
[b] CPZ retention time about 13 min.

excellent results were also achieved using on-column methylation by means of trimethylanilinium hydroxide in methanol ("Meth Elute") (28).

CI-MS, using methane, proved to be highly successful in that the MH$^+$ molecular ion was the largest ion in the spectrum, and this technique was useful in differentiating some of the oxygenated CPZ positional isomers.

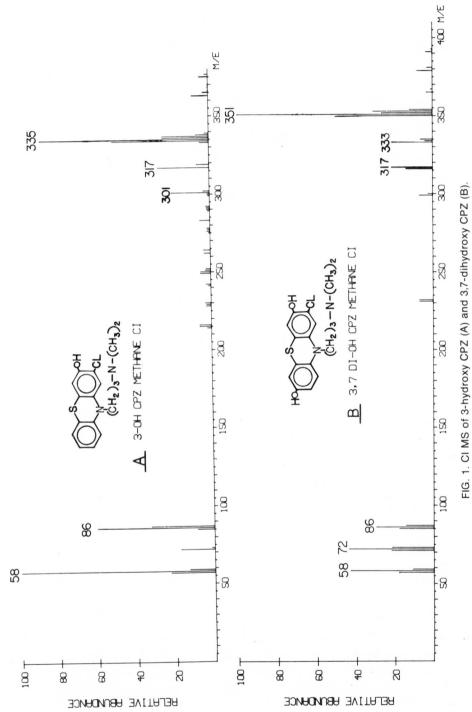

FIG. 1. CI MS of 3-hydroxy CPZ (A) and 3,7-dihydroxy CPZ (B).

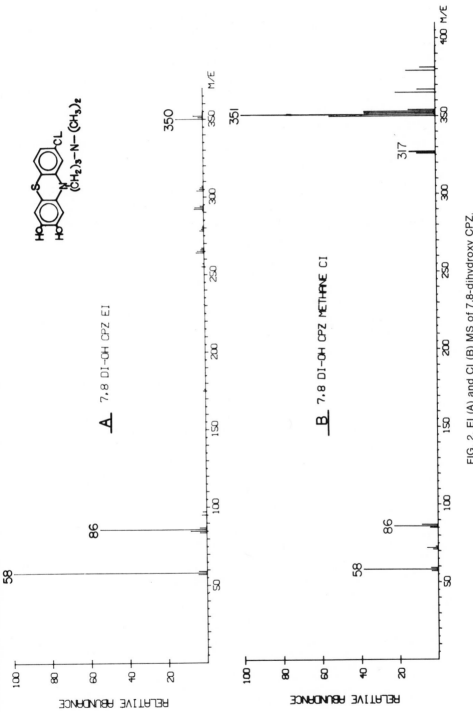

FIG. 2. EI (A) and CI (B) MS of 7,8-dihydroxy CPZ.

Substitution of a hydroxy at C-3 was easily recognized by a phenomenon which appears to be unique for the 2-chloro-3-hydroxy phenothiazine system, i.e., the loss of H_2O from the MH^+ ion (Fig. 1). This water loss also serves to differentiate the 3,7-dihydroxy from the 7,8-dihydroxy compound (Fig. 2) in their CI mass spectra using methane.

Since most metabolic reactions of CPZ involve demethylation as well as ring hydroxylation, it was of interest to prepare CPZ with fully deuterated methyl groups, as well as with deuterium substitution at C-1' and C-3' of the side chain. Application of this deuterated substance in biological work should give the ratio of demethylation, deamination, and dealkylation in CPZ.

In conclusion, it has been demonstrated that CI-MS can immediately identify a 3-hydroxy CPZ, whereas GC under carefully defined conditions, is capable of separating and identifying every possible hydroxylated or dihydroxylated CPZ metabolite, both techniques operating on a 1-μg scale.

SUMMARY

It is demonstrated that GC under carefully defined conditions, preferably used in conjunction with both EI and CI-MS, is capable of identifying and separating every possible hydroxylated or dihydroxylated CPZ metabolite, using about 1 μg of material.

ACKNOWLEDGMENTS

We are greatly indebted to Dr. A. A. Manian, National Institute of Mental Health, for many of the reference samples used. This investigation was supported in part by U.S. Public Health Service Grant No. MH-10450 and MH-14321 (from the National Institute of Mental Health).

REFERENCES

1. Usdin, E., *CRC Crit. Rev. Lab. Clin. Sci.,* **2,** 347 (1971).
2. Fishman, V., and Goldenberg, H., *Proc. Soc. Exptl. Biol. Med.,* **104,** 99 (1960).
3. Johnson, D. E., Rodriguez, C. F., and Burchfield, H. P., *Biochem. Pharmacol.,* **14,** 1453 (1965).
4. Gillette, J. R., and Kamm, J. J., *J. Pharmacol. Exptl. Therap.,* **130,** 262 (1960).
5. Fishman, V., Heaton, A., and Goldenberg, H., *Proc. Soc. Exptl. Biol. Med.,* **109,** 548 (1962).
6. Manian, A. A., Efron, D. H., and Goldberg, M. E., *Life Sci.,* **4,** 2425 (1965).
7. Huang, C. L., Sands, F. L., and Kurland, A. A., *Arch Gen. Psych.,* **8,** 301 (1963).
8. Turano, P., Canton, C., Turner, W. J., and Merlis, S., *Agressol.,* **9,** 193 (1968).
9. Huang, C. L., *Int. J. Neuropharmacol.,* **6,** 1 (1967).
10. Posner, H. S., Culpen, R., and Levine, J., *J. Pharmacol. Exptl. Therap.,* **141,** 377 (1963).
11. Manian, A. A., Watzman, N., Steenberg, M. L., and Buckley, J. P., *Life Sci.,* **7,** 731 (1968).
12. Daly, J. W., and Manian, A. A., *Biochem. Pharmacol.,* **16,** 2131 (1967).
13. Goldenberg, H., and Fishman, B., in *Principles of Psychopharmacology,* Clark, W., and Del Giudice, J. (eds.), Academic Press, New York, 1970, chap. 14.

14. Coccia, P. F. and Westerfeld, W. W., *J. Pharmacol. Exptl. Therap.,* **157,** 446 (1967).
15. Daly, J. W. and Manian, A. A., *Biochem. Pharmacol.,* **18,** 1235 (1969).
16. Turano, P. and Turner, W. J., *J. Chromatog.,* **75,** 277 (1973).
17. Manian, A. A., *Psychopharm. Bull.,* **6,** 44 (1970).
18. Posner, H. S., Hearst, E., Taylor, W. L., and Cosmides, G. J., *J. Pharmacol. Exptl. Therap.,* **137,** 83 (1962).
19. Posner, H. S., and Hearst, E., *Int. J. Neuropharmacol.,* **3,** 635 (1964).
20. Manian, A. A., Efron, D. H. and Harris, S. R., *Life Sci.,* **10,** 679 (1971).
21. Watzman, N., Manian, A. A., Barry, H., and Buckley, J. P., *J. Pharm. Sci.,* **57,** 2089 (1968).
22. Buckley, J. P., Steenberg, M. L., Barry, H., and Manian, A. A., *J. Pharm. Sci.,* **62,** 715 (1973).
23. Turano, P., and Turner, W. J., *J. Chromatog.,* **64,** 347 (1972).
24. Curry, S. H., *Anal. Chem.,* **40,** 1251 (1968).
25. Hammar, C. G., and Holmstedt, B., *Experientia,* **24,** 98 (1968).
26. Craig, J. C., Mary, N. Y., and Roy, S. K., *Anal. Chem.,* **36,** 1142 (1964).
27. Craig, J. C., and Kray, L. R., *Agressol.,* **9,** 3 (1968).
28. Pierce Chemical Company, Rockford, Illinois 61105.
29. Duffield, A. M., Craig, J. C. and Kray, L. R., *Agressol.,* **9,** 111 (1968).
30. Duffield, A. M., Craig, J. C., and Kray, L. R., *Tetrahedron,* **24,** 4267 (1968).
31. Garland, W. A., Craig, J. C. and Trager, W. F., *Unpublished data.*

The Phenothiazines and Structurally Related Drugs, edited by I. S. Forrest, C. J. Carr, and E. Usdin. Raven Press, New York © 1974.

Autoradiography of ^{35}S-Chlorpromazine: Accumulation and Retention in Melanin-Bearing Tissues

Nils Gunnar Lindquist and Sven Ullberg

Department of Toxicology, Uppsala University, S-751 23 Uppsala, Sweden

INTRODUCTION

The melanin affinity of the phenothiazines is generally believed to be the most important factor in the etiology of the toxic retinopathy caused by these drugs. The chlorpromazine-induced hyperpigmentation of the skin has also been related to accumulation of the drug on melanin (1).

Investigations performed in our laboratory indicate that the melanin affinity of the phenothiazines may be a more important and general mechanism of toxicity than was previously believed. Not only toxic retinopathy and hyperpigmentation of the skin, but also pigmentation of the cornea and lens, general melanosis, and irreversible extrapyramidal disorders might be a manifestation of the melanin affinity of the phenothiazines.

The general distribution of ^{35}S-chlorpromazine was investigated in pigmented and albino experimental animals by means of whole-body autoradiography. Mice and monkeys were injected with ^{35}S-chlorpromazine intravenously, each animal receiving a single dose. After various predetermined intervals, the animals were rapidly frozen, and sagittal sections were prepared at different levels through the whole frozen body of the mouse, or through the head of each monkey. The sections were freeze-dried and pressed against a photographic film. After exposure, the films were separated from the sections and developed (2, 3).

In addition, sections through noninjected mice and human brainstems were incubated in an aqueous solution of ^{35}S-chlorpromazine and then rinsed, dried, and autoradiographed.

Electron microscopy and standard histochemical methods for melanin were used to identify the heavy deposits of pigment found constantly in the superficial cervical lymph nodes of adult pigmented mice.

RESULTS

The most conspicuous feature in the distribution of labeled chlorpromazine was the very strong and selective accumulation and retention in the

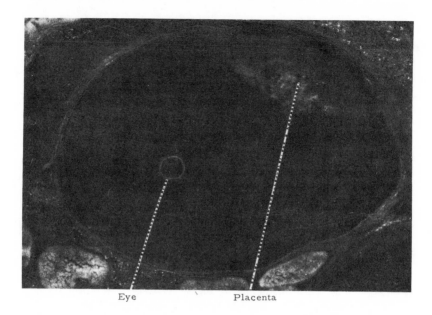

Eye   Placenta

Eye   Placenta

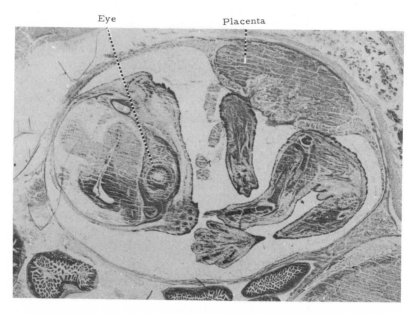

FIG. 1. Detail of an autoradiogram (upper) with the corresponding section (lower) of a pregnant pigmented mouse 5 min after an intravenous injection of ³⁵S-chlorpromazine. There is high accumulation in the fetal eye (hematoxylin-eosin).

melanin-containing tissues. In the albino animals, there was a very low concentration in the corresponding tissues.

The accumulation in the melanin structures was observed as early as 5 min after injection, which is too soon to make it likely that any metabolism of the substance had occurred (Fig. 1). It is therefore very probable that at least part of the substance bound to the melanin was unchanged chlorpromazine.

In pigmented mice at a late gestation stage, accumulation was observed in the fetal eye immediately after the drug had entered the fetal circulation, and the eye uptake was seen before the radioactive substance was observable elsewhere in the fetal body (Fig. 1). After 1 hr, accumulation could be seen in the brain and adrenal glands, but by far the highest uptake was present in the eye (Fig. 2 *top*). No accumulation or retention was found in the albino eye (Fig. 2 *bottom*). After 2 days, when the labeled substance had left the rest of the fetus, it was retained in the fetal eye.

The accumulation was very high in the eye of the early embryos of pigmented mice (on the 12th day of pregnancy).

Phenothiazines are frequently used as antiemetics and tranquilizers during pregnancy. An accumulation of these drugs on the fetal ocular melanin may result in fetal ocular injury. If damage (which gives a slight reduction of vision) has occurred, it may not be observed until long after birth, and may then be difficult to relate to medication given during pregnancy. There thus seems to be a need for carefully controlled studies of children whose mothers were taking these compounds during pregnancy.

In adult pigmented mice, the concentration in the uveal tract was higher than in any other tissue as early as 5 min after injection. The activity was still very high 90 days after administration of labeled chlorpromazine. No accumulation was observed at any survival time in the cornea, aqueous humor, or lens.

The accumulation in the uveal tract of one monkey was very high at 4 hr (Fig. 3) and in another monkey at 4 days (Fig. 4) after injection of labeled chlorpromazine. As in the mice no accumulation was observed in the cornea, aqueous humor, or lens.

The pigmentation of the cornea and lens following long-term therapeutic use of the phenothiazines has not been related to the affinity of the drugs for melanin. It has been suggested that the pigment deposits in the ocular tissues might arise from the influence of ultraviolet light on metabolites of chlorpromazine accumulated in the cornea and lens (4). In the present investigation, however, the accumulation in the eye was always restricted to the pigmented layers and no uptake was seen in the cornea, aqueous humor, or lens. It therefore seems more likely that the drug-induced pigmentation of the cornea and lens is caused by melanosomes released from the iris into the aqueous humor.

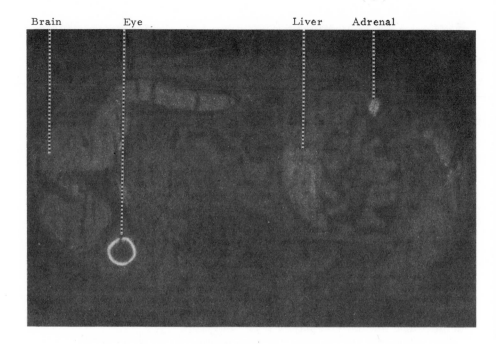

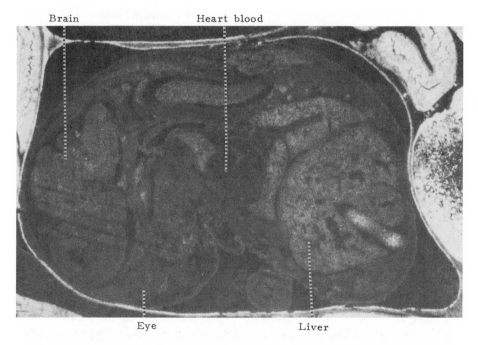

FIG. 2 (top). Autoradiogram of a pigmented mouse fetus 1 hr after intravenous injection of ^{35}S-chlorpromazine to the mother. The fetus was removed surgically. Note slight accumulation in fetal brain and adrenal cortex and very marked accumulation in the uvea of the eye. *(Bottom)* Detail of an autoradiogram of a pregnant albino mouse 1 hr after an intravenous injection of ^{35}S-chlorpromazine. Very little radioactivity can be observed in the fetal eye.

Uveal tract   Optic nerve   Brain   Hair follicles

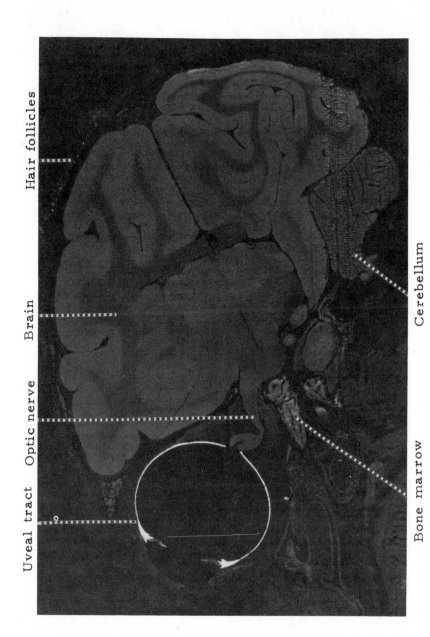

Bone marrow   Cerebellum

FIG. 3. Autoradiogram of a monkey (*Macaca irus*) 4 hr after an intravenous injection of ^{35}S-chlorpromazine. There is high accumulation in the uveal tract.

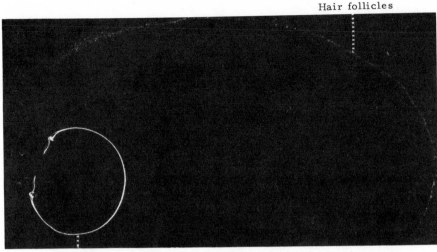

Hair follicles

Uveal tract

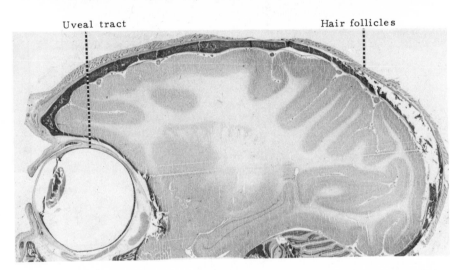

Uveal tract   Hair follicles

FIG. 4. Autoradiogram (upper) with the corresponding section (lower) of a monkey (*Cercopithecus aethiops*) 4 days after an intravenous injection of ³⁵S-chlorpromazine. There is high accumulation in the uveal tract and hair follicles (hematoxylin-eosin).

High accumulation was observed in the superficial cervical lymph nodes of pigmented mice (Fig. 5). The activity was mainly localized in a peripheral zone of the nodes. High uptake was also observed in other superficial lymph nodes such as the axillar and inguinal nodes, but the accumulation was much more marked in the superficial cervical lymph nodes. No accumulation or retention was found in any lymph nodes of the albino mice investigated.

Histochemical and electron-microscopical investigations revealed that

Harder's gland   Hair follicles

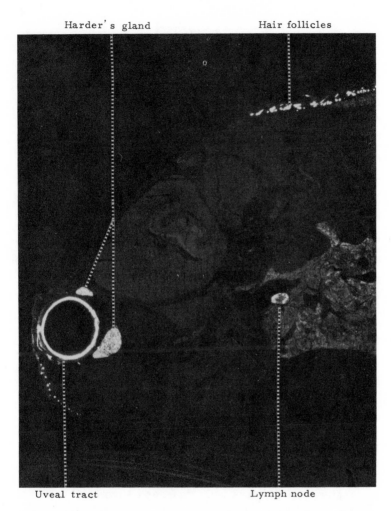

Uveal tract   Lymph node

FIG. 5. Detail of an autoradiogram of a pigmented mouse 24 hr after an intravenous injection of ^{35}S-chlorpromazine. There is high accumulation in the uveal tract, Harder's gland, hair follicles, and superficial cervical lymph node.

melanin is normally found in macrophages in the superficial cervical lymph nodes of pigmented mice (Fig. 6).

No similar pigment was observed in the corresponding lymph nodes of albino mice of the same age. The lymph nodes were found to lack tyrosinase activity, indicating that melanin is not formed in these cells but transported there from other tissues, probably the skin (5). Melanin has earlier been found in the lymph nodes draining the skin in Bantu negroes and in Caucasians (6, 7). If abnormally high amounts of melanin are produced in the body —as in patients with malignant melanoma (8) or a phenothiazine-induced

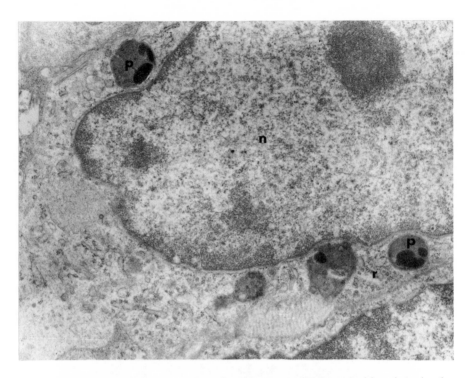

FIG. 6. Electron micrograph of a macrophage in a superficial cervical lymph node of a pigmented mouse showing phagosomes (p) containing melanosomes (n = nucleus, r = ribosomes). × 21,000

hyperpigmentation of the skin (9, 10) – this migration of melanosomes seems to increase, leading to a general melanosis.

Labeled chlorpromazine was selectively accumulated *in vitro* in the melanin structures of the eyes, skin, hair, and superficial cervical lymph nodes. The accumulation appears to be due simply to a chemical affinity. Special physiological conditions such as body temperature and glucose in the medium were not needed. Potts (11) demonstrated that the uptake of chlorpromazine by melanin was very little influenced by the pH and NaCl concentration in the incubation medium.

Following incubation of tape-mounted frozen sections from human midbrain and pons in an aqueous solution of ³⁵S-chlorpromazine, a very high and selective uptake was observed in the pigmented nerve cells in both the substantia nigra (Fig. 7) and locus coeruleus. It was possible to identify the pigmented neurons by light microscopy both in unstained sections and in sections stained with hematoxylin and eosin or toluidine blue. No specific uptake was seen in unpigmented cells, either in the midbrain or in the pons.

The pigmented neurons in the substantia nigra and locus coeruleus are known to be involved in the extrapyramidal control of muscle activity. The

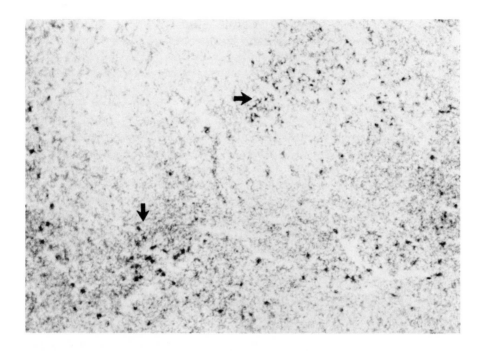

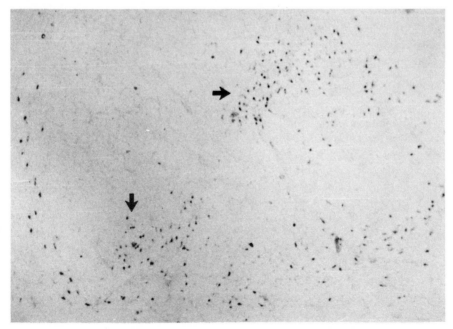

FIG. 7. Autoradiogram (upper) with the corresponding unstained section (lower) of an adult human substantia nigra showing accumulation of ^{35}S-chlorpromazine in pigmented cells. × 15

affinity of the phenothiazines for neuromelanin has not been reported in the literature, probably because neuromelanin is not found in small laboratory animals such as the guinea pig, mouse, rat, or rabbit (12). In human adults (even albinos) and children at adolescence, neuromelanin has constantly been found in both the substantia nigra and locus coeruleus (13–15).

Extrapyramidal disorders are known to be the most common adverse effects of the phenothiazines, and are mainly of three categories: akathisia, dyskinesia, and parkinsonism. The drug-induced akathisia and Parkinson's disease are usually reversible, but irreversible cases have been reported (17). The phenothiazine-induced tardive dyskinesia is known to be irreversible, and symptoms may become apparent after drug withdrawal or reduction of dosage (18). Christensen et al. (19) found degeneration of the pigmented nerve cells in the substantia nigra of patients with phenothiazine-induced tardive dyskinesia. Phenothiazines do not induce extrapyramidal disturbances of this type in small laboratory animals that lack melanin in their substantia nigra (20, 21).

The accumulation of 35S-chlorpromazine on neuromelanin *in vitro* strongly implies an accumulation also *in vivo*. Chlorpromazine has been found to pass readily the blood–brain barrier and reach a high concentration in the brain (5, 22). The affinity of phenothiazines for neuromelanin may lead to their accumulation in the melanin-containing neurons in the substantia nigra and locus coeruleus, and this in turn may result in extrapyramidal disorders.

In conclusion, melanin affinity may be an important factor in the development of phenothiazine-induced lesions in the eye, skin, reticuloendothelial system, and brainstem.

SUMMARY

By means of whole-body autoradiography, the general distribution of 35S-chlorpromazine was studied in experimental animals. The labeled substance was rapidly localized in the melanin-bearing tissues of the eye, superficial cervical lymph nodes, skin, and hair follicles. The concentration in the melanin structures was very high 90 days after injection. There was no accumulation or retention in the corresponding tissues of albino mice. No accumulation or retention was observed in the cornea, lens, or aqueous humor of either pigmented or albino animals. The concentration in all non-melanin structures rapidly decreased, and no long-term retention was observed in any other tissues than the melanin structures.

The labeled substance rapidly passed the placenta and accumulated in the eyes of pigmented mouse fetuses from the 12th day of development. 35S-chlorpromazine was also taken up *in vitro* by melanin structures in sections from pigmented mice. No accumulation was observed in the corresponding tissues of albino mice.

Since neuromelanin is not found in small laboratory animals, frozen sections from human brainstems were incubated in an aqueous solution of ^{35}S-chlorpromazine and then rinsed, dried, and autoradiographed. High accumulation was observed in the melanin-containing nerve cells in both the substantia nigra and locus coeruleus.

If drugs with melanin affinity, such as the phenothiazines, are administered for a long period, one might expect to find side effects in all the melanin-bearing tissues. Melanin affinity may be an important factor in the development of phenothiazine-induced lesions in the eye, skin, reticuloendothelial system, and brainstem.

ACKNOWLEDGMENTS

This investigation was supported by grants from The Swedish Board for Technical Development and The Swedish Medical Research Council (B73–14X–2876–04A).

REFERENCES

1. Satanove, A., *J.A.M.A.*, **191**, 263 (1965).
2. Ullberg, S., *Acta Radiol. (Stockh.) Suppl.* 118 (1954).
3. Ullberg, S., *Proceedings of the Second United Nations International Conference on the Peaceful Uses of Atomic Energy*, Geneva, **24**, 248 (1958).
4. Perry, T. L., Culling, C. F. A., Berry, K., and Hansen, S., *Science*, **146**, 81 (1964).
5. Lindquist, N. G., *Acta Radiol. (Stockh.) Suppl.*, 325 (1973).
6. Baker, W. De C., *East Afr. Med. J.*, **41**, 15 (1964).
7. Gail, D., *Frankfurt. Z. Path.*, **68**, 64 (1957).
8. Goodall, P., Spriggs, A. I., and Wells, F. R., *Br. J. Surg.*, **48**, 549 (1961).
9. Greiner, A. C., and Nicolson, G. A., *Can. Med. Assoc. J.*, **91**, 627 (1964).
10. Hashimoto, K., Wiener, W., Albert, J., and Nelson, R. G., *J. Invest. Dermatol.*, **47**, 296 (1966).
11. Potts, A. M., *Invest. Ophthalmol.*, **3**, 405 (1964).
12. Marsden, C. D., *J. Anat.*, **95**, 256 (1961).
13. Foley, J. M., and Baxter, D., *J. Neuropathol. Exp. Neurol.*, **17**, 586 (1958).
14. Bazelon, M., Fenichel, G. M., and Randall, J., *Neurology*, **17**, 512 (1967).
15. Fenichel, G. M., and Bazelon, M., *Neurology*, **18**, 817 (1968).
16. Marsden, C. D., *Pigments in Pathology*, Wolman, M. (ed.), Academic Press, New York, 1969, p. 395.
17. Hershon, H. I., Kennedy, P. F., and McGuire, R. J., *Br. J. Psychiatry*, **120**, 41 (1972).
18. Crane, G. E., *Psychopharmacol. Bull.*, **8**, 63 (1972).
19. Christensen, E., Møller, J. E., and Faurbye, A., *Acta Psychiatr. Scand.*, **46**, 14 (1970).
20. Cotzias, G. C., Papavasiliou, P. S., van Woert, M. H., and Sakamoto, A., *Fed. Proc.*, **23**, 713 (1964).
21. Dreyfuss, J., Beer, B., Devine, D. D., Roberts, B. F., and Schreiber, E. C., *Neuropharmacology*, **11**, 223 (1972).
22. Sjöstrand, S. E., Cassano, G. B., and Hansson, E., *Arch. Int. Pharmacodyn.*, **156**, 34 (1965).

The Phenothiazines and Structurally Related Drugs, edited by I. S.
Forrest, C. J. Carr, and E. Usdin. Raven Press, New York © 1974.

Imipramine Protein Binding and Pharmacokinetics in Children

B. G. Winsberg, J. M. Perel, M. J. Hurwic, and A. Klutch

Division of Child Psychiatry, Downstate Medical Center, and Child Psychiatric Evaluation Research Unit of the New York State Department of Mental Hygiene, Brooklyn, New York 11203 and Department of Psychiatry, Columbia University and New York State Psychiatric Institute, New York, New York 10032

The relationship between plasma protein binding and the therapeutic efficacy of various pharmacological agents has been a focus of recent interest (1). Since the activity of a drug is dependent both on the amount of free or active drug and the affinity of that drug for its receptor sites, it has been suggested that protein binding will be an important parameter to consider in relationship to a number of other pharmacokinetic variables in the evaluation of psychotropic drug effects (2, 3).

In an earlier report (4) on the effectiveness of imipramine in attenuating the frequency of hyperactive/aggressive behaviors among children, we noted a number of issues common to the clinical pharmacotherapy of behaviorally deviant children. These include: (a) the relative immediacy of the clinical response to a single oral dose of imipramine, i.e., 1 to 2 hr for children as compared to the few weeks usually required for response in adult depressive patients; (b) nonresponsivity to imipramine pharmacotherapy among many of our pediatric patients; and (c) the appearance of sudden imipramine tolerance in children who had previously evidenced a behavioral response.

In a subsequent communication (5) we reviewed our preliminary work on the pharmacokinetics of imipramine in hospitalized behaviorally deviant children — which is part of our ongoing research program designed to explore the indicated issues.

In our recent research, we have found blood levels of imipramine — and of its demethylated metabolite desmethylimipramine — in children receiving medication in the 5 mg/kg therapeutic dosage range to vary from 50 to 500 ng/cc. This is substantially higher than might be anticipated from previous reports (6, 7), which have compared adults and children as to blood levels of other drugs. The plasma half-life of imipramine has been found to be multiphasic and variable in children — ranging from 25 to 60 hr. Absorption of imipramine seems to be quite rapid and complete. Substantially high blood levels (e.g., 150 ng/cc) are in evidence as soon as 30 min after a single 50-mg oral dose. Additionally, and perhaps of importance to the problem of imipramine tolerance, there is preliminary evidence (5) that imipramine plasma levels decline over a period of 3 months on the same oral dose. Whether this decline is a function of autoinduction, increased renal clearance, or a combination of these factors is presently under investigation by our unit along with other clinical behavioral correlates.

It has been recently shown that there are age-related changes in plasma protein binding of imipramine which is independent of plasma protein concentration (8). Imipramine binding in cord and adult plasma have been found to average 74 and 86%, respectively—indicating approximately 26% free drug in the neonate and 14% free medication in the adult. Binding in depressed adult patients with normal protein concentrations has been found to range from 77% to 94.6% ($\bar{X} = 86$, SD $= 3.7$), indicating a fourfold variation in a free-drug concentration. The clinical correlates of these findings are presently undergoing assessment by the above investigators (9).

The work on protein binding may also have immediate implications on dosage regulation among children. For example, the literature on imipramine pharmacotherapy in children indicates that most investigators favor the administration of medication as a single evening dose (10).[1,2] In that connection, Saraf[2] in a recent literature review on imipramine toxicity, has reported a death in a child on a 300 mg (17 mg/kg) h.s. dosage schedule. Since our observations (11), as well as those of Fromm and associates (12), indicate that imipramine has epileptogenic toxicity, and since its widespread use for the treatment of eneuresis requires evening administration, it is of great importance to investigate protein binding as well as the pharmacokinetics of imipramine under various dosage schedules.

The purpose of the present study was (a) to determine the extent of protein binding of imipramine in children with behavior disorders, (b) to investigate the influence of varying concentrations of imipramine on protein binding, and (c) to examine these findings in conjunction with other biochemical and behavioral determinations obtained under conditions of chronic imipramine administration in a representative case.

METHOD

Subjects

Subjects for protein-binding determinations were 16 children of both sexes, ranging in age from 7 to 10 yr admitted to Downstate Medical Center—Kings County Hospital in Brooklyn, New York, for neuropsychiatric behavior disorders. Plasma protein concentrations on all children were in the normal range (6 to 8 g). At the time blood samples were drawn, one-half the group had been pretreated with imipramine (5 mg/kg) for no

---

[1] Waizer, J., Hoffman, S. P., Polizoes, P., and Engelhardt, D. M., *unpublished ms.*

[2] Saraf, K. R., Klein, D. F., Gittelman-Klein, R., and Groff, S., *unpublished ms.*

less than 1 week; the other half had been off all medication for at least 3 weeks prior to the time specimens were obtained. Additionally, a number of samples of cord blood and blood from children at various ages were obtained from the blood bank at Columbia Presbyterian Medical Center.

Procedure

The procedures for imipramine determination and protein binding radioassay are described in detail elsewhere in this volume (9). Blank plasma is incubated with 100 ng of benzyl-methylene ^{14}C imipramine (BM^{14}C) with 400 ng cold carrier. This concentration was chosen since our previous work has indicated that it is in the generally expected range of values obtained in children receiving chronic imipramine pharmacotherapy. For children who received imipramine, plasmas were incubated with a tracer dose of 100 ng of BM^{14}C imipramine only.

RESULTS

Binding

Since previous work in our laboratories had demonstrated no differences in binding between plasmas obtained from both children and adults prior to and after treatment with imipramine using the two methods, the data for both treated and blank plasmas were pooled. Binding was found to range from 78 to 86% ($\overline{X} = 81.3$, SD = 1.66).

Binding at Varying Concentrations

Five blank plasmas were incubated with varying concentrations of BM^{14}C imipramine to determine the percent of binding as a function of varying plasma levels. The incubation concentrations used were 40, 80, 200, 300, 500, 600, 900, 1,300, 1,600 and 2,000 ng/ml. The binding curves thus obtained are *flat* for the five subjects through concentrations of up to 600 ng/ml and ranged from 78 to 85% for individual subjects. A modest decline in binding was evidenced at concentrations greater than 600 ng/ml, e.g., range of 78 to 79%.

DISCUSSION AND IMPLICATIONS

Plasma protein binding of imipramine among children shows far less variability (range 78 to 86%) than that reported in adults (range 77 to 94.6%). A Mann Whitney U Test comparison between our pediatric data and the adult data supplied by Glassman et al. (9) revealed a significant difference ($p = <0.001$). Adults have significantly higher binding values (86%) than do children (81.3%).

The binding values of 7- to 10-year-old children are intermediate between those found in the neonate (8)[3] and adults (9). Preliminary data from our laboratory further suggest that at age 13, adult-like binding values are obtained. Such age related differences in protein binding are of considerable scientific and clinical interest. Current work directed towards this issue in our laboratories centers around developmental changes in protein structure and composition as suggested by Dayton et. al. (2).

Further, our findings show that within the concentration range studied, binding is constant and characteristic for each patient. Assuming that absorption is not affected by oral dosage, this consistency in binding indicates that with increased dosage, the amount of available free drug will be greater. Considering that absorption is quite rapid in children, it might be anticipated that the before-bedtime schedule generally advocated by other investigators is accompanied by increased toxicity risks. This risk is further emphasized by the fact that, in humans, the ratio of tissue to blood concentrations is much greater than 1 (as high as 100:1). It follows that an increased amount of free drug in the plasma will result in a much greater net amount of drug in the brain. In our opinion the bedtime administration of imipramine for behavior disorders, where large doses are involved, should be discouraged.

Since in the child the adipose compartment is smaller than in the adult, imipramine (a highly fat-soluble compound) will be more readily available to saturate nervous system tissue; i.e., children will have a smaller volume of distribution. The relative immediacy of the clinical response in behaviorally disturbed children may be in part accounted for by the greater amount of free drug, the rapidity of absorption, and the greater amount of highly perfused lean body mass in children, as well as by yet unspecified biochemical differences in the disorders and in brain metabolism.

Since protein binding is only one aspect of the total pharmacokinetic and clinical picture, we would like to present some of our findings concerning the relationship between pharmacokinetic and behavioral variables in hospitalized behaviorally disordered children. Plasma levels of imipramine and desmethylimipramine, their urinary metabolites, and changes in various behavioral measures are depicted graphically for a representative case in Fig. 1. Baseline measures were obtained on Day 1 of the graph and medication (5 mg/kg) in divided doses every 8 hrs, began on Day 2 (7 A.M., 3 P.M., and 11 P.M.). Bloods and/or urines were obtained on Days 2, 3, 4, 7, 9, and 10 at 3 P.M.

Classroom behaviors were evaluated using a behavioral rating scale (BRS) which we have previously found sensitive to drug effects (4). Time-sampling (TS) observations were conducted using a procedure developed by this unit. Although the complete TS procedure samples a number of

---

[3] Hurwic, M. J., *unpublished observations.*

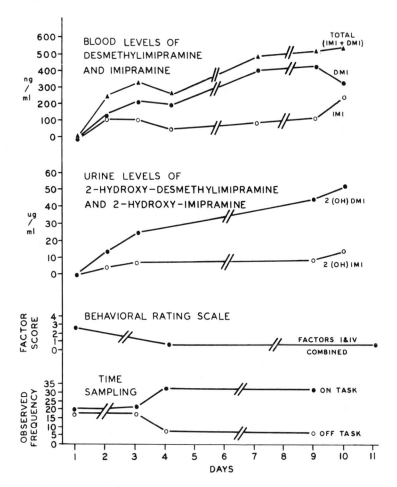

FIG. 1. Graphic representation of the relationship between plasma imipramine and des-methylimipramine, their respective hydroxylated urinary metabolites, and behavioral change in a representative case.

relevant behaviors, Fig. 1 represents observations only on On-Task and Off-Task behaviors.

Inspection of Fig. 1 indicates a consistent relationship among all measures that proceeds concomitantly in the anticipated direction. As plasma levels of imipramine and desmethylimipramine increase, classroom deviance decreases, while On-Task behaviors increase and Off-Task behaviors decrease. Up to Day 10, the quantity[4] of urinary 2-hydroxy metabolite of desmethylimipramine increases as plasma desmethylimipramine increases,

---

[4] The chromatographic analysis used in this investigation is presently being modified so as to yield more precise quantitative data. The values reported here are estimated.

while both plasma imipramine and its urinary 2-hydroxy metabolite show no increase. At Day 10, a decrease in desmethylimipramine and an increase in imipramine is in evidence, while the total concentration remains constant. Rapid fluctuations in the relative proportions of imipramine and desmethylimipramine, while their summed values remain constant, are not infrequently observed in our work with both children and adults. The pattern of urinary and plasma determinations suggests a rapid turnover of imipramine to desmethylimipramine in these particular children. *In vitro* plasma–protein binding in this case was found to be 86% bound and 14% free across all clinical concentrations studies. How such total and proportional plasma values and binding data relate to the clinical response pattern, as well as to nonresponsivity and tolerance among children, constitute the major problems under investigation by this unit in planned programmatic investigations.

SUMMARY

We have reported on imipramine protein binding among neuropsychiatrically ill children and discussed these findings in relation to a number of clinical problems. Our results show that children have substantially less binding and higher blood levels of imipramine than do adults and consequently may be expected to be more prone to toxicity reactions. We have presented additional pharmacokinetic data which may be expected to clarify the dose response and tolerance problem. We strongly recommend that such pharmacokinetic data be gathered along with other behavioral measures in clinical psychopharmacological investigations. Rapidity of response, along with tolerance to and toxicity of medication, should be investigated using paradigms such as those reported above.

ACKNOWLEDGMENTS

The authors extend their appreciation to Dr. Jose Rodriguez who assisted in the conduct of this investigation and to Dr. Irv Bialer who participated in the design of the project and the preparation of this manuscript. This project was supported in part by a grant from Ciba-Geigy Pharmaceuticals.

REFERENCES

1. *Drug Protein Binding, Annals of the New York Academy of Sciences,* **226,** 172 (1973).
2. Dayton, P. G., Israili, Z. H., and Perel, J. M., in *Drug Protein Binding, Annals of the New York Academy of Sciences,* **226,** *in press* (1973).
3. Glassman, A. H., and Perel, J. M., *Arch. of Gen. Psychiat.,* **28,** 649 (1973).
4. Winsberg, B., Bialer, I., Kupietz, S., and Tobias, J., *Am. J. Psychiat.,* **130,** 1425 (1972).
5. Winsberg, B., Bialer, I., Klutch, A., and Perel, J. M., *Psychopharmacol. Bulletin,* **9,** 45 (1973).
6. Jalling, B., Boreus, L. O., Rose, A., and Sjöqvist, F., *Pharmacologia Clinica,* **2,** 200 (1970).
7. Chignell, F. C., Vesell, E. S., Starkweather, D. K., and Berlin, C. M., *Clin. Pharmacol. and Therap.,* **12,** 897 (1971).

8. Pruitt, A. W., and Dayton, P. G., *Europ. J. Clin. Pharmacol.,* **4,** 59 (1971).
9. Glassman, A., Hurwic, M. J., and Perel, J. M., *This volume.*
10. Hussey, R. H., and Wright, A. L., *Acta Paedopsychiatrica,* **37,** 194 (1970).
11. Brown, D., Winsberg, B., Bialer, I., and Press, M., *Am. J. Psychiat.,* **130,** 210 (1973).
12. Fromm, G. H., Amores, C. Y., and Thics, W., *Arch. Neurol.,* **27,** 198 (1972).

The Phenothiazines and Structurally Related Drugs, edited by I. S.
Forrest, C. J. Carr, and E. Usdin. Raven Press, New York © 1974.

The Pharmacokinetics of Butaperazine in Serum

John M. Davis, David S. Janowsky,* H. Joseph Sekerke,*
Hal Manier,* and M. Khaled El-Yousef*

*Illinois State Psychiatric Institute, Department of Psychiatry, University of Chicago,
Chicago, Illinois 60637 and Department of Psychiatry, School of Medicine, Vanderbilt
University, Nashville, Tennessee 37203 and *Cooper Building, Central State Hospital,
Nashville, Tennessee 37217*

INTRODUCTION

Clinically, there are patients who do not respond to low or moderate doses
of antipsychotic drugs but who do respond to higher doses. Conversely,
there are individual patients who respond quite well to low drug doses, but
who do poorly when they receive moderate or high doses. We have previously proposed a hypothesis to explain these findings based on studies relating blood chlorpromazine levels to therapeutic improvement and side effects (1–9). In these previous studies, different patients manifested widely
differing blood levels of chlorpromazine while receiving comparable oral
doses. One patient whose dose was reduced by 50% had a comparable reduction in his chlorpromazine blood level and became more psychotic.
When the dose was increased, he again improved. Another patient receiving
a moderate dose of chlorpromazine and remaining psychotic was found to
have an extremely high blood level. When this patient's dose was reduced,
the patient improved remarkably. This patient may have had a deficit in his
ability to metabolize chlorpromazine, and may thus have built up a high
level of blood chlorpromazine which caused psychotoxicity. In contrast to
this, patients were evaluated and found to have extremely low blood levels
even when they received very high doses. These patients did poorly on
chlorpromazine; they may have metabolized or absorbed chlorpromazine
in such a way that, even while receiving high doses, adequate amounts of
chlorpromazine did not reach the brain.

This type of information offers the potential for providing the clinical
pharmacological background which may help to explain clinically observed
cases of idiosyncratic responses to antipsychotic agents. Such idiosyncracies

of drug metabolism or absorption may affect one drug, but may or may not affect members of similar or different classes of drugs.

The purpose of the experiments described in this chapter is to study the clinical pharmacology of the phenothiazine derivative butaperazine (Repoise®), in an effort to gain basic information which would be relevant to eventually relating butaperazine blood levels to clinical efficacy and side effects. Another intention of the current studies is, therefore, to develop an assay for the measurement of serum butaperazine and to determine if prediction of chronic steady-state butaperazine levels can be made from the study of changes in blood butaperazine levels following administration of an acute single dose. In addition, we intended to define the pharmacokinetic parameters of butaperazine in man. This basic information is needed as a prerequisite to designing further studies relating clinical efficacy and side effects to blood butaperazine levels.

We chose to study butaperazine because (a) butaperazine is a commonly used antipsychotic medication, (b) the possibility exists that a relatively simple butaperazine fluorometric analysis could be developed, and (c) a simple assay for butaperazine would have ready application in the clinical laboratory, if such assay were to prove clinically relevant.

In contrast, many technical difficulties are encountered in the measurement of chlorpromazine. These relate to difficulties inherent in using the electron-capture gas-chromatograph detector (1, 6–9), and problems relating to the fact that in the clinical situation blood levels of chlorpromazine are at the lower levels of sensitivity for the chlorpromazine assay.

METHOD

General Procedure

Nineteen schizophrenic patients were used as subjects in the study. Studies were performed following acute and chronic oral administration of butaperazine. In the acute studies, patients who had been receiving no other psychotropic drugs were fasted overnight, and a baseline or blank blood sample was drawn. To study the serum levels of butaperazine following acute administration, at 9 A.M., patients were given tablets of butaperazine (10, 20, 30, 40, 50, or 60 mg). Ten-cc blood samples were then drawn at 2, 4, 6, 8, 12, 15, 24, 36, and 48 hr after butaperazine administration. Forty-eight to 72 hr after the initial butaperazine dose was administered, the experiment was repeated, with another dose of butaperazine. In general, patients receiving one dose of butaperazine initially received a subsequent dose of one-half or twice the initial dose. Blood samples were again drawn at baseline, 2, 4, 6, 8, 12, 15, 24, 36, and 48 hr after butaperazine administration. Data were analyzed to compare the changes in blood levels following each dose of butaperazine in a given patient.

In studies after chronic administration, various patients were placed on a constant dose of butaperazine of 10, 20, 30, or 40 mg every 12 hr, for a period of 1 or more weeks. Ten-cc blood samples were drawn each day at 9 A.M. just before the morning butaperazine dose. After butaperazine was given for 1 or more weeks, the nature of the changes over time was obtained by drawing a baseline blood sample just prior to butaperazine administration, followed by the drawing of blood samples at 2, 4, 6, 8, 12, 15, 24, 36, 48, and 72 hr. During the time that these samples were being drawn, drug administration was discontinued. Butaperazine administration was then resumed at a dose of either one-half or twice the initial daily dose for a period of 1 or more weeks; then a second butaperazine curve, as described above, was obtained.

Changes in blood levels following different doses of butaperazine were evaluated in the same patient and in different patients. Problems investigated included: (a) definition of whether or not proportional doses of oral butaperazine given acutely or chronically produce proportional increases in butaperazine serum levels in the same patient; (b) definition of what range of blood levels exists between patients receiving the same dose of butaperazine; (c) evaluation of whether prediction of chronic steady-state butaperazine blood levels can be made on the basis of blood-level changes following acute butaperazine administration; (d) evaluation of whether the disappearance rate from plasma of butaperazine following different administered doses remains the same in a given patient; (e) evaluation of how reliable the disappearance from plasma of butaperazine for a given dose is from experiment to experiment; and (f) evaluation of the nature of the curve of the butaperazine disappearance from blood following acute and chronic administration.

Serum butaperazine levels were measured using the following technique. To a 15-ml tapered glass centrifuge tube containing 2 ml of plasma sample (or plasma containing a known amount of butaperazine) were added 1 ml of 2 N NaOH and 5 ml heptane:2-propanol. After shaking at high speed on an Eberbach reciprocal shaker for 30 min and centrifugation, 4 ml of the organic layer was removed to another 15-ml glass centrifuge tube containing 1 ml of 0.1 N HCl. The butaperazine was extracted into the aqueous layer and 0.9 ml of the HCl layer was transferred to a 3-ml tapered glass centrifuge tube containing 0.1 ml 5 N NaOH and 0.2 ml heptane:2-propanol. The final extraction step was performed by mixing at high speed for 2 min on a Vortex mixer. The sample was then centrifuged and the aqueous layer removed. The organic layer was transferred to a fluorometer cell with a pathlength of 3 mm and a capacity of approximately 0.2 ml. The sample was then ready for analysis.

Reagents and apparatus used were as follows:

(1) "Chromatoquality" *n*-heptane and A.C.S. grade 2-propanol (obtained from Matheson, Coleman, and Bell and Fisher Scientific, respectively).

(2) A *n*-heptane: 2-propanol solution, 90:10 (v/v), (used in the extraction procedure).
(3) A sample of butaperazine dimaleate (produced by A. H. Robins Research Laboratories).

A butaperazine stock solution was prepared by dissolving butaperazine dimaleate in water containing just enough HCl to bring about dissolution. This solution was stable when stored in the dark at 4°C.

Analyses were done using an Aminco Bowman Spectrophotofluorometer containing 3/16″ slits in position 2 and the photomultiplier. The activation wavelength was 286 nm, and the fluorescent wavelength was 520 nm.

The fluorometric spectra of serum butaperazine were identical with that of stock butaperazine.

The specificity of the method was confirmed by countercurrent distribution studies of serum from patients on butaperazine versus blank plasma with stock butaperazine added. The same standards were run on each of 26 different assay days, and the results were highly reproducible. The reproducibility of these standards yielded an SEM of 1.6% (standard deviation = 7.6%).

RESULTS

Our initial analysis of the data was devoted to a demonstration of the changes in pharmacokinetic parameters and serum butaperazine levels following different doses of acutely and chronically administered butaperazine (Fig. 1). The serum butaperazine level shown in Fig. 1 peaked soon after administration of the oral doses, and then decreased in level in two phases.

Figure 1 also shows patient #1's serum butaperazine curves following the chronic ingestion of first 20 and then 40 mg butaperazine, given twice daily. The serum butaperazine level curve following the chronic administration of butaperazine is similar in shape to that following acute administration.

In Fig. 2, we have presented the average composite curves of patients receiving both acute and chronic doses of butaperazine. The slope of the decrease in butaperazine levels from serum following two different acute doses and one chronic dose is essentially the same. Furthermore, the peak butaperazine level following the acutely administered 20-mg dose is approximately one-half the height of those peaks following the 40-mg dose. Thus, there appears to be a proportionality between different doses of butaperazine and different blood levels at a given time after administration. The curves observed following acute or chronic administration of other doses of butaperazine were similar in configuration to those in Figs. 1 or 2.

The acute administration of 20 mg butaperazine to 13 subjects resulted

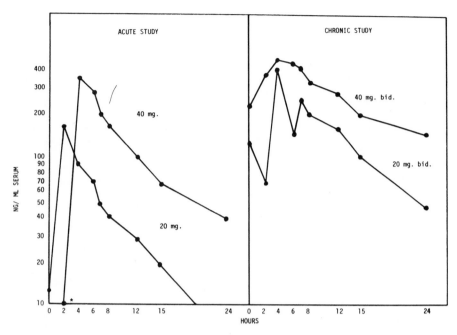

* Butaperazine serum level at 0 hours = 2 ng/ml serum.

FIG. 1. Serum levels of butaperazine in patient #1 after receiving acute and chronic 20- and 40-mg doses.

in an average peak serum level ± SEM of 215 ± 45 ng/ml. Average serum butaperazine levels ± SEM measured 12 hr after the chronic administration of 20 mg butaperazine doses, given to five patients, was essentially the same as the corresponding acute blood level peaks (20 mg = 229 ± 124). Since chronic levels represent the level at 12 hr following oral ingestion, as opposed to the peak level following oral ingestion in the acute studies, there is obviously some buildup of butaperazine in blood over time.

We further investigated the relationship between serum butaperazine and dose. With chlorpromazine, higher doses give higher blood levels, but the relationship is far from linear (1–3). In Fig. 3, we have presented the data from several patients who received 20- and 40-mg acute and chronically administered doses of butaperazine. Peak serum heights after acute butaperazine administration, area under the curve after acute butaperazine administration, and steady-state serum levels after chronic butaperazine administration are approximately double on a 40-mg dose what they are on a 20-mg dose. Since each subject was studied following receipt of two different doses, the relationship between dose and each pharmacokinetic parameter (acute peak height, area under the acute curve, and chronic steady-state level) could be plotted, and the slope of the line computed. The

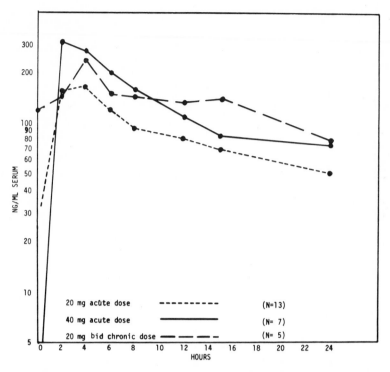

FIG. 2. Average serum butaperazine levels in patients following acutely administered 20- and 40-mg doses and chronically administered 20-mg butaperazine doses.

resultant slopes were averaged and SEM computed. The average slope of the acute peak height was 1.05 ± 0.13; of area under the curve in the acute studies 1.15 ± 0.08; and of the chronic steady-state level 0.99 ± 0.15; i.e., the nanograms butaperazine per milliliter serum per milligram butaperazine ingested was computed. If the relationship of serum level to dose is linear, with a slope of 1, then the ng/ml/mg butaperazine should be constant for any dose ingested, and, indeed, this occurred as shown in Fig. 3, part 2. This latter manner of expressing this relationship is the formal equivalent of the slope. Since serum levels are directly proportional to the dose ingested, one may be able to predict from a single acute dose what the steady-state levels for a given chronic dosage will be.

The data were analyzed to evaluate statistically whether or not correlations existed between various pharmacokinetic parameters. Also, data were analyzed to determine if correlations existed between acutely and chronically administered butaperazine parameters. A high correlation ($r = 0.90$) was found to exist between the serum butaperazine peaks following the 20 and 40 mg acutely administered doses in a given patient. Similarly, the area under the curve following acute 20 and 40 mg butaperazine doses in a given

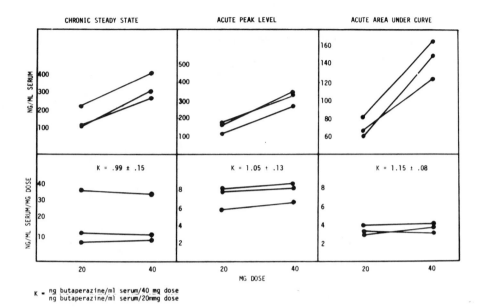

FIG. 3. Demonstration of chronic steady-state butaperazine levels, serum-butaperazine peak levels following acute butaperazine administration, and area under the curve following acute butaperazine administration, following 20- and 40-mg butaperazine doses in three patients expressed as ng/ml serum/mg butaperazine dose.

patient correlated highly ($r = 0.96$), as did the half-life of the decrease in blood levels following acute administration of 20 and 40 mg of butaperazine ($r = 0.82$). Also, as would be expected, peak height in the chronic studies was highly correlated with area under the curve (20 mg dose: $r = 1.00$; 30 mg dose: $r = 0.94$; 40 mg dose: $r = 1.00$), and steady-state butaperazine levels (20 mg dose: $r = 0.97$; 30 mg dose: $r = 0.93$; 40 mg dose: $r = 1.00$). Also, area under the curve in the chronic studies correlated with chronic steady-state serum levels (20 mg dose: $r = 0.97$; 30 mg dose: $r = 0.93$; 40 mg dose: $r = 1.00$). As would be expected, the acute butaperazine peak height correlated highly with the area under the curve (20 mg dose: $r = 0.92$; 40 mg dose: $r = 0.77$).

Since evaluation of steady-state blood levels may have clinical importance, we wanted to determine if the serum-butaperazine levels noted after an acute dose of butaperazine could be used to predict steady-state butaperazine levels. We therefore correlated the height of the serum-butaperazine peak following a given acute dose with the steady-state serum levels. As shown in Table 1, a high degree of correlation was found (20 mg dose: $r = 0.96$; 30 mg dose: $r = 0.95$; 40 mg dose: $r = 0.87$). This suggests that the steady-state level of butaperazine could be calculated from the acute peak height in a given patient.

TABLE 1. *Correlations between various pharmacokinetic parameters for different administered doses of butaperazine*

	Acute peak level versus steady-state level	
Dose (mg)	*n*	*r*
20	5	0.96
30	3	0.95
40	8	0.87
	Acute peak level versus acute area under curve	
	n	*r*
20	12	0.92
30	—	—
40	7	0.77
	Chronic area under curve versus steady state levels	
	n	*r*
20	5	1.00
30	6	0.94
40	5	1.00
	Chronic peak level versus chronic steady state level	
	n	*r*
20	5	0.97
30	6	0.93
40	6	1.00
	Chronic peak level versus chronic area under the curve	
	n	*r*
20	5	1.00
30	6	0.94
40	5	1.00

The time required for the serum butaperazine level to decrease by 50% ($t_{1/2}$) following the attainment of the peak serum level was evaluated in patients receiving both the acute and chronically administered butaperazine.

In both the acute and the chronic studies, butaperazine serum levels appeared to peak between 1 and 3 hr and subsequently to decrease in level in at least two phases. The initial decrease in butaperazine levels was rapid and lasted for about 4 hr after the initial serum peak was attained. The second phase was slower. It lasted from between 4 hr after the peak level has been attained and 24 hr after the ingestion of butaperazine. Table 2 demonstrates that, for the various acute and chronic doses of butaperazine administered,

TABLE 2. *Rapid and slow phase half-lives of the decline in serum butaperazine following acute and chronic administration of different doses of butaperazine*

Dose	n	Rapid phase[a] (Peak–4 hrs. post peak)	Slow phase (4 hrs. post peak–24 post admin.)
Acute studies			
20 mg	13	4.1 ± 0.5	13.1 ± 2.1
30	2	6.0 ± 0.5	11.5 ± 7.0
40	8	3.5 ± 0.6	9.9 ± 1.9
60	2	3.2 ± 1.4	15.0 ± 3.0
Chronic studies			
20 mg	6	4.8 ± 1.1	11.4 ± 3.6
30	6	5.8 ± 1.3	14.6 ± 6.2
40	6	5.02 ± 0.8	12.6 ± 1.8

[a] All values expressed as the half-life of the decline in serum butaperazine levels (average $\pm$ SEM).

the rapid phase half-life was about 4 hr, while the slower phase was about 12 hr. For example, the rapid-phase $t_{1/2}$ for the acute 20-mg dose was 4.1 ± 0.5 hr. The slower phase $t_{1/2}$ for this dose was 13.1 ± 2.1. Little difference in these parameters existed between the same acutely and chronically administered doses. Thus, the results outlined in Table 2 suggest that ingestion of butaperazine chronically for 1 or 2 weeks does not lead to marked changes in butaperazine metabolism.

A moderate degree of variability was found to exist (a) between serum butaperazine peaks in different patients following acute drug administration, (b) between the half-life of the decrease in serum butaperazine levels following an acutely administered dose, (c) between the steady-state levels obtained following administration of butaperazine dosage (corrected for variation in dose), and (d) between the half-life of the decrease in serum-butaperazine levels following chronic drug administration. In plotting this variability, we adjusted the various parameters to conform to a standard 1-mg butaperazine dose (ng butaperazine/ml serum/1.0 mg dose) by dividing the ng butaperazine/ml serum by the administered dose. Figure 4 demonstrates that there is a range of butaperazine peak levels from 4 to 32 ng/ml/ 1.0 mg dose for the acutely administered doses. The range of half-lives for the decrease in serum butaperazine levels following acute administration is from 4 to 30 hr for the second phase of the serum level decline. The chronic steady-state serum butaperazine levels ranged from 1 to 36 ng/ml/mg dose administered. The $t_{1/2}$ of the second-phase decrease in serum butaperazine after chronic administration ranged from 5 to 33 hr. Thus, there is moderate variation for the parameters measured. However, there is considerably less interpatient variation in butaperazine serum levels than in chlorpromazine

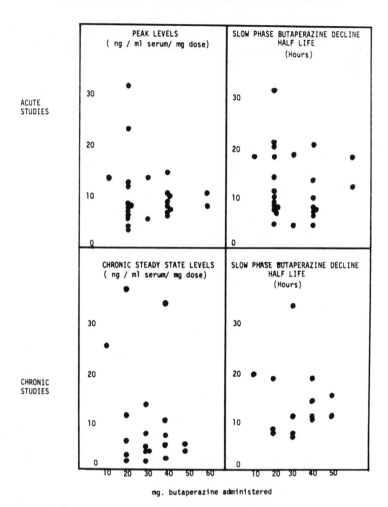

FIG. 4. Interpatient variability of various pharmacokinetic parameters following buta-perazine administration.

levels as described previously (1–9). It is obvious that a correlation between blood levels and efficacy or side effects would be more likely to occur, if there were an extremely large variation in blood levels in patients on a similar dose than if a less marked variation occurred.

DISCUSSION

The above data demonstrate that serum butaperazine levels are directly proportional to the dose ingested. Furthermore, the decrease in serum butaperazine levels following an oral dose is at least biphasic, showing a rapid early decline, followed by a slower later decline. This biphasic decline is not related to dose administered nor to whether the butaperazine has been administered acutely or chronically.

Since the above data indicate that serum levels are highly correlated with dose, it may be possible to predict with modest accuracy, from the serum levels of butaperazine following a single, acutely administered butaperazine dose, the steady-state serum levels following chronic butaperazine administration. If a correlation is eventually found between side effects of butaperazine and/or clinical efficacy and serum butaperazine levels, it may be possible to predict whether a given dose of butaperazine will be useful or toxic by applying the above findings; i.e., the serum levels of butaperazine following an initial acute butaperazine dose may be useful in predicting eventual serum levels following any chronic dosage schedule.

The data in the above studies represent essentially pilot data, and thus should be interpreted with a certain degree of caution. Interpretation of the pharmacokinetic data should take into account the fact that these are studies based on the oral ingestion of butaperazine. The speed of absorption of butaperazine from the gastrointestinal tract, its distribution throughout body stores, and its disappearance from plasma as it is excreted and/or metabolized may all contribute to the variety of plasma levels observed.

More studies, using a greater number of patients, are needed to delineate further the nature of butaperazine's pharmacokinetics. It would be most important to determine if a relationship exists between serum butaperazine levels and side effects or clinical efficacy, either between patients or in the same patient. The data presented above may help to allow such relationships to be defined.

ACKNOWLEDGMENTS

This research was supported in part by U.S. Public Health Service grants GM 15431 and MH 11468 (from the National Institute of Mental Health), and by research support from the State of Tennessee, Department of Mental Health, and the State of Illinois, Department of Mental Health.

REFERENCES

1. Curry, S. H., *Anal. Chem.,* **40,** 1251, (1968).
2. Curry, S. H. and Marshall, J. H. L., *Life Science,* **7,** 9 (1968).
3. Curry, S. H., Davis, J. M., Janowsky, D., and Marshall, J. H. L., *Neuropsychopharmacology,* **5,** 72, (1969).
4. Curry, S. H., Janowsky, D. S., Davis, J. M., and Marshall, J. H. L., *Arch. Gen. Psychiat.,* **22,** 209 (1970).
5. Curry, S. H., Marshall, J. H. L., Davis, J. M., and Janowsky, D. S., *Arch. Gen. Psychiat.,* **22,** 289, (1970).
6. Sekerke, H. J., Davis, J. M., Janowsky, D. S., El-Yousef, M. K., and Manier, H. D., *Psychopharm. Bull,* **9,** 23 (1973).
7. Davis, J. M., Sekerke, H. J., and Janowsky, D. S., *Psychopharm. Bull.,* **9,** 28 (1973).
8. Fann, W. E., Davis, J. M., Janowsky, D. S., and Schmidt, D., *Clin. Pharm. Therap.,* **14,** 135 (1973).
9. Christoph, G. W., Schmidt, D., Janowsky, D. S., and Davis, J. M., *Clin. Chem. Acta.,* **38,** 265 (1972).

The Phenothiazines and Structurally Related Drugs, edited by I. S. Forrest, C. J. Carr, and E. Usdin. Raven Press, New York © 1974.

Metabolic and Clinical Observations on Metiapine in Humans

George J. Wright, Robert H. Hook, and Barry Blackwell*

Merrell-National Laboratories, Division of Richardson-Merrell Inc., 110 East Amity Road, Cincinnati, Ohio 45215, and *University of Cincinnati College of Medicine, Cincinnati, Ohio 45219

INTRODUCTION

Metiapine (Fig. 1) is a dibenzothiazepine derivative possessing the pharmacological characteristics of a major tranquilizer. Independent studies in schizophrenic patients have indicated that metiapine is a potent antipsychotic medication (1–3). These clinical studies have demonstrated that metiapine has about double the potency of chlorpromazine as an antipsychotic agent with somewhat similar sedative actions. Reports on the preclinical toxicology and metabolism of metiapine have been given previously (4–7).

Attempts to correlate the physiological changes due to drugs with blood levels or metabolite patterns are still in their infancy. In the area of psychotropic drug use, this kind of information could prove invaluable in understanding the wide range of individual susceptibility to both therapeutic and unwanted effects, as well as result in more logical therapeutic regimens with regard to dosage and timing of drug ingestion. The work presented in this chapter was undertaken to determine some of the pharmacokinetics of metiapine in normal humans and to relate, if possible, some of the pharmacological responses observed to the kinetics of drug absorption and elimination.

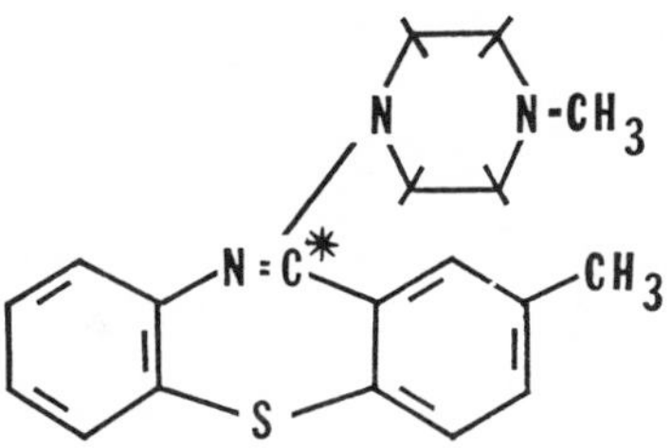

FIG. 1. Structure of metiapine. The asterisk indicates the position of the radiolabel.

445

METHODS AND MATERIAL

Metiapine-14C

Metiapine-14C,   (2-methyl-11-(4-methyl-1-piperazinyl)-dibenzo   [b,f]
[1,4] thiazepine-11-14C), was synthesized by New England Nuclear Corp.
The chemical and physical properties of the sample agreed with those of
authentic metiapine. The specific activity of the undiluted metiapine-14C
was 20.2 μCi/mg. Thin-layer chromatography and autoradiography showed
that the sample was essentially radiochemically pure.

Capsule Preparation

Metiapine-14C was recrystallized after dilution with authentic nonradioactive metiapine, to a specific activity of 0.205 μCi/mg. Capsule fill material
was prepared by mixing diluted metiapine-14C with appropriate excipients
comparable to standard clinical dosage forms. Each batch was sampled
to determine the specific activity of the capsule fill material. Capsules were
prepared from these fill materials and were individually weighed and the
weights recorded.

Subject Selection

Volunteers were selected for the study following comprehensive physical
examinations including electrocardiograms and clinical laboratory tests to
determine their state of health. Those who had clinical evidence or history
of any serious medical or surgical problem were excluded. Six healthy,
normal, male volunteers, ranging in age from 23 to 35 yr (mean 29.5 yr),
were admitted to the study and entered the Cincinnati General Research
Unit on the evening prior to drug administration. They remained in the
Research Unit for 10 days.

Experimental Protocol

After a minimum overnight fast of 12 hr, the drug (50 mg or 100 mg of
metiapine-14C containing 10 or 20 μCi, respectively) was administered
orally in capsules. Four subjects received 50 mg of metiapine and two subjects received 100 mg. Frequent blood samples were taken during the first
24 hr and at least daily for the next 4 days. Total urine and fecal collections
were made for 10 days following dosing. Food was allowed at noon on the
first day and at regular meal times on the days following. Blood pressure
and pulse rates were recorded hourly for the first 18 hr after drug administration and at 4-hr intervals for the next 9 days. Electrocardiograms were
taken daily for 6 days. Respiration rates and oral body temperature were

frequently monitored, and hourly notes were made by the attending nurse. Comprehensive physical examinations were repeated after completion of the study.

Sample Preparation and Liquid Scintillation Counting

Urine was prepared for counting by mixing an aliquot with 15 ml of liquid scintillation solution. Two ml of absolute ethanol was added when aliquots were greater than 0.2 ml. All samples were routinely counted in triplicate.

Feces were homogenized in deionized water to give homogenates with approximately 10% (w/v) solids. After homogenization, a few drops of isoamyl alcohol were added as a defoaming agent. A 0.5-ml aliquot of the homogenate was added to 3.0 ml of hydroxide of Hyamine® (Rohm and Haas, Phila., Pa.) and heated in a capped scintillation vial at 50 to 60°C for 16 to 24 hr. The resulting solution was bleached for 4 to 24 hr at room temperature by the addition of 0.2 ml of 30% hydrogen peroxide. Finally, 0.25 ml of concentrated hydrochloric acid, 2.0 ml of absolute ethanol, and 15 ml of liquid scintillation solution were added to the vial. Triplicate samples were prepared.

Plasma samples were prepared from whole blood with EDTA as anti-coagulant by centrifugation at 1,800 rpm. Plasma (0.2 ml) was placed in vials with 3.0 ml of hydroxide of Hyamine®, heated at 50 to 60°C for 16 to 24 hr, and further processed as described for the fecal samples.

Analyses of radioactivity were performed on a Packard Tri-Carb Liquid Scintillation Counter equipped with an automatic external standard. The counting data were processed on an IBM Model 360/40 computer using an automatic external standard calibration technique that has been described previously (8). The scintillation fluid consisted of 40 ml/liter of Liquifluor® (New England Nuclear, Pilot Chem. Div., Boston, Mass.) in a 2:1 solution of toluene and ethanol (v/v).

Extraction and Thin-Layer Chromatography of Metabolites from Urine

Selected urine samples from one of the subjects who had received 100 mg were examined for unchanged metiapine and metabolite patterns. One urine sample collected 2 to 8 hr after dosing was made basic with either Tris buffer (pH 8.8) or sodium hydroxide (approx. 0.3 N) and extracted with either dichloroethane or chloroform. The organic layers were sampled for assay of radioactivity and subsequently evaporated. Residues were taken up in ethanol for thin-layer chromatography. Also, three urine samples, collected 2 to 8, 8 to 18, and 18 to 24 hr after dosing, were chromatographed without prior preparation. The respective samples were chromatographed on Quanta/Gram LQD thin-layer plates using chloroform-methanol-ammonia (100:10:1, v/v/v) as the developing solvent. Radioactive spots were detected by autoradiography.

RESULTS

Elimination of radioactivity from the six volunteers was nearly complete within 10 days. Table 1 lists the quantitative recovery from each of the subjects at 72 hr and 10 days after administration of drug. The major route of elimination was the urine (a mean of $78.05 \pm 7.01\%$ of the dose) with the remainder of the drug excreted in the feces. Total recovery was $93.32 \pm 6.81\%$ of the dose.

The cumulative recoveries of radioactivity from the urine and feces are shown in Figs. 2 and 3. Absorption of metiapine occurred rapidly as measured by appearance of radioactivity in the urine and by the rapid onset of sedation. It is likely that absorption was complete and that the radioactivity found in the feces was secreted into the intestine via the bile after absorption in a manner similar to that found in the rat and dog (7).

Rapid absorption was confirmed by the early appearance and attainment of peak concentrations of radioactivity in the plasma (Figs. 4 and 5). As a group, the four subjects who received a dose of 50 mg had lower blood levels of radioactivity than those who received 100 mg of metiapine; but, within the 50-mg group, there was no obvious correlation with dose on a weight basis (0.54 to 0.81 mg/kg). Between 8 and 36 hr postdose, the kinetics of disappearance of radioactivity from the plasma approximated first order with a half-life of approximately 20 hr in five of the six volunteers, regardless of dose level given. The disappearance of radioactivity from plasma of one of the subjects (JS) obviously did not conform to first-order kinetics. Post 48 hr, the concentration of radioactivity in plasma dropped below the level which could be reliably measured, although there was some indication that other mechanisms were coming into play to cause a departure from simple first-order kinetics (see Fig. 6).

TABLE 1. *Recovery of radioactivity in urine and feces from normal male volunteers*

Volunteer	Dose (mg)	Percent dose recovered					
		72 hr			10 days		
		Urine	Feces	Total	Urine	Feces	Total
R.E.	100	61.28	7.82	69.10	72.46	12.73	85.19
R.B.	100	57.29	12.15	69.44	71.68	19.14	90.82
C.N.	50	70.57	3.20	73.77	84.08	17.27	101.35
L.L.	50	69.69	2.77	72.46	83.35	15.68	99.03
J.S.	50	74.33	8.67	83.00	85.73	11.37	97.10
W.R.	50	55.79	4.62	60.41	70.97	15.43	86.40

Quantitative recovery of radioactivity in urine and feces after oral administration of metiapine-^{14}C to normal male volunteers.

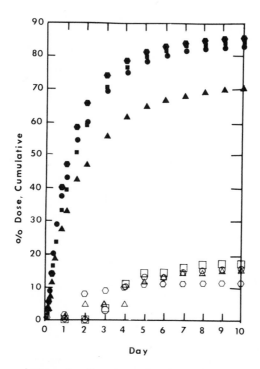

FIG. 2. Cumulative excretion of radioactivity following oral administration of 50 mg of metiapine-^{14}C. Solid sumbols—urinary excretion. Open symbols—fecal excretion. ○ Subject L.L., □ Subject C.N., ◌ Subject J.S., △ Subject D.R.

Preliminary studies of the urinary metabolites of metiapine were done on selected urine samples from subject RE (100 mg). Extraction of radioactivity with dichloroethane or chloroform (2 to 8 hr postdose) made basic with Tris (pH 8.8) or NaOH (approx. 0.3 N) allowed 10.7 to 15.7% of the activity to be extracted into the organic phase. Thin-layer chromatography of three additional urine samples without prior extraction and chromatography of the extracts described above produced evidence of eight radioactive zones. Only a trace of the radioactivity in urine could be attributed to unchanged metiapine (< 1%).

Sedation and hypotension were regularly observed in the volunteers in this study. Table 2 shows the onset and duration of sedation as well as the onset, degree, and duration of systolic hypotension in each of the six individuals. The peak blood levels of radioactivity, time necessary to attain peak level, and dosage per body weight are also given. The data illustrates the wide range of variability between individuals.

Despite the fact that medication was given at 8 A.M. after a normal night of sleep, all subjects experienced marked sedation. However, the sedation varied in time of onset from 1 to 2 hr following ingestion and varied in

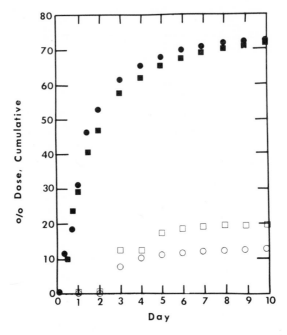

FIG. 3. Cumulative excretion of radioactivity following oral administration of 100 mg of metiapine-[14]C. Solid symbols — urinary excretion. Open symbols — fecal excretion. ○ Subject R.E., □ Subject R.B.

duration from 8 to 23 hr. The two subjects who took longest to fall asleep were also sedated for the shortest time period.

There was even more individual variability in blood pressure change. In two subjects hypotension was immediate, but in one it never occurred. It is particularly interesting that the two subjects who experienced quite marked and immediate hypotension were also the same two who showed least sedation. The hypotension occurred while the subjects were supine suggesting that body position did not play a significant role.

In order to study further these wide variations between and within individuals, rank-order correlations were carried out. Table 3 shows the matrix for Spearman Rank Correlation Coefficients between the eight variables studied. None of these reached the 5% level of significance (coefficient above 0.829) although there were some strong trends. Correlations over 0.50 were noted between the following parameters: (a) onset of sedation was correlated with its duration and also with dose and peak blood level of drug; (b) the onset, degree, and duration of blood pressure drop were also positively related to one another but there was no relationship with dose or blood level of radioactivity; and (c) there was no clear relation between the measures of sedation and hypotension, which suggests

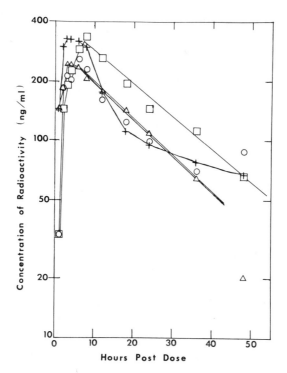

FIG. 4. Concentration of radioactivity in the plasma of normal volunteers after oral dosing with 50 mg of metiapine-^{14}C. Values are expressed as ng/ml equivalents of metiapine. ○ Subject C.N., △ Subject L.L., + Subject J.S., □ Subject W.R.

that the hypotension is not simply a result of the sedation and recumbency.

The onset of sedation and hypotension frequently anticipated the time taken to reach peak blood level of radioactivity and persisted well beyond it. For instance, in subject RB peak blood level occurred at 6 hr but sedation persisted for 23 hr, whereas in subject LL peak blood level occurred at 3 hr and hypotension lasted for 24 hr.

It is noteworthy that almost all physiological changes were of short duration compared to excretion or plasma half-life of radioactivity.

Electrocardiographic changes from baseline were noted on only one of the six volunteers. In this individual, sinus bradycardia was observed on the first day and a sinus arrhythmia was noted on the fifth day. Electrocardiograms taken before and after these episodes were not different from his baseline recordings.

No effect that could be attributed to drug was noted on pulse rate, respiration, or body temperature. No significant changes in clinical laboratory findings were noted. No subjective responses which could be described as extrapyramidal symptoms occurred in these subjects.

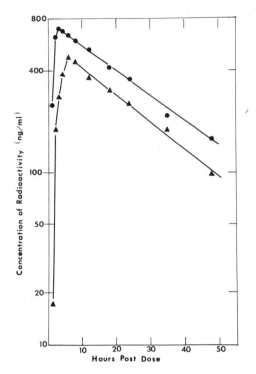

FIG. 5. Concentration of radioactivity in the plasma of normal volunteers after oral dosing with 100 mg of metiapine-^{14}C. Values are expressed as ng/ml equivalents of metiapine. ○ Subject R.E., △ Subject R.B.

DISCUSSION

The absorption of metiapine and elimination of metabolites occurs rapidly with relatively little variation from subject to subject. Figure 6 is a combined plot of the urinary excretion rates of radioactivity normalized to percent of dose for all subjects. The mean percent of dose excreted for each time interval is shown and the segments of the curve have been calculated by subtracting the contribution of the "tail" of the excretion curve from the earlier time points. The excretion half-life of the early segment (A) was 19 hr and represented in excess of 90% of the excreted radioactivity. The half-life of the more slowly excreted material (B) was 55 hr. The disappearance half-life of radioactivity from plasma was very similar to the excretion half-life in urine. The similarity of the curve from all six volunteers demonstrated that urinary excretion was dose dependent and that the capacity to metabolize metiapine had not been exceeded.

Despite the closely comparable excretion kinetics of radioactivity from metiapine, a wide range of physiological response from individual to individual was noted. Sedation was more closely correlated with dose and

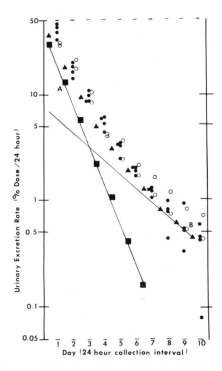

FIG. 6. Urinary excretion rate of radioactivity from normal volunteers dosed with metia-pine-^{14}C. ● Subjects receiving 50 mg, ○ subjects receiving 100 mg, ▲ Mean percent of dose excreted for the inclusive time interval regardless of dose given the volunteer, ■ Data points derived by subtracting line B from actual data points to obtain line A.

TABLE 2. *Physiological changes, dosage, and blood levels*

Change noted	Subject					
	R.E.	R.B.	C.N.	L.L.	J.S.	W.R.
Onset sedation (hr)	1	1.2	1.2	2	1.2	1.8
Duration sedation (hr)	11.8	23	13.7	8	10	9.3
Onset B.P. drop (hr)	1	1	0	Immed.	1	Immed.
Maximum B.P. drop (mm Hg)	25	40	0	27	18	27
Duration B.P. drop (hr)	14	9	0	24	7	9
Peak blood levels (ng/ml)	708	473	257	248	328	334
Time to peak levels (hr)	3	6	6	3	3	8
Dose of drug (mg/kg)	1.3	0.94	0.81	0.63	0.56	0.54

Summary of changes observed after oral administration of metiapine-^{14}C. The dose of drug was expressed in terms of mg/kg to eliminate the effect of differences in body weight.

454 METABOLISM OF METIAPINE IN HUMANS

TABLE 3. *Rank order correlations (Spearman rank correlation coefficients)*

	2	3	4	5	6	7	8
1	0.71	−0.50	−0.27	−0.18	0.71	0.33	0.71
2		−0.67	−0.04	−0.47	0.48	−0.16	0.66
3			0.66	0.73	−0.04	0.11	−0.41
4				0.61	0.30	−0.14	0.04
5					0.13	0.44	0.21
6						−0.04	0.48
7							0.38

1 = Onset sedation
2 = Duration sedation
3 = Onset blood pressure fall
4 = Maximum blood pressure fall
5 = Duration blood pressure fall
6 = Peak blood level
7 = Time to peak blood level
8 = Mg/kg drug

The variables listed in Table 2 were compared to detect consistent trends in the data. A positive value indicates a trend toward a positive correlation; a negative value indicates a trend toward a negative correlation. A coefficient above 0.829 is necessary to reach a 5% level of significance.

blood level of drug than was hypotension. Furthermore, sedation and hypotension were not clearly correlated. These findings are of practical and theoretical significance since they show that hypotension is not a purely postural effect secondary to sedation or recumbency.

Further studies using metabolite identification techniques can be expected to shed light on the differences noted between individuals and between physiological endpoints. Presumably, the differences will be accounted for by rates and routes of transformation which elude detection when only total radioactivity can be measured. The final product of further studies might be the isolation of metabolites responsible for both therapeutic and individual unwanted effects.

SUMMARY

Metiapine-^{14}C was administered as a single oral dose to six normal male subjects: four subjects received 50 mg, and two received 100 mg. Radioactivity was measured in plasma and total urine and fecal samples for a period of 10 days. Peak plasma concentrations of radioactivity were reached from 3 to 8 hr postdose. Urinary excretion in 10 days accounted for 78.05 ± 7.01% of the dose with the remainder of the total 93.32 ± 6.81% recovered excreted in the feces. The plasma half-life measured over an interval of 8 to 36 hr postdose was 19 hr; urinary excretion half-life was approximately 20 hr regardless of dose for most of the material. A minor component had an excretion half-life of approximately 55 hr. Dose appeared to be related to onset and duration of sedation, but was unrelated to hypotension. The data on sedation and hypotension do not indicate a clear relationship between the two effects.

REFERENCES

1. Gallant, D. M., Bishop, M. P., and Guerrero-Figueroa, R., *Curr. Ther. Res.*, **12,** 794 (1970).
2. Simpson, G. M., Croll, D., and Lee, J. H., *Curr. Ther. Res.*, **13,** 257 (1971).
3. Gallant, D. M., Bishop, M. P., and Guerrero-Figueroa, R., *Curr. Ther. Res.*, **13,** 734 (1971).
4. Gibson, J. P., and Newberne, J. W., *Toxic. Appl. Pharmacol.*, **25,** 212 (1973).
5. Gibson, J. P., Rohovsky, M. W., Newberne, J. W., Larson, E. J., *Toxic. Appl. Pharmacol.*, **25,** 220 (1973).
6. Leeson, G. A., Kandel, A., Kuhn, W. L., and Wright, G. J., *Toxic. Appl. Pharmacol.*, **17,** 288 (1970).
7. Hook, R. H., Williams, J. M., and Wright, G. J., *Toxic. Appl. Pharmacol.*, **25,** 445 (1973).
8. Lang, J. F., in *Organic Scintillators and Liquid Scintillation Counting,* Harrocks, D. L., and Peng, C. T. (eds.), Academic, New York, 1971, p. 823.

The Phenothiazines and Structurally Related Drugs, edited by I. S. Forrest, C. J. Carr, and E. Usdin. Raven Press, New York © 1974.

Imipramine Steady-State Studies and Plasma Binding

Alexander H. Glassman, Maria J. Hurwic, Maureen Kanzler, Michael Shostak, and James M. Perel

Department of Biological Psychiatry, New York State Psychiatric Institute, and Department of Psychiatry, College of Physicians and Surgeons, Columbia University, 722 West 168 Street, New York, New York 10032

In 1967, Hammer and Sjoqvist (1) were able to demonstrate that identical oral doses of tricyclic drugs could produce markedly different plasma steady-state levels from one individual to another. This raised the question of how these variable plasma levels affected clinical outcome. During the last 2 yr, four studies have attempted to answer this question. The first, by Asberg (2), revealed a curvilinear response with good responses at mid-range plasma levels and poor responses at both low and high levels. Braithwaite (3) then published data showing a simple linear relationship in which increasing plasma levels were associated with increasing response. Meanwhile, Burrows (4), examining the same question, found no significant correlation between plasma levels and clinical outcome. Most recently, Kragh-Sorensen (5) found an inverse linear relationship with increasing plasma levels associated with decreasing clinical improvement. Thus, the four studies have yielded four different results (see Fig. 1).

These contradictory results may not be as surprising as they first appear. After examining the methodology of the studies, one might be more surprised if they had agreed. Asberg studied 30 patients for 2 weeks. Most clinicians experienced with tricyclic drugs would agree that a significant number of drug-sensitive depressives would not have responded in 2 weeks.

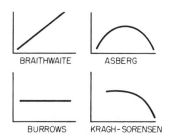

FIG. 1. Schematic representation of four published studies. Outcome (*y*-axis) versus blood level (*x*-axis).

457

Burrows studied 30 patients for 4 to 6 weeks; however, he selected his sample from 70 depressives, choosing only the milder cases. Hospitalized depressed patients are a heterogenous population and drug response is related to depressive subtype (6). By choosing only the milder cases, it is likely that Burrows weighted his sample with neurotic depressive reactions and as a result increased significantly his spontaneous remissions. Such spontaneous remissions would reduce the possibility of finding any drug-related correlation. In addition, his laboratory results would appear suspicious. His plasma levels for nortriptyline were twice the usually reported values and more than one-third of his patients came nowhere near steady-state values.

What all four studies are doing, in essence, is looking for a correlation between plasma steady-state levels and clinical outcome. By examining the inherent variability in these parameters, an estimate of the theoretically necessary sample size can be made. The variability of these parameters governs the correlation describing the relationship between these parameters. Having an expected correlation, sample size can easily be determined.

Most recent data would indicate that interindividual differences in steady-state level range from 5- to 10-fold after 4 weeks on tricyclic drugs (5). The variability in clinical response would be predicted to run between a placebo response improvement rate of 33% and a maximum response of 90 to 95% to electroconvulsive therapy (ECT) (7). Thus, assuming that, under ideal conditions, drugs are as effective as ECT, one would expect a sample of somewhere near 100 patients to demonstrate a correlation with 95% confidence. Obviously, none of these studies approached this sample size. Braithwaite studied only 15 patients; however, his results are statistically significant. Under ordinary circumstances one would accept Braithwaite's measured data rather than talk about an estimated sample size. No matter how sound the assumptions appear, an estimated sample size is based on assumptions, and is not a very solid base from which to dispute hard data. However, when Kragh-Sorensen, studying almost the identical situation as Braithwaite, found essentially opposite results, one wonders if there might not be some merit in the application of "estimated" sample size.

There is also a common assumption underlying all four studies that we have recently brought into question (8). Asberg, in her original study, referring to the work of Borga et al. (9), said that the total plasma level of a tricyclic drug can be assumed to bear a direct relationship to the amount available at the receptor because the binding does not vary from one individual to another. Our data shows that whereas binding for a given individual remains constant over time ($SD^2 = 1.84$), the binding among individuals varies over a range of greater than fourfold ($SD^2 = 21.2$) (Fig. 2).

In order to show that this variability in plasma protein binding is not the result of variation in plasma level, a series of control experiments were

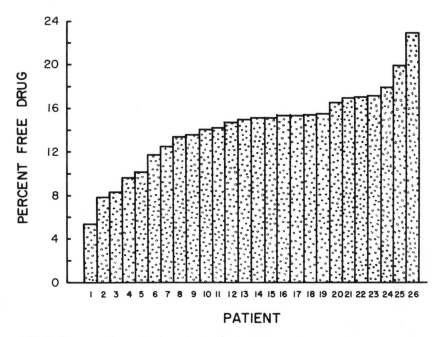

FIG. 2. Percent unbound imipramine from the plasma of 25 consecutive patients.

run. In 12 patients, plasma samples were drawn during a drug-free period prior to the administration of imipramine as well as multiple samples during the period of drug administration. The binding of imipramine in samples drawn during the drug period was examined. In addition to this, imipramine, in concentrations normally present during treatment, was added to the patients' drug-free plasma. All samples were examined by equilibrium dialysis at body temperature as previously described (10). The results were compared, and no significant difference between the *in vivo* and *in vitro* measurements was found.

On the basis of these results, varying concentrations of imipramine were added to human plasma and the effects on binding were measured. The results are expressed in Fig. 3. In concentrations ranging from 15 to 3,000 ng, there was no change in binding. When studies were carried out beyond this range, a moderate decrease in binding occurred between 3 and 10 μg, which is probably due to binding to α-lipoproteins. Dayton et al. (11) have reported that imipramine is almost one-third bound to globulin.

In view of this interindividual variability in binding, it becomes clear that all four of the earlier-mentioned blood-level studies with tricyclic drugs are based on an assumption that, in fact, is not correct. Under *in vivo* conditions, the binding of imipramine varies up to fourfold from one individual to another and is apparently not related to variability in plasma levels. The clinical significance of this finding is not yet clear. Curry (12) has pointed out that in a

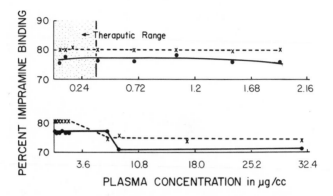

FIG. 3. Plasma binding in two subjects at varying imipramine concentrations.

drug with a large apparent volume of distribution, binding changes over a rather wide range may have only small effects on tissue concentration. Curry's hypothetical model is based on a changing plasma binding while tissue binding is held constant. At this point, it is not possible to say whether the variability in binding from one individual to another is limited to plasma proteins or if it reflects individual differences that exist in tissue binding as well. In this latter situation there would be very major effects on the antidepressant concentration actually available at the receptor. Such variability in tissue binding would have major clinical significance and would be crucial to any attempt to correlate plasma level and clinical outcome.

SUMMARY

Publications on the correlation of plasma levels of tricyclic antidepressants and clinical response are reviewed. The significance of required sample size in relation to anticipated interpatient variation is pointed out.

Various factors such as diagnostic criteria and variability of plasma- and tissue-binding characteristics of individual patients are discussed.

ACKNOWLEDGMENTS

This work was supported in part by U.S. Public Health Service grants MH-17044 and MH-21133 (from the National Institute of Mental Health).

REFERENCES

1. Hammer, W., and Sjoqvist, F., *Life Sci.,* **6,** 1895 (1967).
2. Asberg, M., Cronholm, B., Sjoqvist, F., and Tuck, D., *Brit. Med. J.,* **3,** 331 (1971).
3. Braithwaite, R. A., Goulding, R., Theano, G., Bailey, J., and Coppen, A., *Lancet,* **1,** 1297 (1972).

4. Burrows, G. D., Davies, B., and Scoggins, B. A., *Lancet*, **11,** 619 (1972).

5. Kragh-Sorensen, P., Asberg, M., and Eggert-Hansen, C., *Lancet*, **1,** 113 (1973).

6. Greenblatt, M., Grosser, G. H., and Wechsler, H., *Amer. J. Psychiat*, **120,** 935 (1964).

7. Klein, D. F., and Davis, J. M., *Diagnosis and Drug Treatment of Psychiatric Disorders*, Williams and Wilkens, Baltimore, 1969.

8. Glassman, A. H., Hurwic, M. J., and Perel, J. M., *Amer. J. Psychiat.*, **130,** 1367 (1973).

9. Borga, O., Azarnoff, D. L., Forshell, G. P., and Sjoqvist, F., *Biochem. Pharmacol.*, **18,** 2135 (1969).

10. Perel, J. M., Snell, M. M., Chen, W., and Dayton, P. G., *Biochem. Pharmacol*, **13,** 1305 (1964).

11. Pruitt, A. W., and Dayton, P. G., *Europ. J. Clin. Pharmacol.*, **4,** 59 (1971).

12. Curry, S. H., *J. Pharm. Pharmacol.*, **22,** 753 (1970).

The Phenothiazines and Structurally Related Drugs, edited by I. S. Forrest, C. J. Carr, and E. Usdin. Raven Press, New York © 1974.

Session V: Discussion

Reporter: M. A. Spirtes

1. *P. H. Kaul et al.*

Q. Spirtes: I would like to ask two questions. First, after you extract your sera, do the extracted compounds remain stable, or do they disappear after storage for a number of hours or overnight?

A. Kaul: We have not been keeping the extracts for any length of time. We begin our determinations immediately after extraction, rigidly timing each step of the operation. Evaporation of the solvents is accomplished with the same constant rate of nitrogen flow.

A. Conway: We did determine CPZ-Nor$_1$ after it had been placed in an appropriate solvent at room temperature for 24 hr and we didn't appear to have lost any. It is therefore stable in some solvents but not in others.

Spirtes: My second question concerns the CPZ-Nor$_1$ which disappears after it is injected into humans. Have you by any chance investigated whether or not some of this compound entered the erythrocytes?

A. Kaul: No. As you know, our method of analysis for phenothiazines involves the use of whole blood. Three years ago, we found that about 50% of all phenothiazines were in the erythrocytes and therefore we felt that whole blood would give about the same values as either serum or erythrocytes.

Q. Chan: I have often noted the instability of chlorpromazine and its metabolites in solvents such as heptane, hexane, benzene, and dichloromethane. Have you any data concerning the mechanism involved in this destruction?

A. Kaul: We have been able to confirm the loss of CPZ to the extent of 90 to 100% in dichloromethane. While working on the loss of CPZ-Nor$_1$ in ethyl acetate, we performed thin-layer chromatography (TLC) and found evidence via mass spectrometry that early in the reaction chlorine is lost. At least four products appeared after TLC and eventually chlorine was lost in all four products isolated. The loss of chlorine appeared to transpire during the evaporation of the solvent aided by N$_2$ gas flow.

Chan: I would have hoped for further explanation of these changes. I am glad however to hear of these data.

Kaul: I believe we are at a stage in the technology of phenothiazine determinations at which the many laboratories involved should cooperate with one another in an attempt to reach an understanding as to the best method to use. A suggestion for such a cooperative venture has been put forward during this meeting by Drs. Turner and Forrest and arrangements are being discussed for such a study.

2. M. A. Spirtes

Q. Gorrod: I have just published a review about nitrogen oxidation involving the role of Ziegler's enzyme. I notice that you performed your microsomal incubations at pH 6.7, whereas his enzyme is maximally activated at pH 8.3.

A. I did many of these determinations at pH 8.2.

Q. Gorrod: It is the pK_a of the nitrogen atom which is important. Ziegler's enzyme only works if the nitrogen compound has a pK_a greater than 7. If you involve the oxidation of a compound with pK_a lower than 7, with one or two exceptions, the compound would then be attacked by the cytochrome P-450 system. If you lower the pK_a to 2 or 3, the nitrogen-containing compound would definitely be attacked by the cytochrome P-450 system. This is true for N-oxide or N-hydroxide formation. Thus, during the purification process, a change in ratio of Ziegler's enzyme activity to cytochrome P-450 activity could be expected from the fact that you are purging one enzyme and preserving the other.

A. Yes, I agree.

Gorrod: I agree with your comments on the relative importance of the two N-oxidizing enzyme systems.

Q. Gabay: Most probably the Ziegler enzyme is a flavin enzyme. If FAD is added to the oxidation system, would the oxidative specific activity be increased?

A. Possibly, I haven't tried. I wouldn't be surprised.

W. Z. Potter: Dr. Ziegler has indicated that α-naphthylthiourea is a possible *(in vitro)* inhibitor of the amine oxidase which he has purified. One must be careful with its use, but it may be helpful to those who are working with the differential metabolism of tertiary amines *in vitro*.

Gorrod: Cysteamine would be another such inhibitor.

Potter: When comparing routes of metabolism involving Ziegler's amine oxidase and cytochrome P-450-dependent reactions, an understanding of certain interrelationships may be helpful. Using an *in vitro* microsomal system with or without some "purification" of the amine oxidase one should have a steady-state condition whereby a phenothiazine with its dialkylamine side chain is undergoing P-450-dependent metabolism with rate K_1 and amine oxidase-dependent metabolism with rate K_2. Manipulations altering only K_1 (e.g., inhibition of P-450 with SKF-525A) would not be expected to affect K_2 under these conditions. In fact, however, one does see an increase in the amount of N-oxide after inhibition of P-450 activity. This may be due to the fact that alkylamine oxides are themselves substrates for a P-450-dependent dealkylase as shown for aryl-alkylamine oxides by Ziegler's laboratory [*Biochemistry*, **5,** 2939 (1966)]. Moreover, that same laboratory has just reported at the 1973 Federation Meeting in Atlantic City that purified amine oxidase has activator as well as substrate sites. We have also been personally told that phenothiazines are good activators of the amine oxidase enzyme as well as substrates for it. Thus, in evaluating the relative roles of amine oxidase and P-450-dependent metabolism in the biotransformation of phenothiazines one must perform his experiments under kinetic conditions so that contribution of three factors may be separated:

1. The activation of the amine oxidase by the phenothiazine.
2. The actual rates of the amine oxidase and P-450-dependent pathways.
3. The further biotransformation of the dialkylamine oxide via P-450-dependent dealkylation.

Breyer: There is another possibility described by Ziegler in 1966. One can *incubate* the microsomal mixture under air without the addition of NADPH or NADPH-producing systems. N-oxidation is reduced sharply after such treatment of oxidizing mixtures.

Q. Wright: Could you differentiate between N-hydroxylation and N-oxidation? With a "Cope" elimination reaction during gas chromatography, you would end up with the same final product.

A. I have not tested N-hydroxylation. It would be interesting to perform such experiments and to check the final products appearing after gas chromatography.

Wright: One way of getting at the problem is by reducing the N-oxide back to the amine. The N-hydroxylated compound will not be reduced under the same conditions.

3. *J. C. Craig*

Q. Spirtes: During mass spectrometry, why are the positively charged ions produced used to produce the measured peaks and not the negatively charged ions?

A. This is the way the method developed. I am sure Dr. Duffield, who has contributed to the development of mass spectrometry, could give us further information.

Duffield: Negative-ion mass spectrometry is about 10,000 times less sensitive than positive-ion mass spectrometry.

Spirtes: Thank you, this must mean that the production of negative ions is that much lower than that of positive ions.

4. *G. Lindquist*

Gutmann: In 1964 Dr. I. Forrest and I isolated and proved the existence of a melanin-CPZ charge-transfer complex.

Q. I. Forrest: The complexes to which Dr. Gutmann refers were formed *in vitro* and we certainly have not isolated them from the eyes of animals fed CPZ. Moreover, as you pointed out, Dr. Lindquist, there is no melanin in the lens or cornea, nor do the pigmented particles which we can see with the naked eye look like the CPZ-melanin complexes. They are sort of yellowish to brownish specks. Very often they can be just white opacities. I doubt that they are really melanin-containing particles. What makes you so sure they are?

A. I am not sure at all. To the best of our knowledge no histochemical or electron-microscopic investigations have been carried out on the cornea or lens from a patient showing CPZ-induced pigment deposits in these tissues. Depigmentation of the iris stroma and of the pigmented epithelium of the iris in combination with pigment deposits on the posterior cornea and the anterior capsule of the lens are known to be common senile changes in human eyes.

Grant: From *in vitro* photochemical studies, we know it is possible to complex CPZ to proteins in any biological substrates containing nucleophilic groups by permanent covalent binding and not charge transfer. Thus, there is an alternative to charge-transfer binding, and since this can be photocatalyzed, it could possibly explain retinal effects.

A. Investigations performed by Dr. Potts have shown that the melanin molecule is mainly responsible for the binding of chlorpromazine in the cell and not proteins.

F. Forrest: Children up to the 3rd to 5th years of age do not have melanin in their basal ganglia. It has also been reported that children do not suffer much dyskinesia. Despite the statement of Dr. Crane who sees dyskinesia in everyone, neuromelanin is late in its ontogenetic development. It should be very interesting to investigate whether or not children can develop dyskinesia before the development of neuromelanin, i.e., before the 3rd to 5th years of life. If dyskinesia is not found to develop before this age, then this would support the idea that no CPZ could be bound to neurons until they develop neuromelanin.

A. I believe it is not quite established as yet that children lack neuromelanin, but it is a fact that melanin does accumulate in certain neurons up to about the 20-yr age period, at which time the cells are maximally pigmented. It is however very difficult to determine exactly when pigmentation starts. There have been reports showing the existence of neuromelanin even in the fetus.

Conway: It seems to me that the two possible modes of covalent bonding of CPZ (charge transfer and covalent photonucleophilic) examined as *in vitro* models have not been documented sufficiently to enable us to draw any conclusions as to *in vivo* events.

Q. from floor: Do melanin-storing cells break down after CPZ accumulates in them? I was wondering whether CPZ could be developed as a remedy for melanoma.

A. It has been tried as a melanoma therapeutic agent and it has an inhibiting effect in melanoma growth.

Q. from floor: Is it curative?

A. No, it only has an inhibitory effect on the growth of melanomas.

F. Forrest: In 1963 I published the results of an autopsy which indicated that all the pigmented neurons were destroyed and had been phagocytized. The melanin complex was found outside the cells. This happens only when large doses of CPZ have been given. When smaller doses of CPZ are given to patients, the neuromelanin complex remains inside the neurons, the dopamine content of the cells increases and a dyskinetic syndrome may appear.

Craig: I am sure that Dr. Lindquist is aware of the work of Clare in New Zealand on the accumulation of phenothiazines or their metabolites in the retina of young sheep. He found the drugs mainly in the form of sulfoxide in the retina.

A. The accumulation of the phenothiazines in the melanin structures was observed as early as 5 min after injection of the drugs. This short time lapse is probably too soon to make it likely that any metabolism of the drugs has occurred. It is therefore probable that at least a part of the substance bound to melanin was unchanged CPZ.

6. *J. Davis*

Q. Goodwin: Was there a correlation of drug effects with the half-life or with peak heights of chlorpromazine blood levels?

A. The correlation with the acute half-life was 0.32 and the chronic half-life 0.68. I do not know for what reasons, but the half-lives came out to be less highly predictive than the peak heights.

Q. Goodwin: Does drug absorption or distribution play a more important role in your results than drug metabolism?

A. I can't answer that. Maybe someone who is more knowledgeable about pharmacokinetics could help. One is limited with our type of *data* that *result* from the ingestion of oral tablets. Further data collection and subsequent calculation of pharmacokinetic parameters are planned in the near future. It is perhaps appropriate to defer such speculation until these studies are complete since this is a moderately complex question and more information is needed. It is relevant to note that accuracy of measurement as well as theoretical meaning is important in considering the effectiveness of prediction. For example, if half-life is measured after an oral drug dose, the following determinants of drug disappearance must be considered:

1. variability in speed and amount of absorption,
2. gut motility,
3. metabolism inside the lumen of the intestine,
4. drug metabolism inside the gut wall,
5. drug metabolism in the liver,
6. drug metabolism at all other body sites,

7. drug distribution
8. plasma binding, and
9. error variance in the drug-assay method.

Thus, the consequent variation in the disappearance of the drug from the plasma may not necessarily be the critical pharmacokinetic parameter one should use to predict the amount of drug at important receptor sites.

Perel: If the relationship of drug effect to peak height remains valid, then distribution or absorption could be the controlling factors in the attainment of steady-state levels for a period of at least 2 to 4 weeks. When butaperazine is used, you notice there is a down slope later on and this could be due to drug metabolism. All this is, of course, purely conjectural.

Cooper: We have been doing studies with butaperazine for the last couple of years and I am interested in several areas of your presentation. You have a third component in your blood-level decay curve and this area is very difficult to estimate. I would like to know how you are handling the situation. Are you extrapolating from the last or third slow component, or are you taking the second component and going straight down to the base?

A. The area under the curve was based on the first and second components. The half-lives shown here are based on the second component. The third component was ignored.

Cooper: We have performed correlations by peak-height and steady-state determinations and we do not find them as high as you do. We do find, however, a very high correlation with the area under the curve. However, we are using the third component.

My next question is: Have you any evidence at all for enzyme induction in your patients? I ask this because we have two patients of 20 or 30 investigated to date who had very large peak heights. After 3 to 4 weeks of drug treatment, the peak height fell to levels lower than any other patients in spite of the fact that they were getting 100 mg daily of butaperazine. After 8 to 10 weeks, we find that they have no measurable levels of drug in the blood whatsoever. We were highly pleased with our early results, but these last two patients are beginning to bother us.

A. I haven't made any effort to study enzyme induction.

Q. from floor: Do you have the half-life of the third component?

A. The acute half-life was about 20 hr and the chronic half-life about 40 hr.

From floor: Oates has postulated that the third component might be due to neuronal uptake or release of the drug.

8. *A. H. Glassman*

Q. Fenner: By which method did you determine these plasma concentrations?

A. The method for steady-state levels was that of Dr. Perel. This is a modification of the Moody-Patrick Method. It is a fluorescence technique.

Q. Fenner: What is the specificity of the method?

Perel: This method is very specific, but laborious.

Q. Fenner: A question on the binding itself. Was that measured by an equilibrium-dialysis method?

A. Yes.

Fenner: What is the rate of attainment of equilibrium with imipramine?

A. Equilibrium is attained in 19 hr. We do runs of 24 hr.

Grover: You made one statement which I believe should be taken with a grain of salt. This concerns the relative amounts of bound and free drugs. You stated that the free unbound drug is the portion which is psychoactive. I believe bound drug is also important in determining mode of action. Most of the binding is of a hydrophobic, low-energy type which is easily reversible. If you have drug bound to red blood cells, and these approach a tissue with a higher binding affinity for the drug, there could be an exchange between the red cells and the tissue.

A. Of course, binding has significance. The matter is obviously not as simple as stated. As a matter of fact, in this type of system where an obviously high distribution volume is present, it is the tissue-binding capacity that may be most important rather than plasma binding.

Q. Walkenstein: I am not clear about the dose which was given to children. You gave 5 mg every 8 hr?

A. 5 mg/kg every 8 hr.

Q. Walkenstein: Did I hear you say you gave 50 mg in a single bolus to a child? Wasn't that rather a staggering amount?

A. It appears that a dosage of 25 to 50 mg for a child is generally necessary to produce a positive clinical response in these children. This has been reported now by three or four independent investigators. I am not concerned about the oral dose in terms of the staggering amount given, but I am disturbed about the blood levels attained. They are enormously high. From investigators who gave 150 mg as a bolus dose just before bedtime, there has been a report of toxic symptoms in some of the children.

From floor: I would like to mention Kline's report of a death under these circumstances. I am absolutely certain that we are dealing with very dangerous and noxious compounds and certainly high doses must be carefully avoided.

Davis: My remarks are perhaps more directed to clinicians who often view pharmacologists with the attitude of "so what." In patients who take an overdose of tricyclic antidepressant, it is not uncommon to see fatalities after 1.5 to 2 g of drug have been ingested. This is 10 times the equivalent of a single bolus dose of 200 mg. If the child has a volume distribution which is $\frac{2}{3}$ that of the adult, if the child attains twice the drug blood level as an adult and three times the free uncombined drug level, this would amount to a 9- to 10-fold dose or a 1.5- to 2.0-g bolus dose for a child. Such doses have been known to cause death in adults. It is worthwhile thinking of such things when one is dealing with such dangerous drugs as tricyclics.

A. Just to extend your point I would like to think that the indication for which I gave the drug was important. I could really defend that, since lower doses were ineffective. But one does wonder about clinical toxicity when dealing with inocuous symptoms such as enuresis.

Davis: My remarks were in no way directed against the use of this drug in children for hyperactive behavior. My remarks were rather directed to the idea of thinking of such toxicities when single doses are given. It is when drugs are used in a different manner than usual that difficulties may arise as far as toxicity is concerned.

Q. from floor: What analytical methods did you use?

A. The same as Dr. Perel.

Davis: To continue my comment, I forgot to add something which might conceivably be of importance. The mechanism of death due to an overdose of tricyclic drug is almost always involved with cardiac arrhythmias. Another phenomenon sometimes seen among the toxicities is the occurrence of death 2 to 3 days after the overdose. The coma due to tricyclics is a relatively rapid appearing event. It may last for 12 to 24 hr but the patients do awaken following this period. Then occasionally, a patient may die after 38 hr. It is not known why they get arrhythmias at that time and die. If there were some interaction between a stress such as physical exercise and the overdose symptoms, one might see the same late-death phenomenon in a child.

A. The reason for involving ourselves with this problem is the question of clinical titration. The patient involved was extremely disruptive, totally uncontainable in his situation. He was hospitalized and placed on the drug. You can see that the blood levels were extremely high. They ranged from 575 to 610 ng per ml of blood serum and were accompanied by a remarkable improvement in behavioral responses, sufficiently good so that the mother wished to take the child home. I did not like the blood levels and took this child off imipramine since I wished to avoid any possible toxicities. Whenever we tried to decrease the dose however, the behavioral responses disappeared. We did not monitor the blood levels further and switched to the use of dextroamphetamine on which the child is doing well.

Session VI

Thioxanthenes

Chairmen: Nathan Kline and Herman C. B. Denber

The Phenothiazines and Structurally Related
Drugs, edited by I. S. Forrest, C. J. Carr, and
E. Usdin. Raven Press, N. Y. copyright 1974

Chemical, Pharmacological, and Metabolic Considerations on Thiothixene

Albert Weissman

Pfizer, Inc., Groton, Connecticut 06340

INTRODUCTION: CHEMICAL AND PHARMACOLOGICAL RELATIONSHIP OF THIOXANTHENES AND PHENOTHIAZINES

The thioxanthene nucleus is a 6,6,6-tricyclic system closely related to the phenothiazine nucleus (Table 1). Like phenothiazine derivatives, all thioxanthenes in therapeutic use as antipsychotics have a 3-carbon side chain terminating in an amine grouping, and are substituted in the 2-position of the nucleus. Certain structural features of thioxanthenes differ significantly from those of phenothiazines because free rotation of the side chain is prohibited by the double bond at the Δ-9 position. This provides for a separation of thioxanthene derivatives into *cis* and *trans* spatial isomers (Fig. 1). Of considerable theoretical interest regarding the configurational requirements for antipsychotic drugs (3) is the fact that *cis* and not *trans* isomers are the active compounds (2, 7, 9).

The psychopharmacological activities of thioxanthenes generally parallel those of the analogous phenothiazines. One likely difference lies in the magnitude of extrapyramidal effects seen in the two series. For example, thiothixene (Navane®) is the thioxanthene analog of the phenothiazine, thioproperazine (marketed in England as Majeptil®). This phenothiazine is an active antipsychotic, but one that produces marked extrapyramidal side effects. Probably on that account, thioproperazine has never been developed for use in the United States. In animal studies (9) as well as in clinical experience, thiothixene appears to be less potent than thioproperazine in producing this class of side effects.

No proof exists that animals can become psychotic and hence the efficacy of antispsychotic drugs can be documented only by clinical studies. Nevertheless, some prototypical psychopharmacological features of known antipsychotic drugs in animal studies have been identified. These include (a) selective suppression of conditioned avoidance behavior, (b) blockade of the behavioral effects of amphetamine, and (c) antiemetic effects against apomorphine-induced emesis in dogs. In each of these respects thiothixene exerts outstanding activity as compared with other antipsychotic drugs.

471

TABLE 1. *Relationship between phenothiazine and thioxanthene nuclei and derivatives active in psychotic patients*

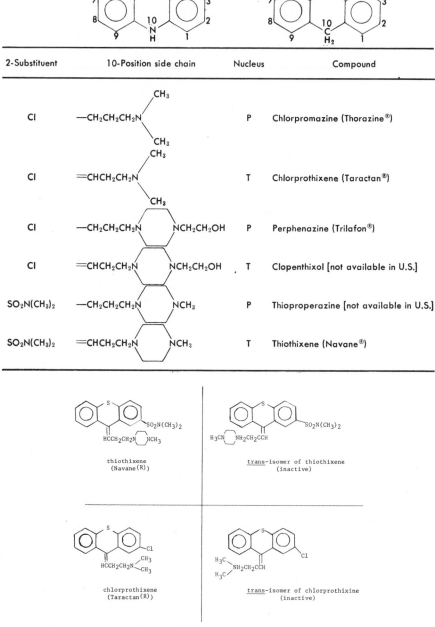

2-Substituent	10-Position side chain	Nucleus	Compound
Cl	—CH$_2$CH$_2$CH$_2$N(CH$_3$)(CH$_3$)	P	Chlorpromazine (Thorazine®)
Cl	=CHCH$_2$CH$_2$N(CH$_3$)(CH$_3$)	T	Chlorprothixene (Taractan®)
Cl	—CH$_2$CH$_2$CH$_2$N⟨⟩NCH$_2$CH$_2$OH	P	Perphenazine (Trilafon®)
Cl	=CHCH$_2$CH$_2$N⟨⟩NCH$_2$CH$_2$OH	T	Clopenthixol [not available in U.S.]
SO$_2$N(CH$_3$)$_2$	—CH$_2$CH$_2$CH$_2$N⟨⟩NCH$_3$	P	Thioproperazine [not available in U.S.]
SO$_2$N(CH$_3$)$_2$	=CHCH$_2$CH$_2$N⟨⟩NCH$_3$	T	Thiothixene (Navane®)

thiothixene
(Navane(R))

trans-isomer of thiothixene
(inactive)

chlorprothixene
(Taractan(R))

trans-isomer of chlorprothixine
(inactive)

Fig. 1. Structures of thiothixene, chlorprothixene, and their inactive *trans* isomers.

SELECTIVE SUPPRESSION OF CONDITIONED AVOIDANCE BEHAVIOR

Perhaps the simplest test of this type performed with thiothixene is one in which rats were first trained to avoid foot shock by leaping onto a platform mounted above the floor of a shock box and extending outwards from the box. During each trial the conditioned stimulus consisted of cues from the box itself for 10 sec and a tone plus these cues for the next 10 sec. If a rat failed to avoid during these 20 sec, foot shock was delivered for 10 sec, or until the animal escaped by leaping onto the platform. Following training, rats were divided into groups and exposed to drug treatment.

In a direct comparison of thiothixene with two other thioxanthenes, chloroprothixene and clopenthixol, thiothixene disrupted conditioned avoidance behavior in most animals at doses of 3.2, 10, and 32 mg/kg (Fig. 2; Ref. 10). The peak effects of thiothixene occurred between 2 and 6 hr after administration. Avoidance disruption after thiothixene was selective; with very few exceptions, rats continued to escape shock when it was presented following the 20-sec avoidance period. After chlorprothixene or clopenthixol, on the other hand, there was a loss of both escape and avoidance behavior. While the onset of action of chloroprothixene and clopenthixol was more rapid, the duration of action of thiothixene was considerably longer.

In a direct comparison against three phenothiazine derivatives (9), the data from thiothixene were virtually identical to those in Fig. 2, and closely resembled data after thioproperazine. Chlorpromazine and prochlorperazine

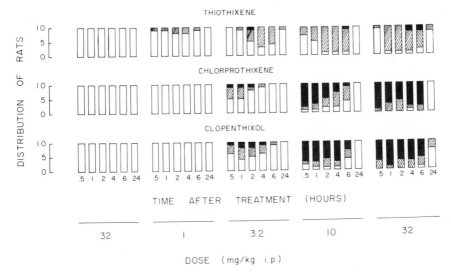

Fig. 2. Effect of thiothixene, chlorprothixene, and clopenthixol on discriminated avoidance behavior. Each bar shows the distribution of avoidance scores among the 10 rats exposed to that dose at the time after treatment shown. Open areas: number of rats unaffected; striped areas: number of rats exhibiting loss of avoidance behavior but retention of escape behavior; black areas: number of rats exhibiting loss of both avoidance and escape behavior.

were distinctly less selective. Additional confirmation of the potent, selective disruption of conditioned avoidance behavior by thiothixene has been published (1, 8, 11).

Thus, thiothixene can be shown to block avoidance behavior in rats over a wide dose range, while animals do not fail to escape the shock when it is presented. This type of selectivity is interpreted to mean that the action of thiothixene is not accompanied by pronounced sedation, muscle weakness or analgesia.

What is the meaning of this selective disruption of conditioned avoidance behavior? The neurological basis for avoidance behavior and its blockade has been studied for many years, but conclusions at the neurological level are still so tenuous and complex that it is probably better to stress psychological explanations which have been proposed. In avoiding the shock when the signal is presented, the animal may be exhibiting a specialized anxiety or fear response; antipsychotic drugs may act to dissipate this fear reaction. A second explanation focuses on the possibility that psychotic behavior in humans itself represents avoidance of life's realities, and a drug which blocks avoidance responses in animals may serve to block such irrational "avoidance responses" as psychotic behavior in man. Still another explanation is that drugs may block the attention paid by animals to emotion-provoking signals such as the tone, and serve to correct attentional deficits in schizophrenics. It should be stressed, however, that the major known antipsychotic drugs have repeatedly been demonstrated to exert a suppressing effect on this type of behavior in animals, and that the test thereby enjoys good empirical validity.

BLOCKADE OF THE BEHAVIORAL EFFECTS OF AMPHETAMINE

Thiothixene is particularly potent in blocking the motor stimulant and stereotyped behavioral effects of amphetamine (9, 10). It also blocks the lethal effects of high doses of amphetamine given to grouped mice. In each case, effective doses of thiothixene are less than 1 mg/kg. It is of interest that the effect of thiothixene in blocking stereotyped symptoms is relatively greater than that in blocking aggregation toxicity, as compared with chlorpromazine (Table 2). This may be attributed to the relatively slight peripheral

TABLE 2. Antiamphetamine effects of thiothixene and related compounds (9)

Compound	Antiamphetamine ED_{50} (mg/kg i.p.)		
	Aggregation-mortality in mice	Hyperactivity in mice	Stereotyped symptoms in rats
Thiothixene	0.3	0.8	0.1
Thioproperazine	0.3	0.5	0.1
Chlorpromazine	1.6	8.6	6.0
Prochlorperazine	0.9	5.6	1.2
P-4657A	10–32	>32	>32

adrenergic blocking properties of thiothixene (6). Here again, these effects of thiothixene are important primarily because known antipsychotic drugs also exert the effect. It is worth recalling, however, that in humans amphetamine in high doses is known to produce psychotic side effects and mania, and perhaps this is why blockade of amphetamine in animals remains a useful way to select antipsychotic drugs. Indeed, the stimulant effect of amphetamine in animals looks very much like uncontrolled mania.

ANTIEMETIC EFFECTS

Thiothixene is among the most potent known antiemetic drugs in blocking the vomiting response to apomorphine (Tables 3 and 4; Refs. 4 and 9). This

TABLE 3. Antiapomorphine effects of thiothixene and related drugs in dogs (9)

Drug	ED_{50} (mg/kg)	
	i.v.	p.o.
Thiothixene	0.0022	0.07–0.1
Thioproperazine	0.0034	0.07–0.1
Chlorpromazine	$\sim$0.7	10–32
Prochlorperazine	0.122	$\sim$1.5

effect, seen in dogs, is of importance not only because other antipsychotic drugs, with very few claimed exceptions, are also effective in preventing apomorphine-elicited emesis, but because apomorphine is widely reported to stimulate dopamine receptors in the brain.

EFFECTS ON DOPAMINE METABOLISM IN BRAIN

Much evidence suggests that the above effects common to known antipsychotic drugs of the phenothiazine, thioxanthene, or 4-phenylbutylamine types, and achieved with great potency by thiothixene, are in large part caused by blockade of dopamine receptors in the brain. Biochemical evidence supports this contention. As one example, thiothixene has been shown by Dr. B. K. Koe (*unpublished data*) in our laboratories to greatly enhance the accumulation of DOPA in the dopamine-rich corpus striatum of the rat brain, when decarboxylase activity is blocked by a known drug inhibitor (Table 5). This biochemical effect is believed to be caused by an enhancement of the dopamine synthetic machinery in the dopaminergic neuron, a compensatory feedback mechanism for the blocked activity at the dopamine receptor. Another resulting effect is seen in the data of Lahti et al. (5), who showed that thiothixene profoundly increases the amount of homovanillic acid in the mouse

TABLE 4. Antiemetic potency of analogous thioxanthenes and phenothiazines in dogs (4)

2-Position	Side Chain Amine	Compound and Class T = Thioxanthene P = Phenothiazine B = Butyrophenone	Minimal Antiemetic Dose in Dogs (mg/kg s.c.)
$SO_2N(CH_3)_2$	N⎯⎯NCH₃	Thiothixene (T) Thioproperazine (P)	0.00125 0.00250
Cl	N⎯⎯NCH₂CH₂OH	Perphenazine (P) Clopenthixol (T)	0.01 0.02
CF₃	N⎯⎯NCH₂CH₂OH	Fluphenazine (P) Flupenthixol (T)	0.005 0.02
Cl	N (CH₃)(CH₃)	Chlorpromazine (P) Chlorprothixene (T)	0.31 0.63
	Haloperidol (B)		0.01

TABLE 5. DOPA accumulation in rat corpus striatum
after inhibition of decarboxylase activity[a]

Treatment	Dose (mg/kg i.p.)	DOPA[b] (% of control)
Thiothixene	17.7	477
Reserpine	5.0	218
Apomorphine	15.7	33

[a] By 2 doses of NSD-1024.
[b] Control DOPA level was 0.728 $\mu g/g$.

brain (Table 6). This acid is the end product of dopamine degradation. Its elevation by thiothixene can be blocked by apomorphine, which is believed to stimulate dopamine receptors, and thus to counter the action of receptor blockers. The blockade of dopamine receptors by antipsychotic drugs probably accounts for the extrapyramidal symptoms they cause. In common with

TABLE 6. *Effect of various doses of apomorphine on the thiothixene-induced elevation in homovanillic acid in mouse brain (5)*

Treatment	Dose (mg/kg)	HVA (μg/gm)
Saline		0.09
Thiothixene	2.0	0.37
Thiothixene + apomorphine	2.0 + 10.0	0.20
Apomorphine	10.0	0.05

other neuroleptics, thiothixene does exert cataleptic effects in animals and humans although less than does its phenothiazine analog, thioproperazine (9).

SIDE EFFECTS OF ANTIPSYCHOTIC DRUGS

Among the side effects other than extrapyramidal effects commonly produced by many neuroleptics in man (particularly chlorpromazine and thioridazine), and readily seen in animal studies as well, are sedative and muscle relaxant effects (sometimes reflected as analgesia), disturbances in thermoregulation, antiadrenergic effects, and anticholinergic effects. These side effects have been progressively reduced with the more modern, selective neuroleptic drugs, and thiothixene is among the very most selective of these recent agents. In other words, despite its marked potency in disrupting conditioned avoidance behavior, in blocking amphetamine-elicited stimulation, and in antagonizing apomorphine emesis, thiothixene is exceedingly weak in producing sedative, thermoregulatory antiadrenergic, anticholinergic, and related effects. We have already mentioned how the failure of thiothixene to disrupt avoidance behavior over a wide dose range may be interpreted as a lack of sedative effectiveness. Let us examine some of the other relevant animal data bearing on side effects common to chlorpromazine.

RELATIVE ABSENCE OF SEDATIVE AND MUSCLE WEAKNESS EFFECTS AFTER THIOTHIXENE

In one study (9), thiothixene was distinctly weaker than chlorpromazine and prochlorperazine in prolonging the duration of sleep after both hexobarbital and ethanol. For example, a dose of 100 mg/kg s.c. of thiothixene caused mice treated 2 hr later with hexobarbital to sleep for a median of 88 min. Only 10 mg/kg of chlorpromazine, given prior to hexobarbital, caused sleep for 114 min. Thiothixene also failed to potentiate ethanol-induced sleep. Analogous results from ether- and thiopental-induced sleep in mice have been reported by Ueki et al. (8). These authors also reported that thiothixene, even at 100 mg/kg in mice, exerted no muscle relaxant effect on an inclined plane test in mice; chlorpromazine, perphenazine, and diazepam showed a marked relaxant effect. On a mouse rotorod test of muscle coordination as well, thiothixene was far less effective than comparison standards.

RELATIVE ABSENCE OF ANTIADRENERGIC AND THERMOREGULATORY EFFECTS

Unlike chlorpromazine, thiothixene exerts virtually no ptotic effect in mice (8) or rats (4). Even at a dose of 10 mg/kg orally to conscious dogs, thiothixene lowered blood pressure by an average of only 8 mm/Hg (Scriabine, *unpublished data*). Unlike chlorpromazine, prochlorperazine, chlorprothixene, or clopenthixol, thiothixene exerts only slight effects on thermoregulation. At room temperature (21°C) thiothixene produces only a mild hypothermia in mice, and when mice are placed in a cold environment, they do not rapidly die of hypothermia after thiothixene, as they do after less selective agents (9, 10).

RELATIVE ABSENCE OF ANTICHOLINERGIC ACTIVITY

The *in vitro* spasmolytic activity of thiothixene and chlorpromazine has been evaluated on guinea pig ileum suspended in Tyrode solution (Table 7).

TABLE 7. *In vitro spasmolytic effect of thiothixene and chlorpromazine on guinea pig ileum (data from J. W. Constantine, unpublished)*

Compound	EC_{50} (μg/cc) in antagonizing contractions of guinea pig ileum induced by:			
	Barium chloride (100 μg/cc)	Histamine (2.5 μg/cc)	Serotonin (1.5 μg/cc)	Acetylcholine (0.2 μg/cc)
Thiothixene	2.4	2.4	3.4	8.7
Chlorpromazine	1.4	0.05	0.7	1.8

Thiothixene was a weak, nonspecific spasmolytic agent and considerably less effective than chlorpromazine in antagonizing histamine-, serotonin-, and acetylcholine-induced muscle contractions (Constantine, *unpublished results*).

DOES THIOTHIXENE RESEMBLE TRICYCLIC ANTIDEPRESSANTS IN ANIMAL STUDIES?

One beneficial clinical effect of thiothixene that has frequently been reported is an activating component sometimes even termed stimulation, or antidepressant activity. It should be made clear that in the usual animal tests for antidepressant activity, however, thiothixene essentially lacks the behavioral and biochemical properties of tricyclic antidepressants. Thus, thiothixene does not reverse the behavioral depression or hypothermia caused by reserpine-like drugs, and thiothixene does not block the uptake of norepinephrine into noradrenergic neurons (Table 8). Similarly, at no dose does

TABLE 8. Inhibiting effect of various tricyclic drugs on the uptake of H^3-norepinephrine into rat heart (data from B. K. Koe, unpublished)

Compound	Dose (mg/kg i.p.) required for 50% inhibition of uptake
Desipramine	0.4
Imipramine	1.7
Amitriptyline	7
Doxepin	7
Chlorpromazine	7
Thiothixene	>56

thiothixene exert stimulant effects in such devices as photocell cages, jiggle cages or operant conditioning chambers. If pressed to extrapolate from animal studies to explain the activating or energizing action of thiothixene, I would do so as follows: thiothixene exhibits potent psychopharmacological effects prototypical for antipsychotic drugs, but does so with great selectivity. There are virtually no sedative, antiadrenergic or anticholinergic effects. Extrapolating to man, it appears that the proven antipsychotic action of thiothixene is not achieved by means of debilitation, and that the energizing effects represent a move towards normal activity.

METABOLISM OF THIOTHIXENE

The pharmacokinetics and metabolism of thiothixene in laboratory animals has been studied by Hobbs with the use of drug labeled with Sulfur-35. Thiothixene is rapidly absorbed from the gastrointestinal tract as determined by a comparison of tissues and excreta following intraperitoneal doses with those after oral doses. Following single doses, radioactivity is primarily excreted in the feces, in most part within two days. This fecal elimination is the result of extensive biliary secretion as determined in animals bearing implanted bile cannulas.

In the rat thiothixene and its metabolite are widely distributed throughout a number of tissues from which they are then removed with varying half-lives. The pigmented rat eye contains higher concentrations than a number of other tissues examined and drug and metabolites are removed with a half-life somewhat greater than that of other tissues. *In vitro* experiments, however, show that thiothixene is less strongly bound to melanin than are a number of other tricyclic psychotherapeutic drugs including chlorpromazine.

Numerous metabolites of thiothixene, most of them currently unidentified, are seen in extracts of bile feces and liver. In contrast, extracts of rat brain contain unchanged drug only.

In summary the disposition of thiothixene is basically similar to that of the other tricyclic psychotherapeutic drugs in that it is rapidly absorbed and distributed, extensively metabolized, and excreted via urine and feces within a relatively short interval.

CONCLUSIONS

Thiothixene exerts several potent actions in animals long recognized to be characteristic for antipsychotic drugs. It selectively blocks conditioned avoidance behavior, blocks amphetamine-induced stimulation, and blocks apomorphine emesis. Biochemical findings suggest that thiothixene blocks dopamine pathways. On the other hand, thiothixene exhibits marked selectivity, as exemplified by its lack of pronounced sedative, adrenolytic, or anticholinergic side effects. Based on animal studies, extrapyramidal effects would be expected after thiothixene, but clinical experience reveals that these are controllable at therapeutic doses. Despite frequent clinical reports of "activating" and "antidepressant" effects of thiothixene, animal studies reveal that thiothixene does not share key pharmacological properties of tricyclic antidepressants.

REFERENCES

1. Cahen, R., Pham-Ba, T., and Hue, M., *Thérapie, 23,* 591 (1968).
2. Dunitz, J. D., *Helv. Chim. Acta,* **47,** 1897 (1964).
3. Horn, A. S., and Snyder, S., *Proc. Nat. Acad. Sci. U.S.A.,* **68,** 2325 (1971).
4. Janssen, P. A. J., in *Modern Problems of Pharmacopsychiatry, Vol. 5: The Neuroleptics,* Bobon, D. P., et al. (Ed.), Karger, Basel, 1970.
5. Lahti, R. A., McAllister, B., and Wozniak, J., *Life Sci.,* **11 (I),** 605 (1972).
6. Leslie, G. B., and Maxwell, D. R., *Brit. J. Pharmacol.,* **22,** 301 (1964).
7. Schaefer, J. P., *Chem. Comm.,* **15,** 743 (1967).
8. Ueki, S., et al., *Igaku Kenkyu (Acta Medica),* **39,** 433 (1969).
9. Weissman, A., *Psychopharmacologia,* **12,** 142 (1968).
10. Weissman, A., in *Modern Problems of Pharmacopsychiatry, Vol. 2: The Thioxanthenes,* Freyhan, F. A., et al. Ed., Karger, Basel, 1969.
11. Muren, J. F., and Weissman, A., *J. Med. Chem.,* **14,** 49 (1971).

The Penothiazines and Structurally Related Drugs, edited by I. S. Forrest, C. J. Carr, and E. Usdin. Raven Press, N. Y. copyright 1974

Thiothixene and the Thioxanthenes

T. A. Ban and H. E. Lehmann

Department of Psychiatry, McGill University, Montreal, Quebec, Canada

INTRODUCTION

In the 21 years following the introduction of chlorpromazine, a large number of neuroleptic drugs have been synthesized. By 1973, there were 10 chemical classes of neuroleptics known, at least 50 neuroleptics had been clinically investigated and one half of those which had been studied were used in clinical practice. Besides the phenothiazines and the butyrophenones, the thioxanthenes are the most important of the various neuroleptics.

Since the synthesis of chlorprothixene (the first psychoactive thioxanthene preparation) 14 years have passed during which period well over 60 thioxanthene preparations have been studied; more than five have been clinically investigated; and at least four, i.e., chlorprothixene, clopenthixol, flupenthixol, and thiothixene, are marketed in one or another country for clinical use. Nevertheless, only two of these drugs, i.e., chlorprothixene (Taractan®; Tarasan®) and thiothixene (Navane®), are available in the United States and Canada for clinical use (Fig. 1).

ACTION MECHANISM

The therapeutic effects of thioxanthenes cannot be reduced to a single psychophysiological, neurophysiological, or biochemical concomitant of drug action. Like other neuroleptics, the thioxanthenes interfere with conditional reflex activity, leaving unconditional reflex activity virtually unaffected; increase limbic system activity together with an inhibition of proprioceptive arousal reactions; and produce catecholamine receptor blockade with an increase in dopamine turnover rate (9, 14).

Although psychoactive thioxanthenes resemble the phenothiazines in most of their actions, there is at least one test in which they are similar to some of the tricyclic antidepressants, e.g., imipramine, desmethylimipramine. In this context, Kato and his collaborators (5) were able to demonstrate that subeffective doses of three thioxanthenes, i.e., chlorprothixene, clopenthixol, and thiothixene, were potentiated by imipramine but not by tranylcypromine when tested against the vasodilating effect of histamine. On the basis of these findings, they suggested that psychoactive thioxanthenes may share some of the properties of tricyclic antidepressants.

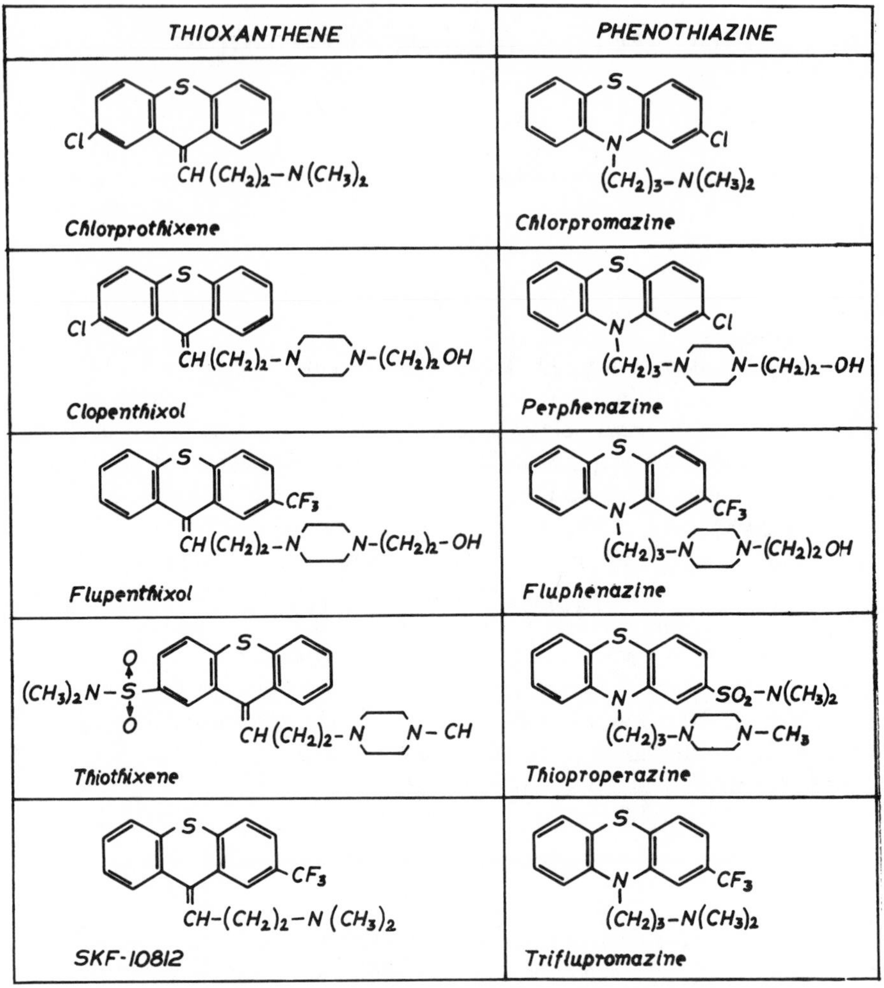

THIOXANTHENE	PHENOTHIAZINE
Chlorprothixene	Chlorpromazine
Clopenthixol	Perphenazine
Flupenthixol	Fluphenazine
Thiothixene	Thioproperazine
SKF-10812	Triflupromazine

Fig. 1. The thioxanthene derivatives and their phenothiazine analogues.

CLINICAL PSYCHOPHARMACOLOGICAL FINDINGS

In a human pharmacological study, St. Jean et al. (13) found that chlor-prothixene in a single 75 mg dosage lowered Critical Flicker Fusion Frequency and decreased performance on psychomotor tests. The decrease in Tapping Speed and the increase in Track Tracer Time with chlorprothixene was less than with chlorpromazine (75 mg) but more than with haloperidol (5 mg), whereas the increase in Auditory Reaction Time and the decrease in Word Association Time were less with the thioxanthene preparation than with the phenothiazine or the butyrophenone drug. The same drug, chlorpro-thixene, in an uncontrolled clinical pharmacological study, when given in a dosage range of 50 to 1,400 mg daily to schizophrenic patients, produced significant improvement within 3 weeks in excitement and suspiciousness and within 6 weeks in depressive psychopathology (6).

In another uncontrolled clinical pharmacological study, thiothixene (the other commercially available thioxanthene preparation) produced significant improvement in emotional withdrawal, blunted affect, suspiciousness, unusual thought content, and hallucinations on the Brief Psychiatric Rating Scale (BPRS); in sociability, delusions, and hallucinations on the Verdun Target Symptom Rating Scale (VTSRS); and in retardation, social interest, social competence, and manifest psychosis on the Nurses' Observation Scale for Inpatient Evaluation (NOSIE) in the dosage range of 5 to 80 mg daily in schizophrenic patients over a 12-week period (1).

RESULTS OF SYSTEMATIC INVESTIGATIONS

The most systematically investigated thioxanthene preparation is thiothixene, the thioproperazine analogue of the series. In view of the favorable therapeutic findings in the initial clinical trials with this drug, a comprehensive clinical study was designed and conducted in two collaborating hospitals (Douglas Hospital and Hôpital des Laurentides) to reveal the range of therapeutic activity of thiothixene, the place of thiothixene in the treatment of schizophrenics, and the place of thiothixene among the thioxanthenes.

The range of therapeutic activity of thiothixene was studied in 60 hospitalized psychiatric patients belonging to four different diagnostic groups (Table 1) (7). Analysis of data revealed that the total population showed a signifi-

TABLE 1. *Breakdown of the experimental population*

Diagnostic category	No.	Type		Sex		Age (yr)		
		Acute	Chronic	Male	Female	Mean	Median	Range
Schizophrenic reactions	20	10	10	16	4	34.11	34.5	19–53
Psychotic depressive reactions	10	10	0	6	4	39.2	44.0	16–53
Geriatrics with psychoses	20	0	20	20	0	66.0	65.5	60–81
Psychoneurotic reactions	10	10	0	7	3	41.5	38.5	27–55

cant improvement—as measured on the BPRS—already after the first week of treatment and that improvement continued until the termination of the clinical study. The therapeutic changes in the schizophrenic and the psychoneurotic group paralleled those of the total population. On the other hand, very few therapeutic changes were seen in geriatric patients and the therapeutic effects seen in depression patients were mainly due to the beneficial action of the drug on psychotic traits, as measured by the Zung Self-Rating

Scale. Furthermore, in the psychoneurotic group, in which both the speed and degree of overall therapeutic improvement paralleled that of the schizophrenic group, after maximal improvement was reached, there was a gradual increase in scores on certain symptoms (e.g., excitement, somatic-hysterical) on the Wittenborn Psychiatric Rating Scale. Since a consistent and continuous therapeutic activity was seen in the schizophrenic population, it was suggested that the primary indication of thiothixene is for schizophrenia. This does not exclude the possibility that under certain conditions thiothixene may also be useful in the treatment of some psychoneuroses and/or depressions.

The place of thiothixene in the treatment of schizophrenic patients was studied in 60 hospitalized schizophrenic patients in four clinical trials (11). Analysis of data revealed that thiothixene is significantly superior to an inactive placebo and comparable in therapeutic efficacy to at least two standard neuroleptic phenothiazines, i.e., chlorpromazine and thioproperazine. In the total thiothixene population of the four clinical studies, statistically significant improvement was seen in the global scores of the three rating scales used as well as in symptoms primarily reflecting cognitive psychopathology (e.g., conceptual disorganization, unusual thought content) after 4 weeks of treatment. Probably most important, however, was the significant improvement in blunted affect already at the time of the one-month assessment.

Finally, the place of thiothixene among the thioxanthenes was studied in a 12-week clinical trial in schizophrenic patients (11). As a result, differences in therapeutic indications between thiothixene (10 to 40 mg/day), clopenthixol (50 to 200 mg/day), and chlorprothixene (150 to 600 mg/day) were revealed. Analysis of the individual items and symptom clusters of the BPRS, VTSRS, and NOSIE revealed significant improvement in delusions on the VTSRS with thiothixene and significant improvement in excitement on the BPRS with clopenthixol. There was significant improvement also in social competence, social interest, and retardation with thiothixene; in irritability, manifest psychoses, and retardation with clopenthixol; and in the total scores with chlorprothixene on the NOSIE. Findings in this study are in agreement with results in other clinical trials in which thiothixene was found to be an active antipsychotic drug with particular effectiveness on affective psychopathology and with particular usefulness for patients who are socially withdrawn (3, 4).

NATURE AND FREQUENCY OF ADVERSE EFFECTS

The thioxanthenes are the result of systematic investigations to develop new drugs with at least equal therapeutic action to the phenothiazines, but with fewer adverse effects. This was achieved by replacing the nitrogen atom (position 10) of the phenothiazine nucleus by a carbon atom (position 9) of the thioxanthene nucleus by Petersen and his collaborators (8) (Fig. 2). It is the general impression to date that the relative frequency of adverse

THIOXANTHENE   PHENOTHIAZINE

Fig. 2. Similarities and difference in the chemical structure of the thioxanthene and the phenothiazine nucleus.

effects to the two commercially available preparations, i.e., thiothixene and chlorprothixene, is lower than to their corresponding phenothiazine analogues, and Ravn (10) suggests that the lack of phenolic metabolites explains why thioxanthenes do not show the same sensitivity to ultraviolet light as the phenothiazines.

Among the behavioral adverse effects, fatigue and drowsiness are the most frequent. Nevertheless, they are more often encountered with chlorprothixene than with thiothixene.

More frequently discussed among the neurological adverse reactions are extrapyramidal manifestations. The incidence of these is considerably lower, and their severity considerably less than that seen with the corresponding phenothiazine preparations. Extrapyramidal signs are more frequently induced by thiothixene than by chlorprothixene. Another neurological adverse reaction is cerebral seizure, which has been reported in the course of chlorprothixene and/or thiothixene treatment. The same applies to ocular changes, i.e., bilateral and symmetrical deposits in the central portions of the anterior lens capsule, which occurs in 7 to 8% of thiothixene-treated patients (2).

Among the endocrinological adverse effects, amenorrhea and galactorrhea have been reported. Among the cardiovascular reactions, hypotension, tachycardia, and electroencephalographic changes have been infrequently seen. Adverse hematological (leucopenia or leucocytosis) and hepatobiliary (elevation of alkaline phosphatase, bilirubin, and transaminase estimates) reactions are rare.

SUMMARY

It has been 14 years since the chemical synthesis of chlorprothixene, the first thioxanthene preparation; during this period at least four other thioxanthene compounds, i.e., clopenthixol, flupenthixol, SKF-10812, and thiothixene, have been clinically investigated.

The most systematically investigated among the thioxanthene preparations is thiothixene, the thioproperazine analogue of the series. In a comprehensive clinical study with thiothixene, its range of therapeutic activity was revealed and its place in the treatment of schizophrenics as well as a choice among the thioxanthenes was established. Thiothixene was found to be an active antipsychotic agent with at least comparable effectiveness to other phenothiazine and thioxanthene neuroleptics in the treatment of schizophrenics and with particular usefulness for patients who are socially withdrawn. There are indications that thiothixene may also be therapeutically useful in some forms of psychoneuroses and in the control of "psychotic traits" in depressions.

It was noted that the relative frequency of adverse effects with the commercially available thioxanthene preparations is lower than with their corresponding phenothiazine analogues. The lower incidence of side effects in general and extrapyramidal signs in particular during long-term maintenance treatment are advantages which should not be ignored.

ACKNOWLEDGMENTS

This study was partially supported by U.S. Public Health Service grant MH-05202-11.

REFERENCES

1. Ban, T. A., Lehmann, H. E., Sterlin, C., and Saxena, B. M., in *Proceedings of the 6th International Congress of the C.I.N.P. (Tarragona 1968): The Present Status of Psychotropic Drugs,* Excerpta Medica International Congress Series No. 180.
2. Bishop, M. P., Gallant, D. M., and Steele, C. A., *Psychiat. Dig.,* **5,** 15 (1968).
3. DiMascio, A., and DeMirgian, E., *Psychosomatics,* **13,** 105 (1972).
4. Gardos, G., Finerty, R. J., and Cole, J. O., *Psychosomatics,* **11,** 36 (1970).
5. Kato, L., Gözsy, B., Roy, P. B., and Trsik, T., in *The Thioxanthenes,* Lehmann, H. E., and Ban, T. A. (eds.), Karger, Basel, 1969.
6. Lehmann, H. E., Ban, T. A., Matthews, V., and Garcia-Rill, T., in *The Butyrophenones,* Lehmann, H. E., and Ban, T. A. (eds.), Quebec Psychopharmacological Research Association, Montreal, 1964.
7. Oliveros, R. T., Ban, T. A., Lehmann, H. E., Sterlin, C., and Saxena, B. M., *Int. J. Clin. Pharmacol. Therap. Toxicol.,* **3,** 26 (1970).
8. Petersen, M. C., McBrayer, J. W., Kopf, R., and Nielsen, I. M., *Arzneimittel Forschung,* **8,** 395 (1958).
9. Pletscher, A., Gey, K. F., and Burkard, W. P., presented at a Symposium on *Toxicité et Effects Secondaire des Medicaments Psychotropes,* Paris, 1967.
10. Ravn, J., in *Discoveries in Biological Psychiatry,* Ayd, F., and Blackwell, B. (eds.), Lippincott, Philadelphia, 1970.
11. Sterlin, C., Ban, T. A., and Jarrold, L., *Curr. Ther. Res.,* **14,** 205 (1972).
12. Sterlin, C., Ban, T. A., Lehmann, H. E., and Saxena, B. M., *Canad. Psychiat. Ass. J.,* **15,** 3 (1970).
13. St. Jean, A., Lidsky, A., Ban, T. A., and Lehmann, H. E., in *The Butyrophenones,* Lehmann, H. E., and Ban, T. A. (eds.), Quebec Psychopharmacological Research Association, Montreal, 1964.
14. Ueki, S., Ogawa, N., Watanabe, S., Gowita, Y., Fukuda, T., and Araki, Y., *Igaker Kenkyu,* **39,** 327 (1969).

The Penothiazines and Structurally Related
Drugs, edited by I. S. Forrest, C. J. Carr, and
E. Usdin. Raven Press, N. Y. copyright 1974

Electrocardiographic Evaluation of Thiothixene: A Double-Blind Comparison with Thioridazine

Robert L. Dillenkoffer, Ronald B. George, Melvin P. Bishop,
and Donald M. Gallant

*Medical Service, Veterans Administration Hospital, Departments of Psychiatry and Neurology
and of Medicine, Tulane University School of Medicine, New Orleans, Louisiana*

INTRODUCTION

Thiothixene (Navane®) is a thioxanthene derivative which has been shown to possess antipsychotic efficacy in the treatment of schizophrenic patients and which can apparently be administered with relative safety in regard to clinical and laboratory evaluations (1–3). The purpose of this study was to evaluate further the safety of thiothixene by comparing it with another commonly used agent, thioridazine (Mellaril®), with special attention to the effects upon the electrocardiogram (EKG).

PROCEDURE

In a controlled double-blind study (medication was prepared by one of the nonparticipant ward personnel), the effects of thiothixene were compared with the effects of thioridazine in a group of 26 chronically schizophrenic men and women (13 patients in each drug group). The median age was 48 yr (range 28 to 57), the average duration of hospitalization 19 yr for the thiothixene group; the average age was 53 yr (range 31 to 60) and the average duration of hospitalization 21 yr for the thioridazine group. The subjects were free of significant disabilities of the cardiovascular, renal, and hepatic systems. All drugs, including prior psychotherapeutic agents, were discontinued for a minimum period of 20 days prior to initiation of the study.

Dosages were 5 mg daily of thiothixene and 100 mg daily of thioridazine for the first week; 10 mg daily of thiothixene and 200 mg daily of thioridazine for week 2; 20 mg daily of thiothixene and 400 mg daily of thioridazine for week 3; and 40 mg daily of thiothixene and 800 mg daily of thioridazine for weeks 4–6 of the study. Effects of the drugs were measured by means of independent global ratings of improvement by two psychiatrists and a special research aide at baseline, midway (week 3), and termination of the study. In addition, weekly brief mental status examinations and evaluations for side effects were performed. EKG tracings were recorded at baseline, during weeks 2, 3, 4, and 6 of medication, and 2 weeks after termination of drug adminis- tration. A control group of 13 personnel, working on the Tulane Research Unit, with an average age of 33 yr (range 23 to 54) had EKG tracings per- formed at the same time intervals as the patients. All of the tracings were evaluated by two of the authors in a "blind" manner. They had no knowledge as to the type or dosage of drug being administered, or even whether patients were in a treatment or control group.

RESULTS

Psychologic Measurements

The independent global ratings of improvement at midway and termination provided by the two psychiatrists and research assistant were averaged (as is our usual policy) to provide a more stable measure. On those pooled global ratings obtained at the time of midway evaluation (week 3 when the dosage of thiothixene was 20 mg daily and that of thioridazine 400 mg daily), thio- thixene appeared to show a slight superiority over thioridazine. Of the 13 patients who received thiothixene, five were rated slightly improved ($+1$), two as moderately improved ($+2$), and the remaining six as unchanged. In the thioridazine group, only four patients were judged to be slightly improved ($+1$) with the remaining nine rated as unchanged. However, the final pooled global ratings (week 6 when dosage of thiothixene was 40 mg daily and of thioridazine 800 mg daily) showed thioridazine to have slight superiority over thiothixene. Of the 13 patients receiving thiothixene, two were rated as slightly improved, three moderately improved, and eight unchanged. In the thioridazine group, seven patients were judged to be slightly improved, two moderately improved, one markedly improved, and three unchanged. It is worth noting that three patients in the thiothixene group who were rated as improved at midway evaluation were judged to be unchanged (i.e., had re- turned to baseline clinical status) upon final examination.

Adverse Extracardiac Effects

Side effects were only mildly inconvenient to the patients in both drug groups. Three of the thiothixene patients had mild but insignificant orthostatic hypotension, and three displayed mild extrapyramidal phenomena. Of the 13 patients in the thioridazine group, seven developed mild orthostatic hypoten- sion, three showed mild extrapyramidal phenomena, four exhibited daytime somnolence, and two displayed a dry mouth.

Electrocardiographic Results

Of the 13 patients in the thiothixene-treated group, 11 had no changes from their baseline EKGs throughout the study period (Fig. 1). One patient had equivocal changes at week 2, while taking 10 mg daily, but these changes

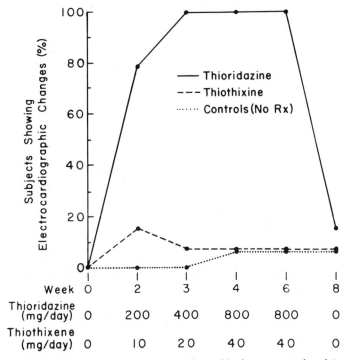

Fig. 1. Percent of subjects showing electrocardiographic changes at various intervals.

disappeared in subsequent tracings although drug dosage was increased (Case A, Fig. 2). The remaining patient had an abnormal tracing at the beginning of the study, with inverted T waves in Leads V_1 through V_3, and subsequent electrocardiograms revealed further T wave changes without any changes in QT intervals, in the precordial leads which did not revert to normal after cessation of the drug (Case B, Fig. 2). Such changes are compatible with ischemic or metabolic effects upon the myocardium, and thus are not specific for phenothiazine-related abnormalities.

The thioridazine group also consisted of 13 patients, of whom all exhibited EKG changes by week 3 of therapy, when they were receiving 400 mg daily in divided doses (Table 1). More significantly, 10 of these 13 patients had changes at the end of the second week, when the dosage was only 200 mg daily (Fig. 3). These consisted of lengthening of QT (and corrected QT)

CASE A, RR 48 ♂

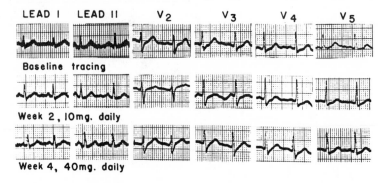

CASE B, VF 31 ♀

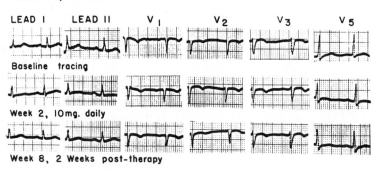

Fig. 2. QT interval and T wave changes seen in two of the 13 patients treated with thiothixene. Changes were not seen in any of the remaining 11 patients.

TABLE 1. *Presence of electrocardiographic changes at various intervals and dosages during therapy with thioridazine*

Patient	Age, sex	Week 2 200 mg daily	Week 3 400 mg daily	Week 4 800 mg daily	Week 6 800 mg daily	Week 8 2 wks post-therapy
F T	51, M	+	+	+	+	0
D A	46, F	+	+	+	+	0
V L	51, M	0	+	+	+	0
M L	50, F	0	+	+	+	0
J C	39, M	+	+	+	+	0
E E	54, M	+	+	+	+	0
P P	50, M	+	+	+	+	0
H H	33, F	+	+	+	+	0
E P	49, F	0	+	+	+	0
J H	31, M	+	+	+	+	0
N A	50, M	+	+	+	+	+
J C	56, F	+	+	+	+	0
R D	48, F	+	+	+	+	+

JC 39 ♂

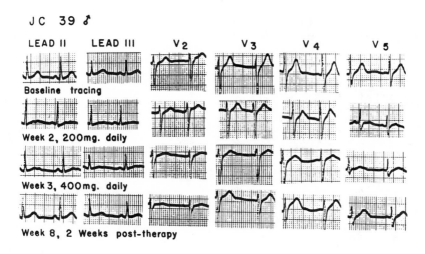

JH 31 ♂

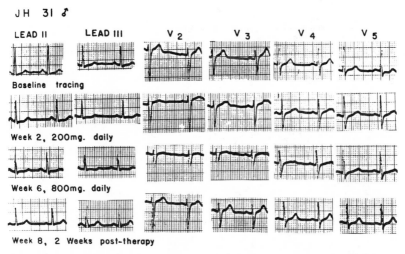

Fig. 3. Typical electrocardiographic changes seen during thioridazine therapy. Note progressive flattening, broadening, and notching of T waves and prolongation of QT intervals. These changes were present in all 13 patients in this group.

intervals (Tables 2 and 3), and moderate to marked lowering and flattening of T waves resulting in varying degrees of QRS-T angle changes (Table 4). Pulse rates increased, decreased, or remained the same without any consistent pattern (Table 3). These abnormalities had disappeared in all but two patients 2 weeks after stopping the medication.

One of the 13 subjects who acted as controls had some nonspecific changes, consisting of flattening and rounding of T waves in the precordial leads, at weeks 4, 6, and 8, without QT prolongation (Fig. 4). This subject was a

TABLE 2. QT interval (sec) during therapy with thioridazine

Patient	Control	Week 2 200 mg daily	Week 3 400 mg daily	Week 4 800 mg daily	Week 6 800 mg daily	Week 8 2 wks post-therapy	QT interval change
F T	0.36	0.34	0.36	0.42[a]	0.40	0.32	0.06
D A	0.34	0.42	0.44[a]	0.42	0.36	0.34	0.10
V L	0.30	0.31	0.36[a]	0.36	0.36	0.34	0.06
M L	0.32	0.34	0.41	0.43[a]	0.42	0.34	0.11
J C (♂)	0.36	0.36	0.40	0.40	0.42[a]	0.38	0.06
E E	0.32	0.34	0.38	0.36	0.40[a]	0.34	0.08
P P	0.30	0.30	0.35	0.36[a]	0.34	0.33	0.06
H H	0.36	0.42	0.40	0.44[a]	0.43	0.42	0.08
E P	0.32	0.32	0.35	0.36[a]	0.34	0.30	0.04
J H	0.36	0.40	0.39	0.38	0.43[a]	0.38	0.07
N A	0.36	0.38	0.40[a]	0.40	0.40	0.37	0.04
J C (♀)	0.28	0.36	0.38	0.40[a]	0.40	0.36	0.12
R D	0.38	0.38	0.40[a]	0.38	0.40	0.38	0.02

[a] Maximum QT interval.

TABLE 3. Rate changes and corrected QT interval changes (sec)
during therapy with thioridazine

Patient	Pulse rate, control	Pulse rate at max. QT interval	$QT_{(c)}$,[a] control	$QT_{(c)}$ at max. QT interval	Increase in $QT_{(c)}$
F T	72	78	0.375	0.445	0.070
D A	75	68	0.360	0.440	0.080
V L	115	100	0.390	0.440	0.050
M L	90	75	0.355	0.430	0.075
J C (♂)	85	80	0.390	0.445	0.055
E E	92	65	0.385	0.390	0.005
P P	112	105	0.370	0.440	0.070
H H	70	70	0.335	0.435	0.100
E P	120	115	0.415	0.445	0.030
J H	75	82	0.360	0.465	0.105
N A	78	80	0.380	0.415	0.035
J C (♀)	102	72	0.335	0.410	0.075
R D	70	72	0.388	0.400	0.012

[a] $QT_{(c)} = QT$ corrected for rate $= \dfrac{QT}{\sqrt{RR\ interval}}$

healthy but somewhat obese 33-yr-old man who had no clinical evidence of
cardiac disease.

The differences in incidence of EKG changes among the three groups were
highly significant. Analysis of results from all three groups yields a *chi*-square
of 16.6 which, with two degrees of freedom, is statistically significant at the
0.001 level. Comparison of the thiothixene and thioridazine groups yields
a *chi*-square of 15.6 which, with one degree of freedom, also shows a probability level of 0.001.

TABLE 4. QRS-T angle changes during therapy with thioridazine

Patient	QRS-T angle in degrees, control	QRS-T angle at maximum T wave change	Change in degrees of QRS-T angle
F T	13.5	19.5	6.0
D A	28.5	22.0	−6.5
V L	15.0	20.0	5.0
M L	35.0	11.5	−23.5
J C (♂)	9.0	21.0	12.0
E E	18.5	19.5	1.0
P P	12.0	16.5	4.5
H H	73.5	27.0	−46.5
E P	26.0	46.5	20.5
J H	5.0	5.0	0
N A	35.0	39.0	4.0
J C (♀)	79.0	103.5	24.5
R D	18.5	30.0	11.5

W P   33   ♂

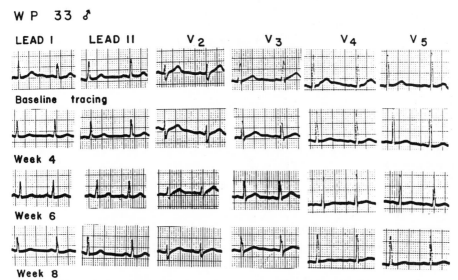

Fig. 4. Nonspecific T wave changes seen in one member of the control group. These appeared at week 4 and persisted thereafter.

DISCUSSION

The findings reported here suggest that the optimal dosage of thiothixene for chronic schizophrenics was close to 30 mg daily, and the optimal therapeutic dosage of thioridazine for the population studied was about 800 mg daily. At these dosages, the extracardiac side effects were mild in both drug groups, with orthostatic hypotension occurring more frequently in the thioridazine-treated patients.

Serial EKGs taken at various dose levels indicated a significant difference between the two drugs, in that all of the patients who received thioridazine developed changes consisting of prolongation of QT intervals, and lowering, flattening, and notching of T waves. These effects have been described previously during treatment with thioridazine (4, 5), and cases of fatal arrhythmia during thioridazine therapy have been reported (5, 6). In the present study, changes were seen in most cases when patients were on 200 mg of thioridazine daily, well below the dose that yielded optimum psychotherapeutic effects.

The findings reported here suggest that thioridazine, when given in recommended doses, is commonly associated with systemic side effects and is uniformly associated with abnormalities of myocardial repolarization. These changes occur even when dosage is well below the optimum therapeutic level, and may persist after the drug is discontinued, as noted in two of our patients 2 weeks after cessation of therapy. Patients who are treated with thioridazine should be followed with serial EKGs even when drug dosage is low.

Electrocardiographic changes during thiothixene therapy and among the controls were less impressive and might have been caused by other factors as discussed above. Thiothixene, when used for treatment of schizophrenic patients, was associated with significantly fewer adverse effects, especially on the myocardium, than thioridazine.

SUMMARY

Thiothixene (Navane®) is a thioxanthene derivative which is used in the treatment of schizophrenia. Clinical and laboratory evaluations have shown the drug to be relatively safe in comparison with other available antipsychotic agents. This study analyzes the electrocardiographic effects of thiothixene as compared with those of the phenothiazine thioridazine (Mellaril®).

EKGs taken before, during, and after therapy were interpreted without knowledge of the type or amount of drug the patient was receiving. Two patients had mild, transient changes while taking thiothixene, whereas treatment with thioridazine was associated with changes in every patient that often appeared while they were on low doses. The difference in incidence of electrocardiographic changes between the two drugs was statistically significant.

ACKNOWLEDGMENTS

This research was partially supported by U.S. Public Health Service grant MH-03701-12 from the Psychopharmacology Research Branch of the National Institute of Mental Health, and by the Behavioral Science Research Foundation, New Orleans, Louisiana. Thiothixene (Navane®) was supplied by the Clinical Research Department of Charles Pfizer and Co., Inc., Groton, Conn.

REFERENCES

1. Sugerman, A. A., Stolberg, H. H., Hermann, J., *Curr. Ther. Res.,* **7,** 310 (1965).
2. Gallant, D. M., Bishop, M. P., Shelton, W., *Am. J. Psychiat.,* **123,** 345 (1966).
3. Gallant, D. M., Bishop, M. P., Timmons, E., et al., *Curr. Ther. Res.,* **8,** 153 (1966).
4. Ban, T. A., St. Jean, A., *Canad. Med. Assoc. J.,* **91,** 537 (1964).
5. Kelly, H. G., Fay, J. E., Laverty, S. G., *Canad. Med. Assoc. J.,* **89,** 546 (1963).
6. Giles, T. D., Modlin, R. K., *JAMA,* **205,** 98 (1968).

The Phenothiazines and Structurally Related Drugs, edited by I. S. Forrest, C. J. Carr, and E. Usdin. Raven Press, N. Y. copyright 1974

Double-Blind Comparison of Thiothixene and Trifluoperazine in Acute Schizophrenia[†]

Herman C. B. Denber and Danielle Turns*

*Department of Psychiatry, College of Medicine, University of Florida, J. Hillis Miller Health Center, Gainesville, Florida 32601 and *Epidemiology Research Division, Hudson River State Hospital, Poughkeepsie, New York*

SUMMARY

Thiothixene was compared with trifluoperazine in a double-blind treatment trial in female, acute schizophrenic patients. Although the drugs are considered to be equipotent, the final average dose of thiothixene was lower than that of trifluoperazine. Despite this dosage difference, the overall improvement rate for thiothixene was better than for trifluoperazine. Side effects were similar in both groups. The IMPS data analyses indicated a greater number of favorable changes with thiothixene.

---

† *This chapter was published in full in* Psychosomatics, *13:100-104, 1972.*

The Phenothiazines and Structurally Related
Drugs, edited by I. S. Forrest, C. J. Carr, and
E. Usdin. Raven Press, N. Y. copyright 1974

Comparison of Phenothiazine and Nonphenothiazine Neuroleptics According to Psychopathology, Side Effects and Computerized EEG

T. M. Itil, C. D. Patterson, A. Keskiner, and J. M. Holden*

*Missouri Institute of Psychiatry, University of Missouri
School of Medicine, St. Louis, Missouri 63139*

INTRODUCTION

Despite the development of a series of new neuroleptics (major tranquilizers), there still remains a group of schizophrenic patients who do not show significant response to the drug treatment. These so-called "therapy-resistant" or "therapy-refractory" patients belong to the group of schizophrenics who were described by Kraepelin (9) as "dementia praecox." The present study was designed to determine psychopathological, social, somatic, and neurophysiological characteristics of therapy-resistant schizophrenics in comparison to responsive patients. In order to establish prognostic subclassification, patients have been treated with the well-established representatives of the three major groups of neuroleptics (major tranquilizers), namely, haloperidol (a butyrophenone), fluphenazine hydrochloride (a phenothiazine), and thiothixene (a thioxanthene). As a by-product of these projects, we were able to compare the clinical and CNS effects of these three neuroleptics.

MATERIAL AND METHOD

Sixty-two male and female chronic schizophrenic patients in the age range of 20 to 50 yr were included in this study. The diagnostic schizophrenic groups were hebephrenic, catatonic, paranoid, simple, and undifferentiated type. Patients were divided into three matched groups of 20, 20, and 22 (Fig. 1). Each group of patients first received the placebo medication for a period of 2 months. After the placebo, the patients belonging to group one received thiothixene, group two fluphenazine, and group three haloperidol, for a period of 3 months. Medically dischargeable patients were dropped from the study and continued on the medication they responded to at the end of the 3-month treatment period. In other patients the ineffective drug was discon-

---

* Present address: Yorkshire, England.

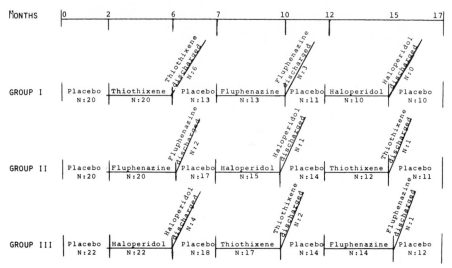

Fig. 1. TRP II—Design of three-drug study in chronic schizophrenics.

tinued, and after 2 months of placebo the next drug was given. With this kind of crossover study design, medically nondischargeable patients received all three major tranquilizers for a period of 3 months each, with 2-month placebo intervals.

In the first 6 weeks of the treatment, patients received drug with a fixed dosage schedule according to mg/kg body weight per day (Fig. 2). During this treatment period the maximum dosage was kept within the ranges recommended by the manufacturer. All three drugs started with 0.1 mg/kg/day and increased within 1 week from 0.1 to 0.3 mg/kg fluphenazine, from 0.1 to 0.5 mg/kg thiothixene, and from 0.1 to 0.15 mg/kg haloperidol. In the

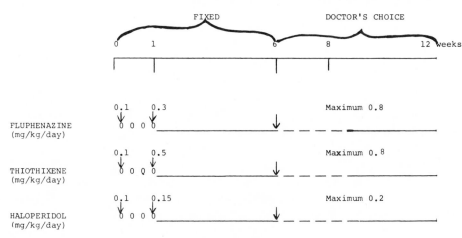

Fig. 2. Dose schedule of three-drug study.

second half of the treatment, for a period of 6 weeks, patients received Doctor's Choice dosages. In patients who did not show appreciable response to the first week of treatment, the dosage was increased up to 0.8 mg/kg/day with fluphenazine and thiothixene, and up to 0.2 mg/kg/day with haloperidol (haloperidol could not be increased further since the drug manufacturer did not want to file an IND for the use of a higher dosage). Based on this schedule, fluphenazine was given in dosage ranges of 16 to 36 mg (mean: 24.8 mg daily) in the first month, 20 to 80 mg (mean: 56.7 mg daily) in the second month, and 20 to 80 mg (mean: 64 mg daily) in the third month. Thiothixene was given in ranges of 16 to 50 mg (mean: 30 mg daily) in the first month, 40 to 80 mg (mean: 58.8 mg daily) in the second month, and 48 to 80 mg (mean: 66.7 mg daily) in the third month. Haloperidol dosages ranged from 4.5 to 12 mg (mean: 8 mg daily) in the first month, from 7 to 15 mg (mean: 11.5 mg daily) in the second month, and from 7.5 to 15 mg (mean: 13.7 mg daily) in the third month.

Except for procyclidine, no additional medication was administered. Forty-one of the 48 thiothixene-treated patients (84%), 42 of the 47 fluphenazine-treated patients (91%), and 39 of the 47 haloperidol-treated patients (83%) had to be given procyclidine as antiparkinsonian medication. Any patient who had to be given more than 3 consecutive days of any other medication was dropped from the study.

A total of 48 subjects (29 males and 19 females; mean age, 36.5; mean length of present hospitalization, 10 yr; mean length of illness, 13.1 yr) completed thiothixene treatment; 47 subjects (29 males and 18 females; mean age, 37; mean length of present hospitalization, 9.9 yr; mean length of illness, 13 yr) completed fluphenazine treatment; and 47 subjects (29 males and 18 females; mean age, 36.3; mean length of present hospitalization, 9.7 yr; mean length of illness, 13.3 yr) completed haloperidol treatment.

The study was double-blind and lasted 28 months.

RESULTS

Psychopathological Evaluations

Global Ratings. Global evaluation was made in monthly intervals during pre- and postdrug placebo periods and during active drug treatment using a seven-point rating scale (1 = no symptoms at all, 7 = the most seriously ill patients). The mean of the scores determined by the research group, composed of two psychiatrists, two nurses, and an occupational therapist, was taken as the global score for that period for the statistical evaluations. At the end of the placebo period, before drug treatment, patients who later received haloperidol and those who received thiothixene were more seriously ill (mean scores were 5.9 and 5.8, respectively), while those treated with fluphenazine were less seriously ill (mean score: 5.6) (Table 1). In all treat-

TABLE 1. Comparison of effects of major tranquilizers in a group of chronic schizophrenics

DRUG	PRE VS PERIOD	MEAN VALUE	+6	+5	+4	+3	+2	+1	0	-1	-2	-3	T-TEST	ANOV
FLUPHENAZINE PRE-5.6 N:47	I	4.8				3	4	20	17	3			--	--
	II	4.5				3	12	20	11	1			--	--
	III	4.7				1	11	20	12	3			--	--
	IV	5.6					2	5	26	17				
THIOTHIXENE PRE-5.8 N:48	I	4.5				2	3	10	23	8	2		--	--
	II	4.3			1	3	6	9	18	9	2		--	--
	III	4.2	1			2	10	6	19	10			--	--
	IV	5.5					1	13	19	5			-	
HALOPERIDOL PRE-5.9 N:47	I	5.3					4	21	22				--	--
	II	4.9			1	1	11	19	14	1			--	--
	III	4.7			2	4	11	16	13		1		--	--
	IV	5.7							11	23	5			

Key:
- = P < .05 Decrease
-- = P < .01 Decrease

ment evaluations (first month, second month, and third month) and under each drug treatment, the patients showed statistically significant ($p < 0.01$, Wilcoxon Test) improvement in comparison to predrug evaluations. A slightly greater (but not statistically significant) improvement was seen with thiothixene during the first and third month of treatment in comparison to fluphenazine and haloperidol. The greatest number of medically dischargeable patients occurred with thiothixene treatment (nine patients), followed next by fluphenazine treatment (six patients), and then by haloperidol treatment (five patients). After the discontinuation of each drug, patients showed worsening of symptoms. Maximum worsening was observed with fluphenazine treatment, followed by haloperidol and then by thiothixene, although these differences were not at the level of statistical significance. This observation may suggest that fluphenazine hydrochloride has the shortest duration of therapeutic effects in comparison to haloperidol and thiothixene.

Brief Psychiatric Rating Scale (BPRS). The BPRS ratings were done at monthly intervals based on interviews by a psychiatrist from a different ward. Sixteen of 18 symptoms were significantly improved during fluphenazine treatment, 14 significantly improved with thiothixene, and nine significantly improved with haloperidol treatment (Table 2). Symptoms such as conceptual disorganization and hallucinatory behavior were significantly ($p < 0.05 - <0.01$, Wilcoxon Test) improved with all three drugs in all treatment periods in comparison to predrug treatment. Symptoms such as anxiety, guilt feelings, and grandiosity were statistically influenced only by fluphenazine; emotional withdrawal, tension, hostility, suspiciousness, and excitement

TABLE 2. *Brief psychiatric rating scale*

| | Total population | | | | | |
| | Fluphenazine (N = 47) | | Thiothixene (N = 48) | | Haloperidol (N = 47) | |
Rating period	Pre- 1 MO	Pre- 3 MO	Pre- 1 MO	Pre- 3 MO	Pre- 1 MO	Pre- 3 MO
Mean daily dosage (mg)	24.8	64.0	30.4	66.8	8.1	13.7
Symptom						
Somatic concern	— —	—			— —	— —
Anxiety	—	— —				
Emot. withdrawal	— —	— —	— —	— —		
Concep. disorg.	— —	— —	— —	— —	—	—
Guilt feelings		—				
Tension	— —	— —	— —	— —		
Mannerisms & posturing	— —	— —		— —	—	—
Grandiosity	— —	—				
Depressed mood			— —	— —		— —
Hostility	— —	— —	— —	— —		
Suspiciousness	— —	— —	— —	— —		
Hallucin. behav.	— —	— —	— —	— —	—	— —
Motor retardation				—	—	—
Uncooperative	— —	— —	— —	— —		
Unusual thought	— —	— —	—	— —		
Blunted affect	— —	— —	—	— —		—
Excitement	— —	— —	— —	— —		
Disorientation	— —	— —	— —	— —	—	

LEGEND:

— = significantly decreasing at 5% level ⎫ Wilcoxon test
— — = significantly decreasing at 1% level ⎭

were influenced only by fluphenazine and thiothixene; somatic concern improved only after fluphenazine and haloperidol; and depressive mood and motor retardation were statistically improved only after thiothixene and haloperidol.

Side Effects

Clinical Side Effects. Clinical side effects were scored every 2 weeks, based on a psychosomatic rating scale (6). For the statistical evaluations, the means of two evaluations of the first month and two evaluations of the third month were used.

Eleven of the 50 symptoms showed significant changes during the first and third month of the treatment with these three neuroleptic drugs (Table 3).

TABLE 3. *Psychosomatic rating scale (side effects)*

	Total population					
	Fluphenazine (N = 47)		Thiothixene (N = 48)		Haloperidol (N = 47)	
Rating period	Pre-1 MO	Pre-3 MO	Pre-1 MO	Pre-3 MO	Pre-1 MO	Pre-3 MO
Mean daily dosage (mg)	24.8	64.0	30.4	66.8	8.1	13.7
Symptom						
Hyperkinesia	+		++		++	
Tremor	++	+	++	++	++	++
Akathisia	++	++	++	++	++	++
Rigidity	++	++	++	+	++	++
Parkinsonian	++	+	++	++	+	++
Miosis	+	+				
Incr. appetite			++	++		
Decr. appetite			− −	−	−	
Weakness			+			
Insomnia				−		−
Sedated					+	

LEGEND:

+ = significantly increasing at 5% level
++ = significantly increasing at 1% level } *t-test*
− = significantly decreasing at 5% level
− − = significantly decreasing at 1% level

Three more symptoms, akathisia, rigidity, and parkinsonism, were significantly increased during all three drug treatments at all time periods. Hyperkinesia was increased only during the first month of the treatment with each drug. Miosis increased only after fluphenazine, and sedation was observed only after haloperidol. Insomnia was observed during the third month with thiothixene and haloperidol. Appetite was increased only with thiothixene and was decreased in some subjects by thiothixene and haloperidol. An increase of weakness was observed only with thiothixene. The alterations in side effects from predrug- to drug-treatment periods of the three drugs were similar, and no statistically significant differences could be detected.

Physical and Laboratory Side Effects. Statistically significant increase of weight was observed with all three drugs (Table 4). An increase of white-blood-cell count was seen with thiothixene and haloperidol, increase of cholesterol was seen only with thiothixene, and an increase of hematocrit was seen only with haloperidol. Bilirubin and SGOT decreased significantly only with fluphenazine. Alkaline phosphatase and thymol turbidity significantly decreased with fluphenazine and increased with haloperidol. Systolic blood pressure decreased with fluphenazine, and diastolic blood pressure decreased with thiothixene.

TABLE 4. *Physical and laboratory data*

| | Total population | | | | | |
| | Fluphenazine (N = 47) | | Thiothixene (N = 46) | | Haloperidol (N = 47) | |
Rating period	Pre- 1 MO	Pre- 3 MO	Pre- 1 MO	Pre- 3 MO	Pre- 1 MO	Pre- 3 MO
Mean daily dosage (mg)	24.8	64.0	30.4	66.8	8.1	13.7
Measure						
Bilirubin	− −					
SGOT	− −					
Alk. phos.	−				++	++
T. T.		− −				++
Syst. blood pres.		−				
Dias. blood pres.				−		
Weight		+	+	++		+
Choles.			+	++		
WBC			++	+		++
Hct.						+
Lymphs.						
Monos.						

LEGEND:

+ = significantly increasing at 5% level ⎫
++ = significantly increasing at 1% level ⎬ *t*-test
− = significantly decreasing at 5% level ⎪
− − = significantly decreasing at 1% level ⎭

Computerized EEG Findings

During Resting Time. A 10-min resting EEG was recorded from the left and right frontal, central, parietal, and occipital regions with the reference electrodes at the ears. The right occipital to right ear lead was recorded on tape (Ampex FR-1300) and was analyzed offline utilizing computerized (IBM 1620–1710) period analysis programs (1, 10). This method determined the percentage of time spent in several frequency bands of both the primary wave and first derivative, the frequency deviation from the primary wave, as well as the average absolute amplitude and amplitude variability. A minimum total of 60×10 sec artifact-free EEG epochs was analyzed in each EEG evaluation. The computer-analyzed EEG (CEEG) measurements of pre- and postdrug periods were compared using *t*-test statistics in order to obtain CEEG profiles of each compound.

CEEG profiles of drugs demonstrated that thiothixene produces a decrease of very slow waves (1.5 to 3.5 cps), an increase of theta (3.5 to 7.5 cps) and alpha activity (7.5 to 13 cps), and a decrease of very fast beta activity (about 26 cps) during the third month of the treatment in comparison to predrug treatment (Fig. 3). Computer EEG profiles of fluphenazine and haloperidol showed close similarities to that of thiothixene.

EEG During All-Night Sleep Time. Because short, 10-min resting EEG recordings may not reflect the true effects of psychotropic drugs on the CNS,

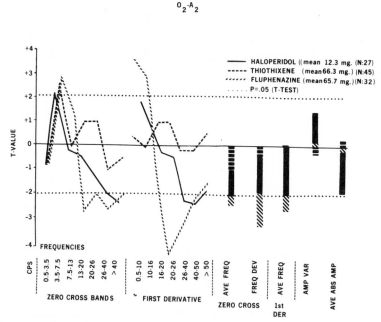

Fig. 3. Computerized EEG changes in chronic schizophrenics after 3 months of treatment with neuroleptics (based on digital-computer period analyses). Abscissa: 21 measurements of the EEG analyses. Ordinate: *t*-values of the third month of drug treatment in comparison with predrug treatment. As seen, an increase of the slow waves and decrease of fast activity in both zero cross (primary waves) and first-derivative measurements are the characteristic changes of all three major tranquilizers. Changes reached the level of statistical significance most after fluphenazine treatment, followed by thiothixene and haloperidol.

in recent years we have carried out systematic investigations with psychotropic drugs during all-night sleep. In this procedure, we analyze 6- to 8-hr continuous EEG recordings (30-sec recording and 4-sec computation time) while the patients sleep. At the end of all-night sleep, the computer gives a set of 22 CEEG measurements in terms of mean and standard deviations. The all-night sleep EEG profiles (predrug CEEG measurements minus postdrug measurements in terms of *t*-values) demonstrate again that all three neuroleptics have very similar profiles (Fig. 4). These are characterized by a decrease of 1.3 to 5 cps waves and a significant increase of 8 to 12 cps alpha waves. The other EEG variables did not reach the level of statistical significance (except the decrease of amplitude variability after haloperidol).

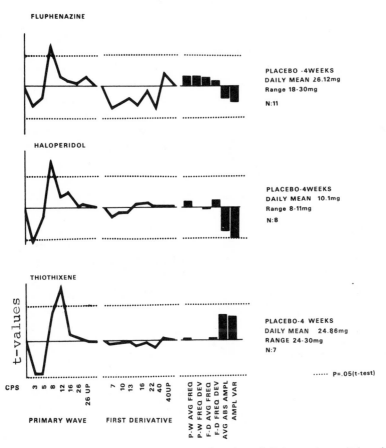

Fig. 4. All-night sleep EEG profiles of neuroleptics (based on digital-computer period analysis). Abscissa: 22 EEG measurements. Ordinate: *t*-values of the changes of 4 weeks drug treatment in comparison with the predrug placebo period. Major changes with all three tranquilizers are the decrease of very slow waves (1.3 to 5 cps) and increase of 5 to 8 and 8 to 12 cps waves in primary wave measurements. The increase of theta and alpha activity reached the level of statistical significance with all three drugs. According to these data, neuroleptics decrease very slow waves of sleep (decrease of deep sleep stages) and increase slow spindle activity (fast theta and alpha).

CONCLUSIONS

Using a double-blind, crossover study design, the clinical effectiveness of three well-known major tranquilizers was demonstrated in a large group of chronic schizophrenic patients. The most striking aspect of the study is the tremendous similarity of effects of the three neuroleptics, not only in the subjective evaluated areas such as psychopathology and side effects, but also in objective areas such as blood chemistry, hematology, and, particularly, computer-analyzed awake and sleep EEGs. The improvement of the psychopathology was seen most after fluphenazine and thiothixene and least after haloperidol. This may be due to the fact that haloperidol was given only in recommended dosages, whereas the other two compounds were administered in higher than recommended dosages. Previously, we recommended administering higher than recommended dosages of neuroleptics in chronic schizophrenic patients (2, 8). This study confirms our previous findings. As far as side effects are concerned, these were observed in very similar quality and quantity after all three neuroleptics. It was interesting, however, that haloperidol produced side effects similar to those of the other two neuroleptics, although at the lower dosages and with less therapeutic benefit.

As previously reported, a slight stimulatory property (slight increase of slow beta activity in EEG) of thiothixene was seen. This was reflected not only in the appearance of insomnia, but also in improvements of emotional withdrawal, motor retardation, blunted affect, and improved depressive mood. Only thiothixene influenced all these four symptoms at the level of statistical significance. The similarity of the CNS effects of all three neuroleptics during resting and sleeping time was most striking. The CEEG profiles of three neuroleptics confirmed our previous findings. An increase of slow waves and alpha activity and a decrease of fast waves have been considered "specific" for neuroleptics (major tranquilizers), and these types of EEG alterations have been called "chlorpromazine-type EEGs" (4, 5), or "major tranquilizer reaction types" (3). The amazing similarity of the CEEG profiles during sleep time is a further confirmation of the significant role of CEEG in classification of psychotropic drugs based on the quantitative EEG. As previously reported, there were significant clinical and EEG correlations in this population: an increase of slow waves and, particularly, a decrease of very high frequency fast activities that were significantly correlated with a decrease of total psychopathology (7).

SUMMARY

Sixty-two male and female chronic schizophrenics resistant to drug therapy were treated in a double-blind crossover study with representatives of three groups of antipsychotics—butyrophenones, thioxanthenes, and phenothiazines. The patients were treated with each drug for 3 months with a 2-month pre- and post-treatment placebo interval. Ratings of psychopathology and clinical side effects, blood chemistries, and computerized awake and sleep EEGs were done at intervals throughout the study, which lasted 28 months.

The global ratings indicated significant improvement in symptoms with all three drugs in comparison to placebo. The BPRS showed 16 of 18 symptoms significantly improved with fluphenazine compared to placebo, 14 of 18 significantly improved with thiothixene, and nine of 18 significantly improved with haloperidol. Alterations in clinical side effects from placebo to drug treatment were similar for the three drugs, and no statistically significant differences among the three drugs were detected.

CEEGs showed that the thioxanthene produced a decrease of very slow waves, an increase in theta and alpha activity, and a decrease in very fast beta activity. The profiles of the phenothiazine and the butyrophenone showed close similarities to that of the thioxanthene.

The findings are discussed in relationship to differences in clinical characteristics of the three groups of antipsychotic drugs and the role of the CEEG in classifying psychotropic drugs.

ACKNOWLEDGMENT

This research was supported in part by U.S. Public Health Service grant MH-11381 and by the Psychiatric Research Foundation of Missouri.

REFERENCES

1. Burch, N. R., Nettleton, W. H., Sweeney, J., and Edwards, R. J., *Ann. N.Y. Acad. Sci.,* **115,** 827 (1964).
2. Itil, T. M., in *The World Biennial of Psychiatry and Psychotherapy,* Vol. II, Arieti, S. (Ed.), *in press,* 1973.
3. Itil, T. M., in *Clinical Psychopharmacology, Modern Problems of Pharmacopsychiatry,* Vol. I, Freyhan, F. A., Petrilowitsch, N., and Pichot, P. (Eds.), Karger, Basel, New York, 1968.
4. Itil, T. M., *Elektroencephalographische Studien Bei Psychosen und Psychotropen Medikamenten,* Ahmet Sait Matbaasi, Istanbul, 1964.
5. Itil, T. M., *Med. Exp. (Basel),* **5,** 347 (1961).
6. Itil, T. M., and Keskiner, A., *Psychiatric Research Foundation of Missouri, Publication No. 12,* 1966.
7. Itil, T. M., Saletu, B., Marasa, J., and Mucciardi, A., *American Journal of Psychiatry* (in press, 1973).
8. Itil, T. M., Keskiner, A., Heinemann, L., Han, T., Gannon, P., and Hsu, W., *Psychosomatics* **II (5),** 456 (1970).
9. Kraepelin, E., *Allg. Ztschr. J. Psych.,* 56 (1899).
10. Shapiro, D. M., and Fink, M., *Psychiatric Research Foundation of Missouri, Publication No. 1,* 1966.

The Phenothiazines and Structurally Related
Drugs, edited by I. S. Forrest, C. J. Carr, and
E. Usdin. Raven Press, N. Y. copyright 1974

Double-Blind Comparison of Thiothixene and Protriptyline in Psychotic Depression

Ari Kiev

Cornell Program in Social Psychiatry, 525 East 68th Street, New York, New York 10021

INTRODUCTION

The use of available psychotropic agents in the treatment of patients with psychotic depression poses a challenge to the physician in that many of the potentially useful drugs, chiefly the tricyclic antidepressants, are known, on occasion, to trigger previously dormant schizophrenic symptoms. Moreover, even the most useful of these agents often requires protracted periods of administration before any beneficial effects can be noted in patients with psychotic depressive reactions. Several recent studies (1–3) have reported on the usefulness of thiothixene, a widely used antipsychotic agent of the thioxanthene series, in the treatment of depressive states. The present double-blind study was undertaken to compare the antidepressant activity of thiothixene to that of an established tricyclic antidepressant, protriptyline, in psychotically depressed patients in a private psychiatric practice.

DIAGNOSTIC CONSIDERATIONS

Psychotic depressions generally manifest themselves as either psychotic depressive reaction (Amercan Psychiatric Association Diagnostic Code 298.0) or manic-depressive illness, depressed type (American Psychiatric Association Diagnostic Code 296.2). In both cases, the important differentiation from depressive neurosis depends upon the degree of impact of the reaction on reality testing or functional adequacy. Thus, according to American Psychiatric Association nosology (4), patients are described as psychotic when their mental functioning is sufficiently impaired to interfere grossly with their capacity to meet ordinary demands of life. Such impairment may result from a serious distortion in capacity to recognize reality; hallucinations and delusions may distort perceptions. Alterations in mood may be so profound that the patient's capacity to respond appropriately is grossly impaired. Deficits in perception, language, and memory may be so severe that the patient's capacity for mental grasp of his situation is effectively lost. Patients with neuroses, by contrast, manifest neither gross distortion or misrepresentation of external reality, nor gross personality disorganization. Even when severely handicapped by their symptoms, neurotic patients, unlike psychotic patients, are usually aware that their mental functioning is disturbed.

Psychotic depressive reaction can be distinguished from manic-depressive illness, depressed type, by the absence of a history of repeated episodes of depression or cyclothymic mood swings (including mania and hypomania), a lack of periodicity to the episodes, and by the evidence, on occasion, of specific precipitating stresses.

METHOD AND MATERIALS

Fifty adult patients in a private psychiatric practice with a diagnosis of psychotic depression were selected for inclusion in this double-blind study. All but three fulfilled the requirements of psychotic depressive reaction as listed in the American Psychiatric Association Diagnostic and Statistical Manual of Mental Disorders (DSM-II) (4); the remaining three were classified as manic-depressive illness, depressed type. Patients with severe cardiac conditions and women of childbearing potential were excluded. Patients were to have received no psychotropic medication for a period of at least 3 months prior to their inclusion in this study, although most had been treated with chemotherapy at an earlier date, largely with less than optimum results. The study was designed to be of 6 weeks' duration.

The patient population was divided by random design into two drug groups. The groups were closely matched with regard to severity and duration of illness, and age. Among the thiothixene group, there were 11 patients classified as moderately ill and 14 as severely ill. Among the protriptyline group, there were seven patients classified as moderately ill and 18 as severely ill. The mean duration of illness among the thiothixene group was 2.0 yr, and among the protriptyline group 3.1 yr. There were 15 males and 10 females in the thiothixene group, nine males and 16 females in the protriptyline group. The mean age of the thiothixene group was 37.6 yr, and of the protriptyline group 34.2 yr.

Medication was provided in identical capsules containing 5 mg of either thiothixene or protriptyline. The drug code was unknown to patients and investigator. The starting dose of the assigned drug was one capsule b.i.d., with dosage to be raised or lowered depending upon patient response. The mean duration of therapy among the thiothixene group was 5.7 weeks with a mean optimum dosage of 13.5 mg per day (range: 10 to 30 mg). The duration of therapy among the protriptyline group was 6.4 weeks with a mean optimum dosage of 22.9 mg per day (range: 10 to 30 mg). The maximum dosage among the thiothixene group was 30 mg per day, and among the protriptyline group, 40 mg per day.

Clinical efficacy was evaluated utilizing the following measures: Hamilton Depression Scale at baseline, weekly, and at the conclusion of the study; Brief

Psychiatric Rating Scale (BPRS) at baseline, midpoint, and conclusion of the study; and Clinical Global Impression of improvement at the conclusion of the study.

Observations for side effects were made at the time of routine office visits.

RESULTS

Both drug groups showed significant improvement as measured by the BPRS and the Hamilton Depression Scale. However, as shown in Table 1,

TABLE 1. Comparison: thiothixene versus protriptyline group

Scale	(Baseline—Final) Mean difference	*t* Statistic	d of f	Significance level
BPRS				
Depressive weights	11.389	1.232	41	>0.10
Sum of scores	4.885	1.210	41	>0.10
Hamilton Depression Scale				
Factor 1	0.988	1.461	45	0.12
Factor 2	0.934	2.085	45	0.035
Factor 3	0.558	1.081	45	>0.20
Factor 4	0.366	1.420	45	0.12

there was a statistically significant difference between the two groups, the thiothixene group showing greater improvement than the protriptyline group in Factor 2 of the Hamilton Scale (agitated depression). Moreover, symmetry analysis indicated that the thiothixene group had a greater continuing effect in response to Factor 3 (anxiety) than the protriptyline group, the difference being statistically significant at the $p < 0.01$ level.

Table 2 shows the item analysis for those parameters on the BPRS whose mean change over the period of the trial was greater than 0.55 in either drug group. The improvement among the thiothixene group was significant for all 12 items shown; among the protriptyline group, improvement was significant for nine of the 12 items. The greatest improvement among the thiothixene group was shown for the items depressed mood, guilt, and tension, while the protriptyline group showed greatest improvement for the items guilt, depressed mood, and emotional withdrawal.

Table 3 shows the item analysis for those parameters on the Hamilton Depression Scale whose mean change was greater than 0.55 in either group. The improvement among both groups was significant for all 13 items shown. The greatest mean improvement for both drug groups was recorded for the items anxiety, work and activities, guilt feelings, and depressed mood.

TABLE 2. Item analysis: BPRS[a]

Item	Mean baseline—Final change		Sign test—Significance level		Comparison—Significance level[b]
	Thiothixene	Protriptyline	Thiothixene	Protriptyline	
Depressed mood	2.421	2.318	<0.001	<0.001	0.76
Guilt	2.368	2.591	<0.001	<0.001	0.72
Tension	2.316	1.591	<0.001	<0.001	0.052
Emotional withdrawal	1.895	1.818	<0.001	<0.001	0.68
Anxiety	1.842	1.546	<0.001	<0.001	0.43
Suspiciousness	1.789	1.273	<0.001	<0.001	0.14
Motor retardation	1.632	1.091	<0.001	0.004	0.31
Blunted affect	1.632	1.364	<0.002	<0.004	0.51
Somatic concern	1.421	1.091	0.004	0.001	0.36
Hostility	0.947	0.455	0.002	0.212	0.36
Conceptual Disorganization	0.842	0.545	0.004	0.145	0.32
Excitement	0.632	−0.046	0.031	>0.50	0.19

[a] Items with mean changes greater than 0.55 in either group.
[b] Per Wilcoxon Rank Sum Test.

TABLE 3. Item analysis: Hamilton Depression Scale[a]

Item	Mean baseline—Final change		Sign test—Significance level		Comparison—Significance level[b]
	Thiothixene	Protriptyline	Thiothixene	Protriptyline	
Anxiety-psychic	2.143	1.458	<0.001	0.001	0.23
Work and activities	1.762	1.292	<0.001	<0.001	0.08
Guilt feelings	1.571	1.167	<0.001	<0.001	0.19
Depressed mood	1.524	1.333	<0.001	<0.001	0.54
Anxiety somatic	1.429	0.958	<0.001	<0.001	0.16
Suicide	1.095	1.042	<0.001	<0.001	0.38
Hypochondriasis	1.095	0.833	<0.001	<0.001	0.45
Insomnia-early	0.952	0.708	<0.001	<0.002	0.36
Agitation	0.905	0.833	<0.001	<0.001	0.72
Insomnia-middle	0.857	0.542	<0.001	0.002	0.23
Insomnia-late	0.714	0.417	<0.001	0.029	0.29
Somatic-general	0.619	0.458	<0.002	<0.001	0.35
Genital symptom	0.286	1.042	0.033	<0.001	0.42

[a] Items with mean changes greater than 0.55 in either group.
[b] Per Wilcoxon Rank Sum Test.

The Overall Global Evaluation by diagnosis for the two drug groups is presented in Tables 4 and 5. Among the patients diagnosed according to the APA criteria for psychotic depressive reaction, 17 of 20 (85%) in the thothi-xene group who completed the study were rated as markedly or moderately improved. In the protriptyline group, 15 of 23 (65%) of the patients with

TABLE 4. Overall global evaluation by diagnosis—thiothixene

Diagnosis	Improvement					
	Marked	Moderate	Slight	No change	Worse	Unable to evaluate
Manic depressive illness, depressed type	1	0	0	0	0	0
Psychotic depressive reaction	9	8	3	0	0	4

TABLE 5. Overall global evaluation by diagnosis—protriptyline

Diagnosis	Improvement					
	Marked	Moderate	Slight	No change	Worse	Unable to evaluate
Manic depressive illness, depressed type	1	1	0	0	0	0
Psychotic depressive reaction	6	9	6	1	1	0

TABLE 6. Overall global evaluation—by severity of illness

Drug administered	Severity of illness	Improvement					
		Marked	Moderate	Slight	No change	Worse	Unable to evaluate
Thiothixene	Markedly ill	6	3	2	0	0	3
	Moderately ill	4	5	1	0	0	1
Protriptyline	Markedly ill	6	8	3	0	1	0
	Moderately ill	1	2	3	1	0	0

psychotic depressive reaction were so rated. Table 6 shows the Overall Global Evaluation as related to baseline severity of illness.

In comparing results obtained in this trial with previous therapy, thiothixene produced moderate or marked improvement among 18 patients who had previously experienced no change or only slight improvement on treatment with other psychotropic agents. Use of protriptyline resulted in improved response among 11 patients when compared to their previous drug therapy, equal response among five, and an inferior response in two cases.

Side effects associated with the two drugs were quantitatively comparable and predominantly mild to moderate in degree; 15 of the 25 patients in the thiothixene group reported side effects compared to 12 of the 25 in the protriptyline group. Principal side effects in the thiothixene group were restlessness and tremor; in the protriptyline group, dry mouth was the single most frequent complaint. Two patients in the thiothixene group discontinued their medication because of restlessness. Two patients in the protriptyline group also had to discontinue their medication because of side effects, one because of a rash and the other because of a paranoid reaction.

DISCUSSION

Many depressed patients present the clinician with a problem in diagnosis (and, therefore, in management) because of the presence of severe agitation or the suggestion of an underlying schizophrenic process. Such patients are often classified as borderline schizoaffective or pseudoneurotic schizophrenics, despite the predominance of the depressive mood in their presenting symptomatology. The choice of a psychotropic agent for such patients is a difficult one. In the case of an underlying schizophrenic process, phenothiazines have failed to demonstrate any antidepressant effects; in fact, they often act as depressants. The tricyclic antidepressants are frequently contraindicated because of their potential to trigger psychotic episodes; indeed, this phenomenon was observed in one of the patients in the current study.

The results of this study point to the value of thiothixene in the management of psychotic depression. In particular, the statistically significant differences between thiothixene and protriptyline in terms of scores on agitated depression and anxiety are suggestive of specific indications for the use of the drug in patients with agitation and severe anxiety accompanying the psychotic depression. This finding is consistent with the previous use of the drug as an antipsychotic agent.

This suggestion is further supported by certain additional findings which approached statistical significance and which show a clear tendency in favor of thiothixene, particularly for the psychotic manifestations of psychotic depression. Specifically, the thiothixene-treated group showed greater mean improvement in Factors 1, 3, and 4 of the Hamilton Depression Scale; respectively, retarded depression, anxiety, and somatization; in mean response to tension as measured on the BPRS; and, on the Hamilton Scale, with regard to work and activities.

Thus, although thiothixene appears similar to protriptyline in terms of its effect on depressive symptoms, it quite clearly can be differentiated by its effects on agitation, tension, and anxiety. To the extent that a patient's functioning is impaired by such symptoms, the use of thiothixene may well enable the agitated depressive, who may also exhibit schizophrenic features or elements, to function again more rapidly. Indeed, where the patient's impairment stems more from agitation and anxiety than from loss of energy and retardation, the use of thiothixene may well be the wiser clinical choice.

Given the difficulties inherent in psychiatric diagnosis, which often preclude our ability to distinguish between depressive reaction of psychotic proportions and a psychotic schizophrenic reaction with depressive features, a drug such as thiothixene which appears to have both antidepressant and antipsychotic effects becomes a valuable therapeutic tool.

SUMMARY

In a double-blind controlled study comparing the clinical efficacy of thiothixene to protriptyline in psychotic depression, thiothixene, a widely used antipsychotic agent, was shown to be at least as effective as the established tricyclic antidepressant.

In a number of ratings there were statistically significant differences between the two groups. The thiothixene group showed greater improvement in Factor 2 of the Hamilton Scale (agitated depression) and a greater continuing effect in response to Factor 3 (anxiety) than the protriptyline group.

Side effects associated with the two drugs were quantitatively comparable and predominantly of mild to moderate degree. Two patients in each group discontinued their medication because of side effects.

REFERENCES

1. Pennington, V. M., *Psychosomatics,* **9,** 346 (1968).
2. Overall, J. I., Hollister, L. E., Shelton, J., Kimbell, I., Jr., and Pennington, V., *Clin. Pharm. and Therap.,* **10,** 36 (1969).
3. McLaughlin, B. E., *Dis. Nerv. Syst.,* **30** (Suppl. 2), 85 (1969).
4. American Psychiatric Association, *Diagnostic and Statistical Manual of Mental Disorders, DSM-II,* 1968, pp. 23, 39.

The Phenothiazines and Structurally Related
Drugs, edited by I. S. Forrest, C. J. Carr, and
E. Usdin. Raven Press, N. Y. copyright 1974

Thiothixene in Childhood Psychoses

J. Simeon, B. Saletu, M. Saletu, T. M. Itil, and J. DaSilva

*Department of Psychiatry, St. Louis Division, Missouri Institute of Psychiatry,
University of Missouri-Columbia, School of Medicine, St. Louis, Missouri 63139*

INTRODUCTION

Clinical research experience with psychotropic drugs in psychotic children is still limited and treatment is based mostly on extrapolation from adult psychopharmacology. In spite of the administration of a large number of psychotropic drugs in childhood psychoses (1), in a review (2) of recent developments in the study of early childhood psychoses only four psychotropic drugs (including LSD) with therapeutic effects were reported. The conclusions were reached that drug studies have shown mixed results with no consistent or marked improvement, but that they further indicated the possibility of neurobiological factors. Studies indicating antipsychotic effects in children have been reported for trifluoperazine (3), chlorpromazine and diphenhydramine (4), a combination of thioridazine and diphenylhydantoin (5), fluphenazine (6), haloperidol (7), and triiodothyronine (8). Thiothixene was selected for this study because of its potential antipsychotic and anxiolytic properties (9, 10), broad therapeutic index, and absence of oversedation, as well as its excellent results in children with schizophrenia, psychosis, severe mental retardation, chronic brain syndromes (11, 12), and behavior disorders (13).

SUBJECTS

Criteria for selection included children with prolonged or recurring psychotic disorders (infantile autism, childhood schizophrenia, and organic psychoses) who showed no satisfactory response to previous treatment; excluded were those with severe physical or neurological illnesses.

Ten psychotic boys, 5 to 15 yr old (mean, 10 yr), hospitalized in a 12-bed research ward, were included in this study. Clinically they could be classified as infantile autism (B.P., M.M., J.Ma., P.M.), childhood schizophrenia (F.P., S.P., S.H., D.R.), and organic psychosis (R.W., J.Mo.) (Table 1). Nine of the 10 children had been under therapy for more than 2 yr, and seven had received drug therapy prior to admission, showing no apparent improvement. All had shown their first symptoms of behavioral disorder, not necessarily typical of psychosis, at an age ranging from 1 to 5 yr (mean,

520

Table 1

CHARACTERISTICS OF PSYCHOTIC CHILDREN TREATED WITH THIOTHIXENE

Pts.	Age of First Symptoms	Previous Therapy	Age on Admission	I.Q.	M.A.	Degree of Illness** On Admission	Degree of Illness** End of Placebo
1. R.W.	2	>2 yrs.*	14-10	105	15-7	5	5
2. F.P.	2	>2 yrs.*	8-8	110	10-0	5	5
3. S.P.	5	>2 yrs.*	10-8	76	8-1	5	5
4. B.P.	1	5 mos.	5-2	70	3-7	5	4
5. M.M.	2	>2 yrs.*	10-10	65	7-0	6	6
6. S.H.	1	>2 yrs.	10-5	92	9-7	4	4
7. J.Mo.	1	>2 yrs.*	7-7	76	5-9	5	4
8. J. Ma.	1	>2 yrs.*	10-3	30	2-9	7	7
9. P.M.	4	>2 yrs.*	10-8	46	4-11	6	6
10. D.R.	1½	>2 yrs.	10-7	83	8-9	5	5
Mean:	2.1		10-0	75	7.6	5.3	5.1

* including previous drug therapy

** Degree of Illness:
1 Normal
2 Borderline
3 Mild
4 Moderate
5 Marked
6 Severe
7 Most Severe

2.1 yr). On admission their mental ages ranged from 3 to 16 yr (mean, 7.6 yr) and their I.Q.s (WISC) from 30 to 110 (mean, 75); the degree of illness was evaluated as moderate in one boy, marked in six, severe in two, and most severe in one. Behavioral characteristics at any time during their lives are shown in Table 2. Their psychopathology was characterized by inappro-

Table 2.

BEHAVIORAL CHARACTERISTICS* OF PSYCHOTIC CHILDREN: PATIENT PROFILE

BEHAVIORAL CHARACTERISTICS \ PATIENTS	1 RW	2 FP	3 SP	4 BP	5 MM	6 SH	7 J.Mo.	8 J.Ma.	9 PM	10 DR
1. Extreme self-isolation, aloofness, or withdrawal, noticeable in infancy					+			+	+	
2. Do not anticipate being picked up, unresponsive to mother					+			+	+	
3. Insensitivity to pain							+		+	+
4. Lack or avoidance of eye contact, looking through or past people				+	+	+	+	+	+	+
5. Try to maintain sameness in a) objects and their placement b) behavior patterns	+	+		+	+				+	+
6. Pay more attention to objects than to people				+	+			+		
7. Repetitive manipulation of objects. Little recognition of function					+			+		
8. Fail to develop speech, mute					+			+		
9. Limited speech or echolalia, without communication. Immediate and delayed echolalia			+	+				+	+	
10. Pronominal reversal					+			+		
11. Repetitive body movement, rocking, hand flapping, posturing	+	+		+	+	+		+	+	
12. Self-mutilation, head banging		+			+	+		+	+	
13. Laughing or smiling, crying or tantrums for no apparent reason	+	+		+	+	+		+	+	+
14. Impression of normal intelligence. Retardation with islets of normal functioning			+	+	+		+			+
15. In some cases, short period of normal development followed by regression									+	
16. Normal motor development	+		+		+	+		+	+	+
17. Empty clinging				+		+		+		
18. Difficulty in playing with other children	+	+			+	+		+	+	+
19. Abnormal responses to stimuli. Avoidance, hypo-or hyper-sensitivity, especially to sound					+			+	+	
20. Little or no comprehension of language				+	+			+	+	
21. Use people as objects or tools								+		
22. Problems with feeding, sleeping, toileting refusals, fads	+	+		+		+		+	+	
23. Abnormal fears or lack of appropriate sense of fear	+	+	+	+	+	+	+	+	+	
24. Unusual abilities, e.g., rote memory, musical, reading, spatial					+					+
25. Hyperkinesis, hypokinesis	+	+	+	+	+		+	+	+	
26. Serious or sad facial expression					+	+		+	+	+
27. Extreme negativism, no imitation of others	+			+		+			+	+
28. Short attention span with less distractibility				+	+	+		+	+	

*(Hingtgen Bryson 1972)

priate and bizarre behavior and by language, thought, emotional, mood, motor, and perceptual disorders (Table 3).

Table 3.

SYMPTOMS OF PSYCHOTIC CHILDREN DURING PLACEBO

SYMPTOMS \ PATIENT	1 RW	2 FP	3 SP	4 BP	5 MM	6 SH	7 J.Mo.	8 J.Ma.	9 PM	10 DR
1. Hyperkinesis	3	3	2	2	1	1	1	3	2	
2. Inappropriate overt behavior	3	3	2	3	3	2	1	3	3	2
3. Mood lability	2	2	2	1	2	2		3	1	
4. Manifest anxiety	1	1	2	1	1	1	1		3	
5. Lack of appropriate fears or anger			1		2		2	3		
6. Anger	2	2	2	1		2	1		3	
7. Emotional unresponsiveness	3	3	3	1	3	3	2	3	3	2
8. Poor response to environment	3	3	2		2			3	3	
9. Poor relationship to children	3	3	2		2	2	3	3	2	2
10. Poor relationship to adults	3	2	3		2	2	2	3	2	2
11. Assaultiveness	2	2	1		+1 −3		1	+1 −3	−3	
12. Poor attention span	3	3	3	1	3			3		
13. Hypodistractibility				2	3			3	2	
14. Mutism					3			3		
15. Poor communication	1		2	3	3			3	3	2
16. Poor speech	1			1	3			3		2
17. Thought disorder (content)	2	2				2	2			2
18. Overtalkativeness	3	3	2	1			1		3	
19. Lying	3	3	3			1				
20. Tearfulness	3	3	1	2	1	1		3	1	
21. Enuresis					1			1		
22. Insomnia		1	2		1			3		
23. Feeding problems	3	3	1	3		1	1	1	1	1
24. Dressing problems				2				3		

Degree of disorder: 1 slight
2 moderate
3 marked

METHOD

After admission, any prior drugs were discontinued and the children were given a complete diagnostic evaluation, including pediatric, neurological, psychological, and language examinations; X-rays of chest, skull, and carpal bone age; clinical EEG and laboratory tests (CBC, liver function test, FBS, BUN, VDRL, urinalysis, T_4); and plasma amino-acid analysis.

The patients first received placebo for 3 to 9 weeks (mean, 5.2 weeks) and then trihexyphenidyl (2.0 mg daily) for 1 to 3 weeks (mean, 1.6 weeks). Trihexyphenidyl was initially given alone and then concurrently with thiothixene at a fixed dose to prevent the emergence of any extrapyramidal symptoms and to minimize variability during chronic neurophysiological investigations. Thiothixene was given for 6 to 46 weeks (mean, 16.5 weeks). The maximum daily dosage ranged from 6 to 60 mg (mean, 27 mg) and the optimum daily dosage from 6 to 30 mg (mean, 14 mg) (Table 4).

Table 4

CLINICAL GLOBAL IMPROVEMENT AND DAILY DOSAGES (in mg.)
WITH THIOTHIXENE IN CHILDHOOD PSYCHOSES

Patient	Improvement	Maximum Dosage	Optimum Dosage
B.P.	+++	20	10
J.Mo.	+++	6	6
R.W.	++	40	30
S.H.	++	50	10
P.M.	++*	20	12
F.P.	+	20	20
S.P.	+	30	15
M.M.	+	15	15
J.Ma.	+	60	15
D.R.	+*	10	6
Mean		27	14

*   Treatment interrupted by parents

Note: Improvement compared to the two week pre-drug placebo period.

Thiothixene dosages were individually adjusted, starting with 1 mg daily and increasing rapidly. The drug was given in a liquid preparation providing flexibility of dosage and ease of administration and monitoring. The study called for thiothixene to be given for at least 4 weeks unless worsening or toxic symptoms occurred. Throughout their treatment, the children also received educational, occupational, recreational, and speech therapy as indicated.

A clinical global impressions rating scale (ECDEU) (14), a 27-item psychiatric rating scale for children[1] and a treatment emergent symptoms scale (ECDEU) were completed nonblindly at weekly intervals. The ratings on admission, at the end of the placebo and trihexyphenidyl periods, and weekly during thiothixene treatment were statistically analyzed. Parent's questionnaires (15) and school reports (16) were completed weekly, or whenever a child went home or to school. Body weight, heart rate, and blood pressures were recorded weekly, and clinical laboratory tests monthly.

Neurophysiological investigations included quantitatively analyzed EEG and visual evoked potentials (VEP) in the placebo period and during trihexyphenidyl administration alone, as well as during the first day and fourth week of thiothixene treatment. A 10-min resting EEG was recorded utilizing the 10×20 system. The right occipital-right ear lead was analyzed off line based on period analysis (17) using a digital computer (PDP-12) (18). This program permits analysis of the primary wave and its first derivative in 10-sec epochs at the sampling rate of 320 points per sec. Twenty-two EEG measurements were obtained from each EEG epoch [eight different frequency bands, average frequency, and frequency deviation of both the primary wave and the first derivative, as well as the average amplitude and amplitude variability (Drohocki)].

VEPs were elicited by light flashes produced by a Grass TS-2 photic stimulator at dial intensity 4, which is equivalent to 375,000 candle power at a distance of 10 inches (25 cm) with an assumed square pulse of 10 μsec. The lamp face was centered 6 inches in front of the glabella. The rate of the stimulus presentation was randomized (six stimuli over 20 sec). Electrodes were placed over the right and left occipital regions with the reference electrodes 7 cm anterior to the left. VEPs were amplified with two Tektronix type 122 preamplifiers in series with two transistorized postamplifiers and were fed into a CAT 400B for summation. The analysis time was 500 msec. A squared-wave calibration of 9.5 μV in series with the recording electrodes was fed into the input of the preamplifiers ahead of the evoked responses. Each average VEP of 50 stimuli was finally plotted on a Mosely X–Y plotter (five times per session). The subject's vigilance level was maintained by arousing him as soon as an EEG drowsiness pattern appeared. After each set of responses, the trial was interrupted and the children were interviewed in order to maintain their vigilance.

RESULTS

Clinical Findings

With placebo and with trihexyphenidyl alone, clinical global improvements were moderate in one patient and slight in two, while one was worse (Table 5). With thiothixene, clinical global improvements were marked in two pa-

---

[1] Modified from M. Pritchard (40).

Table 5

CLINICAL GLOBAL SCORES OF PSYCHOTIC CHILDREN TREATED WITH THIOTHIXENE

Patient	Pre-Thiothixene			Thiothixene											
	Admission	Placebo	Trihexyphenidyl	Week:1	2	3	4	5	6	7	8	9	10	11	12
R.W.	5*	5	5	5	5	4	4	4	4	3	3	3	4		
F.P.	5	5	5	5	4	4	4	4	5						
S.P.	5	5	5	5	5	5	4	4	4	5	5				
B.P.	5	4	4	5	4	3	3	3	4	3	3	4	2	3	2
M.M.	6	6	6	6	6	6	6	6	6						
S.H.	4	4	5	4	3	4	4	4	3	3	3	4	4	4	3
J.Mo.	5	4	3	3	3	3	2	2	1	1	1	1	1	1	1
J.Ma.	7	7	7	7	6	6	6	6	6	6	6	6	6	6	6
P.M.	6	6	5	5	5	5	5	4	4	4	4	**	**	6	5
D.R.	5	5	5	5	4	4	4	4	4	4	4	4	4	4	4
Mean:	5.3	5.1	5.0	5	4.5	4.4	4.2	4.1	4.1	3.6	3.6	3.7	3.5	4	3.5

* Legend: Severity of Illness
    1 Normal
    2 Borderline
    3 Mild
    4 Moderate
    5 Marked
    6 Severe
    7 Most Severe

** patient on vacation

tients, moderate in three, and slight in five (Table 4). In two patients—one with moderate and the other with slight improvements—drug therapy was interrupted by the parents after 8 and 12 weeks, respectively. The clinical global impression seven-point rating scale (1 = normal to 7 = most severely ill) demonstrated a slight decrease from a mean score of 5.3 at the time of admission to 5.1 during the placebo period, and a further decrease to 5.0 during the trihexyphenidyl treatment (Table 5). These changes did not reach the level of statistical significance ($p < 0.05$, Wilcoxon). With subsequent thiothixene treatment, a significant and persistent improvement started in the second week of the neuroleptic drug administration, and the mean global score dropped to 3.6 at the seventh week of thiothixene and concurrent trihexyphenidyl therapy (Table 5).

Statistical analysis of the psychiatric rating scale for children showed deterioration in 16 of 27 items during the placebo period as compared to admission; nine items showed improvement. However, none of these changes was statistically significant ($p < 0.05$, Wilcoxon). Nor were there any statistically significant changes during trihexyphenidyl administration, although a slight improvement in emotional expression (mood lability, anger, or anxiety) occurred in eight patients. Insomnia increased in one patient, and nocturnal enuresis stopped in another.

During thiothixene therapy, 10 symptoms showed marked and significant improvement as compared to predrug placebo, and to trihexyphenidyl treatment ($p < 0.01$ to 0.05, Wilcoxon) (Table 6). Specifically, improvements occurred in the quantity and quality of motor activity, quantity of speech,

Table 6.

STATISTICALLY SIGNIFICANT CHANGES IN CLINICAL SYMPTOMATOLOGY OF PSYCHOTIC CHILDREN

DURING TREATMENT WITH TRIHEXYPHENIDYL AND THIOTHIXENE

(Based on the Psychiatric Rating Scale for Children)

PERIODS / SYMPTOMS	TRIHEXY-PHENIDYL	PLACEBO TO THIOTHIXENE AND TRIHEXYPHENIDYL — WEEKS								TRIHEXYPHENIDYL TO THIOTHIXENE AND TRIHEXYPHENIDYL — WEEKS							
		1	2	3	4	5	6	7	8	1	2	3	4	5	6	7	8
Quantity of Motor Activity When Stationary			*				*		*	*							*
Quantity of Speech														*			
Mood Lability						*		*						*			
Social Relationship to Adults							*								*		
Anger			*	*	*			*									
Feeding Difficulties													*		*	*	
Motor Activity (Abnormality of Quality)													*	*		*	
Speech Abnormality (Content)									*		*				*	*	
Emotional Unresponsiveness			❋	❋	*	❋	❋	❋	❋					*	*	❋	❋
Attention Disorder													*	❋	*	*	*

* Improvement P<.05
❋ Improvement P<.01

(Wilcoxon Matched Pairs Test)
N:10

content of thought, social relationships with adults, anger, mood lability, emotional unresponsiveness, feeding difficulties, and attention disorder. The therapists and teachers working with these children found that learning, behavioral therapy, speech therapy, and occupational therapy were greatly facilitated in those patients whose symptoms improved with drug therapy. Following thiothixene withdrawal, seven children showed behavioral relapses, two being worse than during the prethiothixene placebo (D.R., J.Ma.), while three patients (R.W., J.Mo., S.P.) showed no worsening.

Adverse Effects

No adverse effects were noted during trihexyphenidyl administration except for insomnia in one patient. During thiothixene treatment there were mild, transient adverse symptoms which did not significantly interfere with the patients' functioning (Fig. 1). These consisted of drowsiness in five patients; tremor, rigidity, nausea, and vomiting in two each; and akathisia, dystonia, salivation, constipation, enuresis, and fever in one each. Drowsiness occurred at daily dosages ranging from 5 to 15 mg (mean, 8.8 mg) at periods of 1 to 22 weeks after the start of thiothixene administration. Worsening of symptoms was observed in four patients: insomnia and tearfulness increased in two patients each, and anxiety, enuresis, depression, and nightmares increased

	DR	J.Mo	RW	J.Ma	MM	SH	SP	FP	PM	BP
drowsiness	+	+	+		+	+				
tremor	+					+				
rigidity	+					+				
akathisia					+					
dystonia		+								
salivation					+					
nausea					+	+				
vomiting					+	+				
constipation					+					
enuresis				+						
fever				+						
weight gain (lbs)	+10	+4	+2	+12	+2	+20	+2	+6	+8	+20

Fig. 1. Adverse effects associated with thiothixene administration in psychotic boys. Behavioral adverse effects (+) during thiothixene and trihexyphenidyl therapy were mild and transient. Drowsiness occurred in five patients at daily doses ranging from 5 to 15 mg (mean, 8.8 mg) at periods of 1 to 22 weeks after the start of drug administration. Tremor, rigidity, nausea, and vomiting occurred in two patients each, and akathisia, dystonia, salivation, constipation, enuresis, and fever in one each.

in one patient each. In five patients, weight gain showed no deviation from the predrug percentile position; duration of thiothixene therapy was 6 to 25 weeks (mean, 13 weeks), maximum daily doses 6 to 40 mg (mean, 22 mg), and weight gain 2 to 8 lbs (mean, 4 lbs) (Fig. 2). The weights of the remaining five patients showed deviations from the predrug percentile position; they received thiothixene for 11 to 46 weeks (mean, 20 weeks), maximum daily doses 10 to 60 mg (mean, 32 mg), and gained 6 to 20 lbs (mean, 14 lbs). In six children there were slight and transient decreases of systolic and/or diastolic blood pressures during the third to sixth week of thiothixene therapy, but without any apparent clinical manifestations. Determinations of CBC, liver function tests, and urinalysis did not demonstrate any serious abnormalities attributable to thiothixene. WBC values below 5,000 cc/mm were observed in D.R. (4,800) during placebo; in B.P. (4,400) and J.Mo. (4,200) during trihexyphenidyl; in J.Mo. (lowest: 3,200) and F.P. (4,800) during thiothixene; and in J.Mo. (4,300), P.M. (4,700), and F.P. (4,700) after thiothixene withdrawal. In J.Mo., WBC decreased from 4,400 to 3,200 cc/mm in the fifth month of thiothixene and returned to 4,500 2 weeks later; concurrent with thiothixene this child was also receiving a hyposensitizing vaccine weekly for allergies. During placebo the alkaline phosphatase values ranged from 119 to 280 mU/ml (mean, 192 mU/ml). The three patients who had received no drug therapy prior to admission (D.R., B.P., S.H.)

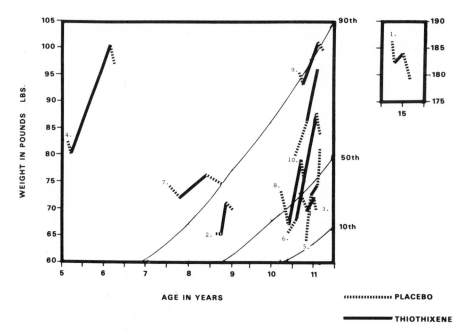

Fig. 2. Body weight changes in psychotic boys treated with thiothixene. Weight changes during placebo and after thiothixene withdrawal are also indicated. All patients gained weight with thiothixene but five only showed deviations from the predrug percentile position (mean gain, 14 lbs); the mean daily maximum dose was 32 mg and mean duration 20 weeks, as compared to those whose mean gain was 4 lbs, with a mean daily maximum dose of 22 mg during a mean of 13 weeks of therapy.

showed placebo values of 210, 175, and 135, respectively. During thiothixene, five patients showed increases ranging from 25 to 80 mU/ml (mean, 49 mU/ml) compared to placebo. Although still within normal limits,[2] these increases occurred after 2 to 3 months of thiothixene administration. Standard alkaline phosphatase values at our laboratory for normal children 5 to 7, 8 to 10, and 11 to 13 years old are 55 to 170, 55 to 285 and 30 to 330 mU/ml, respectively. During placebo, SGOT values were above 50 units in M.M. (85), J.Mo. (75), and R.W. (68), and during thiothixene in F.P. (90). During placebo LDH values were above 200 units in five patients, during thiothixene in three, and after thiothixene withdrawal in five. All other laboratory values during thiothixene administration remained within normal limits.

Neurophysiological Findings

Quantitative analysis of the EEG by means of digital computer period analysis demonstrated an increase of fast theta and slow alpha activity, as well

---

[2] The only exception was B.P., whose maximum 220 mU/ml during thiothixene decreased to 194, 3 weeks after drug withdrawal.

as a decrease of fast alpha and beta activity in the primary wave measurements during thiothixene treatment as compared with placebo (Fig. 3). The decrease in the slow beta frequencies (13 to 18 cps) reached the level of statistical significance ($p < 0.05$, t-test). Similarly, an augmentation of slow and attenuation of fast activity in the first derivatives occurred. There was a trend toward a decrease in average frequency and frequency deviation as

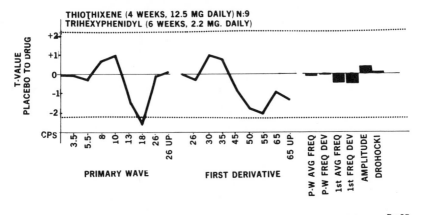

Fig. 3. Changes in computer EEG measurement of psychotic children during treatment with trihexyphenidyl and thiothixene. Twenty-two computer EEG measurements are shown in the abscissa; drug-induced changes as compared with placebo are expressed in terms of t-values (t-value is directly proportional to change value; inversely proportional to variance) and are indicated in the ordinate. As one can see, fast theta and slow alpha activity increases while fast alpha and beta activity decreases. The decrease in the 13 to 18 cps band reaches the level of statistical significance. In the first derivatives an augmentation of the slower frequencies and attenuation of the fast frequencies can also be seen. There was a trend toward decreased average frequency and frequency deviation in both primary wave and first deviative measurements as well as an increase in amplitude and amplitude variability (Drohocki).

well as an increase in average absolute amplitude and amplitude variability (Drohocki). These changes, which will be discussed in more detail elsewhere (19), represent a shift toward normalization of the children's brain function. There was a significant correlation between clinical improvement and changes in computer EEG measurements. The greater the clinical improvement, the greater the decrease in frequency deviation and the greater the increase in fast theta activity in the EEG.

Evaluation of visual evoked potentials demonstrated a significant increase in both latencies and amplitude measurements (Fig. 4). Interestingly, the amplitude augmentation was more pronounced over the right than over the left hemisphere. The findings, which will be described in detail elsewhere (20), indicate a normalization of the psychotic children's brain function over the right hemisphere. Moreover, the correlation analysis of clinical and VEP measurements showed a significant ($p < 0.01$ to 0.05) correlation between clinical improvement, and latency and amplitude changes during thiothixene

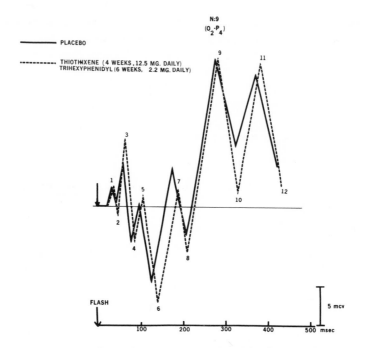

VEP CHANGES FROM PLACEBO TO THIOTHIXENE AND TRIHEXYPHENIDYL

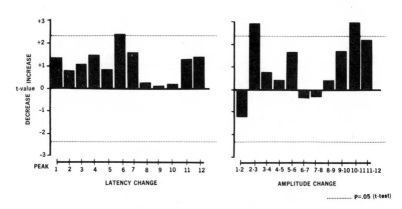

Fig. 4. Changes in the visual evoked potential of psychotic children during treatment with trihexyphenidyl and thiothixene as compared with placebo (right side). The average VEP of the total patient population on placebo as well as after 4 weeks of thiothixene treatment (this is with concomitant trihexyphenidyl treatment) is shown in the upper part of the figure. Generally a latency increase and amplitude augmentation can be seen after drug treatment. In the lower part, the latency and amplitude changes for each peak from placebo to drug are expressed in form of *t*-values (*t*-value is directly proportional to the change value; inversely proportional to the variance). The abscissa indicates peaks; the ordinate represents changes. Thiothixene treatment and concomitant antiparkinsonian drug treatment increases the latencies of all peaks, which reaches the level of statistical significance in peak 6. The amplitudes are also augmented, which was significant in the amplitudes of peaks 2 to 3 and peaks 10 to 11.

treatment: the greater the improvement in the overall clinical symptomatology, the more augmented were the latencies and amplitudes.

DISCUSSION

The results of this study indicate the usefulness of thiothixene in the therapy of childhood psychoses and corroborate similar findings by others (12, 13). Although the improvements we observed were not as marked as often reported for adult schizophrenics, even slight symptomatic improvements in the severely ill children facilitated other nondrug therapies. This beneficial effect was recognized by teachers, nurses, and occupational and speech therapists, especially during relapses following drug withdrawal. In general, improvements of hyperactivity, anger, and emotional unresponsiveness occurred first, followed by those of thought and attention disorders and the quality of motor activity. Severe language and intellectual impairments appeared to be the crucial factors limiting the therapeutic drug effects. The maximum and optimum dosages in this study are much higher than those previously reported in children.

The minimal or transient adverse effects may have been due to the prophylactic use of trihexyphenidyl. The absence of oversedation even with very high dosages might have been due to the stimulatory effect of the concurrent antiparkinsonian medication. That trihexyphenidyl has indeed a stimulatory effect was recently described by us based on significant latency decreases in VEPs of psychotic children during treatment with this drug alone (21). Such a significant attenuation of latencies was noted as characteristic for stimulatory compounds such as methylphenidate, dextroamphetamine, or monoamine oxidase inhibitors (22, 23). In addition to the probability of a rapid determination of optimal dosages, the concurrent use of antiparkinsonian agents can help avoid adverse effects at a time when the child is most disturbed; if improvement occurs, the real need for an antiparkinsonian agent can easily be determined by its gradual discontinuation.

No clinically significant changes in laboratory values were observed during thiothixene treatment. The interpretation of drug-induced clinical laboratory changes, short of marked abnormalities, can be extremely difficult, owing to a lack of normative data for children with and without psychiatric disorders and lack of norms for specific ages and developmental stages for the laboratory performing the tests. Further factors such as prior drug administration, conditions unrelated to the drug, and laboratory errors complicate interpretations. Transient hematologic changes in children receiving neuroleptic drugs have been reported (24); thus regular monitoring of blood and liver function values in any child receiving psychotropic medication would seem to be good medical practice. In our study, body weight gain appeared to be related to both dose levels and duration of drug therapy.

Quantitative computerized EEG analysis demonstrated an increase of fast theta and slow alpha and decrease of fast alpha and beta activity. These alterations have been described by us as characteristic for the "EEG major tranquilizer reaction type" (25–27). The significant correlation between clinical improvement and decrease of beta activity confirms previous findings indicating a direct relationship between drug-induced changes in computer-analyzed EEG and psychopathology: the greater the drug-induced attenuation of fast CNS activities, the greater the improvement in psychopathology (28, 29). Furthermore, such changes represent a shift of brain functions toward normality. As we have recently demonstrated, the differences between adult chronic schizophrenics and matched normals (30, 31), psychotic children and matched normals (19), and children with "high risk" of becoming schizophrenics and matched normals (32) are characterized by a greater amount of very slow and fast activity as well as less alpha waves in the former groups as compared with the latter ones.

The latency increase in VEPs during thiothixene treatment of psychotic children is characteristic for neuroleptic drugs, as described in chronic schizophrenics (33–35) and normals (36). However, the amplitude changes (increase) are unlike those observed in adults (decrease), possibly due to trihexyphenidyl effects or to a different mode of action of psychotropic agents in children. The augmentation of latency and amplitude represents a shift of the children's brain functions toward normality, as psychotic children have shorter latencies and smaller amplitudes than normal controls (20). Similar differences were observed between adult schizophrenics and normals (37, 38), as well as between "high risk" children and normals (32). The significant correlations between latency and amplitude changes and clinical ones further demonstrated that drug-induced behavioral alterations are directly related to changes in brain function, as has been postulated (39). The use of psychotropic drugs as tools in exploring behavioral-neurophysiological associations may provide a more scientific basis for the classification of mental illnesses and selection of biological therapy.

SUMMARY

Ten hospitalized psychotic boys, 5 to 15 years old, received thiothixene in maximum daily doses 6 to 60 mg (mean maximum, 27 mg; mean optimum, 14 mg). Trihexyphenidyl was given concurrently. Clinical improvements were marked in two patients, moderate in three, and slight in five. Motor activity, speech, thought content, social relationship, mood, emotion, feeding, and attention improved significantly. Adverse effects were transient and mild, except for weight gain in five patients. EEG computer analysis demonstrated an increase of fast theta and slow alpha activity, as well as decrease of fast alpha and beta activity during thiothixene as compared to placebo. Quantitative evaluation of VEPs showed an increase in both latency and amplitude measurements. These neurophysiological changes were significantly correlated with improvement in clinical symptomatology and indicate a normalization of the pathoneurophysiology.

ACKNOWLEDGMENT

The authors would like to express their thanks to Shirley Davis, R.N., and Susie Hearst, R.N., study coordinators; Verdell Lockett, EP technician; Charles Coffin, computer programmer and statistician; Carla Utech, research assistant; Carla Lane, editorial assistant; Barbara McKinney and Gloria Llanas, secretaries; and to the entire staff of the Child Psychiatry Section and the EEG laboratories for their most valuable assistance. This research was supported in part by the Psychiatric Research Foundation of Missouri.

REFERENCES

1. Simeon, J., and Itil, T. M., *Psychopharmacology Bulletin,* **9,** 50 (1973).
2. Hingtgen, J. N., and Bryson, C. Q., *Schizophrenia Bulletin,* **5,** 8 (1972).
3. Fish, B., Shapiro, T., and Campbell, M., *Amer. J. Psychiat.,* **123,** 32 (1966).
4. Fish, B., and Shapiro, T., *J. Amer. Acad. Child. Psychiat.,* **4,** 35 (1965).
5. Itil, T. M., Rizzo, A. E., and Shapiro, D. M., *Dis. Nerv. Sys.,* **28,** 731 (1967).
6. Engelhardt, D. M., *Resumé of Findings in the Use of Psychotropic Agents in Outpatient Children, Annual Report to Early Clinical Evaluation Drug Unit,* 1969.
7. Faretra, G., Dooher, L., and Dowling, J., *Amer. J. Psychiat.,* **126,** 146 (1970).
8. Campbell, M., Fish, B., David, R., Shapiro, T., Collins, P., and Koh, C., *J. Autism and Childhood Schizophrenia,* **2,** 343 (1972).
9. Simeon, J., Keskiner, A., Ponce, D., Itil, T. M., and Fink, M., *Curr. Therap. Res.,* **9,** 10 (1967).
10. Simeon, J., Nikolovski, O. T., and Spero, M., *Curr. Therap. Res.,* **12,** 369 (1970).
11. Fish, B., Campbell, M., Shapiro, T., and Weinstein, J., in *The Thioxanthenes, Mod. Probl. Pharmacopsychiat.,* Vol. 2, Karger, Basel, 1969, pp. 90–99.
12. Campbell, M., Fish, B., Shapiro, T., Floyd, A., Jr., *Arch. Gen. Psychiat.,* **23,** 70 (1970).
13. Wolpert, A., Quintos, A., White, L., and Merlis, S., *Curr. Therap. Res.,* **10,** 566 (1968).
14. *ECDEU Assessment Manual for Psychopharmacology, Pediatric and Revised Adult Batteries* (2nd Revision), January, 1973, Department H.E.W., N.I.M.H.
15. Conners, C. K., *Child Development,* **41,** 667 (1970).
16. Conners, C. K., *Amer. J. Psychiat.,* **126,** 152 (1969).
17. Burch, N. R., Nettleton, W. H., Sweeney, J., and Edwards, R. J., *Ann. N.Y. Acad. Sci.,* **115,** 827 (1964).
18. Shapiro, D., Hsu, W., and Itil, T. M., in *The Nervous System and Electric Currents,* Vol. 2, Wulfsohn, N. L., and Sances, A., Jr., (eds.), Plenum Press, New York, 1971, p. 59.
19. Itil, T. M., Saletu, B., Simeon, J., and Coffin, C., *in preparation.*
20. Saletu, B., Saletu, M., Itil, T. M., and Simeon, J., *in preparation.*
21. Saletu, B., Simeon, J., Saletu, M., and Itil, T. M., *Biol. Psychiat., in press.*
22. Saletu, B., Saletu, M., Itil, T. M., and Coffin, C., *Pharmakopsychiat.,* **5,** 129 (1972).
23. Saletu, B. in *Modern Probl. Pharmacopsychiat., Psychotropic Drugs and the Human EEG,* Vol. 7, Itil, T. M. (ed.), Karger, Basel, 1973.
24. Baldwin, R. L., and Peters, J. E., *Southern Medical J.,* **61,** 1072 (1968).
25. Itil, T. M., *Med. Exp. (Basel),* **5,** 347 (1961).
26. Itil, T. M., in *Psychopharmacology: A Review of Progress, 1957–1967,* Efron, D. H., Cole, J. O., Levine, J., and Wittenborn, R. O., (eds.), U.S. Government Printing Office, Washington, D.C., 1968, pp. 509–522.

27. Itil, T. M., Güven, F., Cora, R., Hsu, W., Polvan, N., Ucok, A., Sanseigne, A., and Ulett, G. A., in *Drugs, Development, and Brain Functions*, Smith, W. L., (ed.), Charles C Thomas, Springfield, Ill., 1971, pp. 145–166.
28. Itil, T. M., Saletu, B., Marasa, J., and Mucciardi, A., Presented at the American Psychiatric Association Annual Meeting, May 7–11, 1973, Honolulu, Hawaii.
29. Saletu, B., Itil, T. M., Arat, M., and Akpinar, S., *Int. Pharmacopsychiat.*, 148 (1973).
30. Itil, T. M.. Saletu, B., and Davis, S., *Biol. Psychiat.*, **5**, 1 (1972).
31. Itil, T. M., Hsu, W., Klingenberg, H., Saletu, B., and Gannon, P., *Biol. Psychiat.*, **4**, 3 (1972).
32. Itil, T. M., Hsu, W., Saletu, B., Rudman, S., Saletu, M., Ulett, G., Mednick, S., and Schulsinger, F., Presented at the 126th Annual Meeting of the American Psychiatric Association, May 7–11, 1973, Honolulu, Hawaii.
33. Saletu, B., Saletu, M., Itil, T. M., and Jones, J., *Psychopharmacologia (Berl.)*, **20**, 242 (1971).
34. Saletu, B., Saletu, M., Itil, T. M., and Hsu, W., *Pharmakopsychiat.*, **4**, 158 (1971).
35. Saletu, B., Saletu, M., Itil, T. M., and Marasa, J., *Biol. Psychiat.*, **3**, 299 (1971).
36. Saletu, B., Saletu, M., and Itil, T. M., *Psychopharmacologia (Berl.)*, **24**, 347 (1972).
37. Saletu, B., Itil, T. M., and Saletu, M., *Amer. J. Psychiat.*, **128**, 116 (1971).
38. Vasconetto, C., Floris, B., and Morocutti, C., *Electroencephalog. Clin. Neurophysiol.*, **31**, 77 (1971).
39. Saletu, B., Saletu, M., and Itil, T. M., *Biol. Psychiat.*, **6**, 45 (1973).
40. Pritchard, M., *Brit. J. Psychiat.*, **109**, 572 (1963).

The Phenothiazines and Structurally Related
Drugs, edited by I. S. Forrest, C. J. Carr, and
E. Usdin. Raven Press, N. Y. copyright 1974

Session VI: Discussion

Reporter: G. Simpson

1. *A. Weissman*

I. Forrest: One could speculate that the *cis* form is effective because of
the planarity of the molecule of its first metabolic derivative which, having
given one electron, could fit between two strands of DNA or RNA, but this
may not apply to the *trans* structure.

Q. Lomax: Many of the responses described could be due to peripheral
rather than central effects. What is the correlation between relative potencies
in these tests and clinical effectiveness in psychiatric treatment?

A. To my knowledge, it is quite good.

Q. Buckley: You are not eliminating the central adrenergic blocking action
because the peripheral studies suggest slight peripheral adrenergic blocking
activity?

A. No.

Q. Spirtes: Does thiothixene increase the amount of DOPA in the brain?

A. Yes.

Q. Spirtes: Couldn't this increase be due to a blocking of DOPA entrance into neurons?

A. Possibly.

Q. Spirtes: Did you determine dopamine?

A. Yes, the levels are unchanged after thiothixene.

Q. Spirtes: Since homovanillic acid excretion is increased and DOPA
brain levels are higher, couldn't this indicate a blockage of entrance of DOPA
into the neurons and an increase in dopamine turnover and synthesis?

A. Possibly.

2. *T. A. Ban*

Vinar: We performed several controlled double-blind studies to compare
the clinical efficacy of thioxanthenes with phenothiazines. The patient samples
ranged between 40 to 60 for each drug, and they were schizophrenics in a
broad diagnostic sense. We were interested especially in a comparison of the
thioxanthene derivative with its corresponding phenothiazine drug, i.e., chlorpromazine with chlorprothixene, perphenazine with clopenthixol, fluphenazine with flupenthixol, and thioproperazine with thiothixene. Apart from
other differences in their sedative or other actions, generally, it can be said,
that the thioxanthene derivative always induced less frequent and less intensive extrapyramidal side effects which, interestingly enough, were correlated
with the improvement of depressive symptomatology in patients treated with
thioxanthenes, whereas depression did not improve—or sometimes it was induced—in the patients treated by phenothiazines. We do not think that relationship is due to chance only. In another study which is not yet finished,

we compare fluphenazine decanoate injections with flupenthixol decanoate. It seems, that especially in this maintenance treatment, the absence of depression in patients treated with flupenthixol might be advantageous.

3. *R. L. Dillenkoffer*

Ban: In the early 1960's we studied electrocardiographic changes with neuroleptic phenothiazines and found EKG changes significantly more often with thioridazine than with chlorpromazine or trifluoperazine. Our findings correspond with Dr. Dillenkoffer's data, that the thioridazine-induced EKG changes are dose-related and that they occur in a significant number of patients treated with thioridazine at a dose of 300 mg per day.

4. *H. C. B. Denber*

Gardos: Dr. Denber's data on the Lorr Morbidity Scale seems to show differential effects, namely that on Factor 2, which shows paranoid symptomatology, trifluoperazine produced better results while on Factor 1 and other ratings, thiothixene seemed superior. Delay and Deniker pointed out that thiothixene was particularly effective in hebephrenic patients. In a recently completed study we found that nonparanoid schizophrenics improved more on thiothixene while paranoids improved more on chlorpromazine. I wonder if other investigators looked at the diagnoses of their schizophrenic patients for differential effect with thiothixene. It seems that nonparanoid patients do particularly well on thiothixene.

Kaim: V.A. Cooperative Studies (and the NIMH Collaborative Studies) have, on retrospective analysis, apparently indicated differential effects of different phenothiazines on the several clusters of schizophrenic symptoms. However, prospective V.A. studies have never replicated these differences.

5. *T. M. Itil*

Kulkarni: Both these papers (Itil and Simeon) showed their EEG changes in the following fashion:

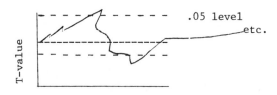

Various frequencies

Although not categorically stated, one gets the impression that there was a greater or smaller change (increase or decrease) obtained with waves of various frequencies.

This is misleading. T-value tells us only the *reliability* of the actual change (and this is not shown at all). The actual magnitude of T-value does not tell us the magnitude of the finding itself.

They should be showing the actual changes and then show which ones are significant depending on the T-value. They could show the T-values for all the changes but the actual changes themselves should appear in the figure.

A. We have been working on this problem for a long time and have published our technique and data-handling procedures which answer this question.

Q. I. Forrest: Has delay in relapse been correlated with prolonged presence of drug metabolites? Perhaps Dr. Weissman would know?

Weissman: All I know is that the half-life is reported as being long, but I do not have this data.

Q. F. Grant: Does thiothixene fulfill the criteria postulated by Janssen for antipsychotic activity?

Kaufman: The postulate is that a 4-atom chain is necessary from the aromatic ring to the alkyl nitrogen. Thiothixene satisfies the criteria.

6. *A. Kiev*

Q. Kline: What was the dosage?

A. Five-mg capsules of each drug.

Q. Simpson: While diagnosis is not a fine art, it can and should be more accurate than this presentation would suggest. I do not know what kind of patients we are talking about. Endogenous or "vital" depressions are not too difficult to diagnose. Were your patients affective disorders or did they show Bleulerian or Schneiderian symptoms? Agitated or involutional melancholic patients responded to amitriptyline in our study and we could not show benefits of thiothixene over this drug. In fact, the trends and the only statistical differences were in favor of the amitriptyline. (The dosage was slightly lower than that used by Doctor Kiev.)

I have seen two agitated depressions this year with severe tardive dyskinesia from their neuroleptic treatment and I would be loathe to prescribe thiothixene or any neuroleptic for this group of patients.

A. They were not schizophrenic patients, they were psychotic depressives.

Gardos: The activating and antidepressant effects of thiothixene have been referred to by most of the speakers. The $64,000 question is how to reconcile these findings with the pharmacologist's report that the drug shows no activity characteristic of tricyclic antidepressants. One clue is provided by Dr. Weissman who mentioned that thiothixene showed weak adrenergic-blocking action. A further important fact is that the antidepressant effect is only seen in the low-dose range. An assumption of dual action may account for these findings. All effective antipsychotics show adrenergic blockade as well as possible amine potentiation in low doses. Thiothixene may show a different ratio of these two actions from the phenothiazines and may, therefore, display more antidepressant effects at low doses before the adrenergic blockade overshadows this effect.

Since antidepressant effect is practically never seen in doses above 30 mg daily of thiothixene, this may account for the contrasting findings of Dr. Denber and Dr. Kiev on depression.

Buckley: Dr. Weissman presented data that thiothixene did not prevent uptake of N.E. Therefore, the antidepressant effects seen at low doses cannot be explained by this mechanism.

7. *J. Simeon*

Winsberg: This report identifies a number of methodological pitfalls in the area of pediatric psychopharmacology. These problems have been well reviewed by Weng, Sprague, and Quoy. Small sample size, subject heterogeneity, e.g., lack of diagnostic specification of subjects, broad range of IQ, and no delineation of pretest behavioral pathology, lack of reliable and validated clinical behavioral measures, and failure to control for order effects render most of the reported results uninterpretable.

Session VII

Specific Chlorpromazine Metabolites

Chairmen: Irene S. Forrest and George J. Cosmides

The Phenothiazines and Structurally Related Drugs, edited by I. S.
Forrest, C. J. Carr, and E. Usdin. Raven Press, New York © 1974.

Phototoxicity and Chlorpromazine Photochemistry

Frederick W. Grant

Research Division, Marcy State Hospital, Marcy, New York 13403

INTRODUCTION

Our premise has been that any understanding of the basic mechanisms
of light-induced pigmentation, allergy, hypersensitivity to burn, ocular
opacity, etc., common in patients receiving phenothiazine therapy, must
incorporate an understanding of the basic photochemistry of these drugs or
their metabolites. In the case of chlorpromazine, generally conceded to be
the chief offender in this area, our knowledge of photodecay mechanisms is
quite meager. In fairness to chlorpromazine, it should be pointed out that
it has been difficult to rank the phenothiazine drugs as to phototoxic effect
when the dosages commonly prescribed in this class vary over a wide range.
Thus, the phototoxicity associated with chlorpromazine has possibly been
exaggerated because of the higher dosage levels common to this therapy.

To our knowledge, Ippen (1) was the first investigator to suggest an intrinsic photolability for chlorpromazine and associated this with an increased
incidence of phototoxic effect. He devised a simple colorimetric test implicating 2-chlorophenothiazine drugs (chlorpromazine, prochlorperazine,
perphenazine, etc.) as especially phototoxic. I am not aware that any attempt has been made to verify this conclusion in a clinical setting. We are
attempting to determine the molecular mechanism of *in vitro* chlorpromazine photodecay with the expectation that this will lead to an increased
understanding of *in vivo* phototoxicity.

The Anaerobic Photochemistry of Chlorpromazine

Huang and Sands (2, 3) appear to be among the few that have made some
effort to establish the end products of chlorpromazine photodecay in contrast to much interest in the radical and charge-transfer species that ac-
company these transformations. Since their results under aerobic conditions
(2) led to anticipated oxidation products difficult to implicate in phototoxic
effects, we turned our attention to their anaerobic study (3). In this instance,
under ultraviolet irradiation at 310 nm in water, promazine and 2-hydroxy-

promazine were identified among a variety of unidentified products. Unchanged chlorpromazine persisted after days of irradiation under these conditions. An increasing accumulation of blue "polymeric" material was observed and implicated as a possible source of drug-related skin pigmentation. The two "identified" photoproducts were presented without comment or inference.

In a recent paper (4) we clarified this anaerobic situation with the following procedural changes: (a) we utilized solar irradiation as more closely approximating the natural environment of the patient; (b) this, together with the use of glass test containers, permitted us to excite chlorpromazine at its 303-nm absorption peak and not at the environmentally less accessible 255-nm peak; and (c) we reduced the chlorpromazine concentration to 0.1 mM to minimize filtering and quenching effects (5). These changes had a dramatic effect on decay rate and product composition. Chlorpromazine was no longer evident after 15 min of irradiation, and promazine and 2-hydroxypromazine were the only organic products formed at this time and in combined quantitative yield. The known unreliability of solar irradiation as a reference standard in photochemical studies did not influence our results over the winter and summer seasons in upstate New York. It had the unexpected result of establishing a temperature dependence of product composition favoring 2-hydroxypromazine over promazine with an increase in temperature.

There are important implications arising from the formation of promazine and 2-hydroxypromazine as primary photodegradation products of chlorpromazine. Photolyses in the presence of alcohols and amines demonstrated that chlorpromazine is subject to photonucleophilic aromatic substitution of chloride ion. Since nucleophiles are associated with carbohydrates, proteins, and nucleic acids, any of these substrates are subject to permanent covalent bonding with photoexcited chlorpromazine and one might logically anticipate a change in biological properties of a toxic nature. Colin Chignell of the National Heart and Lung Institute has established a permanent covalent bonding of chlorpromazine to serum albumin under *in vitro* conditions with light catalysis *(unpublished observations)*, and we know of no other extant mechanism of photocatalyzed drug-protein interaction that can account for this effect other than the photonucleophilic substitution mechanism described here. Photoexcited chlorpromazine is a rare example of a transient hapten which combines with protein to form antigen by mechanisms precisely analogous to the classical studies of Landsteiner (6) with dinitrochlorobenzene.

Although not stressed in our initial paper (4), the formation of promazine as the other primary photodegradation product implies that photoexcited chlorpromazine can function as an oxidizing agent. The photoreduction of chlorpromazine to promazine must be accompanied by the appearance of an oxidized substance not observed among the organic photoproducts. In a recent analogy (7) involving the photoreduction of another phenothiazine—methylene blue—water was established as the reducing agent while being oxidized to hydrogen peroxide. This suggests a role for photoexcited chlorpromazine in promoting melanin deposition and pigmentation at sites of excessive drug accumulation.

Analogous Photolyses of Aryl Halides

Photoreduction and photonucleophilic substitution have been observed in certain aryl halides and, in some instances, act competitively as in the case of chlorpromazine. They are subject to the following influences.

Substituent Effects

Havinga (8) has observed that many heterolytic photosubstitutions are subject to "meta-activation" by substituents that are normally ortho-para activating in their ground states. An increase in temperature is reported to minimize this effect in certain instances. These results were predictable from electron-density calculations of the first excited singlet state.

Solvent Dependence

As expected, a decrease in solvent polarity favors homolytic mechanisms (photoreduction) over heterolytic substitution (9–11), where solvent stabilization of departing halide ion becomes increasingly difficult. Pinhey and Rigby (12) found evidence for radicals in the photolysis of halophenols conducted in pure isopropyl alcohol by isolating pinacol. Halogen has been found to be consistently lost as halide ion rather than as a radical in aqueous media (10).

Nature of the Substituted Halogen

Photoreduction increasingly predominates over photosubstitution in going from aryl chloride to bromide to iodide. This was found to be the case for metachloro- and metabromophenol (9) and has been associated with changes in intersystem crossing efficiency from the singlet to the triplet state (11). The photoreduction of a number of haloquinolines was found to take place efficiently with the bromo derivatives but not at all in the chloro series (13). No photosubstitution was observed in either case.

Influence of Oxygen

The ability of oxygen to act as a radical scavenger or quencher is often used as an indicator of excited triplet or radical involvement in photochemical mechanisms. By this, and other criteria, there appears common agreement that most photosubstitutions in polar or aqueous media involve an excited singlet species. This includes "meta-activated" substitution (8), chlorobenzene photolysis (11), and others. Appropriately, the photolysis of bromoquinolines (13) leading to reduction and no substitution, is quenched by oxygen-implicating triplet or radical intermediates.

Other Mechanistic Considerations

Photoexcitation of electrons to antibonding orbitals may change a ground-state electron donor to an electron acceptor (14). Halides, such as monochloroacetic acid, are also very effective electron scavengers (15). A combination of these properties in photolabile aryl halides suggests that the primary photochemical event from the excited singlet state may be the acceptance of an electron from solvent or other donor forming a transient "radical-anion" which offers a low-energy path for the polarization of the carbon-halogen bond making it susceptible to substitution or elimination as halide ion. The rapidity of these events is illustrated in the photohydrolysis of 5-chlorophenylphosphate (16) which shows no evidence of hydroxide ion attack even in 0.1 N sodium hydroxide. Radical anions have been postulated in a variety of photosubstitution and photoreduction mechanisms (17, 18) and in related reactions (13, 19, 20).

METHODS

We have essentially utilized the techniques described in our previous publication (4). Chlorpromazine at 0.1 to 0.2 mM was exposed to solar irradiation through glass under conditions of pH, solvent polarity, oxygen tension, and in the presence of reducing or oxidizing agents designed to bring chlorpromazine photochemistry within the scope of our present knowledge of aryl halide photolyses as described above. Our results are based on the qualitative or semiquantitative evaluation of photoproducts determined by thin-layer chromatography and chemical or spectroscopic analysis.

For example, promazine and 2-hydroxypromazine were established as photoproducts of the solar irradiation of aqueous solutions of chlorpromazine by the following criteria: (a) the organic photoproducts present immediately after the disappearance of chlorpromazine gave a negative Beilstein test; (b) promazine and 2-hydroxypromazine were identified by comparison of R_f against authentic standards in thin-layer chromatography in three different solvent systems (4); and (c) these assignments were confirmed by ultraviolet spectroscopy (promazine: 252 nm, 302 nm; 2-hydroxypromazine: 250 nm, 307 nm), and visible absorption spectra in 50% aqueous sulfuric acid (promazine: 515 nm; 2-hydroxypromazine: 548 nm). These photoproducts had also been authenticated by Huang and Sands(3) by comparison of infrared spectra with standards.

We have ruled out the possibility that the hydroxylated photoproduct is 1-, 6-, 7-, 8-, or 9-hydroxychlorpromazine, or 3-hydroxypromazine (kindly supplied by Dr. A. Manian of the N.I.M.H.) by the criteria described above.

To minimize the effect of unstable environmental light and temperature, every irradiation was carried out simultaneously with an aqueous deoxygenated chlorpromazine solution. Test results were evaluated against the product composition of this standard.

RESULTS AND DISCUSSION

Ultraviolet Absorption

Aqueous solutions of chlorpromazine selectively absorb ultraviolet irradiation at 255 nm and 303 nm. Since photochemistry and phototoxicity necessarily follow the absorption of light energy, it is important to appreciate that far-ultraviolet irradiation from the sun is effectively filtered out by the ozone layer. We have not been concerned here with the possible photosensitization of the 255-nm absorption maximum by available solar energy. Laboratory studies attempting to relate the light sensitivity of drugs to phototoxicity have often been overzealous in using light sources that cover the entire ultraviolet range, exciting all absorbing peaks, and resulting in a confusing mixture of photoproducts and an unreliable assessment of drug photostability. Our previous study (4) demonstrated that the photodechlorination of chlorpromazine is associated with 303-nm excitation.

Photoexcitation of ground state "basic" electrons to antibonding states often results in differences in polarity between these states. Changes in absorption maxima in solvents of different polarity reflect the compatibility of the excited state in a polar or nonpolar environment. We have observed that the 303-nm peak of chlorpromazine in aqueous media shifts to 310 nm in benzene, indicating that the excited state is less polar than the ground state. This, in turn, is characteristic of localized *n-pi** excitation (21). However, since this type of absorption is normally weaker than the 303-nm maxima observed for chlorpromazine (possibly being a component of a poorly resolved peak), this assignment must be tentative.

Solvent Polarity

Acetone was found to be a suitable water-miscible, nonsensitizing, nonnucleophilic solvent for the study of polarity effects. Fisher spectranalyzed acetone contains 0.3% water which proved sufficient to promote the photodechlorination of chlorpromazine to promazine and 2-hydroxypromazine, however, at about one-third the rate observed in water. Of equal interest was the absence of any profound change in the ratio of photosubstitution to photoreduction that one might have expected in a mixed ionic-radical mechanism. However, oxygen effectively quenched both of these reactions in acetone, but had a barely perceptible inhibiting effect in water. This suggests that photodechlorination may involve an excited triplet state which is very short-lived in water. It seems less likely that solvent is affecting intersystem crossing efficiency, since a change in product composition would be expected.

A new photoproduct was isolated from irradiations in acetone or benzene and identified as 2-chlorophenothiazine. Phenothiazine and trifluoromethylphenothiazine were also found in photolyses of promazine and triflupromazine, respectively.

In nucleophilic solvents such as alcohols, the rate was also decreased as water content was reduced, and photosubstitution was evident in the isolation of 2-hydroxy- and 2-alkoxypromazine, but not at the expense of the photoreduction product. Photosubstitution was remarkably insensitive to any measure of nucleophilicity in mixed aqueous solvents, products being found in proportion to their concentrations. It has not as yet been established whether this is true in less aqueous solvents at reduced photolysis rate.

Oxidizing and Complexing Agents

As pointed out above, oxygen has a slight inhibiting effect on aqueous chlorpromazine photodechlorination suggestive of a nonradical or very short-lived radical mechanism for this reaction. None of the obvious products of chlorpromazine oxidation, such as the sulfoxide or 7-hydroxy derivative, was found under these conditions.

A profound change in photoproduct composition was noted in the presence of silver, mercuric, and ferricyanide ions and in strong acid in an oxygen environment. For instance, photolyses under nitrogen in 1% aqueous mercuric chloride were much slower than in pure water, yielding chlorpromazine sulfoxide as a major product with no evidence of photodechlorination. Since no oxygen was available, the oxygen of the sulfoxide must have arisen from water. Mercuric ion was reduced in this process.

We interpret these results as describing the photodecay mechanism of chlorpromazine in electron-deficient or radical-cation (22) form rather than any oxidation subsequent to photoexcitation. It is reasonable to assume a large activation energy for the loss of chloride ion from such a cation. Photoexcitation could further accentuate this positive charge in the ring system diverting water from nucleophilic substitution of chloride ion to nucleophilic attack at sulfur.

Reducing Agents and Nucleophiles

We have previously observed (4) that nucleophiles such as alcohols and amines are also capable of photosubstituting the chloride ion of chlorpromazine-forming products in proportion to their concentrations. The unimportance of nucleophilic strength in these substitutions is further illustrated by the absence of any noticeable effect on decay rate or product composition in aqueous alcoholic 0.1 N sodium hydroxide. This is reminiscent of the experience of De-Jongh and Havinga (16) with another substrate. The photoexcited species is apparently very reactive and short-lived accepting nucleophiles on a first-come, first-served basis.

Photolyses carried out in the presence of reducing agents such as ascorbic acid, various catechols, and ferrocyanide, were also without effect in favoring photoreduction or in altering the photoproduct profile in any significant way. Since promazine is unavoidably a reduction product, water must be the reducing agent even in the presence of added reducing agents! Apparently the photoexcited species is equally indiscriminate in accepting nucleophiles or electrons. We have not as yet established that water is oxidized to hydrogen peroxide in this reaction although Usui and co-workers (23) have detected hydrogen peroxide during the photoreduction of methylene blue, another phenothiazine.

The potential formation of hydrogen peroxide in surface tissues containing chlorpromazine as a result of light exposure, is a new concept perhaps most directly applicable to pigmentation effects by accelerating the oxidative conversion of DOPA to DOPAquinone and ultimately to melanin.

The high degree of susceptibility of photoexcited chlorpromazine to nucleophiles leads to a rational theory of antigen formation in photoallergy, a point brought out previously (4).

Clearly, much work is required in implicating these laboratory findings in clinical manifestations of chlorpromazine phototoxicity.

SUMMARY

The solar irradiation of aqueous solutions of chlorpromazine results in a very rapid photodechlorination via two pathways—photosubstitution and photoreduction. These pathways are remarkably insensitive to changes in solvent polarity, oxygen, and added nucleophiles suggesting that the photoexcited species is either a singlet or a short-lived triplet. Precedent exists for a subsequent rapid uptake of an electron from water to form a radical-anion which provides a low-energy pathway for the elimination of chloride ion. Since these photoreactions are congenial to physiological conditions of pH, oxygen tension, ionic strength, etc., we suggest photodechlorination as the initiator and molecular basis for many, if not all, of the phototoxic effects experienced by individuals under chlorpromazine therapy. We specifically suggest substitution mechanisms in antigen formation and photoallergy, and the hydrogen peroxide logically accompanying photoreduction as a cause of excessive melanin deposition and pigmentation.

Preliminary evidence points to a different photodecay mechanism for chlorpromazine involved in ground-state charge-transfer complexing.

Chlorpromazine sulfoxide is a prominent photoproduct here and, interestingly, arises not from an oxygenation but from water as a source of oxygen.

REFERENCES

1. Ippen, H., in *Proc. Int. Congress on Photobiology,* 1960, p. 509.
2. Huang, C. L., and Sands, F. L., *J. Chromatogr.,* **13,** 246 (1964).
3. Huang, C. L., and Sands, F. L., *J. Pharm. Sci.,* **56,** 259 (1967).
4. Grant, F. W., and Greene, J., *Toxic. Appl. Pharmacol.,* **23,** 71 (1972).
5. At the suggestion of Prof. E. White, Johns Hopkins University.
6. Landsteiner, K., *The Specificity of Serological Reactions,* 2nd ed., Harvard Univ. Press, Cambridge, Mass., 1945.
7. Somer, G., and Green, M. E., *Photochem. Photobiol.,* **17,** 179 (1973).
8. Havinga, E., and Kronenberg, M. E., *Pure Appl. Chem.,* **16,** 137 (1968).
9. Pinhey, J. T., and Rigby, R. D. G., *Tetr. Letters,* 1271 (1969).
10. Omura, K., and Matsuura, T., *Chem. Comm.,* 1394 (1969).
11. Robinson, G. E. and Vernon, J. M., *J. Chem. Soc. (C),* 3363 (1971).
12. Pinhey, J. T., and Rigby, R. D. G., *Tetr. Letters,* 1267 (1969).
13. Parkanyi, C., and Lee, Y. J., *Abstr. 165th Am. Chem. Soc. Mtg.,* Dallas, Texas, April, 1973, Organic Div., paper No. 11.
14. McCall, M. T., Hammond, G. S., Yonemitsu, O., and Witkop, B., *J. Am. Chem. Soc.,* **92,** 6991 (1970).
15. Ayscough, P. B., Collins, R. G., and Dainton, F. S., *Nature,* **205,** 965 (1965).
16. De-Jongh, R. O., and Havinga, E., *Rec. Trav. chim.,* **87,** 1318 (1968).
17. Nasielski, J., Kirsch-Demesmae, A., Kirsch, P., Nasielski-Hinke, R., *Chem. Comm.,* 302 (1970).
18. Tosa, T., Pac, C., and Sakurai, H., *Tetr. Letters,* 3635 (1969).
19. Van-Vliet, A., Cornelisse, J., and Havinga, E., *Rec. Trav. chim.,* **88,** 1339 (1969).
20. Yonemitsu, O., Nakai, H., Okuno, Y., Naruto, S., Hemmi, K., and Witkop, B., *Photochem. Photobiol.,* **15,** 509 (1972).
21. Dyer, J. R., *Applications of Absorption Spectroscopy of Organic Compounds,* Prentice-Hall Inc., Englewood Cliffs, N.J., 1965, p. 8.
22. Piette, L. H., and Forrest, I. S., *Biochim. Biophys. Acta,* **57,** 419 (1962).
23. Usui, Y., and Koizumi, M., *Bull. Chem. Soc. Japan,* **34,** 1651 (1961).

The Phenothiazines and Structurally Related Drugs, edited by I. S. Forrest, C. J. Carr, and E. Usdin. Raven Press, New York © 1974.

Activation of L-Amino Acid Oxidase by Phenothiazines: Thermodynamic and Physical Chemical Studies

D. V. Siva Sankar, Barry Fireman, Joel Littman, and M. V. Subba Rao

Division of Research Laboratories, Queens Children's Hospital, Bellerose, New York 11426

INTRODUCTION

Chlorpromazine is unique in its ability to inhibit many diverse metabolic, molecular, and membrane reactions (1). This is probably due to the resemblance between the flavin (alloxazine) and phenothiazine rings, even though inhibition of NAD^+-dependent enzymes by phenothiazines may invoke analogy with the purine ring systems as well.

We have previously reported (1) on the oxygen-dependent activation of L-amino acid oxidase by chlorpromazine (CPZ). Gabay and Harris (2) have reviewed the inhibitory effect of phenothiazines on D-amino acid oxidase. The importance of our present work lies in the areas of the action of CPZ and also of the mechanism of action of amino acid oxidases. Our previous findings show that the substrate inhibition by L-leucine of the enzyme decreases as the partial pressure of oxygen increases, and that the specific effect of CPZ in enhancing oxygen uptake increases with increasing oxygen tension. These data implicate an effect of CPZ in making the function of oxygen more effective and of oxygen in rendering the specific effect of CPZ larger.

The work from the laboratories of Gabay (2), Yagi (3), and their associates shows that the inhibition of D-amino acid oxidase [D-AAO, D-amino acid: O_2 oxidoreductase (deaminating) E.C. 1.4.3.3] by CPZ was construed as competitive with the flavin adenine dinucleotide (FAD) using mixtures of FAD and purified apoenzyme. However, the fact that FAD does not dissociate from the enzyme in the course of the reaction with CPZ (see below) eliminates the binding of CPZ at the same site as FAD. The reaction

$$(E\text{-FAD}) + CPZ \rightleftharpoons (E\text{-CPZ}) + FAD,$$

does not occur. While

$$(E\text{-}FAD) + CPZ \rightleftharpoons (E\underset{FAD)}{\overset{CPZ)}{\diagup\diagdown}} \quad \text{may occur.}$$

The work of Kunio Yagi (3) and his associates shows the following reaction in the formation of a purple complex on reacting neutral amino acids with D-AAO.

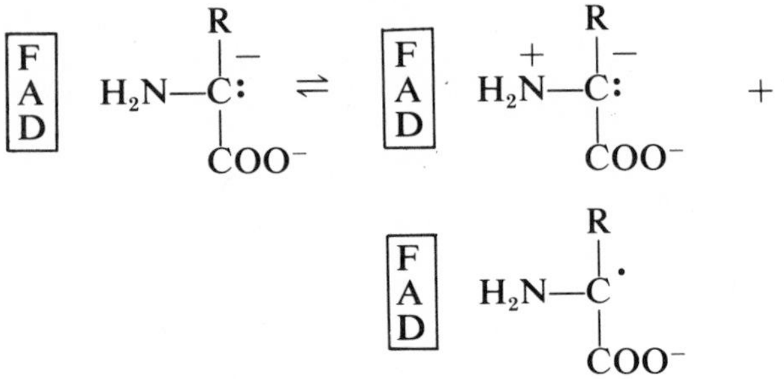

$$\boxed{\begin{matrix}F\\A\\D\end{matrix}}\ \ H_2N{-}\overset{\overset{R}{|}}{\underset{\underset{COO^-}{|}}{C}}\!\!:^{-} \ \rightleftharpoons\ \boxed{\begin{matrix}F\\A\\D\end{matrix}}\ \ \overset{+}{H_2N}{-}\overset{\overset{R}{|}}{\underset{\underset{COO^-}{|}}{C}}\!\!:^{-} \ +$$

$$\boxed{\begin{matrix}F\\A\\D\end{matrix}}\ \ H_2N{-}\overset{\overset{R}{|}}{\underset{\underset{COO^-}{|}}{C}}\!\!\cdot$$

They support the concept of an α, β unsaturated enamine intermediate not being formed (4). There are still other reports (5–8) that have to be justified in mechanistic terms. In the work on characterization of the borohydride-reduced (E-S) complex between D-AAO and D-alanine, Hellerman and Coffey (5) implicated the epsilon-amino group on lysine in the enzyme as the site of combination of D-AAO with D-alanine. On the other hand the work of Page and VanEtten (6, 7) suggests a histidyl group as the most likely active center in L-amino acid oxidase action. In a recent and interesting finding from Massey's group (8) the product of the action of D-AAO on α-amino-β-chlorobutyrate was α-ketobutyrate but not α-keto-β-chlorobutyrate. This finding suggests an early formation of an enamine with protonation on the enzyme to form an amino acid, which is then released and further hydrolyzed into α-ketobutyrate. The relative extent to which enamine protonation and release occur is temperature dependent.

A few other findings are also relevant to our present study on the action of phenothiazines on L-amino acid oxidase from *Crotalus adamanteus*. The enzyme from *Neurospora crassa* (9) also is subject to substrate inhibition. In a study on the inhibitory site on Na⁻ and K-activated ATPase, Tai, and Brody (10) reported that chlorpromazine per se affected neither free −SH concentration nor enzymatic activity, while the free radical of CPZ inhibited this enzyme by interacting with the −SH groups. Again, it was not CPZ, but its sulfoxide that competitively inhibited (11) lipoamide dehydrogenase (not the transhydrogenase or diaphorase) activity. In keeping with our concept that CPZ may bind with L-AAO on a site different from FAD, but still capable of affecting the reductive conformational change, Segatchian (12) found the interaction between CPZ and aldolase (an enzyme with lysine as active center) to be associated with quenching of aldolase fluorescence emission and other spectral changes.

Finally, Horowitz (13) showed in 1965 that in *Neurospora crassa* mutants, there is a common control for tyrosine oxidase and L-AAO, using L-phenylalanine as a substrate. This may suggest location of these two enzymes on the same operon. The value of this finding in human genetics in terms of the epidemiology of PKU, tyrosinosis, albinism, etc. and of maple-syrup-urine disease is worth exploring.

MATERIALS AND METHODS

The L-amino acid oxidase was obtained from Sigma Chemical Co. The chlorpromazine was a gift from Smith Kline and French, Philadelphia, Penn. L-Leucine and all other chemicals used were of reagent grade. The different mixtures of oxygen and nitrogen were obtained as cylinders from Matheson Co., New York.

L-Amino acid oxidase activity was determined manometrically in a Warburg apparatus at 38°C with the use of air or different oxygen tensions as the gas phase. The center well contained 0.2 ml of 20% KOH. The main compartment of the flask contained 0.1 ml of 0.3 M buffer (varying type and pH). Varying amounts of amino acids as substrates, and varying amounts of chlorpromazine (CPZ) were also in the main compartment. The side arm contained crude or purified enzyme dissolved in 0.02 M K-PO$_4$ buffer of pH suitable to the experiment being carried out. The total volume was brought to 2.2 ml with distilled water.

Different oxygen tensions were fed into the vessel during the 15-min temperature equilibration through the manometer escape vent. The system was closed off after equilibration. (Where oxygen was flushed into the system, the fluid pressure in the flask was adjusted to a reading of 150 mm in the closed side of the manometer through the use of a hypodermic syringe through the stopcock exhaust.) The flasks were tipped after a 10- to 15-min equilibration period and readings (started 1 to 10 min later) were taken at 10-min intervals for 30 min.

Spectral studies in the visible range were carried out with a Beckman spectrophotometer DU model 2400. Each microcuvette contained purified enzyme, CPZ (1 mM), amino acid (10 mM), 0.2 ml of K-PO$_4$ buffer (pH 7.0), and additional water to make the final volume equal to 0.6 ml. One-hundred percent nitrogen was bubbled into each microcuvette. This was followed by the addition of a thin layer of isooctane (0.1 ml) to each microcuvette to keep changes in the oxygen tension level minimal. The enzyme, substrate, CPZ, and oxygen were added sequentially (a reading was taken 10 sec after each addition) in different orders and combinations.

Methylene blue studies were conducted in Thunberg tubes in the following manner: each lower portion of the vessel contained 0.2 ml of 10 mg % methylene blue, 0.2 ml pH 8.0, 0.3 M K-PO$_4$ buffer, 1 to 50 mM of L-leu, 0–1 mM CPZ and distilled water to bring the total volume to 1.0 ml. The upper portion of the vessel contained the enzyme. The vessel was evacuated of oxygen through the exhaust vent. At the same time 100% N$_2$ was fed into the vessel through a Y tube. After the oxygen level was brought to 0% in the vessel, the system was closed off. The upper and lower contents were mixed and put into a 37°C water bath. The time required for decolorization was noted.

The gram atoms and/or gram moles of oxygen were calculated from gas laws. The K_s value for L-leucine was obtained from the Michaelis-Menten equation at levels where there was no substrate inhibition using the Lineweaver-Burk plots. The K'_s, representing the substrate inhibition constant, was obtained from a plot of $1/v$ versus S, using the equation (14)

$$\frac{1}{v} = \frac{1}{V} + \frac{S}{K'_s V}.$$

The K_{O_2} values are obtained from a plot of $1/v$ versus $1/(O_2)$ at different concentrations of L-leucine and of CPZ. The intercept of the plots on the X-axis was considered as $-1/(K_{O_2})$. The mean K_{O_2} for different levels of L-leu and a given level of CPZ was computed. The Q_{10} for 18°C, 27°C, and 37°C was calculated from the equation shown below, using the ratios of velocities instead of the ratios of rate constants. The Arrhenius plots were made according to Dixon and Webb (14). E'_a, which is really the apparent energy of activation, is the sum (or the difference) between the energy of activation and inhibition.

$$\mathrm{Log}\ Q_{10} = \frac{10}{T_2 - T_1} \times \log \frac{k_2}{k_1},$$

$$E_a = \frac{4.575(T_1 T_2)}{T_2 - T_1} \times \log \frac{k_2}{k_1}.$$

RESULTS

The results of this investigation are presented in Tables 1 through 5 and Figs. 1 through 7. DL-Alanine does not display inhibition of D-AAO at 37°C and with oxygen as electron acceptor, but if methylene blue is used as an electron acceptor, DL-alanine does begin to inhibit the enzyme at higher substrate concentrations (cf. Table 1). Further in this non-oxygen system, CPZ also inhibits the enzyme. The findings show that the time required for decolorization of methylene blue increases continuously with the concentration of DL-alanine increasing from 9.0 to 180.0 mM in the vessels without CPZ. But in the experiments with CPZ (while CPZ itself is inhibiting at a

TABLE 1. *Effect of varying concentrations of* DL-*alanine and of chlorpromazine on the oxidation of* DL-*alanine by* D-*amino acid oxidase*

DL-alanine conc. (mM)	Time (in min) required for decolorization with chlorpromazine at a concentration of:			
	0.0 M	1.2×10^{-3} M	7.2×10^{-3} M	14.4×10^{-3} M
9.0	7.61	12.13	28.00	40.90
18.0	8.00	9.20	19.08	34.00
54.0	9.40	11.40	18.75	25.00
90.0	11.70	12.58	24.00	26.00
180.0	13.45	16.40	27.08	31.60

Each lower portion of the vessel contained 0.2 ml of 10 mg % methylene blue, 0.2 ml pH 8.0, 0.3 M K-PO_4 buffer, varying amounts of 0.3 M DL-alanine and varying amounts of CPZ. L-amino acid oxidase (250 μg) was used per vessel, which is equal to 0.5 units per vessel. Methylene blue was used as the electron acceptor in Thunberg tubes.

TABLE 2. *The relationship of oxygen tension and of chlorpromazine concentration on* V_1 *and* V_2^a *for the oxidation of* L-*leucine by* L-*amino acid oxidase*

PO$_2$ mm Hg	CPZ concentration							
	0.00 mM		15 mM		25 mM		40 mM	
	V_1	V_2	V_1	V_2	V_1	V_2	V_1	V_2
38	3.7	3.62	—	5.0	15.4	8.0	24.8	8.4
76	3.78	3.0	8.0	3.7	12.5	4.1	22.2	7.4
228	6.7	4.0	12.5	5.85	16.6	8.0	22.2	22.2
570	18.2	18.2	25.0	25.0	28.6	28.6	66.0	66.0

[a] Representing maximum velocities disregarding substrate inhibition (V_1), and from intercept on Y-axis with substrate inhibition (V_2).

TABLE 3. *Variation of* K_{O_2} *with respect to variation of concentration of chlorpromazine in the oxidation of* L-*leucine by* L-*amino acid oxidase*

CPZ conc. (mM)	K_{O_2} (mm Hg)	
	Mean	Range
0.00	677.3	294–1000
5.0	482.9	312–833
15.0	394.4	294–695
25.0	354.6	185–625

The K_{O_2} values are obtained from different concentrations of substrate L-leucine in each experiment.

given concentration of DL-alanine), the time required at a given concentration of CPZ decreases first, and then increases again. The largest decrease is found at higher concentrations of DL-alanine as the concentration of CPZ

TABLE 4. *Kinetic constants of* L-*AAO with* L-*leu at different temperatures without and with CPZ*

Temperature (°C)	CPZ	K_s	K'_s
18	No	5.4×10^{-3}	30×10^{-3}
	Yes	22×10^{-3}	20×10^{-3}
27	No	4.4×10^{-3}	27×10^{-3}
	Yes	14.0×10^{-3}	20×10^{-3}
37	No	7.1×10^{-3}	3.3×10^{-3}
	Yes	14.3×10^{-3}	1.0×10^{-3}

TABLE 5. E_a *and* Q_{10} *calculated for temperature effects on* L-*AAO with* L-*leu without and with CPZ*

	Q_{10}		$E'_a (E_a - E_i)$ in calories	
	18–27°C	27–37°C	18–27°C	27–37°C
5 mM L-leu	0.23	7.62	-26.19×10^3	3.76×10^4
5 mM L-leu + CPZ	1.62	1.87	8.34×10^3	1.15×10^4
20 mM L-leu	0.39	2.33	-16.33×10^3	1.6×10^4
20 mM L-leu + CPZ	0.83	2.44	-2.06×10^3	2.08×10^4

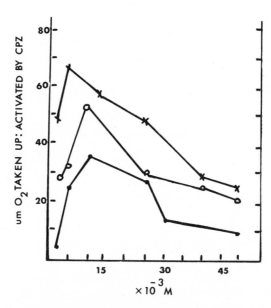

FIG. 1. The activating effect of CPZ on the oxidation of L-leucine (x—x), L-phenylalanine (O—O), and L-methionine (●—●) shown as percentage increase in oxygen over experiments without CPZ. The concentration of CPZ here was 1 millimolar, which explains the relative decrease of the effect of CPZ at higher concentrations of amino acid.

is progressively increased. This may indicate that in D-AAO, there are two sites (i) substrate site and (ii) CPZ (or FAD?) site. The effect of CPZ on substrate site is, as with L-AAO, to inhibit substrate inhibition. The effect of CPZ on the CPZ (or FAD) site in D-AAO is to cause inhibition, whereas with L-AAO, this inhibitory site attachment is not as strong as the effect of CPZ on substrate site.

The results in Table 2 indicate the theoretical maximum velocities with and without substrate inhibition. Thus $(V_1 - V_2)$ will yield an approximation of substrate inhibition. The effect of varying concentration of CPZ and/or of oxygen is also shown. CPZ enhances both V_1 and V_2, although the difference between V_1 and V_2 is still visibly there. On the other hand, the effect of oxygen is to increase V_2 much more than V_1, thus obliterating $(V_1 - V_2)$. The effect of CPZ is overshadowed by higher concentrations of oxygen. The results from Table 3 show that the effect of CPZ on oxygen is to decrease K_{O_2}, thus rendering any possible (E-O$_2$) binding tighter.

The effect of CPZ on the binding of the substrate, L-leucine, by L-AAO is shown in Table 4. K_s refers to the binding at concentrations where there is no substrate inhibition and K'_s to inhibitory binding constant obtained from plots of 1/v versus S. The effect of temperature is also shown. Chlorpromazine increases K_s and decreases K'_s. The ratio of K_s/K'_s undergoes significant change at 37°C under the effect of CPZ. Actually, our unpublished results show that the specific effect of CPZ (1 mM) is maximum at 27°C.

The thermodynamic results are shown in Table 5. Between 18 to 27°C, the Q_{10} values show an increased substrate inhibition, while CPZ rectifies it. Similarly, the apparent E'_a is negative between 18 to 27°C, indicating higher substrate inhibition. The effect of CPZ is to diminish this. As the concentration of L-leucine is raised from 5 to 20 mM, the effect of CPZ decreases. The picture at 27 to 37°C is different. The Q_{10} picks up, showing that enzymatic oxidation increasingly outpaces substrate inhibition. The effect of CPZ, with decreasing substrate inhibition, is less marked.

Figure 1 shows the effect of CPZ on the oxidation of L-leucine, L-phenylalanine, and L-methionine by L-AAO, as percent increase in oxygen uptake. It may be noticed that the activating effect is more pronounced when the amino acid shows more substrate inhibition. The effect of CPZ (1 mM) decreases as the concentration of amino acid increases. Here again, the more potent the substrate inhibition, the lower the concentration of amino acid required, at which the effect of CPZ begins to decrease. This may indicate competition between CPZ and the inhibitory intermediate.

The oxygen uptake (or enzymatic activity) has a pH optimum of approximately 8.0, even in the presence of CPZ (cf. Fig. 2). At this pH, CPZ is not very soluble in aqueous solutions. Previously we (1) showed that the effect of CPZ was not due to increasing the surface area of the enzyme by the fine precipitate. As pointed out before, the effect of CPZ decreases as the oxygen tension increases (cf. Fig. 3). Further, the concentration of L-leucine where

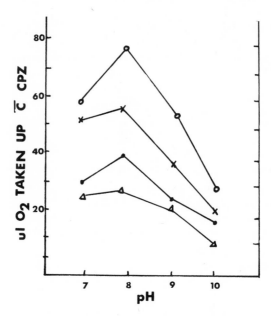

FIG. 2. The activating effect of CPZ on the oxidation of L-AAO as a function of pH. The data shown are percentage increments over experiments without CPZ. The concentration of CPZ was 1 millimolar. The concentrations of L-leucine were —15 mM ($\triangle$—$\triangle$), 25 mM ($\bullet$—$\bullet$), 50 mM (x—x) and 70 mM ($\bigcirc$—$\bigcirc$).

the maximum effect of 1 mM CPZ is shown also increases with oxygen tension. The curve (cf. Fig. 3) reaches a minimum at 30% (or 228 mm Hg) of oxygen tension.

Figure 4 shows the Arrhenius plot at temperatures of 18, 27, and 37°C. As mentioned before, the kinetics change at approximately 27°C. The negative E'_a becomes positive and Q_{10} becomes greater than 1.0. This discontinuity is corrected by CPZ, probably due to its suppression of the inhibitory activity at lower temperatures.

The spectral changes accompanying several alterations of sequential addition of CPZ, AA, and O_2 (bubbling) are shown in Figs. 5–7. The addition of the amino acid brings forth an immediate extinction of the 460 mμ peak. The addition of oxygen restores it. The effect of CPZ is also qualitatively similar to that of oxygen. The effect of CPZ is most pronounced when added to a system already containing enzyme, amino acid, and oxygen.

DISCUSSION

The activating effect of CPZ on L-AAO is in sharp contrast to its inhibitory activity on D-AAO. The experiments in Table 1 indicate that although CPZ is inhibitory to D-AAO, it does protect it partially from substrate inhibition. This may indicate that the action of CPZ is twofold in D-AAO, one inhibitory, and the other a suppressing effect on substrate inhibition. This denotes two sites for the action of CPZ. Yet a third site for the action

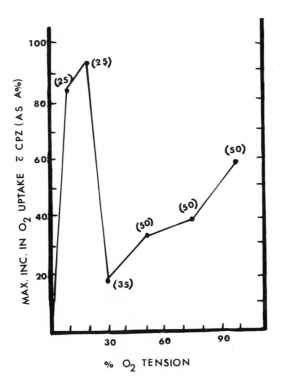

FIG. 3. Maximum increase (as % increase in activity) in oxygen uptake caused by CPZ
$(1 \times 10^{-3}\,\text{M})$ at different oxygen tensions. The values in parentheses indicate the concentration of L-leucine at which the effect of CPZ is maximum at the given percentage of oxygen in the Warburg flask.

of CPZ is indicated in its effect on decreasing K_{O_2} and in its decreasing
activity with increasing oxygen tension.

Thus there are three sites of action for CPZ. These sites may be:

(i) Site responsible for formation of

$$(\text{E-FAD}) + \text{AA} \rightleftharpoons \text{E} \begin{matrix} \nearrow \text{FADH} \\ \searrow \text{IA}^* \end{matrix}$$

$$(\text{ii}) \left(\text{E} \begin{matrix} \nearrow \text{FADH} \\ \searrow \text{IA}^* \end{matrix} \right) \rightleftharpoons (\text{E-FADH}_2) + \text{IA},$$

and

$$(\text{iii}) \ (\text{E-FADH}_2) + O_2 \rightleftharpoons (\text{E-FAD}) + H_2O_2.$$

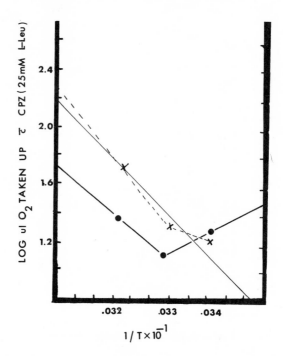

FIG. 4. Arrhenius plot of log velocity (as microliters of oxygen taken up without CPZ (●—●) and with CPZ (x—x). The concentration of L-leucine was 25 mM.

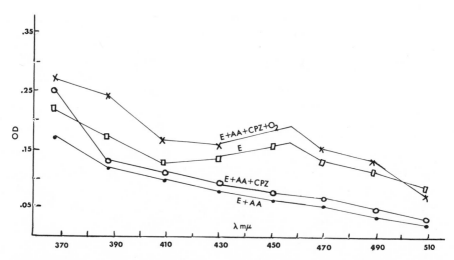

FIG. 5. Spectral changes accompanying addition of several reagents to L-AAO. The sequence of additions to the enzyme at pH 7.0 under oil (anaerobic) was amino acid, CPZ, and bubbling of oxygen.

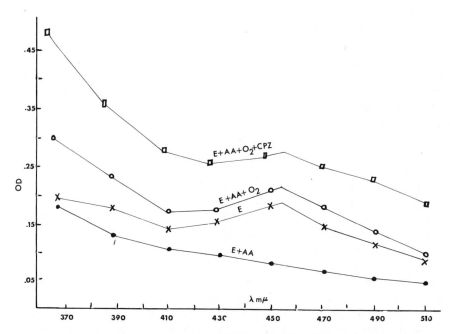

FIG. 6. Spectral changes accompanying addition of several reagents to L-AAO. The sequence of additions to the enzyme at pH 7.0 was amino acid, bubbling of oxygen, and CPZ.

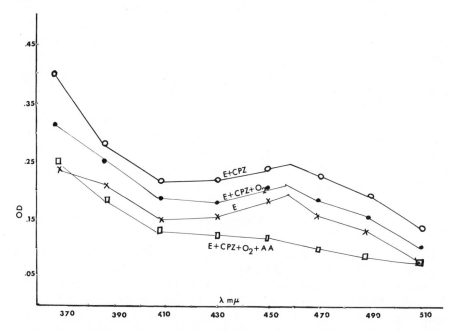

FIG. 7. Spectral changes accompanying addition of several reagents to L-AAO. The sequence of additions to the enzyme at pH 7.0 was CPZ, bubbling of oxygen, and amino acid.

On the other hand, the three sites may be commonly related, with CPZ inhibiting (ii) only and thus effecting (i) and (iii).

Massey and Curti (15) have proposed an essentially similar mechanism for the action of the D- and L-amino acid oxidase. They suggested that the most important difference between the two enzymes is in the rate of formation of the fully reduced enzyme with inhibitory activity. Our present data support a basic hypothesis of this type and also the formation of a ternary complex between (E-FAD), AA, and oxygen (16).

Chlorpromazine may inhibit the formation of both (E-FADH) and (E-FADH$_2$) complexes. Its competition with the formation of (E-FADH$_2$) complex is responsible for its activating effect on L-AAO. At a lower temperature, the reaction between (E-FADH$_2$) and oxygen is less pronounced, leading to a more pronounced accumulation of (E-FADH$_2$). This is the case at lower partial pressures of oxygen also. CPZ probably inhibits formation of (E-FADH$_2$) and renders the oxygen available for oxidation of (E-FADH).

The K_{O_2} values vary with the concentration of the amino acid and CPZ. The fact that this enzyme has an oxygen-dependent substrate inhibition along with its microheterogeneity (17) may suggest that this enzyme may control the availability of keto acids in the tissue milieu by undergoing self-regulation. In the presence of oxygen, more oxidation takes place with release of the (chemically) highly active keto acids, which should be immediately metabolized.

The question of identification of the type of complexes formed and the stage at which these are formed is difficult to answer at present. The evidence that points out the involvement of lysine and histidine as active centers can certainly indicate a ternary complex. The question also remains (1) whether there is formation of a free radical of chlorpromazine which seems to prevent formation of (E-FADH$_2$) and admit oxygen to oxidize (E-FADH). The partial pressure of oxygen has also been found (18) to be important in the oxidation of β-chloroalanine by D-AAO to chloropyruvate or pyruvate. The effect of CPZ on the oxidation of β-chloroleucine is worth studying. Further, chlorpromazine has one double bond between the center ring and the substituted phenyl ring and as such may compete more with FADH$_2$ than FADH.

SUMMARY

Chlorpromazine activates L-amino acid oxidase while it inhibits D-amino acid oxidase. The more effective the inhibition of L-AAO is by substrate, the more effective is the action of CPZ under aerobic conditions. The higher the partial pressure of oxygen, the lower the specific effect of CPZ. Under anaerobic conditions, when DL-alanine inhibits D-AAO, CPZ has two apparent effects—one of enzyme inhibition, and the other of partial suppression of substrate inhibition.

The effect of temperature of reaction at a given oxygen tension indicates more substrate inhibition at lower temperatures, and more effectiveness of CPZ in reversing this inhibition. Oxygen tends to enhance and obliterate the difference between theoretical maximum velocities, whereas CPZ enhances both. The concept that CPZ complexes with a ternary complex of $\{(E\text{-}FAD_r) + AA + O_2\}$ is advanced where $FADH_2$ as the reduced form (FAD_r) is more analogous to chlorpromazine. Some preliminary spectral data are reported.

ACKNOWLEDGMENTS

Parts of this chapter are abstracted from theses submitted by Fireman and Littman to the Biology Department of Long Island University. The authors wish to thank Mr. Robert Goldman and Miss Roberta Hiat for technical assistance in parts of this work, and Drs. Lauretta Bender and Gloria Faretra for their interest in the progress of this work.

REFERENCES

1. Sankar, D. V. S., and Fireman, B. I., *Res. Comm. Chem. Path. and Pharm.*, 1, 288 (1970).
2. Gabay, S., and Harris, S. R., in *Topics in Medicinal Chemistry*, Rabinowitz, J. L., and Myerson, R. M. (eds.), Vol. 3, Wiley, New York, 1970, p. 57.
3. Yagi, K., in *Advances in Enzymology*, 34, Nord, F. F. (ed.), Wiley, New York, 1971, p. 41.
4. Porter, D. J. T., and Bright, H. J., *Biochem. Biophys. Res. Commun.*, 36, 209 (1969).
5. Hellerman, L., and Coffey, D. S., *J. Biol. Chem.*, 242, 582 (1967).
6. Page, D. S., and VanEtten, R. L., *Biochim. Biophys. Acta*, 191, 38 (1969).
7. Page, D. S., and VanEtten, R. L., *Biochim. Biophys. Acta*, 191, 190 (1969).
8. Walsh, C. T., Krodel, E., Massey, V., and Abeles, R. H., *J. Biol. Chem.*, 248, 1946 (1973).
9. Luppa, D., and Aurich, H., *Acta Biol. Med.*, 27, 839 (1971).
10. Brody, T. M., *Mol. Pharmacol.*, 6, 557 (1970).
11. Millard, S. A., *Biochim. Biophys. Acta*, 216, 439 (1970).
12. Seghatchian, M. J., *Biochem. Pharmacol.*, 20, 683 (1971).
13. Horowitz, N. H., *Biochem. Biophys. Res. Commun.*, 18, 686 (1965).
14. Dixon, M., and Webb, E. C., *Enzymes*, Academic Press, New York, 1964.
15. Massey, V., and Curti, B., in *Flavins Flavoproteins, Proc. Conf. 2nd*, Yagi, K. (ed.), Univ. Tokyo Press, Tokyo, Japan, 1967.
16. Massey, V., and Curti, B., *J. Biol. Chem.*, 242, 1259 (1967).
17. Hayes, M. B., and Wellner, D., *J. Biol. Chem.*, 244, 6636 (1969).
18. Walsh, C. T., Schonbrunn, A., and Abeles, R. H., *J. Biol. Chem.*, 246, 6855 (1971).

The Phenothiazines and Structurally Related Drugs, edited by I. S.
Forrest, C. J. Carr, and E. Usdin. Raven Press, New York © 1974.

Hydroxylation of 7-Hydroxychlor-promazine by Mushroom Tyrosinase

Thomas A. Grover, Lawrence H. Piette, and Albert A. Manian*

*Department of Biochemistry and Biophysics, School of Medicine, University of Hawaii,
Honolulu, Hawaii 96822, and *Pharmacology Section, Psychopharmacology Research
Branch, National Institute of Mental Health, Rockville, Maryland 20852*

INTRODUCTION

In previous studies (1, 2), evidence suggests that hydroxy metabolites of chlorpromazine (CPZ) may be of importance in mediating the various physiological responses observed with CPZ therapy. Thus, in a series of pharmacological and behavioral tests (1) 7-hydroxychlorpromazine (7-HO-CPZ) possessed activity similar to its parent compound, CPZ, and recently was shown to appear in the central nervous system of experimental animals (2). We are in the process of studying the influence of particular hydroxy derivatives of CPZ on the activity of tyrosine hydroxylase to better understand the influence CPZ has on catecholamine levels in the brain. This report deals with preliminary experiments in which mushroom tyrosinase was used as a model system in preparation for subsequent experiments with tyrosine hydroxylase.

Mushroom tyrosinase catalyzes the hydroxylation of 7-HO-CPZ to 7,8-diHO-CPZ and 3-hydroxypromazine (3-HO-Pr) to 2,3-diHO-Pr. 8-Hydroxychlorpromazine and 2-HO-Pr are not converted to their dihydroxy derivatives by this enzyme. Evidence for the formation of the dihydroxy derivatives was obtained by monitoring changes in optical absorption at 300 nm and 510 nm, by differences in the electron spin resonance (ESR) spectra of acid-oxidized samples of the mono- and dihydroxy derivatives, and by product identification by thin-layer silica gel chromatography.

EXPERIMENTAL

Materials

Mushroom tyrosinase grade III was purchased from Sigma and used without further purification. CPZ was generously provided by Dr. R. Hoppe of Smith, Kline and French. The hydroxy derivatives of CPZ and promazine used in this study were obtained from the Psychopharmacology Research

Branch, N.I.M.H. 6,7-Dimethyl-5,6,7,8-tetrahydropterine, B grade, was obtained from Calbiochem and L-tyrosine-3,5-^{3}H (29 Ci/mM) from New England Nuclear. Ultraviolet (U.V.) and visible spectra were recorded on a Perkin-Elmer 202 spectrophotometer. A Varian E-4 was used to obtain ESR spectra and counting measurements were performed on a Packard Tri-Carb spectrometer.

Kinetic Assay

The influence of hydroxy derivatives of CPZ and promazine on the rate of conversion of tyrosine to DOPA by tyrosinase was studied by following the rate of tritium release as water from L-tyrosine-3,5-^{3}H (3, 4). Standard reaction mixtures contained, per tube, phosphate buffer, pH 6.5, 50 μmole; L-tyrosine-3,5-^{3}H, 4.4 $\times$ 10^6 dpm, 0.1 to 1.0 μmole; L-dopa, 0.025 μmole; phenothiazine derivative when indicated, 0.01 to 0.1 μmole; enzyme, 10 units; volume 1.01 ml. The reactions were started with enzyme and incubated in the air with shaking for 15 min at 37°C. Following incubation, reactions were terminated immediately. Tritiated water was separated and counted using the methods employed by Pomerantz (3).

Thin-Layer Chromatography

Samples of the compounds to be chromatographed were spotted on Eastman silica gel sheets (6060) in the dark with nitrogen purging and developed using a mixture of chloroform-acetone-diethylamine (87:10:3) (5).

METHODS AND RESULTS

Optical Evidence

The U.V. spectra in Fig. 1 show the changes that occur in absorption during the tyrosinase-catalyzed oxidation of 7-HO-CPZ. The increase in absorption at 300 nm is significant and most probably represents the formation of the quinone of 7,8-diHO-CPZ, since authentic 7,8-diHO-CPZ shows a spectrum identical to that in curve C when oxidized to its quinone and substituted into the assay mixture for 7-HO-CPZ. The shift in the peak occurring at 250 nm to longer wavelength is also evidence for the conversion of 7-HO-CPZ to 7,8-diHO-CPZ (Fig. 2). These changes do not occur in the absence of enzyme and/or hydrogen donor (pterine). Visible evidence for this conversion develops as the reaction proceeds in the form of a red coloration of the assay medium. This change can be monitored at 510 nm and is identical to the visible absorption that occurs when authentic 7,8-diHO-CPZ is oxidized in air to its quinone form (the hydroquinone of 7,8-diHO-CPZ has no visible absorption). This quinone is easily reduced to its hydroquinone form as shown in Fig. 3.

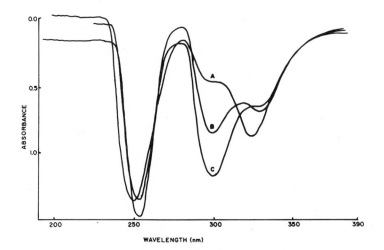

FIG. 1. Course of tyrosinase: 7-HO-CPZ reaction. The sample cuvette contained 7-HO-CPZ (1 μmole), tyrosinase (200 units), pterine (1 μmole), and phosphate buffer (0.4 μmole, pH 6.5) in a volume of 3 ml. The reference cuvette was identical except 7-HO-CPZ was omitted. Temperature was 22°C, (A) spectrum at start of reaction, (B) spectrum after 2 min of reaction, (C) spectrum at end of reaction.

With the observation that the quinone of 7,8-diHO-CPZ forms spontaneously in air, the question arises as to the participation of tyrosinase in this oxidation. A comparison of the rates of oxidation of 7,8-diHO-CPZ in the presence and absence of tyrosinase is shown in Table 1. The increases in rate observed with the addition of enzyme make it apparent that tyrosinase is capable of catalyzing this oxidation. Evidence for the oxidation of 3-HO-

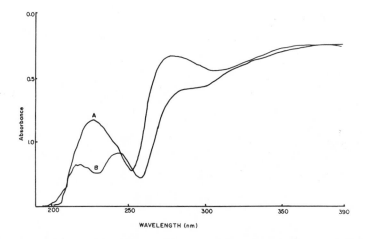

FIG. 2. U.V. spectra of (A) 7-HO-CPZ (3×10^{-5} M) and (B) 7,8-diHO-CPZ (5×10^{-5} M) in water.

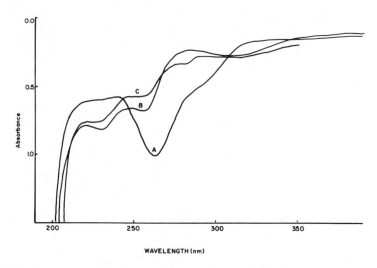

FIG. 3. U.V. spectra of reduced and oxidized forms of 7,8-diHO-CPZ (3×10^{-5} M) in water: (A) O_2 oxidized, (B) N_2 saturated water, (C) sample in (A) following reduction with zinc and HCl.

TABLE 1. *Comparison of spontaneous and tyrosinase catalyzed oxidation of 7-8-diHO-CPZ*

Conditions	Rate of oxidation (change in absorbance @ 510 nm/sec)
O_2 sat. buffer	2.6×10^{-3}
O_2 + 50 units tyrosinase	4.0×10^{-3}
O_2 + 100 units tyrosinase	5.4×10^{-3}
O_2 + 200 units tyrosinase	9.8×10^{-3}
O_2 + 1.3×10^{-4} M DOPA	2.5×10^{-3}
O_2 + ht. denatured tyrosinase	2.6×10^{-3}

7,8-diHO-CPZ concentration at start of oxidation was 6.6×10^{-5} M. Oxidation was carried out at 22°C in 0.1 M phosphate buffer, pH 6.5.

Pr to 2,3-diHO-Pr is identical to that presented for 7-HO-CPZ. When 8-HO-CPZ or 2-HO-Pr are used as substrates for tyrosinase, none of the above changes in absorption is observed.

ESR Evidence

All of the phenothiazine derivatives are easily oxidized to their stable semiquinone free-radical form in 50% hydrochloric or sulfuric acid solutions. These semiquinones give very characteristic ESR spectra. The number of lines and complexity of the ESR hyperfine pattern are dependent upon the degree and place of substitution in the phenothiazine ring. Hydroxy substitution in the 7 position of CPZ and in the 3 position of Pr gives ESR spectra lacking resolvable hyperfine lines; this is most likely due to the alteration of the spin density at positions 8 and 2, and the first methylene of the side chain, respectively, the greatest spin density being at the methylene and the 3 and 7 positions after substitution. The spectra of 2-HO-Pr and 8-HO-CPZ are quite rich in hyperfine as are 2,3-diHO-Pr and 7,8-diHO-CPZ. These latter spectra indicate that substitution in the 2 and 8 positions strongly affects the spin density in the side chain. Differences in spectra between the mono- and dihydroxy derivatives can be used qualitatively then to substantiate formation of the dihydroxy derivatives. In Fig. 4, the ESR spectra of acid-oxidized samples of 7-HO-CPZ and 3-HO-Pr are shown. These are typical of those that would be obtained from an enzymatic reaction mixture with tyrosinase at the start of a reaction with either of these compounds as substrates. When spectra are taken following catalysis, they are found to be identical to the dihydroxy model compounds (Fig. 5). If sequential samples are taken during the course of a reaction, a continuous change in spectra from the mono- to the dihydroxy derivative is observed when either 7-HO-CPZ or 3-HO-Pr is a substrate. However, these changes are not evident for the substrates 8-HO-CPZ and 2-HO-Pr.

Thin-Layer Chromatography Evidence

Further evidence for the formation of 7,8-diHO-CPZ from 7-HO-CPZ was obtained with silica-gel thin-layer chromatography, using a mixture of chloroform-acetone-diethylamine (87:10:3) (5) for development. With this

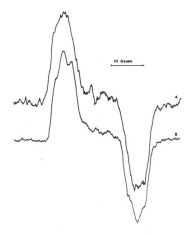

FIG. 4. ESR spectra of acid-oxidized samples of (A) 3-HO-Pr and (B) 7-HO-CPZ at 1×10^{-4} M.

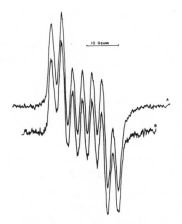

FIG. 5. ESR spectra of acid-oxidized samples of: (A) a sample following reaction of tyrosinase and 7-HO-CPZ under conditions similar to those in Fig. 1, and (B) 7-8-diHO-CPZ (2×10^{-4} M).

system, authentic 7-HO-CPZ and 7,8-diHO-CPZ have R_f values of 0.32 and 0.49 respectively, and samples spotted from a reaction mixture containing tyrosinase and 7-HO-CPZ show spots with similar R_f values of 0.32 and 0.48 confirming the formation of the dihydroxy derivative.

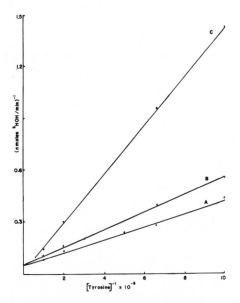

FIG. 6. Reciprocal plot showing inhibition of the conversion of L-tyrosine-3,5-^{3}H to DOPA by tyrosinase: (A) without 7-HO-CPZ, (B) with 1×10^{-5} M 7-HO-CPZ, and (C) with 1×10^{-4} M 7-HO-CPZ.

Kinetics

With the results obtained above demonstrating that 7-HO-CPZ can be oxidized by tyrosinase to 7,8-diHO-CPZ, it became important to study the effect of 7-HO-CPZ on the conversion of tyrosine to DOPA (dihydroxy-phenylalanine) by this enzyme. This conversion is best studied using L-tyrosine-3,5-^{3}H and following the formation of tritiated water, which represents stoichiometrically the amount of DOPA produced (3, 4). Results obtained using this assay procedure suggest that 7-HO-CPZ is a strong competitive inhibitor of tyrosine in this reaction (Fig. 6). 3-Hydroxypro-mazine appears to inhibit the reaction in a similar manner. Chlorpromazine also inhibits this reaction to a significant extent, but doesn't appear to be hydroxylated by tyrosinase. Some inhibition of DOPA formation by 8-HO-CPZ, 2-HO-Pr, and 7,8-diHO-CPZ (quinone) does occur but has not been characterized. In Table 2, a comparison of the relative degree of inhibition of DOPA formation by these compounds is shown.

TABLE 2. *Inhibition of the conversion of -tyrosine-3,5-^{3}H to DOPA by hydroxy derivatives of CPZ and Pr.*

Substrate (1 × 10^{-4} M)	Inhibitor (1 × 10^{-4} M)	Velocity^a (μmoles/min)	% Inhibition
L-Tyrosine	none	1.16 × 10^{-3}	zero
"	CPZ	0.65 × 10^{-3}	44
"	7-HO-CPZ	0.41 × 10^{-3}	65
"	8-HO-CPZ	0.95 × 10^{-3}	18
"	2-HO-Pr	0.96 × 10^{-3}	18
"	3-HO-Pr	0.37 × 10^{-3}	68
"	7,8-diHO-CPZ	0.90 × 10^{-3}	22

^{a} The rate of formation of tritiated water from L-tyrosine-3,5-^{3}H.
Enzyme concentration was 10 units. Duplicate samples were incubated for 15 min at 37°C, pH 6.5.

DISCUSSION

Mushroom tyrosinase is notably less specific than mammalian tyrosinases and tyrosine hydroxylase in its selection of substrates; however, the results reported here support the mechanism for enzymatic hydroxylation of 7-HO-CPZ and 3-HO-PR to 7,8-diHO-CPZ and 2,3-diHO-Pr, respectively. They further demonstrate that dihydroxylation can only take place after the 3 position of Pr or the 7 position of CPZ are first substituted. Hydroxy substitution first in the 2 (Pr) or 8 (CPZ) position precludes further hydroxylation to the dihydroxy derivatives; thus a mechanism such as is the most likely one for dihydroxylation and eventual quinone formation.

7-Hydroxychlorpromazine inhibition of the conversion of tyrosine to DOPA by mushroom tyrosinase appears to be strongly competitive and adds further to existing evidence (1, 2, 6) suggesting a role for this metabolite in mediating some of the diverse effects observed with CPZ.

A possible explanation for a relatively rare but significant side effect of prolonged CPZ therapy, hyperpigmentation, emerges from the results presented in this report. In a few patients (1 to 2%) this side effect manifests itself as the development of purple-grey or blue-black pigmentation of areas of the skin exposed to sunlight. In addition, many other patients (25%) develop corneal and lens opacities. These same patients excrete abnormally high amounts of unconjugated 7-HO-CPZ in their urine (6). Various reports have appeared suggesting this hyperpigmentation may result from light-induced formation of polymers of CPZ (7, 8) or 7-HO-CPZ (6) or may represent the formation of charge-transfer complexes between CPZ or 7-HO-CPZ and melanin (9, 10). From the results reported here an alternative explanation emerges. Tyrosinase ordinarily exists in the skin in an inhibited state that is activated by sunlight, and most polyhydroxyphenyl compounds with ortho or para groups can be oxidized to pigmented polymers. We propose that in patients with high levels of circulating 7-HO-CPZ, upon exposure to sunlight, tyrosinase is activated and forms first 7,8-diHO-CPZ followed by its quinone, which, in the manner of DOPA-quinone, would be expected spontaneously to form "melanin-like" polymers or copolymers with DOPA-quinone. Since the quinone of 7,8-diHO-CPZ is highly colored (deep red at pH 6.5), a polymer of this compound would also be expected to be colored, which may explain the abnormal pigmentation observed with some patients exposed to long-term CPZ therapy.

SUMMARY

The ability of mushroom tyrosinase to catalyze the hydroxylation of particular hydroxy derivatives of chlorpromazine (CPZ) and promazine (Pr) was tested. 7-Hydroxychlorpromazine and 3-HO-Pr were converted to 7,8-diHO-CPZ and 2,3-diHO-Pr, respectively, whereas 8-HO-CPZ and 2-HO-Pr proved to be unusable substrates for the enzyme. The oxidation of 7,8-diHO-CPZ to its orthoquinone was also shown to be catalyzed by tyrosinase. Kinetic studies of the conversion of tyrosine to DOPA by this enzyme demonstrated that 7-HO-CPZ was a strong competitive inhibitor. An interesting mechanism attempting to explain the occurrence of hyperpigmentation in long-term CPZ users is presented.

ACKNOWLEDGMENT

This work was supported in part by funds from the Psychopharmacology Research Branch, National Institute of Mental Health, under Contract No. HSM–42–71–1.

REFERENCES

1. Manian, A. A., Efron, D. H., and Goldberg, M. E., *Life Sciences,* **4,** 2425 (1965).
2. Manian, A. A., Efron, D. H., and Harris, S. R., *Life Sciences,* **10,** 679 (1971).
3. Pomerantz, S. H., *Biochem. Biophys. Res. Comm.,* **16,** 188 (1964).
4. Nagatsu, T., Levitt, M., and Udenfriend, S., *Anal. Biochem.,* **9,** 122 (1964).
5. Coccia, P. F., and Westerfeld, W. W., *J. Pharmacol. Exp. Ther.,* **157,** 446 (1967).
6. Perry, T. L., Culling, C. F. A., Berry, D., and Hanser, S., *Science,* **146,** 81 (1964).
7. Huang, C., and Sands, F., *J. Pharmaceut. Sci.,* **56,** 259 (1967).
8. van Woert, M. H., *Nature,* **219,** 1054 (1968).
9. Bolt, A. G., and Forrest, I. S., *Life Sciences,* **6,** 1285 (1967).
10. Zelickson, A., *J.A.M.A.,* **194,** 670 (1965).

The Phenothiazines and Structurally Related Drugs, edited by I. S. Forrest, C. J. Carr, and E. Usdin. Raven Press, New York © 1974.

Studies on the Metal Chelation of Chlorpromazine and Its Hydroxylated Metabolites

K. S. Rajan, A. A. Manian,* J. M. Davis,** and A. Skripkus

*IIT Research Institute, Chicago, Illinois 60616, *National Institute of Mental Health, Rockville, Maryland 20852, and **Department of Psychiatry and Pharmacology, Vanderbilt University, Nashville, Tennessee 37023*

INTRODUCTION

Manian et al. (1) have reported that 3-hydroxy and 7-hydroxychlorpromazines show pharmacological activity similar to chlorpromazine (CPZ). The toxic reactions noticed in patients exposed to high dosages of CPZ have been attributed to 7-hydroxychlorpromazine or its metabolites by Perry et al. (2). Studies by Daly and Manian (3) have indicated that 7,8-dioxygenated chlorpromazines are potential toxic metabolites of chlorpromazines. It is felt that the toxic side effects might be obviated by stabilizing the 7-hydroxy- and 7,8-dihydroxychlorpromazines against oxidation through their chelation with appropriate metal ions.

It is known that the interactions of chlorpromazines and related phenothiazines with biogenic amines at the presynaptic and postsynaptic sites may be important for their antipsychotic activity. In view of the co-occurrence of metal ions such as Mg^{2+}, Cu^{2+}, Fe^{2+}, Fe^{3+}, and Zn^{2+} in synaptosomes and the possible importance of metal chelates of biogenic amines and adenosinetriphosphate (ATP) in monoamine binding, storage, and transport (4–7), a knowledge of the metal chelation of phenothiazines and their hydroxylated metabolites becomes necessary for an understanding of their interactions with the monoamines.

Borg and Cotzias (8, 9) studied the reactions of bi- and trivalent metal ions with a number of phenothiazine derivatives. They reported that only the trivalent forms of iron, manganese, and cobalt coordinated with the phenothiazines. They characterized the colored reaction product as a semiquinone radical ion. On the basis of fluorescence, ultraviolet (U.V.), and visible spectral studies, Huang and Gabay (10, 11) reported that the strengths of metal binding of chlorpromazine followed the order, $Fe^{3+} > Cr^{3+} > Cu^{2+} > Ni^{2+} > Co^{2+}$. On the basis of surface tension measurements, Ira Blei (12) found that chlorpromazine interacted with ADP and ATP resulting in the formation of a complex.

The metal chelation characteristics of the hydroxylated phenothiazines have not been investigated. Also, quantitative studies on the metal binding of these compounds in the presence and in the absence of ATP and biogenic amines have not been carried out so far. It is therefore the objective of this research to investigate the metal coordination of the chlorpromazines and promazines in aqueous model systems.

MATERIALS AND METHODS

The interactions of the selected phenothiazines and the metal ions were investigated using model systems. The potentiometric pH method was employed to measure the equilibrium H^+ ion concentrations of the ligands, i.e., the phenothiazines and ATP in the presence and in the absence of equimolar ratios of the metal ions.

Reagents

Chlorpromazine · HCl was obtained from Smith Kline and French Laboratories, in Philadelphia. The hydroxy isomers of chlorpromazine and promazine were generously supplied by the Psychopharmacology Research Branch, N.I.M.H. The diprotonated forms of the phenothiazines were prepared in solution. Disodium salt of ATP was obtained from Sigma Chemical Co., St. Louis, Mo. Stock solutions of the metal ions were prepared by dissolving reagent grade metal nitrates in water and standardized by complexometric titrations against EDTA.

Potentiometric Titration Cell and Electrode Calibration

The equilibrium titrations were carried out in a 100-ml jacketed beaker equipped with magnetic stirrer and a tightly fitting rubber stopper through which were inserted inlet and outlet tubes for N_2, a microburette delivery tube, and glass and calomel extension electrodes. The temperature of the experimental solution in the titration cell was maintained constant by circulation of thermostated water at $25.0 \pm 0.05°C$. A radiometer pH meter (type pH M_4), fitted with the glass and calomel electrodes, was used to measure the H^+ concentrations. The electrode system was calibrated to measure H^+ ion concentrations rather than H^+ activity. Details of the titration cell, electrode calibration, and the titration procedure were described earlier (13).

Equilibrium Measurements

A known amount of the individual phenothiazine was weighed into the titration cell and the required volume of standard HCl was added in order to obtain the diprotonated form of the ligand in solution. This was then followed by the addition of a calculated volume of the standardized solution of metal ion while the mixture was agitated with a magnetic stirrer. The solution was then made up to 50 ml with CO_2-free water and appropriate quantities of KNO_3 or KCl solutions to obtain a constant ionic strength of 1.0. Prepurified nitrogen was bubbled through the experimental solution in the cell. When the solution had attained thermal equilibrium, the H^+-ion concentration was determined by a number of successive readings of the pH meter. Increments of standard NaOH were then added from a microburette and the equilibrium pH values were measured until they reached 11.0 to 11.5. In the case of the free ligands (the phenothiazines), the same procedure was followed except that the metal ion solution was not added. On the basis of these equilibrium pH measurements, titration curves were constructed by plotting the $-\log [H^+]$ values as a function of m, the equivalents of base added per mole of the ligand or per mole of metal salt. Consideration of the titration curve provides the basis for rationalizing the acid–base reactions and the postulation of the metal-chelation reactions of the phenothiazines. This is then followed by the appropriate mathematical treatments of the data.

Absorption Spectra

Absorption spectral measurements of solutions of the phenothiazines and metal–phenothiazine systems were made on a Carey 14 Recording Spectrophotometer.

RESULTS

Metal-binding of 7,8-Dihydroxychlorpromazine

Potentiometric equilibrium curves of the systems consisting of the ligands, diprotonated 7,8-di(OH)CPZ, and Na_2H_2ATP and their chelates of Cu^{2+}, Mg^{2+}, and Ca^{2+} ions are presented in Fig. 1. The titration curve for the free ligand, diprotonated 7,8-di(OH)CPZ, shows two inflections at $m = 1$ and $m = 2$, respectively, where m represents the number of equivalents of base added per mole of the ligand. This could be rationalized to indicate the dissociation of two protons from the thiazine nitrogen and the side-chain amino group. The two inflections at $m = 1$ and $m = 2$ in the ATP curve indicate the dissociation of two protons from the phosphate groups in two separate steps. The titration curve of the Cu^{2+}-7,8-di(OH)CPZ system shows inflections at $m = 1$ and $m \approx 3$. The significant pH depression in the buffer range, $m = 0$ to $m = 1$, pH range 3 to 4, could be accounted for by assuming the interaction of the Cu^{2+} ion with the ligand through the dissociation of the thiazine nitrogen. Further, the development of the blue

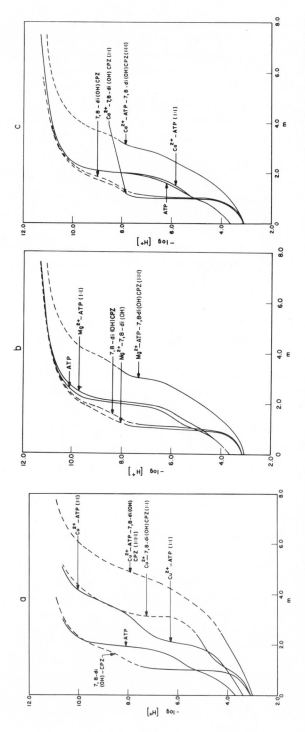

FIG. 1. Interactions of diprotonated 7,8-dihydroxychlorpromazines with metal ions: $I = 1.0$ (KNO$_3$); $T = 25°$C; (a) Cu^{2+}-7,8-di(OH)CPZ, (b) Mg^{2+}-7,8-di(OH)CPZ, (c) Ca^{2+}-7,8-di(OH)CPZ.

coloration of the solution (similar to that of the Cu^{2+}-ethylenediamine system) is indicative of a predominant coordination of the Cu^{2+} ion through the nitrogens. If the metal binding were only through the orthohydroxyl groups, the development of yellow coloration would have resulted, as in the case of the Cu^{2+}-TIRON chelate system. The equilibrium region between $m = 1$ and $m = 3$ (pH range 4.0 to 7.5) could be rationalized to involve the dissociation of two protons from the Cu^{2+}-bound ligand. The observed separation of solid phase in this pH range may be indicative of a disproportionation reaction resulting in the formation of a binuclear Cu^{2+}-chelate and 1 mole of free ligand. The metal-binding reactions that may be occurring are represented by the following equations:

$$Cu^{2+} + H_3A^+ \rightleftharpoons Cu(H_3A)^{3+},$$

$$Cu(H_3A)^{3+} \rightleftharpoons Cu(HA)^+ + 2H^+,$$

$$2Cu(HA)^+ \rightleftharpoons Cu_2HA^{3+} + HA^-,$$

where H_4A^{2+} represents the diprotonated 7,8-di(OH)CPZ. The titration curve for the system, Cu^{2+}-ATP-7,8-di(OH)CPZ (1:1:1) (Fig. 1a) shows inflections at $m = 4$ and $m = 5$. The depression of the 1:1:1 curve over that of the free ligand is indicative of the involvement of the Cu^{2+} ion in strong coordination with both the ATP and the 7,8-di(OH)CPZ molecules. The observed separation of solid phase above $m = 2.8$ and a significant pH drift above $m = 2.8$ together with the intensification of the blue color could be attributed to (a) the separation of the solid free ligand and (b) the formation of a binuclear copper complex in which 2 moles of copper are attached to 1 mole of 7,8-di(OH)CPZ. Hence in the pH range 3 to 6, the reactions occurring may be represented by the equations:

$$Cu^{2+} + L^{4-} \rightleftharpoons CuL^{2-}, \text{ where } L^{4-} \text{ represents the anion of ATP,}$$

$$CuL^{2-} + H_2A \rightleftharpoons Cu(H_2A)L^{2-},$$

$$2Cu(H_2A)L^{2-} \rightleftharpoons Cu_2(H_2A)L_2^{4-} + H_2A.$$

Values of the proton association constants of the free ligand, 7,8-di(OH)CPZ, and their metal-binding constants which were determined on the basis of the above-assumed reactions are presented in Tables 1 and 2.

Potentiometric curves representing the interactions of Mg^{2+} ion with 7,8-di(OH)CPZ in the presence of ATP are shown in Fig. 1b. An analysis of the titration data indicates that in the pH region 3 to 5, the Mg^{2+} ion is weakly coordinated through the release of the proton from the thiazine nitrogen. Separation of solid phase is observed in the pH range 7 to 8.5 followed by the combined occurrence of a blue-colored solution of the metal complex. In the presence of an equimolar amount of ATP and 7,8-di(OH)-CPZ, the Mg^{2+} ion interacts with both the ligands through the release of

TABLE I

PROTON ASSOCIATION REACTIONS OF PHENOTHIAZINES

Temperature = 25.0 ± 0.05 °C   Ionic Strength = 1.0 (KNO$_3$)

Phenothiazines #	Reactions	Log K*
Chlorpromazine 2HCl (H_2A^{2+})	$A + H^+ \rightleftharpoons HA^+$ $HA^+ + H^+ \rightleftharpoons H_2A^{2+}$	 2.9
7-Hydroxychlorpromazine 2HCl (H_3A^{2+})	$A^- + H^+ \rightleftharpoons HA$ $HA + H^+ \rightleftharpoons H_2A^+$ $H_2A^+ + H^+ \rightleftharpoons H_3A^{2+}$	 8.4 3.3
7,8-Dihydroxychlorpromazine·2HCl (H_4L^{2+})	$A^{2-} + H^+ \rightleftharpoons HA^-$ $HA^- + H^+ \rightleftharpoons H_2A$ $H_2A + H^+ \rightleftharpoons H_3A^+$ $H_3A^+ + H^+ \rightleftharpoons H_4A^{2+}$	 8.2 3.4
Promazine 2HCl (H_2A^{2+})	$A + H^+ \rightleftharpoons HA^+$ $HA^+ + H^+ \rightleftharpoons H_2A^{2+}$	 3.4
2,3-Dihydroxypromazine 2HCl (H_4A^{2+})	$A^{2-} + H^+ \rightleftharpoons HA^-$ $HA^- + H^+ \rightleftharpoons H_2A$ $H_2A + H^+ \rightleftharpoons H_3A^+$ $H_3A^+ + H^+ \rightleftharpoons H_4A^{2+}$	 8.5 3.4
3-Hydroxypromazine 2HCl (H_3A^{2+})	$A^- + H^+ \rightleftharpoons HA$ $HA + H^+ \rightleftharpoons H_2A^+$ $H_2A^+ + H^+ \rightleftharpoons H_3A^{2+}$	 3.2

* Equilibrium constants for the proton associations reactions

\# Diprotonated phenothiazines   9

three protons, i.e., two protons from ATP and one from the thiazine ring nitrogen according to the following equations:

$$Mg^{2+} + L^{4-} \quad \rightleftharpoons MgL^{2-},$$

$$MgL^{2-} + H_3A^+ \rightleftharpoons Mg(H_3A)L^- .$$

In the pH range of 5 to 7.5, therefore, the formation of a ternary chelate is indicated. In the pH range of 7 to 9.5 a possible interaction with the ortho-hydroxyl group is indicated. Disproportionation of the ternary chelate occurs resulting in the formation of a binuclear chelate solution and the solid free ligand base. Values of the metal-binding constants are presented in Table 2.

Figure 1c shows the titration curves of systems representing the interaction of the Ca^{2+} ion with 7,8-di(OH)CPZ and ATP. A weak interaction of 7,8-di(OH)CPZ with Ca^{2+} is indicated in the pH range 3 to 5. In the pH range 7 to 9.5, there is the separation of the solid phase possibly due to the dissociation of the complex. In the combined presence of ATP and 7,8-di(OH)CPZ, the Ca^{2+} ion is bound by both ligands in the pH range 5 to 7.5. In Table 2, the values of the metal-chelate stability constants are presented.

Interactions of 7-Hydroxychlorpromazine with Metal Ions

Potentiometric titration data of the reactions of the Cu^{2+} ion with 7-(OH)CPZ in the presence of and in the absence of ATP are presented in Fig. 2a. The Cu^{2+}-7-(OH)CPZ (1:1) curve shows an inflection at $m = 1.5$, which is indicative of the possible occurrence of a binuclear chelate of the 2:2 type. Dissociation of the Cu^{2+}-7-(OH)CPZ chelate is indicated above pH 6. There is, however, no indication of any disproportionation reaction in the pH range 3 to 6. In the combined presence of an equimolar amount of ATP, the Cu^{2+} ion is bound by both the ligands in one overlapping buffer region between pH 2.7 to 6.0. The reaction may be represented by the equation:

$$Cu^{2+} + L^{4-} + H_2A^+ \rightleftharpoons Cu(H_2A)L^- .$$

In the pH range 6 to 8, a two-proton dissociation equilibrium is indicated by the potentiometric data. This could presumably be from the side-chain amine and the phenolic (OH) in accordance with the following reaction:

$$Cu(H_2A)L^- \rightleftharpoons CuAL^{3-} + 2H^+ .$$

Values of equilibrium constants for the associations of the protons and metal ions are presented in Tables 1 and 2, respectively.

Figure 2b shows the potentiometric curves of the systems consisting of Mg^{2+}-7-(OH)CPZ and Mg^{2+}-ATP-7-(OH)CPZ. A weak interaction of the Mg^{2+} ion with the ligand through the dissociation of a proton from the thiazine nitrogen is indicated. The curve for the Mg^{2+}-ATP-7-(OH)CPZ sys-

TABLE 2. Coordination of phenothiazines with metal ions and metal-ATP chelates

Ligands	Chelation reactions	pH range	Chelate formation constant log K	Remarks
Adenosine 5-triphosphate, disodium salt (Na_2H_2L)	$Cu^{2+} + L^{4-} \rightleftharpoons CuL^{2-}$	3.0–5.0	5.17 ± 0.04	Mononuclear chelate
	$Mg^{2+} + L^{4-} \rightleftharpoons MgL^{2-}$	4.0–7.5	3.22 ± 0.02	
	$Ca^{2+} + L^{4-} \rightleftharpoons CaL^{2-}$	3.0–7.0	2.84 ± 0.06	
Promazine · 2HCl (H_2A^{2+})	$Cu^{2+} + HA^+ \rightleftharpoons Cu(HA)^{3+}$	3.0–5.0	5.0 ± 0.1	Disproportionates
	$Cu(HA)^{3+} \rightleftharpoons CuA^{2+} + H^+$	5.0–7.5	—	Weak binding
	$CuL^{2-} + HA^+ \rightleftharpoons Cu(HA)L^-$	4.0–6.0	—	Protonated chelate
	$Mg^{2+} + HA^+ \rightleftharpoons Mg(HA)^{3+}$	3.0–8.0	4.9 ± 0.3	Weak interaction
	$MgL^{2-} + HA^+ \rightleftharpoons Mg(HA)L^-$	5.0–8.0	—	
3-(OH)Promazine · 2HCl (H_3A^{2+})	$Cu^{2+} + H_2A^+ \rightleftharpoons Cu(H_2A)^{3+}$	3.0–5.0	—	Polymerization
	$Cu(H_2A)^{3+} \rightleftharpoons CuA^+ + 2H^+$	5.0–8.0	—	Deprotonation and disproportionation
	$CuL^{2-} + H_2A^+ \rightleftharpoons Cu(H_2A)L^-$	4.0–6.0	—	Weak interaction
	$Mg^{2+} + H_2A^+ \rightleftharpoons Mg(H_2A)^{3+}$	3.0–8.0	4.9 ± 0.2	Protonated chelate
	$MgL^{2-} + H_2A^+ \rightleftharpoons Mg(H_2A)L^-$	5.0–7.5	—	Weak binding
2,3-di(OH)Promazine · 2HCl (H_4A^{2+})	$Cu^{2+} + H_2A \rightleftharpoons Cu(H_2A)^{2+}$	3.0–4.0	$11.2 + 0.2$	Protonated chelate
	$Cu(H_2A)^{2+} \rightleftharpoons Cu(HA)^+ + H^+$	4.0–8.0	—	
	$CuL^{2-} + H_3A^+ \rightleftharpoons Cu(H_3A)L^-$	3.5–4.5	—	
	$Cu(H_3A)L^- \rightleftharpoons Cu(HA)L^{3-} + 2H^+$	4.5–8.0	—	Weak interaction
	$Mg^{2+} + H_3A^+ \rightleftharpoons Mg(H_3A)^{3+}$	3.0–7.5	6.2 ± 0.3	
	$MgL^{2-} + H_3A^+ \rightleftharpoons Mg(H_3A)L^-$	5.0–7.5	—	Weak interaction
Chlorpromazine · 2HCl (H_2A^{2+})	$Cu^{2+} + HA^+ \rightleftharpoons CuHA^{3+}$	2.5–5.0	4.3 ± 0.1	Protonated chelate
	$CuHA^{3+} \rightleftharpoons CuA^{2+} + H^+$	5.0–7.0	—	Disproportionates
	$CuL^{2-} + HA^+ \rightleftharpoons Cu(HA)L^-$	4.0–6.0	—	Weak binding
	$Ca^{2+} + HA^+ \rightleftharpoons Ca(HA)^{3+}$	2.5–5.0	8.1 ± 0.2	
7-(OH)Chlorpromazine · 2HCl (H_3A^{2+})	$Cu^{2+} + H_2A^+ \rightleftharpoons Cu(H_2A)^{3+}$	3.0–5.5	5.8 ± 0.1	Protonated chelate
	$Cu(H_2A)^{3+} \rightleftharpoons CuA^+ + 2H^+$	5.5–8.0	—	Disproportionates
	$CuL^{2-} + H_2A^+ \rightleftharpoons Cu(H_2A)L^-$	3.5–5.5	—	Weak binding

Reaction	pH range	value	Note
$Mg^{2+} + H_2A^+ \rightleftharpoons Mg(H_2A)^{3+}$	3.0–7.0	6.4 ± 0.1	Protonated chelate
$MgL^{2-} + H_2A^+ \rightleftharpoons Mg(H_2A)L^-$	5.0–7.0	—	Weak binding
$Ca^{2+} + H_2A^+ \rightleftharpoons Ca(H_2A)^{3+}$	3.0–7.0	5.9 ± 0.3	
$CaL^{2-} + H_2A^+ \rightleftharpoons Ca(H_2A)L^-$	5.0–7.0	—	Weak binding

7,8-di(OH)Chlorpromazine · 2HCl
(H_4A^{2+})

Reaction	pH range	value	Note
$Cu^{2+} + H_3A^+ \rightleftharpoons Cu(H_3A)^{3+}$	3.0–4.0	5.2 ± 0.3	Protonated
$Cu^{2+} + HA^- \rightleftharpoons Cu(HA)^+$	4.0–7.5	14.0 ± 0.3	Disproportionates
$CuL^{2-} + H_2A \rightleftharpoons Cu(H_2A)L^{2-}$	4.0–6.0	6.2 ± 0.3	Polymerization
$Mg^{2+} + H_3A^+ \rightleftharpoons Mg(H_3A)^{3+}$	3.0–7.0	6.2 ± 0.4	Protonated chelate
$MgL^{2-} + H_3A^+ \rightleftharpoons Mg(H_3A)L^-$	5.0–7.0	—	Weak binding
$Ca^{2+} + H_3A^+ \rightleftharpoons Ca(H_3A)^{3+}$	3.0–7.5	6.2 ± 0.3	Protonated chelate
$CaL^{2-} + H_3A^+ \rightleftharpoons Ca(H_3A)L^-$	5.0–7.5	—	Weak binding

Temperature = 25.0 ± 0.05; ionic strength = 1.0 (KNO_3); ATP = Na_2H_2L.

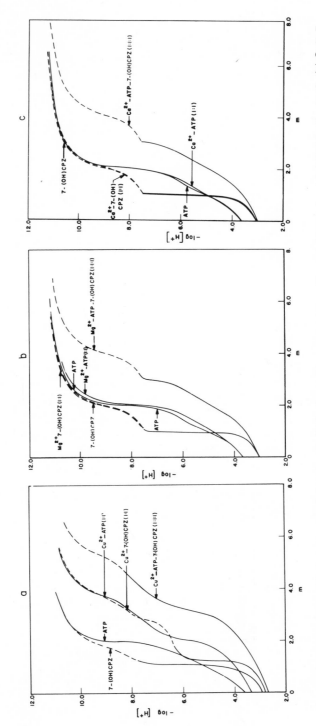

FIG. 2. Potentiometric equilibrium curves of diprotonated 7-hydroxychlorpromazines with metal ions: $I = 1.0$ (KNO$_3$); $T = 25°C$; (a) Cu^{2+}-7-(OH)CPZ, (b) Mg^{2+}-7-(OH)CPZ, (c) Ca^{2+}-7-(OH)CPZ.

tem shows inflections at $m = 2$ and $m = 3$, which is indicative of the coordination of 7-(OH)CPZ with Mg^{2+}-ATP in the pH range 5 to 7.5. Stability constants for the binding of the Mg^{2+} ion by the two ligands are presented in Table 2.

Titration data on the Ca^{2+}-7-(OH)CPZ system indicate a weak binding by the metal. The inflection at $m = 1$ (Fig. 2c) is indicative of the possible involvement of thiazine nitrogen in metal binding. Above pH 7.5, the solid phase separated. In the presence of ATP, the Ca^{2+} ion interacts with both the ligands in the pH range 5 to 7.5. Equilibrium constants calculated for the coordination of the Cu^{2+} ion are presented in Table 3.

TABLE 3. *Absorption spectra of the interactions of chlorpromazines with the Cu^{2+} ion*

Phenothiazine	Concentration (M)	pH	Absorption maxima (mμ)	Optical density
CPZ	1.821×10^{-5}	7.2	305	0.07
			255	0.59
Cu^{2+}-CPZ(1:1)	1.268×10^{-5}	6.9	305	0.30
			255	0.26
Cu^{2+}-ATP-CPZ(1:1:1)	9.646×10^{-6}	5.8	≈305	0.02
			255	0.35
7(OH)CPZ	3.207×10^{-5}	5.3	309	0.16
			252	0.78
Cu^{2+}-7(OH)CPZ(1:1)	3.207×10^{-5}	6.0	≈310	0.02
			252	0.13
Cu^{2+}-ATP-7(OH)CPZ(1:1:1)	3.207×10^{-5}	5.8	≈310	0.02
			253	0.25
7,8-di(OH)CPZ	2.695×10^{-5}	5.4	≈340	0.02
			≈298 shoulder	0.04
			262	0.58
			233	0.06
Cu^{2+}-7,8-di(OH)CPZ(1:1)	2.695×10^{-5}	6.2	≈340	0.01
			≈298 shoulder	0.02
			263	0.17
			233	disappeared
Cu^{2+}-ATP-7,8-di(OH)CPZ(1:1:1)	2.695×10^{-5}	5.7	≈340	disappeared
			≈298 shoulder	0.02
			263	0.21
			233	disappeared

Interactions of Chlorpromazine with Metal Ions

Potentiometric equilibrium data on the reactions of chlorpromazine with Cu^{2+} ions are presented in Fig. 3. The inflection at $m = 1$ in the titration curve of the Cu^{2+}-CPZ system is indicative of metal binding in the pH range

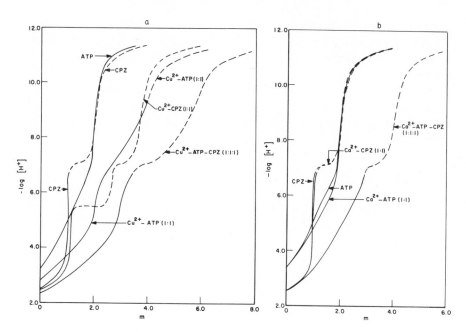

FIG. 3. Equilibrium titration curves of diprotonated chlorpromazines with metal ions: $I = 1.0$ (KNO$_3$); $T = 25°C$; (a) Cu^{2+}-CPZ, (b) Ca^{2+}-CPZ.

2.5 to 5.5. The titration curve for the Cu^{2+}-ATP-CPZ (1:1:1) system shows two inflections at $m = 2$ and $m = 3$, indicating the formation of a ternary chelate in which ATP and CPZ are both bound to Cu^{2+} ion in the pH range 3.8 to 5.5. The chelate undergoes dissociation and hydrolysis above pH 6.5. The titration curves for Ca^{2+}-CPZ and Ca^{2+}-ATP-CPZ presented in Fig. 3b indicate weak interactions.

Metal Binding by the Promazines

The interactions of promazine (PMZ), 3-hydroxypromazine (3-(OH)-PMZ), and 2,3-dihydroxypromazine (2,3-di(OH)PMZ) with Cu^{2+} and Mg^{2+} ions were investigated. The potentiometric titration data are presented in Figs. 4–6. The proton association constants of the promazines were determined by using their diprotonated forms, and the values of the constants are presented in Table 1. Consideration of the titration curves of Cu^{2+}-promazines (Fig. 4a) indicates the possible formation of polynuclear chelates because of the appearance of inflections at nonintegral values of m. The titration curves of the Mg^{2+}-promazine systems show inflections at integral values of m indicating the predominant occurrence of mononuclear chelation. Values of the stability constants calculated on the basis of the titration data are presented in Table 2.

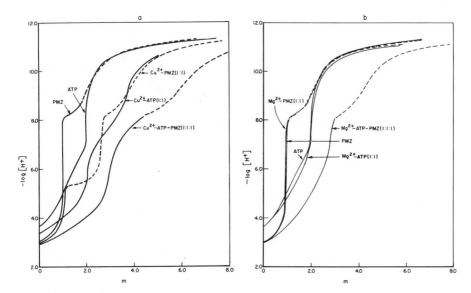

FIG. 4. Potentiometric titration curves of diprotonated promazines with metal ions: $I = 1.0$ (KNO$_3$); $T = 25°C$; (a) Cu^{2+}-PMZ, (b) Mg^{2+}-PMZ.

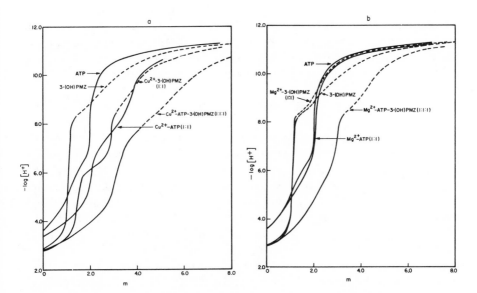

FIG. 5. Coordination of diprotonated 3-hydroxypromazines with metal ions: $I = $ (KNO$_3$); $T = 25°C$; (a) Cu^{2+}-3-(OH)PMZ, (b) Mg^{2+}-3-(OH)PMZ.

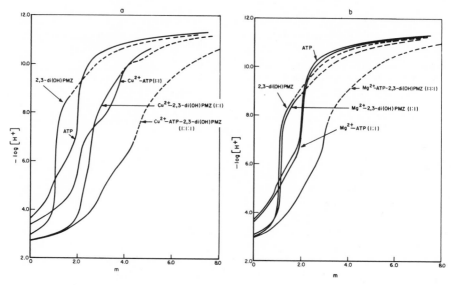

FIG. 6. Potentiometric pH curves of diprotonated 2,3-dihydroxypromazines with metal ions: $I = 1.0$ (KNO$_3$); $T = 25°C$; (a) Cu^{2+}-2,3-di(OH)PMZ, (b) Mg^{2+}-2,3-di(OH)PMZ.

Absorption Spectra of Cu²⁺-Chlorpromazines

The nature of interaction of the Cu^{2+} ion with each of the chlorpromazines, viz., CPZ, 7-(OH)CPZ, and 7,8-di(OH)CPZ, was investigated by means of absorption spectral measurements. Details regarding the concentration of aqueous solutions of the above systems, their pHs, the absorption maxima, and the corresponding optical densities are presented in Table 3.

DISCUSSION

A consideration of the pKs of the chlorpromazines (Table 1) indicates that the basicity of the thiazine-ring nitrogen of each of the hydroxychlorpromazines is only slightly increased over that of CPZ. Values of pK$_2$, representing the dissociation of the proton bound to the side-chain amino nitrogen for the CPZ, PMZ, and 3(OH)PMZ are not included in Table 1 because of the occurrence of precipitation reactions in the respective equilibrium buffer regions. However, the pK$_2$ values of the 7(OH)CPZ, 7,8di(OH)CPZ, and 2,3di(OH)PMZ systems are compared to those of CPZ reported in the literature (14–16) for the purpose of discussion. The pK$_2$ of each of the ligands, viz., 7,8di(OH)CPZ, 7(OH)CPZ, and 2,3di(OH)-PMZ, is found to be significantly affected by the introduction of the hydroxo groups. Such variations in the basicities of the donor nitrogen could be reflected in the extent of metal chelation. It should be noted that, in addition to the two nitrogens, the phenolic-hydroxyl groups provide strong metal-binding sites as illustrated by the structures below:

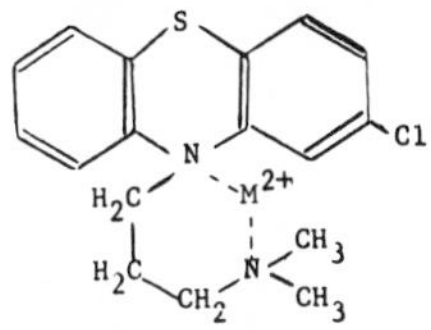

Metal-binding by CPZ

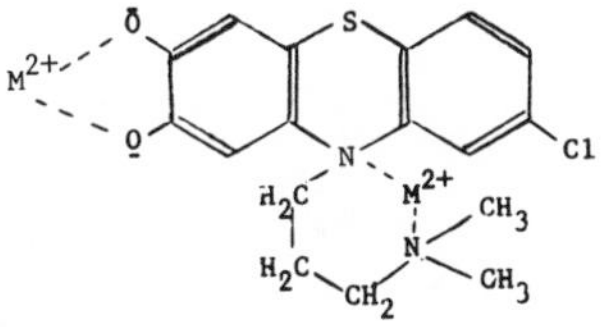

Metal-binding by 7,8-di(OH)CPZ

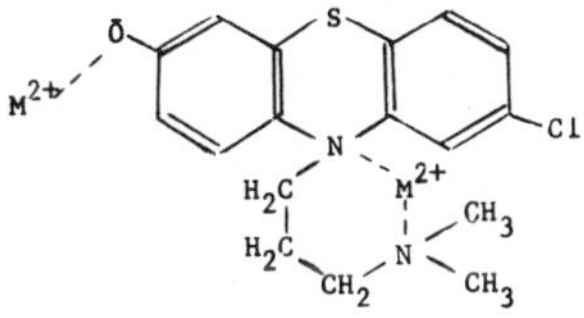

Metal-binding by 7-(OH)CPZ

The diprotonated forms of the phenothiazines were used in solution in order to determine the metal-binding tendency of the thiazine-ring nitrogen and the terminal amino nitrogen.

The metal-chelate stability data presented in Table 2 indicate that the 7,8-di(OH) compound exhibits larger metal-binding affinity than the other two compounds possibly through the involvement of the orthohydroxyl groups, the thiazine nitrogen, and the terminal amino group. In the pH range of 3 to 7.5, both Mg^{2+} and Ca^{2+} ions react with the chlorpromazines through the displacement of one proton from the dihydrochlorides indicating a weak coordination with the two nitrogen donors. The potentiometric curves further indicate that in the presence of ATP, Mg^{2+} and Ca^{2+} ions are coordinated to both the chlorpromazines and the ATP in the pH range 5.0 to 7.5. On the basis of the stability of the equilibrium measurements, it may be stated that the possible oxidative reactions of the hydroxychlorpromazines are considerably suppressed. It should be stated, however, that these reactions are carried out in an atmosphere of nitrogen gas. The equilibrium data on the Cu^{2+}-chlorpromazines indicate that the 7-hydroxy and the 7,8-dihydroxy compounds tend to form binuclear chelates of Cu^{2+} in the pH range 5 to 7.5 through the disproportionation reactions illustrated by the structural formulas in Plate 1. An examination of the absorption spectral

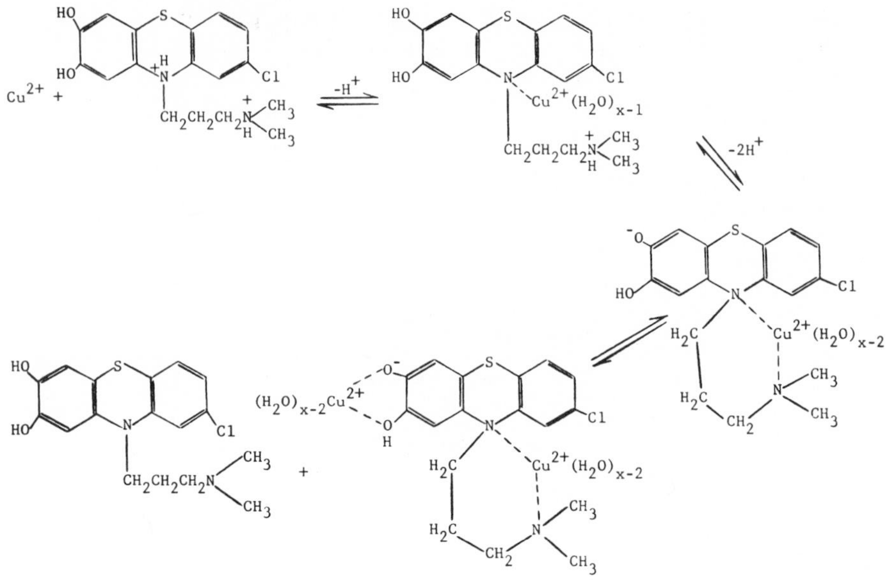

PLATE 1. Interactions of 7,8-di(OH)CPZ with Cu^{2+} in the pH range 3 to 8.

data (Figs. 7–9 and Table 3) indicates that the characteristic band of the chlorpromazines at 255 mμ shows a diminution in intensity when an equimolar amount of the Cu^{2+} ion is added. The absence of any absorption band at 274 mμ reported by Borg and Cotzias (8) in the spectra is indicative of the absence of any oxidation of the metal-bound chlorpromazines as well as the free ligands. It should be noted that the absorption peak at 255 mμ of the chlorpromazine is shifted to 263 mμ in the case of the 7,8-dihydroxy isomer. On the basis of the potentiometric and spectral data, it may be stated that all three chlorpromazines coordinate with the metal ions, viz., Cu^{2+}, Mg^{2+}, and Ca^{2+}, and that the oxidation of the ligands is considerably suppressed through metal chelation. The occurrence of solid particulates in the pH range 6 to 8 in the case of the metal-chlorpromazine systems has been rationalized to be due to a disproportionation of the respective chelates and not due to any oxidative degradation. Exposure of the Cu^{2+}-chlorpromazine solutions to ambient air did not result in any observable oxidation, since the absorption band at 274 mμ was absent in the spectrum.

Among the three promazines investigated in this study, the 2,3-dihydroxy isomer is found to exhibit the strongest binding with the metal ions (see Table 2). It is of interest to note that the presence of the orthohydroxyl group in the promazines and the chlorpromazines considerably enhances their metal-chelating affinities, presumably through the involvement of the hydroxyl groups and through the possible formation of polynuclear chelates.

The fact that the phenothiazines do form stable metal chelates in the presence of ATP may be considered to be quite significant for an under-

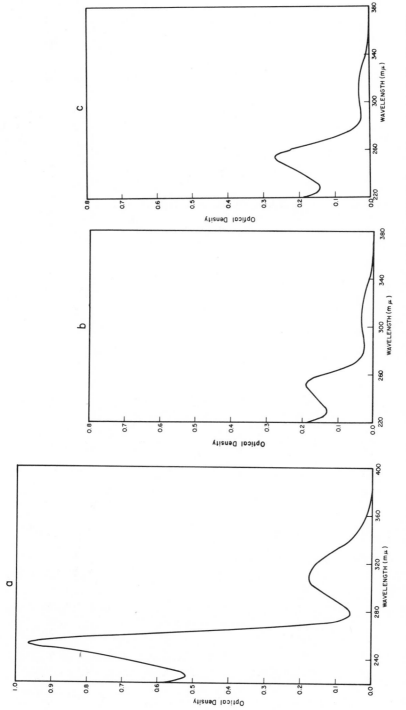

FIG. 7. Absorption spectra of diprotonated chlorpromazines: (a) CPZ at pH = 7.2, (b) Cu^{2+}-CPZ (1:1) at pH = 6.9, (c) Cu^{2+}-ATP-CPZ (1:1:1) at pH = 5.8.

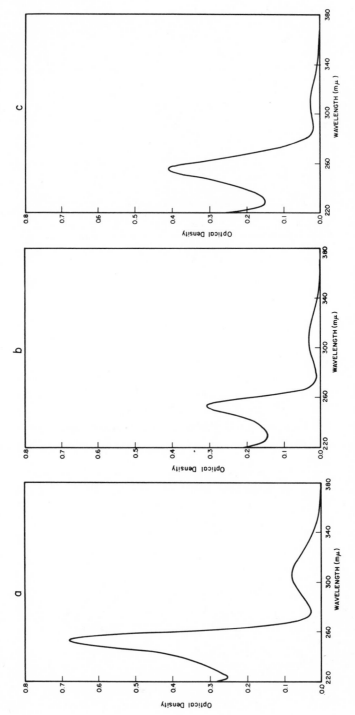

FIG. 8. Absorption spectra of diprotonated 7-hydroxychlorpromazines: (a) 7-(OH)CPZ at pH = 5.3, (b) Cu²⁺-7-(OH)CPZ (1:1) at pH = 6.0, (c) Cu²⁺-ATP-7-(OH)CPZ (1:1:1) at pH = 5.8.

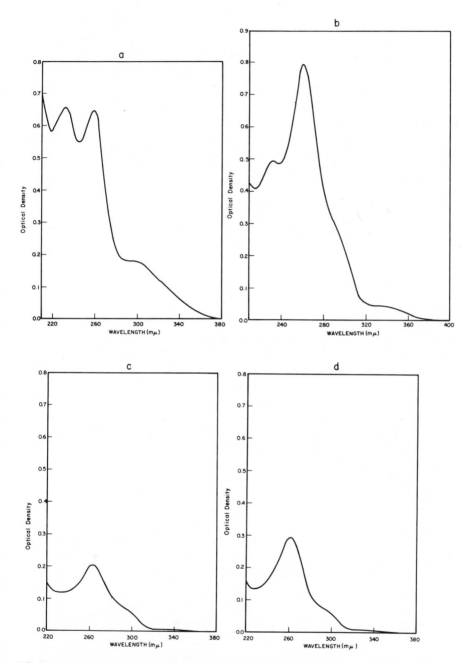

FIG. 9. Absorption spectra of diprotonated 7,8-dihydroxychlorpromazines: (a) 7,8-di(OH)-CPZ, (b) 7,8-di(OH)CPZ at pH = 5.4, (c) Cu^{2+}-7,8-di(OH)CPZ (1:1) at pH = 6.2, (d) Cu^{2+}-ATP-7,8-di(OH)CPZ (1:1:1) at pH = 5.8.

standing of the mechanism of their drug action from the point of view of a metal-coordination hypothesis for biogenic amine activity. The variations in the metal-binding stabilities of the phenothiazines and their hydroxylated metabolites could very well constitute a basis for delineating the nature and extent of interaction with norepinephrine at the presynaptic and postsynaptic sites. The exploratory data generated in this chapter merely indicate (a) the metal-chelating tendencies of a few of the phenothiazines and (b) the absence of any oxidative instabilities. However, a more extensive and detailed study of the following is necessary for an understanding of the molecular mechanisms involved in the action of the phenothiazines:

(1) The metal chelation of a wide range of phenothiazines as a function of their molecular structures and basicities,

(2) their aqueous and lipid soluble characteristics, and

(3) their equilibrium interactions with norepinephrine and other biogenic amines.

SUMMARY

The interactions of phenothiazines with metal ions such as Cu^{2+}, Mg^{2+}, and Ca^{2+} have been investigated in an aqueous electrolyte medium of constant ionic strength (1.0 KNO_3 and KCl) and under nitrogen atmosphere by means of potentiometric equilibrium method and absorption spectral technique. The phenothiazines consisted of (a) 7,8-dihydroxychlorpromazine, (b) 7-hydroxychlorpromazine, (c) chlorpromazine, (d) 2,3-dihydroxypromazine, (e) 3-hydroxypromazine, and (f) promazine. The acid-base characteristics of these phenothiazines have been examined. The strongest metal binding was exhibited by the orthodihydroxy compounds, viz., 7,8-di(OH)-CPZ and 2,3-di(OH)PMZ for the Cu^{2+} ion with thermodynamic stability constants (log K) of 14.0 and 11.2, respectively. In the pH range 3 to 5 all the phenothiazines exhibited significant tendency for metal binding. Above pH 5, the possible formation of binuclear chelate species has been postulated for the systems involving Cu^{2+} and 7-(OH)CPZ and 7,8-di(OH)CPZ. In the combined presence of an equimolar amount of ATP, the phenothiazines exhibited a definite tendency to form ternary chelates. Further, the oxidative instability characteristics appeared to be largely suppressed through metal coordination.

ACKNOWLEDGMENTS

This work was supported by Grant 1R03–MH22208–01–PPR (from the National Institute of Mental Health) and by the Foundation for Neuropsychiatric Research, Bethesda, Maryland.

REFERENCES

1. Manian, A. A., Efron, D. H., and Goldberg, M. E., *Life Sci.,* **4,** 2425 (1965).
2. Perry, T. L., Culling, G. F. A., Berry, K., and Hansen, S., *Science,* **146,** 81 (1964).
3. Daly, J. W., and Manian, A. A., *Biochem. Pharmacol.,* **18,** 1235 (1969).
4. Colburn, R. W., and Maas, J. W., *Nature,* **208,** 37 (1965).
5. Maas, J. W., and Colburn, R. W., *Nature,* **208,** 41 (1965).
6. Rajan, K. S., Davis, J. M., and Colburn, R. W., *J. Neurochem.,* **18,** 345 (1971).
7. Rajan, K. S., Davis, J. M., Colburn, R. W., and Jarke, F. H., *J. Neurochem.,* **19,** 1099 (1972).
8. Borg, D. C., and Cotzias, G. C., *Proc. Nat. Acad. Sci. U.S.A.,* **48,** 617 (1962).
9. Borg, D. C., and Cotzias, G. C., *Proc. Nat. Acad. Sci. U.S.A.,* **48,** 623 (1962).
10. Huang, P. C., and Gabay, S., *Fed. Proc.,* **30,** 629 (1971).
11. Huang, P. C., and Gabay, S., *Pharmacologist,* **13,** 440 (1971).
12. Ira Blei, *Arch. Biochem. Biophys.,* **109,** 321 (1965).
13. Rajan, K. S., and Martell, A. E., *J. Inorg. Nucl. Chem.,* **26,** 1927 (1964).
14. Chatten, L. G., and Harris, L. E., *Anal. Chem.,* **34,** 1495 (1962).
15. Schill, G., *Acta Pharm. Suecica,* **2,** 99 (1965).
16. Green, A. L., *J. Pharm. Pharmac.,* **19,** 10 (1967).

The Phenothiazines and Structurally Related Drugs, edited by I. S. Forrest, C. J. Carr, and E. Usdin. Raven Press, New York © 1974.

Behavioral, Biochemical, and Pharmacological Effects of Chronic Dosage of Phenothiazine Tranquilizers in Rats

Roger P. Maickel, Michael C. Braunstein, Marianne McGlynn, Wayne R. Snodgrass, and Roy W. Webb

Department of Pharmacology, Medical Sciences Program, Indiana University, Bloomington, Indiana 47401

INTRODUCTION

The class of drugs known as major tranquilizers or antipsychotic agents includes a chemical subgroup consisting of a large variety of compounds derived from phenothiazine. Since the introduction of the first of these agents into clinical usage in the early 1950's (1, 2), a proliferation of research and clinical efforts has occurred, the extent of which has not been seen in any other area of pharmacology. Several reviews have described the synthesis (3), structure-activity relationships (4), disposition and fate (5), and clinical efficacy (6) of these agents. In addition, a veritable literature by itself exists in terms of basic and clinical research papers on the various phenothiazine agents.

Despite this voluminous literature, few, if any, reports exist in which detailed correlations have been made of various behavioral, biochemical, and pharmacological effects of these drugs, especially upon chronic dosage. For example, previous reports from this laboratory have indicated that chlorpromazine and other phenothiazine tranquilizers have effects on a variety of behavioral test systems (7, 8), inhibit rat brain acetylcholinesterase (8, 9), accumulate in brain and plasma with chronic dosage (10), and show significant toxicological phenomena (11). All of these studies were done in different groups of animals, with different dosages of drugs; cross-correlation is therefore rather difficult. This chapter is a report on a study of some effects of chronic dosage of chlorpromazine in rats, with correlated studies of promazine and triflupromazine.

MATERIALS AND METHODS

Adult male Sprague-Dawley rats weighing 120 to 200 grams were used in all experiments. The animals were obtained from Murphy Breeding

Laboratories, Plainfield, Indiana, and were maintained on ad lib Purina Lab chow and tap water for 7 to 10 days prior to and during experimental use. The animal room was maintained on a 14 hr on, 10 hr off light cycle at a temperature of 22 to 23°C.

Drugs were administered by subcutaneous injection as solutions in distilled water such that animals received 0.1 ml per 100 g body weight. Placebo doses were distilled water at 0.1 ml per 100 g body weight. Phenothiazines were measured as described by Mahju and Maickel (10), behavioral procedures were as described by Mahju and Maickel (10) and Cox and Maickel (12), brain acetylcholinesterase was determined by the method of Berg and Maickel (9), and liver triglycerides were determined as described by Butler et al. (13).

RESULTS

Effects of Chronic Dosage with Phenothiazine Tranquilizers on Body Weight of Rats

Groups of six to eight rats were given daily dosages of promazine (2×5 mg/kg), chlorpromazine (2×2 mg/kg) or triflupromazine (2×1 mg/kg) at 12 ± 1 hr intervals for 30 days. The animals were weighed just prior to receiving the morning dose (given between 0800 and 0930 hr); the weights were recorded and 5-day interval weights are reported in Table 1. When these data were treated in a computer analysis for line shape in a duration of treatment/percent change in body weight plot, the curves obtained fell into two categories. Placebo- and promazine-dosed animals showed a linear weight increase with time over the entire 30-day treatment period. In contrast chlorpromazine and triflupromazine showed a biphasic response. For

TABLE 1. *Effects of phenothiazine tranquilizers on body weight*

	Body weight (g ± S.D.)			
Day of dosage	Control	Promazine	Chlorpromazine	Triflu-promazine
0	134 ± 4.6 (8)	139 ± 5.3 (8)	136 ± 5.0 (8)	135 ± 3.1 (8)
5	157 ± 9.1 (8)	160 ± 11.3 (8)	153 ± 5.9 (8)	154 ± 9.6 (8)
10	194 ± 10.7 (8)	197 ± 11.9 (8)	188 ± 16.7 (7)	186 ± 11.0 (8)
15	224 ± 17.0 (8)	224 ± 20.6 (8)	211 ± 16.3 (7)	209 ± 13.3 (7)
20	249 ± 23.4 (7)	251 ± 27.8 (8)	226 ± 19.5 (7)	228 ± 20.8 (7)
25	278 ± 20.9 (7)	279 ± 26.1 (8)	234 ± 21.2 (6)	236 ± 19.4 (7)
30	301 ± 27.8 (7)	300 ± 31.4 (8)	250 ± 21.9 (6)	248 ± 27.3 (7)

Each value is the mean ± S.D. of the number of animals indicated in parentheses.

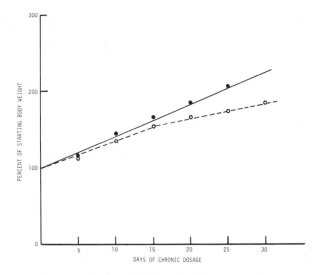

FIG. 1. Effect of chronic administration of phenothiazine tranquilizers on body weight of rats. Data are those shown in Table 1. Placebo and promazine values are indicated by (——●——); chlorpromazine and triflupromazine are indicated by (------○------).

these two drugs, the rate of weight increase was indistinguishable from that of placebo over the first 2 weeks; for the period 15 to 30 days, however, the rate of weight increase was significantly lower than that of the placebo animals. The data for placebo and chlorpromazine are graphically depicted in Fig. 1. Four deaths were observed over the course of the treatment, one each in the placebo and triflupromazine groups and two in the chlorpromazine group. Postmortem examinations did not reveal any obvious drug-induced pathology; three of the animals showed evidence of respiratory infections.

Effects of Chronic Dosage with Phenothiazine Tranquilizers on Rat Liver Glycogen and Triglycerides

Groups of six to eight rats were treated as described in the preceding section and killed after 1, 4, 7, 15, 21, and 30 days of dosage. Livers were removed, examined visually for evidence of lipid accumulation, and assayed for glycogen and triglyceride content. The results, shown in Table 2, indicate that all of the drugs elevate both triglycerides and glycogen in liver. The potency ranking for triglyceride elevation is chlorpromazine > triflupromazine > promazine; for glycogen elevation, the ranking is chlorpromazine > promazine > triflupromazine. In all cases, the rate of increase falls off with time, suggesting some sort of adaptation to these actions of the drugs.

TABLE 2. *Effects of phenothiazine tranquilizers on liver components*

Day of dosage	Control		Promazine		Chlorpromazine		Triflupromazine	
	GLY	TGL	GLY	TGL	GLY	TGL	GLY	TGL
0	37 ± 3.2	3.9 ± 0.7	—	—	—	—	—	—
1	39 ± 4.0	4.3 ± 0.9	35 ± 6.1	4.1 ± 0.9	40 ± 7.1	4.7 ± 1.0	36 ± 3.9	4.3 ± 1.1
4	37 ± 1.6	4.1 ± 1.1	44 ± 3.8	4.7 ± 1.3	48 ± 3.6	6.7 ± 1.1	40 ± 7.2	4.9 ± 0.9
7	34 ± 4.9	4.1 ± 1.0	47 ± 1.7	5.4 ± 0.9	57 ± 7.1	8.3 ± 2.0	47 ± 3.1	5.8 ± 0.7
15	36 ± 3.3	4.0 ± 0.3	50 ± 5.1	5.2 ± 1.0	59 ± 8.4	8.6 ± 1.1	49 ± 9.3	6.2 ± 1.3
21	38 ± 1.7	4.3 ± 0.8	55 ± 5.9	4.8 ± 0.3	64 ± 7.3	9.0 ± 1.7	51 ± 8.6	6.4 ± 1.7
30	35 ± 5.2	4.2 ± 1.2	53 ± 8.0	5.3 ± 1.1	60 ± 8.8	8.5 ± 1.3	50 ± 7.7	6.0 ± 1.1

Each value is the mean ± S.D. of values from six to eight rats, except controls which are 16 to 18. Underlined values are significantly different from day zero values ($p < 0.05$). Animals were killed 12 hr after the last dose.

Effects of Chronic Dosage with Phenothiazine Tranquilizers on Plasma and Tissue Accumulation of the Drugs

Plasma, brain, and liver samples from four rats of each of the groups in the preceding section were assayed for content of phenothiazine tran-

TABLE 3. *Accumulation of phenothiazine tranquilizers in rat tissues*

Day of dosage	Tissue	Tissue content ($\mu g/g$)		
		Chlorpromazine	Promazine	Triflupromazine
1	Plasma	0.27 ± 0.10	0.21 ± 0.07	<0.08
	Brain	1.03 ± 0.17	2.01 ± 0.43	0.83 ± 0.19
	Liver	0.79 ± 0.31	0.69 ± 0.09	0.76 ± 0.27
4	Plasma	0.49 ± 0.09	0.68 ± 0.11	<0.08
	Brain	2.76 ± 0.41	5.55 ± 1.30	1.17 ± 0.18
	Liver	1.95 ± 0.47	1.78 ± 0.84	0.94 ± 0.21
7	Plasma	1.07 ± 0.48	1.48 ± 0.33	0.17 ± 0.08
	Brain	5.71 ± 0.94	11.90 ± 1.79	1.94 ± 0.30
	Liver	2.98 ± 0.49	3.02 ± 0.86	1.94 ± 0.30
15	Plasma	1.52 ± 0.41	2.79 ± 0.48	0.33 ± 0.08
	Brain	9.38 ± 1.77	21.45 ± 3.83	3.90 ± 0.84
	Liver	5.18 ± 1.02	5.17 ± 1.05	2.76 ± 0.19
21	Plasma	2.93 ± 0.77	3.91 ± 1.01	0.51 ± 0.11
	Brain	17.61 ± 2.09	31.76 ± 8.31	5.02 ± 1.01
	Liver	8.77 ± 1.93	7.93 ± 0.99	3.97 ± 0.43
30	Plasma	5.01 ± 1.64	5.46 ± 0.89	0.71 ± 0.31
	Brain	29.73 ± 4.34	50.26 ± 6.04	6.81 ± 1.05
	Liver	12.65 ± 2.70	12.67 ± 1.05	5.02 ± 0.79

Each value is the mean ± S.D. of four animals. Animals were killed 12 hr after the last dose.

quilizers. The results, shown in Table 3, are basically similar to those previously reported by Mahju and Maickel (10) after taking into account the dosage differences. Significant accumulation was seen in plasma, as well as in both tissues. Of particular interest is the apparent greater tendency for promazine to accumulate in brain, and chlorpromazine and triflupromazine to accumulate in liver.

Effects of Chronic Dosage with Phenothiazine Tranquilizers on Open Field Behavior of Rats

Groups of six rats were dosed with each of the three phenothiazine tranquilizers and tested in an open field situation for 15 min just prior to being killed to supply the tissue samples used in sections B and C. All of the animals were thus naive; none was tested more than once. The animals were viewed by a nonbiased observer using a double-blind situation and counting the number of squares entered completely. The results are presented in Table 4. Two points are of specific interest. Both promazine and triflupromazine show a decrease in activity, the former only in the test after 7 days and the latter after 7, 15, and 21 days. An adaptation to the effects of the drug occurred in both cases with a return to normal activity. In contrast, chlorpromazine showed a decrease in activity after 7 and 15 days, with a rebound increase in activity at 21 and 30 days.

TABLE 4. *Effect of phenothiazine tranquilizers on open field exploration*

| Day of dosage | Placebo | Number of squares entered | | |
		Chlorpromazine	Promazine	Triflupromazine
0	31 ± 3	—	—	—
1	34 ± 4	33 ± 5	35 ± 4	32 ± 3
4	30 ± 4	29 ± 3	34 ± 4	29 ± 4
7	30 ± 3	21 ± 2	17 ± 5	17 ± 2
15	31 ± 5	24 ± 1	26 ± 3	18 ± 5
21	29 ± 2	36 ± 4	31 ± 5	24 ± 3
30	33 ± 3	39 ± 3	30 ± 5	34 ± 3

Each value is the mean ± S.D. of six animals. Underlined values are significantly different from placebo ($p < 0.05$).

Effects of Chronic Dosage with Chlorpromazine on Continuous Avoidance Behavior of Rats

The interesting effects of chlorpromazine prompted a more detailed study of this compound using two lever continuous avoidance. Animals were run at weekly intervals for 6 weeks, with daily dosage as described above.

TABLE 5. *Effects of chlorpromazine on continuous avoidance responding*

Day of dosage	Avoidance rate (% of baseline)
0	100 ± 11
7	$\underline{62 \pm 16}$
14	$\underline{28 \pm 12}$
21	$\underline{6 \pm 5}$
28	$\underline{8 \pm 6}$
35	$\underline{12 \pm 10}$
42	$\underline{38 \pm 11}$
Post drug 7	89 ± 12
Post drug 14	$\underline{143 \pm 16}$

Each value is the mean $\pm$ S.D. of 12 rats reported as percent of baseline response rate for each animal. Underlined values are significantly different from baseline responding ($p < 0.05$).

The results are presented in Table 5. Clear evidence for adaptation is seen in the pattern of avoidance responding, as the decrement seen in the first few weeks is significantly attenuated over the final 2 weeks. Of particular interest is the "rebound" increase in avoidance responding seen in the second week after the chronic dosage was discontinued.

Ability of Chronic Dosage with Phenothiazine Tranquilizers to Induce Symptoms of Pseudoparkinsonism in Rats

One of the clinically observed side effects of chronic use of the phenothiazine tranquilizers has been a moderate incidence of drug-induced parkinsonism. This side effect is most often seen with high dosages and/or long-term therapy; it can be reversed by discontinuing the drug, reducing the dosage, or by administration of cholinergic-blocking agents such as atropine. The chronically dosed animals used in the studies reported above have been observed at periodic intervals for evidence of parkinsonism symptoms. The results obtained are shown in Table 6; they clearly indicate that with continuing dosage, some of the symptoms are observed with all three of the agents. In particular, the tremors are most noticeable with chlorpromazine and triflupromazine. Excessive salivation was not seen at all; this may reflect a unique species phenomenon of the rat.

DISCUSSION

Gordon (14), in 1967, stated that at that time there were more than 2,000 papers on chlorpromazine alone, not to mention the other phenothiazine tranquilizers. Since that publication at least an additional 2,000 papers have

TABLE 6. *Parkinsonism symptoms evoked by chronic tranquilizer administration*

Day of dosage	Drug	Symptoms observed (%)				
		Motor retardation	Tremors	Rigidity	Salivation	Shuffling gait
1	PMZ	0	0	0	0	0
	CPZ	0	0	0	0	0
	TFZ	0	0	0	0	0
4	PMZ	0	0	0	0	0
	CPZ	0	0	0	0	10
	TFZ	0	0	10	0	16
7	PMZ	67	0	0	0	24
	CPZ	60	0	10	0	40
	TFZ	60	0	10	0	30
15	PMZ	20	0	0	0	10
	CPZ	63	10	20	0	30
	TFZ	80	10	22	0	33
21	PMZ	20	0	0	0	0
	CPZ	60	30	20	0	25
	TFZ	60	30	24	0	33
30	PMZ	20	0	0	0	0
	CPZ	60	67	25	0	33
	TFZ	40	80	55	0	40

Each value is the percent of animals (out of eight to 12 observed) that showed the appropriate effects. Abbreviations are: PMZ = promazine, CPZ = chlorpromazine, TFZ = triflupromazine.

been published; the fact that there is a *Third* International Phenothiazine Symposium is a confirmation of this continued interest.

Despite this tremendous interest, and despite the widespread clinical usage of these compounds, correlated studies of various biochemical, pharmacological, and behavioral effects of chronic administration of these drugs have not been reported. Numerous studies have been reported covering the various aspects of gross toxicity of the drugs, and a large number of reports on metabolism and excretion have also been published (4, 5, 14).

This laboratory has been interested in the biochemical, behavioral, and pharmacological actions of the phenothiazine tranquilizers for a number of years. Indeed, a previous report of the senior author in 1963 (15) described the effects of several of these drugs on pituitary-adrenocortical function in rats. A dose-dependent hypersecretion of ACTH was observed, correlating with the potency of the drugs as antipsychotic agents: triflupromazine > chlorpromazine > promazine > chlorpromazine sulfoxide, as well as with their ability to potentiate hexobarbital narcosis. Subsequent studies have extended this early work, correlating brain levels of the phenothiazines with their time course of action on various behavioral test systems (7), demonstrating potency rankings on deprivation-induced fluid consumption (7) and showing dose-dependent actions on activity (8, 10) and brain acetylcholinesterase (8, 9).

Here we report on a number of aspects of chronic dosage of chlorpromazine, promazine, and triflupromazine. In Table 1 and Fig. 1, a striking difference is seen in the effects of these three drugs on body weight of rats. Promazine has no effect, even when given 2 × 5 mg/kg per day for 30 days. In contrast, chlorpromazine (2 × 2 mg/kg per day) or triflupromazine (2 × 2 mg/kg per day) had no significant effect for the first 15 days of dosage, then caused a decreased rate of weight gain over the next 15 days. A cursory examination of food consumption at scattered intervals over the test period did not show any significant alterations with any of the drugs as compared to placebo, although the limitations of accuracy of the measurements would have hidden small changes. Of interest is the observation (Table 2) that all three drugs caused increases over control in liver glycogen, and chlorpromazine and triflupromazine evoked significant elevations in liver triglycerides over the latter portion of the test period. At the same time, a continual accumulation of all three drugs was seen in plasma, brain, and liver (Table 3).

When the animals chronically dosed with phenothiazine tranquilizers were tested in various behavioral systems, some interesting adaptation phenomena were seen. For example, the three drugs behaved completely differently in a simple open field exploration test (Table 4). Promazine showed no effects until 7 to 15 days of dosage, when a significant decrease in exploratory activity was noted, followed by a return to normal by the 21st day of dosage. Chlorpromazine showed a similar reduction in activity at 7 to 15 days, followed by a rebound with increased exploratory activity above placebo at 21 and 30 days. Triflupromazine produced only a depression of activity over the period 7 to 21 days, with recovery to normal activity levels at 30 days. This adaptation in exploratory activity was accompanied by a variety of changes in observable behavioral components (licking, biting, rearing, circling, etc.); attempts to correlate these with the continued drug dosage were unsuccessful.

In the area of behavioral adaptations to chronic dosages of the phenothiazine tranquilizers, we have also examined the effects of chlorpromazine on continuous avoidance responding. A portion of these data are presented in Table 5. These results—the avoidance responding component only— demonstrate several interesting phenomena. First of all, the rate of avoidance responding is reduced in a gradual manner over the first 3 weeks of dosage. Maximum reduction in avoidance responding corresponds to that point in time when brain levels of the drug are approaching 15 to 30 μg/g. Despite the fact that brain levels of the drug continue to increase beyond this level, the avoidance rate at 35 to 42 days of dosage begins to return to normal. Preliminary studies of animals carried to 63 to 70 days on a similar regimen indicate that the avoidance response rate continues to increase in a nonlinear manner, approaching 60 to 75% of control as a maximum. However, an inherent problem in these studies is the increasing age and responsivity of the animals. Since the training and predrug baseline periods comprise 30 to 45 days, after 10 weeks of drug runs (an additional 70 days) the animals are approaching 280 to 320 days of age and control performance is beginning to deteriorate.

In the process of examining the continuous avoidance behavior with chronic chlorpromazine dosage, we have also measured the escapes and escape failures (shocks taken) on the second lever of the avoidance system. These data, while most interesting, have not been presented in tabular form since they are also somewhat confusing. Basically, they may be summarized by saying that the animals (12 at each testing point) fall into two distinct classes: seven rats showed little or no adaptation to the chronic dosage, and five others clearly adapted to the regimen. If all of the data were summed and tabulated as a single mean, no significant differences could be measured. Since no correlation was observed with brain or plasma levels of the drug in the individual animals, these differences in behavioral performance would appear to be due to either individual differences in animal behavior, or in metabolism and metabolite accumulation; we have no data as yet on the latter possibility.

Finally, we have also examined the production of extrapyramidal side effects in rats on the chronic treatment regimens. As shown by the data in Table 6, all three drugs elicited some symptoms with the frequency and severity occurring in the potency ranking: triflupromazine > chlorpromazine > promazine. Excessive salivation was not seen in any of the animals, although some chromodactorrhea was occasionally observed.

SUMMARY

The data presented herein indicate that a variety of biochemical, behavioral and pharmacological effects are seen when rats are chronically dosed with phenothiazine tranquilizers. The drugs accumulate in plasma and tissues. Concomitant with this accumulation are moderate elevations in liver glycogen and triglycerides, extrapyramidal symptoms, and various types of behavioral adaptations. Since many of these effects cannot be correlated with brain levels of the drugs themselves, further study of the possible role of active metabolites appears to be a necessity.

ACKNOWLEDGMENTS

This work has been supported by grants MH–18852 and MH–41083 (from the U.S. Public Health Service). We wish to thank the following manufacturers for supplying us with compounds: chlorpromazine (Thorazine®)—Smith Kline and French; promazine (Sparine®)—Wyeth Laboratories; triflupromazine—Smith Kline and French.

REFERENCES

1. Delay, J., Deniker, P., and Harl, J. M., *Ann. Med. Psychol. (Paris)*, **2**, 112 (1952).
2. Laborit, H., and Jaulmes, C., *Toulouse Med.*, **53**, 821 (1952).
3. Zirkle, C. L., and Kaiser, C., In *Medicinal Chemistry*, Part II, Burger, A., (ed.), Wiley-Interscience, New York, 1970, pp. 1410–1469.
4. Domino, E. F., In *Psychopharmacology: A Review of Progress, 1957–1967*, Efron, D. H., (ed.), U.S. Government Printing Office, Washington, D.C., 1968, pp. 1045–1056.
5. Usdin, E., *Psychopharmacol. Bull.*, **6**, 4 (1970).
6. Cole, J. O., and Davis, J. M., In: *Psychopharmacology: A Review of Progress, 1957–1967*, Efron, D. H., (ed.), U.S. Government Printing Office, Washington, D.C., 1968, pp. 1057–1063.
7. Maickel, R. P., Gerald, M. C., Warburton, D. M., and Mahju, M. A., *Agressologie*, **9**, 373 (1968).
8. Maickel, R. P., *Int. J. Neuropharmacol.*, **7**, 23 (1968).
9. Berg, S. W., and Maickel, R. P., *Life Sci.*, **7**, Part II, 1197 (1968).
10. Mahju, M. A., and Maickel, R. P., *Biochem. Pharmacol.*, **18**, 2701 (1969).
11. Maickel, R. P., McGlynn, M., and Snodgrass, W. R., *Toxicol. Appl. Pharmacol.*, **17**, 312 (1970).
12. Cox, R. H., Jr., and Maickel, R. P., *J. Pharmacol. Exp. Therap.*, **181**, 1 (1972).
13. Butler, W. M., Jr., Maling, H. M., Horning, M. G., and Brodie, B. B., *J. Lipid Res.*, **2**, 95 (1960).
14. Gordon, M., In *Psychopharmacological Agents*, Volume II, Gordon, M., (ed.), Academic Press, New York, 1967, pp. 1–198.
15. Smith, R. L., Maickel, R. P., and Brodie, B. B., *J. Pharmacol. Exp. Therap.*, **139**, 185 (1963).

The Phenothiazines and Structurally Related Drugs, edited by I. S.
Forrest, C. J. Carr, and E. Usdin. Raven Press, New York © 1974.

Effects of Hydroxylated Phenothiazine Metabolites on Rat Brain Mitochondria

Sarah A. Tijoe, Albert A. Manian,* and John J. O'Neill

*Department of Pharmacology, College of Medicine, Ohio State University, Columbus,
Ohio 43210, and * Psychopharmacology Research Branch, National Institute of Mental
Health, Rockville, Maryland 20852*

INTRODUCTION

In view of increasing evidence that oxidative metabolism (1–3) and low
intracellular calcium (4) levels are essential to neuronal function, pharmacologic agents which can modify these processes have the potential for
altering neuronal functions *in vivo*. Chlorpromazine is known to exert many
inhibitory effects on mitochondria. These inhibitory actions include inhibition of cytochrome oxidase (5), uncoupling of phosphorylation associated
with the oxidation of reduced cytochrome-*c* (6), inhibition of magnesium and
DNP-stimulated ATPase, inhibition of glutamate dehydrogenase (7) and
succinate dehydrogenase (8), and inhibition of the ^{32}Pi-ATP exchange reaction (9). Recently we have shown marked inhibitory effects by 7,8-dihy-
droxychlorpromazine on both calcium transport and oxygen uptake in
isolated rat brain mitochondria (10). These inhibitory effects differ from
those observed in the presence of chlorpromazine. We will present further
studies concerning the actions of hydroxylated phenothiazines on rat brain
mitochondria.

CALCIUM UPTAKE AND RETENTION

The mitochondria used in these experiments were prepared according to
the method of Ozawa (11) with some slight modifications (10). In experiments involving calcium transport, mitochondria were incubated in the
presence of ^{45}CaCl$_2$. Samples were taken at timed intervals and filtered
through 0.45 micron Millipore filters to remove the mitochondria. Aliquots
of these filtrates were then counted in a gas flow planchet counter in order
to determine the amount of isotope remaining in solution. Figure 1 illustrates
the results of a typical experiment in which mitochondria were allowed to
accumulate calcium with ATP as an energy source in the presence of either
chlorpromazine (CPZ), 7-hydroxychlorpromazine (7-OH-CPZ), or 7,8-

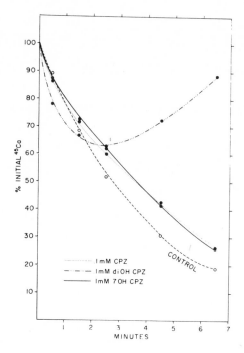

FIG. 1. Percentage of the initial concentration of calcium in filtrate plotted as a function of time of incubation. Composition of reaction mixture: 36 mM HEPES[1] (pH 7.4), 4.5 mM MgCl$_2$, 4.5 mM ATP, 0.1 mM ^{45}CaCl$_2$, 6 mM mannitol, 4 μM histidine, 0.04 mg bovine serum albumin per ml, KCl to 0.25 osmolar, 0.36 mg mitochondrial protein per ml. Drugs present from the beginning of incubation. Temp. = 24°C.

dihydroxychlorpromazine (7,8-diOH-CPZ). Both chlorpromazine and 7-hydroxychlorpromazine decrease the amount of calcium accumulated by the mitochondria slightly. 7,8-Dihydroxychlorpromazine has a more striking effect. In the presence of this metabolite, calcium is accumulated initially at a rate comparable to that of the control for the first 2 or 3 min. At this point, however, an efflux of calcium ions from the mitochondria begins and continues until all of the previously accumulated calcium is released into the medium. Thus, calcium retention by these mitochondria is largely disrupted by 7,8-dihydroxychlorpromazine.

When brain mitochondria accumulate calcium with a respiratory substrate, such as glutamate, as an energy source, somewhat different results are obtained. Under these conditions (Fig. 2A) CPZ, 7-OH-CPZ, and 7,8-diOH-CPZ all exert about the same degree of inhibition of calcium uptake. In a third type of experiment, mitochondria are preloaded with calcium; drugs are not present initially but are added after 6 min. At this time the rapid

[1] HEPES: N-2-hydroxyethylpiperazine-N'-2-ethane sulfonic acid.

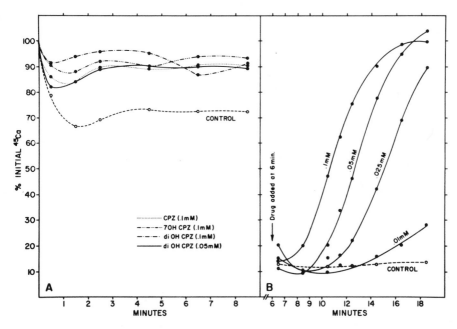

FIG. 2. Effects of CPZ and its hydroxylated metabolites on calcium uptake and retention by rat brain mitochondria. The percentage of initial calcium concentration has been plotted as a function of incubation time. Composition of reaction mixture (A): 38.0 mM HEPES (pH 7.4), 1.9 mM phosphate, 5.7 mM potassium glutamate, 4.75 mM $MgCL_2$, 0.05 mM $^{45}CaCl_2$, 6 mM mannitol, 4 μM histidine, 0.04 mg BSA per ml, KCl to 0.25 osmolar, 0.312 mg mitochondrial protein per ml. (B): 36 mM HEPES (pH 7.4), 4.5 mM $MgCl_2$, 4.5 mM ATP, 0.1 mM $^{45}CaCl_2$, 6 mM mannitol, 4 μM histidine, 0.04 mg BSA per ml, KCl to 0.25 osmolar, 0.326 mg mitochondrial protein per ml. Temp. = 24°C.

phase of calcium uptake has taken place and calcium efflux can then be monitored. Figure 2B illustrates the rate of calcium efflux observed when 0.1 mM 7,8-diOH-CPZ is added to mitochondria preloaded with calcium in the presence of ATP. Again there is a delay in the start of this efflux, but essentially all of the accumulated calcium is eventually lost by the mitochondria. The delay in the onset of this efflux becomes longer as the concentration of this chlorpromazine metabolite is decreased. In experiments of longer duration, concentrations as low as 0.01 mM 7,8-diOH-CPZ were found to promote a loss of essentially all mitochondrial calcium. An efflux with the same time course is also observed if mitochondria are preloaded with calcium in the presence of ATP, glutamate, and inorganic phosphate. This calcium efflux is delayed by about 2 min if 0.6 mM dithiothreitol (DTT), a sulfhydryl reagent, is added with or before 0.1 mM 7,8-diOH-CPZ. This suggests that the phenothiazine metabolite may be reacting with mitochondrial sulfhydryl groups which are temporarily reduced by DTT or that an oxidized form of the drug metabolite is damaging to mitochondria and can be reduced by DTT. Dithiothreitol prevents the red color, seen with solu-

TABLE 1. ^{45}Calcium retention by brain mitochondria: the effects of CPZ-metabolites

	Percent ^{45}Ca in filtrate					
Time (min):	6.5	10.5	12.5	14.5	16.5	18.5
Control	23.6	18.6	24.2	16.5	27.1	16.8
3,7-diOH-CPZ	31.0	49.9	52.4	55.6	63.8	64.1
7,8-diOH-CPZ	26.3	25.0	31.6	41.0	69.0	88.0

Composition of reaction medium: 36 mM HEPES (pH 7.4), 4.5 mM ATP, 4.5 mM MgCl$_2$, 0.1 mM ^{45}CaCl$_2$, 6 mM mannitol, KCl to 0.250 Osm, 0.352 mg mitochondrial protein per ml. Temp. = 24°C. Drugs (0.1 mM) were added at 6.0 min. Percentages based on the amount of ^{45}Ca initially present in the filtrate.

tions of 7,8-diOH-CPZ, from appearing initially, although the red color does eventually return. The calcium efflux begins, however, before the re-appearance of this color.

In order to determine what sites in the structure of 7,8-diOH-CPZ are contributing to these mitochondrial effects, other phenothiazine compounds were studied. 3,7-Dihydroxychlorpromazine was chosen so that the importance of having adjacent hydroxyl groups could be determined. It was found (Table 1) that when 3,7-diOH-CPZ was added to mitochondria pre-loaded with calcium, an efflux of calcium was observed, but this efflux was more linear during the period studied than that observed with 7,8-diOH-CPZ. In addition there did not appear to be a delay in the onset of action with the 3,7-dihydroxy compound. These effects were also studied with 2,3-dihydroxypromazine, which has adjacent hydroxyl groups but lacks the chloro substituent. Promazine, 3-OH-promazine, and 2,3-diOH-promazine were all found to produce very little, if any, calcium efflux when added to preloaded mitochondria. This suggests that a highly electronegative chloro group at position 2 contributes significantly to the ability of phenothiazines to alter calcium retention by brain mitochondria (Table 2).

TABLE 2. Effect of 2,3-diOH-promazine on ^{45}Ca retention

	Percent ^{45}Ca in filtrate				
Time (min):	6.5	10.5	12.5	14.5	16.5
Control	27.2	30.9	15.2	25.8	12.6
2,3-diOH-promazine	10.2	23.6	31.5	28.7	29.8
Promazine	28.1	33.4	27.9	27.0	26.2
7,8-diOH-CPZ	23.9	44.3	75.2	85.6	94.1

Conditions were described previously (Table 1). Percentages based on the amount of ^{45}Ca initially present in the filtrate. Mitochondrial protein: 0.40 mg/ml.

The effects of two other dihydroxylated phenothiazines were studied. These were 7,8-dihydroxyprochlorperazine and 7,8-dihydroxyperphenazine. The effects observed in the presence of these agents were similar to those seen with 7,8-diOH-CPZ. The results of a typical experiment with 7,8-diOH-prochlorperazine are listed in Table 3. There is an initial delay in the onset of the action of this dihydroxy compound, but once calcium efflux begins it is rapid and extensive. Both 7-OH prochlorperazine and the parent compound prochlorperazine caused some release of mitochondrial calcium compared to the control mitochondria with 7-OH-prochlorperazine being slightly more potent. Similar results were also found with the perphenazine series. Perphenazine itself promotes some calcium release, but 7,8-diOH-perphenazine causes a rapid and complete release of accumulated calcium with a delayed onset of action. Likewise, fluphenazine and 7-OH-fluphenazine cause some calcium loss from mitochondria but not the rapid and complete depletion seen with 7,8-diOH-CPZ. The piperazinyl side chain in prochlorperazine, perphenazine, and fluphenazine does apparently increase the effectiveness of these compounds as inhibitors of calcium uptake and retention, since all three of these agents are more potent inhibitors than chlorpromazine. The piperazinyl side chain did not, however, appear to alter the time of onset or the rate of calcium efflux seen with 7,8-diOH-prochlorperazine or 7,8-diOH-perphenazine compared to that seen with 7,8-diOH-CPZ at the concentrations used in these experiments (0.1 mM).

The effects of 7,8-dioxochlorpromazine, the quinone form of 7,8-diOH-CPZ, were also investigated. Again, as was seen with 7,8-diOH-CPZ, a delayed onset was followed by a rapid and complete loss of preloaded calcium from the mitochondria upon the addition of 7,8-dioxo-CPZ. Since there is some evidence from oxygen uptake experiments that 7,8-dihydroxychlorpromazine undergoes oxidation, the oxidized form 7,8-dioxochlorpromazine may contribute significantly to the effects seen (see below). When 7-hydroxy-8-methoxychlorpromazine or 7-methoxy,8-hydroxychlorpromazine are added, however, dissimilar results are obtained. Little or no calcium loss is observed upon the addition of either of these O-methylated derivatives to calcium-loaded mitochondria.

TABLE 3. *Effect of prochlorperazine on ^{45}Ca retention*

	Percent ^{45}Ca in filtrate					
Time (min):	6.5	8.5	10.5	12.5	14.5	16.5
Control	5.9	14.2	5.1	11.4	6.3	12.7
Prochlorperazine	15.5	16.4	18.0	18.2	20.4	31.4
7-OH-prochlorperazine	24.9	14.2	22.1	27.5	27.8	43.6
7,8-diOH-prochlorperazine	24.2	14.6	24.6	55.1	79.3	89.4
7,8-diOH-CPZ	6.4	9.6	26.8	70.6	90.1	95.2

Conditions were as described previously (Table 1). Percentages based on the amount of ^{45}Ca initially present in the filtrate. Mitochondrial protein: 0.257 mg/ml.

ELECTRON MICROSCOPY

An investigation of the fine structure of mitochondria was undertaken in order to determine whether or not the ultrastructure of these organelles was being altered by 7,8-diOH-CPZ. The results of this investigation are illustrated in Fig. 3. Typical control brain mitochondria following a 4-min

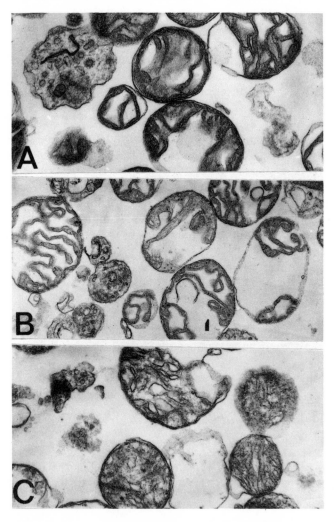

FIG. 3. Conditions were as described previously (Table 1) except that drugs (0.1 mм) were present initially. Samples were taken after 4-min incubations. Mitochondria were fixed with glutaraldehyde in suspension, collected in a pellet, and postfixed with osmium tetroxide. Sections were stained with lead citrate and uranyl acetate. (A): Control mitochondria × 31,500. (B): Chlorpromazine-treated mitochondria × 25,500. (C): 7,8-DiOH-CPZ-treated mitochondria × 31,500.

incubation in the presence of 0.1 mM calcium chloride with ATP as an energy source are shown in panel A. Note that the matrix material is dense and contracted. In panel B, we show brain mitochondria following incubation under the same conditions as those in panel A except that 0.1 mM chlorpromazine was also present. In these mitochondria, the cristae have widened slightly and the matrix appears less dense than in the control mitochondria. Mitochondria incubated for 4 min with 0.1 mM 7,8-diOH-CPZ are illustrated in Fig. 3C. The mitochondria are noticeably inflated causing the matrix material to appear diluted. With longer incubations in the presence of 7,8-diOH-CPZ these mitochondria become extremely swollen and appear to be extensively damaged.

OXYGEN UPTAKE

The effects of 7,8-diOH-CPZ on mitochondrial oxygen uptake are more marked than those seen with either chlorpromazine or 7-OH-chlorpromazine. Both chlorpromazine and 7-OH-chlorpromazine increase the rate of state 4 oxygen uptake and decrease the rate of state 3 respiration slightly. In addition, the state 3 to 4 transition becomes less sharp, indicating an uncoupling effect by these phenothiazines. The results observed on adding 7,8-diOH-CPZ to the incubation mixture are illustrated in Fig. 4. 7,8-DiOH-CPZ causes an immediate stimulation of oxygen uptake, followed by a decline in this rate and finally an inhibition. If ADP is added once this diminished rate has begun, no stimulation of oxygen consumption is observed. The addition of calcium ions, which normally stimulate oxygen uptake, is also without effect, as is the addition of 2,4-dinitrophenol. Adding DTT, however, does produce an immediate increase in oxygen consumption. As in the calcium experiments, this sulfhydryl compound may delay the effects of 7,8-diOH-CPZ by either reducing mitochondrial sulfhydryl groups or by reducing an oxidized form of the phenothiazine compound or both. In oxygen uptake experiments, the appearance of a red-colored product does coincide with the onset of respiratory inhibition and the block of ADP-stimulated oxygen uptake. The red color is removed when DTT is added but the color returns with time.

The inhibition of mitochondrial respiration by 7,8-diOH-CPZ is apparent within 2 min following the addition of the drug, when glutamate is the respiratory substrate. In contrast, with succinate as the substrate the inhibition takes longer to appear and may not be observed until 5 min after adding the phenothiazine. This inhibition of respiration is also released by DTT (Fig. 4C). It has been observed that when glutamate-supported respiration becomes inhibited by 7,8-diOH-CPZ, the addition of succinate results in an increased oxygen uptake, which suggests that this respiratory block can be bypassed at least temporarily by succinate.

It was found that 7,8-dioxo-CPZ has effects on oxygen uptake similar to

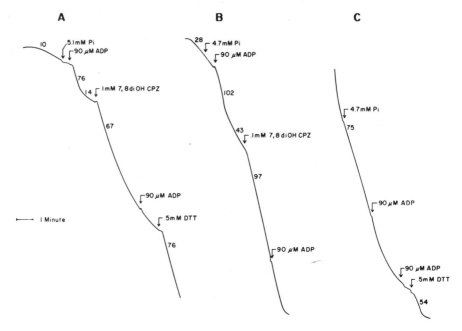

FIG. 4. Effects of 7,8-diOH-CPZ on oxygen uptake. Composition of reaction medium: 32 mM HEPES (pH 7.4), 82 mM KCl, 5 mM glutamate (trace A), or 5 mM succinate (traces B and C), 30 mM mannitol, 0.2 mM EDTA, 0.2 mg BSA per ml, 1.49 mg mitochondrial protein/ml. Temp. = 21°C. In trace C, mitochondria were preincubated for 2 min with 0.1 mM 7,8-diOH-CPZ before oxygen uptake was recorded. Figures next to tracings refer to nanoatoms oxygen per minute per mg.

those seen with 7,8-diOH-CPZ. 7,8-Dioxo-CPZ initially stimulates glutamate-supported respiration, but after 1.5 min state 4 respiration becomes inhibited and no increase in oxygen uptake is observed, when ADP and inorganic phosphate (Pi) are added. Although the dioxo form has the same time course of action as 7,8-diOH-CPZ, the amount of oxygen removed from the medium from the time of drug addition to the onset of state 4 inhibition is less with 7,8-dioxo-CPZ than with 7,8-diOH-CPZ. This observation suggests that part of the initial burst of oxygen uptake seen with 7,8-diOH-CPZ may result from the oxidation of the compound itself. As with 7,8-diOH-CPZ, once respiratory inhibition has occurred, calcium ions and dinitrophenol fail to stimulate oxygen uptake. The addition of DTT also releases this form of inhibition of state 4 respiration.

The failure of ADP to increase mitochondrial oxygen uptake after mitochondria are exposed to either 0.1 mM 7,8-diOH-CPZ or 0.1 mM 7,8-dioxo-CPZ for 2 min suggests that oxidative phosphorylation is being severely compromised by these two agents. In order to examine this possibility more directly, the adenine nucleotide content of the incubation medium plus mitochondria after exposure to 7,8-diOH-CPZ and 7,8-dioxo-CPZ were measured fluorometrically by the method of Lowry et al. (12). Incubations were stopped with perchloric acid 2.6 min after the addition of 0.743 μmoles of ADP. 7,8-DiOH-CPZ (0.1 mM) or 7,8-dioxo-CPZ (0.1 mM) was added 2 min before ADP. The adenine nucleotide content of these mitochondria are listed in Table 4 along with μatoms of oxygen consumed in the 2.6 min after the addition of ADP. As was expected ATP synthesis was almost completely inhibited by both 7,8-diOH-CPZ and 7,8-dioxo-CPZ. The ATP synthesized with 7,8-diOH-CPZ was 7.6% of the control level, and 4.8% of control with 7,8-dioxo-CPZ. In both cases, this inhibition was relieved somewhat if DTT was also present. With the addition of DTT, the ATP synthesized was increased to 30.2% and 14.0% of control with 7,8-diOH-CPZ and 7,8-dioxo-CPZ, respectively. In contrast, control ATP synthesis was decreased slightly when DTT was added. This may have been due to nonspecific ATPase stimulation by DTT.

The effects of several other dihydroxylated phenothiazines on oxygen uptake were also studied. 2,3-Dihydroxypromazine was found to have inhibitory effects similar to those seen with 7,8-diOH-CPZ and 7,8-dioxo-CPZ on oxygen uptake. With glutamate as substrate, oxygen uptake is stimulated upon the addition of 2,3-diOH promazine, followed by a decline in rate and then an inhibition. ADP, calcium, and dinitrophenol all fail to stimulate oxygen uptake after this inhibition has begun. Similar effects are seen with succinate as substrate, except that more time is required before the effects of ADP on respiration are inhibited. 3,7-Dihydroxychlorproma-

TABLE 4. *Nucleotide analysis: effects of chlorpromazine metabolites on ATP synthesis*[a]

	ATP	ADP	AMP	μatoms O	ATP (% of control)
Control	0.584 ± 0.039	$0.117 \pm <0.007$	$0.044 \pm <0.007$	0.344	100
Control + DTT	0.451 ± 0.033	0.248 ± 0.007	$0.110 \pm <0.007$	0.272	77.3
7,8-diOH-CPZ	0.045 ± 0.002	0.660 ± 0.025	0.151 ± 0.012	0.116	7.6
7,8-diOH CPZ + DTT	0.176 ± 0.001	0.480 ± 0.078	$0.122 \pm <0.007$	0.244	30.2
7,8-dioxo-CPZ	0.028 ± 0.001	$0.699 \pm <0.007$	$0.184 \pm <0.007$	0.063	4.8
7,8-dioxo-CPZ + DTT	0.082 ± 0.002	0.655 ± 0.007	0.140 ± 0.016	0.166	14.0
Fresh mitochondria	0.012 ± 0.003	0.269 ± 0.016	0.120 ± 0.010		

[a] Results are expressed as micromoles $\pm$S.E.M.

Conditions: Incubation media: 33.4 mM HEPES buffer, pH 7.4, 79.5 mM potassium chloride, 4.2 mM glutamate, 0.5 mg BSA, 1.13 mg mitochondrial protein, 1.7 mM inorganic phosphate. When present: 0.08 mM, 7,8-dihydroxychlorpromazine or 7,8-dioxochlorpromazine, 0.08 mM dithiothreitol (DTT). Samples were taken 2.6 min after the addition of 0.743 micromoles ADP and inorganic phosphate. Drugs were added 2.0 min before ADP. Oxygen consumed in 2.6 min after ADP addition is listed.

zine has slightly different effects on mitochondrial respiration. This compound does not cause as large an increase in the rate of oxygen consumption when added to mitochondria respiring in state 4, as that seen with other dihydroxylated phenothiazines. In fact, the increase in oxygen consumption seen following 3,7-diOH-CPZ appears to be more like that seen following the addition of chlorpromazine than that following 7,8-diOH-CPZ. In the presence of 0.1 mM 3,7-diOH-CPZ, repeated additions of ADP result in increases in mitochondrial respiration, whereas the mitochondria become more and more uncoupled with time. After about 6 to 8 min, further additions of ADP fail to stimulate respiration, although the mitochondria continue to respire at a rate slightly faster than the control state 4 rate. In contrast, other dihydroxylated phenothiazines decrease oxygen uptake to a rate slower than that of control state 4 respiration, when they block ADP-stimulated respiration. Such differences are illustrated in Table 5 in which the effects of 3,7-diOH-CPZ, 2,3-diOH-promazine, and 7,8-diOH-perphenazine on mitochondrial oxygen uptake are compared. Although all three of these compounds produce an initial increase in oxygen consumption, this initial rate is greater with 2,3-diOH-promazine (0.081 μatoms O/min) and 7,8-diOH-perphenazine (0.051 μatoms O/min) than with 3,7-diOH-CPZ (0.033 μatoms O/min). Also, the time required for ADP-stimulated respiration to be inhibited is shorter for 2,3-diOH-promazine (3 min) and 7,8-diOH-perphenazine (4 min) than for 3,7-diOH-CPZ (8 min). Finally, when ADP-stimulated respiration is blocked, the residual rate of oxygen uptake is greater with 3,7-diOH-CPZ (0.026 μatoms O/min) than the control state 4 respiratory rate (0.016 μatoms O/min). The rate seen with 2,3-diOH-promazine (0.005 μatoms O/min) or 7,8-diOH-perphenazine (0.009 μatoms O/min) is much below control state 4 respiration. It appears that mitochondrial state 4 respiration is not affected to the same extent by 3,7-diOH-CPZ as it is by 7,8-diOH-CPZ, 2,3-diOH-promazine, or 7,8-diOH-perphenazine. Having the hydroxyl groups adjacent to each other on one ring

TABLE 5. Comparison of the effects of dihydroxylated phenothiazes on oxygen uptake

Conditions	Initial μatoms O/min	After ADP inhibited μatoms O/min	Time for inhibition
State 4 respiration (control)	0.016		
3,7-diOH-CPZ	0.033	0.026	8 min
2,3-diOH-promazine	0.081	0.005	3 min
7,8-diOH-perphenazine	0.051	0.009	4 min

Rates of oxygen uptake listed are those immediately after drug addition and after inhibition of ADP-stimulated respiration. Drugs present in 0.1 mM concentration. Composition of incubation medium: 33.3 mM HEPES (pH 7.4), 79 mM KCl, 4.1 mM glutamate, 0.4 mg BSA per ml, 4.1 mM Pi. Temp. = 22°.

of the phenothiazine molecule apparently increases the rapidity with which mitochondrial respiration is altered by these agents. When one of these hydroxyl groups undergoes O-methylation as in 7-hydroxy-8-methoxy-CPZ or 8-hydroxy-7-methoxy-CPZ, progressive uncoupling of the mitochondria is observed. ADP-stimulated oxygen uptake is inhibited by the O-methylated derivatives only at higher drug concentrations, i.e., 0.2 mM.

Fine structure studies were done on mitochondria respiring with glutamate as described in Table 4. The fine structure of mitochondria respiring in the presence of 7,8-diOH-CPZ or 7,8-dioxo-CPZ was not markedly different from controls at a time when oxidative phosphorylation was being inhibited.

DISCUSSION

Much work remains to be done before all of the specific sites of action of the mono- and dihydroxylated phenothiazines on mitochondria can be identified. Several aspects of this question are becoming clear from the studies that we have conducted thus far. 7,8-Dihydroxychlorpromazine is a potent inhibitor of mitochondrial calcium retention and oxidative phosphorylation. Calcium retention is interrupted by this drug metabolite at concentrations as low as 0.01 mM and oxidative phosphorylation is inhibited by concentrations as low as 0.02 mM. However, not all dihydroxyphenothiazine compounds affect both of these mitochondrial processes to this extent. 2,3-Dihydroxypromazine has very little effect on calcium retention by brain mitochondria, even at a concentration of 0.1 mM, while this agent appears to be equally as effective as 7,8-diOH-CPZ in inhibiting oxidative phosphorylation. This suggests that a strongly electronegative chloro group at position 2 plays an important role in allowing these compounds to produce a calcium efflux. On the other hand an electronegative substituent at position 2 is not essential for the inhibition of ADP-stimulated respiration by dihydroxylated phenothiazines. The two adjacent hydroxyls are important in altering mitochondrial respiration, since promazine is not as potent an uncoupler as chlorpromazine, but 2,3-diOH-promazine appears to be as effective as 7,8-diOH-CPZ in blocking oxidative phosphorylation. The results of experiments with 3,7-diOH-CPZ support these suggestions. This compound, which has a chlorine in position 2, is more effective in producing a calcium efflux than 2,3-diOH-promazine, although 3,7-diOH-CPZ, 7-OH-8-MeO-CPZ, and 8-OH-7-MeO-CPZ are all less effective than 2,3-diOH-promazine in inhibiting oxidative phosphorylation. This again indicates that the adjacent hydroxyl groups are important in inhibiting oxidative phosphorylation. The hypothesis that the presence of two hydroxyl groups in the molecule does have some role in the production of a rapid calcium efflux is supported by the fact that the O-methylated compounds do not cause an efflux. It is possible that a quinone form of these agents is active in all of the inhibitory processes described here, since

7,8-dioxo-CPZ produced a calcium efflux; an inhibition of ADP, ^{45}Ca, and DNP-stimulated oxygen uptake; and an inhibition of ATP synthesis with the same time course of action as 7,8-diOH-CPZ.

Since chlorpromazine itself has many inhibitory sites of action in mitochondria, it is likely that the phenothiazine metabolites have many of the same sites of action in their inhibitory effects on mitochondrial calcium transport and respiration. However, the dihydroxylated phenothiazines must have additional damaging effects on mitochondria, since the parent compounds do not cause as rapid a release of calcium or as dramatic a block of ATP synthesis in comparable concentrations. Quinone forms of the dihydroxylated phenothiazines have the potential for acting as electron acceptors which may bypass the electron-transport chain. Quinones may also react readily with mitochondrial sulfhydryl groups. Both of these possibilities are of potential importance and could help explain the inhibitory effects on respiration with these agents. It is known that the number of mitochondrial sulfhydryl groups increases during state 3 respiration over the number present during state 4 (13) and that agents which react with sulfhydryl groups inhibit oxidative phosphorylation (14, 15). Tellurite, such a sulfhydryl reagent, has been shown to inhibit the oxidation of NADH-linked substrates (16). This inhibition is not relieved by the addition of dinitrophenol, but is relieved by the addition of succinate. A number of napthoquinones, on the other hand, have been shown to inhibit succinate-supported respiration (17, 18). Much less is known about the accessibility of sulfhydryl groups during ATP-supported calcium uptake, but high concentrations of sulfhydryl reagents can inhibit this uptake process (19) also. The effects of dihydroxyphenothiazines on mitochondrial calcium transport may involve other mechanisms, however, since mitochondria exposed to 7,8-diOH-CPZ during calcium uptake appear swollen, while those exposed to this agent in the presence of a respiratory substrate show no such alteration in fine structure.

Chlorpromazine is known to undergo hydroxylation (20), resulting in the formation of a number of monohydroxylated metabolites. 7-OH-CPZ possesses pharmacological activity similar to that of CPZ and has been shown to be present in the central nervous system of experimental animals (21, 22). Orthodihydroxy metabolites are formed when monohydroxylated chlorpromazine derivatives are incubated with liver microsomes. This is followed by mono-O-methylation (23, 24). 7,8-DiOH-CPZ and its methoxylated analogues have recently been found in samples taken from chronic schizophrenic patients solely on CPZ therapy (25). These findings suggest that dihydroxylated phenothiazines are formed in vivo. If these metabolites reach—or are formed in—the central nervous system, their effects on brain mitochondrial calcium transport and oxidative phosphorylation might contribute to the pharmacological and/or toxicological effects of the phenothiazines. However, before such contributions can be identified, the role of mitochondria as calcium regulators and energy generators in neurons must be more fully described, especially with regard to the dependence of neuronal function on low intracellular calcium (4, 26) and the need for oxidative metabolism in axonal transport (3).

SUMMARY

The effects of several dihydroxylated phenothiazines on brain mitochondrial calcium transport and oxygen uptake were studied. It was found that 7,8-dihydroxychlorpromazine disrupts retention of calcium by mitochondria, whereas 2,3-dihydroxypromazine has very little effect on calcium transport. In contrast, 7,8-dihydroxychlorpromazine and 2,3-dihydroxypromazine appeared to be equally effective in blocking ADP-stimulated oxygen uptake. 7,8-Dioxochlorpromazine, like 7,8-dihydroxychlorpromazine, prevented both calcium retention and ADP-stimulated oxygen uptake in these mitochondria. An analysis of the nucleotide content of the mitochondria and incubation medium following the addition of ADP to brain mitochondria respiring with glutamate as substrate revealed that 0.1 mM 7,8-dihydroxychlorpromazine or 7,8-dioxochlorpromazine reduced ATP synthesis to 7.6% and 4.8% of control, respectively. This inhibition was partially prevented if dithiothreitol, a sulfhydryl reagent, was also present. The importance of substitutions at position 2 in the phenothiazine nucleus and of quinone formation by orthodihydroxyphenothiazine metabolites in the inhibitory actions of these agents toward brain mitochondria is discussed.

ACKNOWLEDGMENTS

S. Tjioe is a recipient of a Pharmaceutical Manufacturers Association Foundation Fellowship Award in Pharmacology-Morphology. This study was supported by grant No. MH-20309-01 (from the U.S. Public Health Service). We wish to thank Professor J. Cymerman Craig, University of California Medical Center, San Francisco, California, for providing 3,7-dihydroxychlorpromazine and the Squibb Institute for Medical Research, Princeton, New Jersey, for 7-hydroxyfluphenazine.

REFERENCES

1. Wright, E. B., *Amer. J. Physiol.*, **147**, 78 (1946).
2. Wright, E. B., *Amer. J. Physiol.*, **148**, 174 (1947).
3. Ochs, S., *Proc. Nat. Acad. Sci. (U.S.A.)*, **68**, 1279 (1971).
4. Tasaki, I., Watanabe, A., and Lerman, L., *Amer. J. Physiol.*, **213**, 1465 (1967).
5. Abood, L. G., *Proc. Soc. Exptl. Biol.*, **88**, 588 (1955).
6. Berger, M. J., *J. Neurochem.*, **2**, 30 (1957).
7. Fahien, L. A., and Shemisa, O., *Molec. Pharmacol.*, **6**, 156 (1970).
8. Bernsohn, J., Namajuska, J., and Boshes, B., *J. Neurochem.*, **1**, 145 (1956).
9. Dawkins, M. J. R., *Nature*, **182**, 875 (1958).

10. Tjioe, S. A., Manian, A. A., and O'Neill, J. J., *Biochem. Biophys. Res. Comm.*, **48**, 212 (1972).
11. Ozawa, K., Seta, K., Takeda, H., Ando, K., Honda, H., and Araki, C., *J. Biochem.*, **59**, 501 (1966).
12. Lowry, O. H., and Passonneau, J. V., *J. Biol. Chem.*, **239**, 31 (1964).
13. Sabadie-Pialoux, N., and Gautheron, D., *Biochem. Biophys. Acta*, **234**, 9 (1971).
14. Fluharty, A. L., and Sandi, D. R., *Biochemistry*, **2**, 519 (1963).
15. Fonyo, A., and Bessman, S. P., *Biochem. Biophys. Res. Comm.*, **24**, 61 (1966).
16. Siliprandi, D., De Meio, R. H., Toninello, A., and Zoccarato, F., *Biochem. Biophys. Res. Comm.*, **45**, 1071 (1971).
17. Howland, J. L., *Biochem. Biophys. Acta*, **73**, 665 (1963).
18. Howland, J. L., *Biochem. Biophys. Acta*, **77**, 659 (1963).
19. Tjioe, S., Haugaard, N., and Bianchi, C. P., *J. Neurochem.*, **18**, 2171 (1971).
20. Fishman, V., and Goldenberg, H., *Proc. Soc. Exp. Biol. Med.*, **112**, 501 (1963).
21. Manian, A. A., Efron, D. H., and Goldberg, M. E., *Life Sci.*, **4**, 2425 (1965).
22. Manian, A. A., Efron, D. H., and Harris, S. R., *Life Sci.*, **10**, 679 (1971).
23. Daly, J. W., and Manian, A. A., *Biochem. Pharmacol.*, **16**, 2131 (1967).
24. Daly, J. W., and Manian, A. A., *Biochem. Pharmacol.*, **18**, 1235 (1969).
25. Turano, P., Turner, W. J., and Manian, A. A., *J. Chromat.*, **75**, 277 (1973).
26. Godfraind, J. M., Kawamura, H., Krnjevic, K., and Pumalin, R. J., *J. Physiol.*, **215**, 199 (1971).

The Phenothiazines and Structurally Related Drugs, edited by I. S.
Forrest, C. J. Carr, and E. Usdin. Raven Press, New York © 1974.

Pharmacological and Behavioral Effects of Mono- and Disubstituted Chlorpromazine Derivatives

Joseph P. Buckley, Marie L. Steenberg, Herbert Barry III*, and
Albert A. Manian**

College of Pharmacy, University of Houston, Houston, Texas 77004, *Department of
Pharmacology, School of Pharmacy, University of Pittsburgh, Pittsburgh, Pennsylvania
15261, and **Pharmacology Section, Psychopharmacology Research Branch, National
Institute of Mental Health, Rockville, Maryland 20852

INTRODUCTION

Several metabolites of promazine and chlorpromazine (CPZ) have been identified in human urine, including 3-hydroxyphenothiazine and 7-hydroxy-CPZ (1). These and other monohydroxylated and methoxylated derivatives have been found to be pharmacologically active (2–7); and it appears that several metabolites possibly contribute to the total effect of the parent drug. The purpose of this chapter was to evaluate several mono- and disubstituted metabolites of CPZ for their possible effects on the central nervous system and to study further the behavioral effects of the three most potent metabolites: 3,7-dihydroxy-CPZ, 7,8-dihydroxy-CPZ, and 7-hydroxy-CPZ.

EXPERIMENTAL

Nine mono- and disubstituted metabolites of CPZ, CPZ, and 3-(2-chloro-7-hydroxy-10-phenothiazinyl)propionic acid (Table 1) were used in the present investigation.

TABLE 1. Experimental compounds

Compound	
I	8-hydroxy-7-methoxychlorpromazine
II	7-hydroxy-8-methoxychlorpromazine
III	7-hydroxy-8-methoxy-nor$_1$-chlorpromazine
IV	7-hydroxy-8-methoxy-nor$_2$-chlorpromazine
V	3,7-dihydroxychlorpromazine
VI	7,8-dihydroxychlorpromazine hydrochloride
VII	7-hydroxychlorpromazine
VIII	7-hydroxy-nor$_1$-chlorpromazine
IX	7-hydroxy-nor$_2$-chlorpromazine
X	3-(2-chloro-7-hydroxy-10-phenothiazinyl) propionic acid

Subjects and General Procedures

Male Swiss-Webster mice (Carworth Laboratories) weighing 20 to 30 g and male Albino rats (Wistar descendants) supplied by Hilltop Laboratories Animals Incorporated, Scottdale, Pennsylvania, weighing between 200 and 300 g, were used after being acclimated to laboratory conditions for a minimum of 4 to 5 days. The free bases were dissolved in a sufficient amount of 0.1 N HCl and then adjusted to volume with normal saline except for compounds IV and IX which were dissolved in propylene glycol, USP, and compound X which was dissolved in 0.5 N sodium hydroxide. Compound VI, synthesized as the hydrochloride salt, was dissolved in normal saline; however, since this solution changed color almost immediately, 0.1% ascorbic acid was added to prevent oxidation. The solutions were freshly prepared and the injection volume was kept constant at 10 ml/kg for mice and 1.0 ml/kg for rats. The rats used in the behavioral studies were housed in individual cages and all animals were permitted food and water ad lib.

LD_{50}

The acute 72-hr LD_{50} was determined in mice using three dose levels and the LD_{50} determined using probit analysis as described by Goldstein (8).

Gross Behavior in Rats

The compounds were evaluated by a gross observation rating scale described by Watzman et al. (7). The time course of drug effects was determined and the items on the scale checked 15 min prior to and 30, 60, 120, 180, and 240 min following drug administration with special emphasis on the behavioral and autonomic effects.

Spontaneous Motor Activity

Effects of the compounds on the spontaneous motor activity of mice were determined using three photocell activity cages (Woodard Research Corporation) and two animals treated with identical doses of the same compound were placed in each of two photocell cages 0.5 to 1 hr following drug administration and counts recorded every 15 min for a 1-hr period. Each dose was tested in a factorial design in each of the three activity cages, in order to negate the differences in sensitivity among units. Control animals were tested simultaneously in one of the activity cages at the same time intervals following administration of an equal volume of saline or the particular solvent used. The ED_{50} (dose decreasing performance by 50%) was calculated for each compound.

Forced Motor Activity

The effects of the compounds on forced motor activity of mice were studied using the rotarod as described by Watzman and Barry (9). The wooden rod rotated at 4 rpm during the first 30 sec, at 6 rpm during the next 30 sec, and at progressively increasing speed thereafter at 30-sec intervals until the animals fell off (maximum 5 min). Six animals tested simultaneously were given two trials spaced 4 to 6 hr apart on each of 2 consecutive days for a total of four trials. The last trial was preceded at an interval of 30 min to 1 hr by the administration of saline, solvent, or one of the selected doses of CPZ or metabolites. The drug or placebo effects for each animal was computed as the ratio of performance time on the fourth trial divided by performance time on the third trial. Ten min following the initiation for the fourth rotarod trial, the six animals were placed into three photocell activity cages as described under spontaneous motor activity and activity recorded for 15 min.

Antireserpine Activity

Male mice weighing 20 to 25 g were used and each experiment was carried out on five groups, each containing five animals (10). The doses of the metabolites were identical to those used in the spontaneous motor activity studies. The experiment was conducted at a temperature of 18 to 20°C and the animals permitted to stabilize to this temperature for a 1-hr period after which rectal temperature was determined using a Tele-thermometer (Yellow Springs Instrument Company) with the probe inserted 2 cm into the rectum. Five groups were used simultaneously: groups I, II, and III received different doses of CPZ or a metabolite, group IV received desmethylimipramine (20 mg/kg, i.p.), and group V received saline (10 ml/kg, i.p.). One hr after treatment, the rectal temperature was again determined and the animals examined for the development of ptosis, diarrhea, and changes in motor activity. Reserpine, 1 mg/kg, i.p., was then administered and 4 hr later, rectal temperature was obtained and alterations in ptosis, diarrhea, and motor activity were noted using the saline group as control. Hypothermia was calculated as a decrease in rectal temperature from the individual control values of each mouse. The control value was the temperature recorded following CPZ or metabolite administration since these compounds were found to decrease body temperature.

Effects on Barbiturate Sleeping Time

In these studies 448 male mice weighing 20 to 24 g were used. Fifty-six animals were divided into 14 groups of four animals each. Each group received either normal saline, 10 ml/kg; a dose of CPZ; or one of five test compounds i.p. Thirty to 60 min after administration of the compound, either hexobarbital sodium (100 mg/kg, i.p.) or barbital sodium (300 mg/kg, i.p.) was administered. The onset of sleeping time (loss of righting reflex) and duration of sleeping time (recovery from immobility) were determined. Sleeping time is defined as the interval between the loss and return of the righting reflex. The test was terminated if the mouse continued to sleep 4 hr following the loss of the righting reflex. The following day the study was repeated with the remaining five test compounds and CPZ using the other 56 mice. This 2-day experiment was replicated so that a total of eight mice received one dose of each compound. Each metabolite was tested for effects on hexobarbital sleeping time at three dose levels and barbital sleeping time at two dose levels.

Since mice receiving the highest dose of CPZ and some of its derivatives did not recover the righting reflex in less than 4 hr, the problem was approached using the HD_{20} of barbital (11). Male mice, in groups of 10, received selected doses of barbital sodium i.p. in order to estimate the HD_{20} of barbital which according to the method of Litchfield and Wilcoxon (12) was determined to be 147.9 mg/kg. Male mice weighing 20 to 24 g in groups of eight received the highest dose of either chlorpromazine or one of the 10 metabolites, 30 to 60 min prior to the administration of the HD_{20} of barbital sodium.

Continuous Lever-Pressing Shock-Avoidance

Male albino Wistar rats were tested in eight standard operant conditioning chambers (Lehigh Valley Electronics, Incorporated, Fogelsville, Pa.) each with two levers on one wall (13). The animals were trained to perform a continuous avoidance of a painful electric shock (300 V a.c. through 150,-000 ohms resistance in a scrambled pattern to the grid floor) with a duration of 0.5 sec and an interval of 5 sec between shocks. Each press on the right-hand lever turned on a cue light for 0.5 sec and initiated a 20-sec interval until the next shock, so that the animal received a shock only when it allowed 20 sec to elapse after the avoidance response. The programming equipment consisted of transistorized timing and switching modules (Massey-Dickinson, Incorporated) and each shock and each avoidance lever press in each test box was automatically registered on counters and event markers. The totals were recorded every 0.5 hr throughout the 2-hr session. The effects of the compounds were investigated in 32 rats divided into four groups of eight each, tested concurrently. Two groups were tested in the morning and the other two groups in the afternoon. The tests were spaced at least 48 hr apart; the two groups tested at the same time of the day were tested on alternate days, Monday through Saturday. In order to control for any consistent difference among days of the week, the groups tested on Monday,

Wednesday, and Friday of 1 week were tested Tuesday, Thursday, and Saturday of the following week and vice versa.

One group of eight animals tested at each time of day was injected with drug (2 mg/kg, i.p.) or isotonic saline (1 ml/kg, i.p.) 0.5 hr prior to the start of the 2-hr session, the other 0.5 hr following the start of the session. The experiment was designed to equate effects of differences among successive test sessions and test chambers. Accordingly, the four compounds tested were alternated with saline in successive sessions and administered in a Latin Square sequence so that each animal was tested under each drug and each group of eight animals tested concurrently contained one under each of the four drugs in addition to four saline animals. Therefore, four animals were used in the same test chamber during the same session in which two received saline and two received different compounds. The same test sequence was repeated using a higher dose of the compounds (5 mg/kg, i.p.) with a saline test for all the animals intervening between the two series of tests with different dosage levels.

Pole-Climbing Avoidance

Thirty-two rats were tested using apparatus described by Aceto et al. (14) in which four units were utilized simultaneously. The 165-sec cycle was initiated with a warning signal (light) for 15 sec followed by the delivery of an electric shock to the grid floor (2 mA, 250 V a.c.) for a maximum of 30 sec. Both the light and shock were terminated for a minimum of 120 sec prior to the onset of the next cycle. A response of jumping on the pole terminated the light and avoided the shock if prior to shock onset, or terminated both light and shock following shock onset. All response latencies were recorded by means of a pen polygraph in units of 0.1 sec. Each session consisted of 20 trials with the exception that 30 trials were given in the first session. Saline (1 ml/kg, i.p.) or one of the four compounds (2 mg/kg, i.p.) was administered 0.5 hr prior to the start of the session. The animals received saline in sessions, 3, 5, 7, 9, and 11 and drug in sessions 4, 6, 8, and 10. Each compound was administered in a Latin Square sequence, so that each animal was tested under each drug and the four animals tested concurrently were treated with different drugs. Two test sessions were conducted per week allowing 48 hr between the saline session and the next drug session and 120 hr between the drug session and the following saline session.

Discriminative Control by Drug States

Twenty-five rats weighing 200 to 250 g received a daily diet of 12 g of Purina Lab Chow checkers and water ad lib. The tests were conducted shortly before feeding time with an interval of at least 48 hr between successive tests. The drugs used as discriminative stimulus for approach or avoidance response were chlorpromazine for a group of 13 animals (1 mg/kg, i.p., 0.5 hr prior to session) and pentobarbital sodium for a group of 12 animals (10 mg/kg, i.p., 0.25 hr prior to the session).

Initially the animals were trained to press a lever to receive one 45-mg food pellet after each fifty press (FR-5 schedule), in 5-min sessions after i.p. injection of drug for one subgroup of animals and saline for the other subgroup. When performance was well established, each animal was given the alternative treatment (saline or drug) and every fifth lever press was followed by a painful electric shock instead of food. Therefore, drug was associated with food for one subgroup of animals and shock for the other subgroup. The training sessions were conducted over a period of 6 months (15 to 17).

Subsequent tests with CPZ and three of its metabolites provided a measure of the ability of the experimental animals to perceive similarity or dissimilarity to the previously established drug or saline conditions. Both groups of animals were given a series of tests with 2 mg/kg, i.p., 0.5 hr before the session. After an interval of 6 months, the nine surviving animals in the group trained to discriminate CPZ from saline were given further training sessions, using a dose of CPZ of 2 mg/kg, followed by a test with each of the three metabolites at the same dose used previously (2 mg/kg) and then at a higher dose (4 mg/kg). Additional studies were carried out using progressively increasing doses of quaternary CPZ (2, 4, 8 mg/kg). Since this compound is a quaternary ammonium derivative, it is poorly absorbed into the central nervous system and the effects observed are essentially peripheral (18).

RESULTS

LD_{50}

The i.p. 72-hr LD_{50}, ED_{50} (effects on spontaneous motor activity) and safety index (LD_{50}/ED_{50}) in mice are summarized in Table 2. Compound VI

TABLE 2. Acute LD_{50}, ED_{50}, and safety index of the compounds in mice

Compounds	LD_{50} (mg/kg, i.p.)	ED_{50} (mg/kg, i.p.)	Safety index (LD_{50}/ED_{50})
Chlorpromazine	119.7	2.0	59.9
I	114.6	44.5	2.6
II	130.3	27.2	4.8
III	77.8	35.4	2.2
IV	67.5	31.7	2.1
V	52.8	5.1	10.4
VI	24.8	6.6	3.8
VII	119.4	7.5	15.9
VIII	58.1	16.1	3.6
IX	48.2	13.7	3.5
X	133.7	75.3	1.8

was the most toxic of the compounds tested on a mg/kg basis; however, compound X had the lowest safety index and therefore the lowest safety range. CPZ was more potent on a mg/kg basis in depressing spontaneous motor activity and had a greater safety index than any of the metabolites investigated. The 7-hydroxy (VII) and 3,7-dihydroxy derivative (V) had the highest safety index of the metabolites investigated with indices of 15.9 and 10.4, respectively.

Gross Behavior in Rats

CPZ and its metabolites decreased motor activity and rate of respiration within 30 min. Heart rate was decreased by all compounds except III and VIII. The pupil was slightly dilated by all compounds except IX. Body temperature was decreased by all compounds except compound V, and ptosis occurred with all the compounds except III and V.

Spontaneous Motor Activity

Table 3 summarizes the effects of the compounds on spontaneous motor activity in mice Almost all doses of the 10 compounds exhibited a dose-dependent depressant effect on spontaneous motor activity.

TABLE 3. *Effects of the experimental compounds on spontaneous motor activity in mice[a]*

Compound	Dose (mg/kg, i.p.)	% of Control	Dose (mg/kg, i.p.)	% of Control	Dose (mg/kg, i.p.)	% of Control[b]
Chlorpromazine	1	87.0	2	53.8	4	5.2
I	20	122.5	40	68.2	60	11.5
II	13	101.6	26	50.0[b]	39	15.9
III	16	97.2	32	59.4	48	23.4
IV	12.5	85.1	25	61.7	50	30.3
V	5	49.6	10	32.5[b]	20	11.8
VI	3	90.2	5	66.7	10	28.5
VII	6.25	63.8	9	34.1	12.5	9.0
VIII	12	78.9	18	32.0[b]	24	22.8
IX	5	110.4	10	47.1	30	17.3
X	40	94.6	60	87.3	80	37.8

[a] 0.5-hr counting time.
[b] Significantly different from saline-treated control groups ($p < 0.05$).

Forced Motor Activity

Figures 1 and 2 summarize the effects of CPZ and 10 experimental compounds on spontaneous and forced motor activity using data in which effects on spontaneous activity were investigated 10 min following initiation of

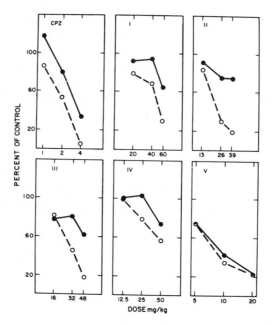

FIG. 1. Effects of chlorpromazine and compounds I to V on spontaneous (O----O) and forced motor activity (●——●) in mice. From (13) with permission.

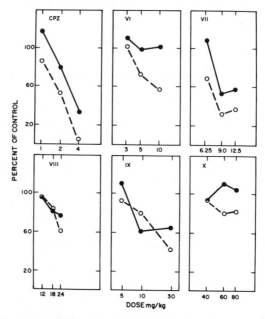

FIG. 2. Effects of chlorpromazine and compounds VI to X on spontaneous (O----O) and forced motor activity (●——●) in mice. From (13) with permission.

the rotarod test. CPZ markedly decreased forced motor coordination in doses of 2 and 4 mg/kg, whereas much higher doses of the experimental compounds were needed to produce detrimental effects both on this parameter and on spontaneous motor activity. CPZ and most of the other compounds had a greater detrimental effect on spontaneous than on forced motor activity and in particular II, III, and VI decreased spontaneous motor activity with minimal effects on forced motor activity. However, compounds V, VIII, and IX produced similar effects on both forced and spontaneous motor activity suggesting that these compounds produced maximal effects on the cerebral cortex. Compound X did not significantly alter either forced motor activity or spontaneous motor activity under these experimental conditions even though it did produce some decrement in spontaneous motor activity in the initial studies (Table 3). This difference in activity could possibly be due to stimulant effects produced during the rotarod portion of this phase of the study.

Antireserpine Activity

CPZ and the metabolites were found to decrease temperature; therefore rectal temperature was obtained following the administration of the test compounds and again 4 hr following administration of reserpine (1 mg/kg, i.p.). Compound VII (7-hydroxy-CPZ) was the only experimental compound that significantly counteracted the decrease in body temperature due to reserpine and then the difference was significant only at the lowest dose used, 6.25 mg/kg, i.p. Reserpine produced a mean $\pm$ S.E. decrease of $3.62 \pm 0.34°C$ in the 25 animals receiving saline compared with a decrease of $1.32 \pm 0.26°C$ in the 25 animals receiving desmethylimipramine (20 mg/kg, i.p.) and $2.10 \pm 0.54°C$ in the 25 animals receiving VII (6.25 mg/kg, i.p.). None of the 11 compounds tested showed any effect on the reserpine-induced ptosis and only desmethylimipramine was capable of blocking this effect.

Effects on Barbiturate Sleeping Time

CPZ, VII, and VIII significantly increased hexobarbital sleeping time in the lowest dosage level used. Compound VII (6.25 mg/kg) increased hexobarbital sleeping time from 38.6 ± 1.5 to 52.0 ± 7.3 min (34.7%) and VIII (12.0 mg/kg) increased sleeping time from 38.6 ± 1.5 to 57.9 ± 5.1 min (50.0%). Chlorpromazine (1 mg/kg) increased sleeping time 80% and at all doses was much more potent than any of the compounds investigated. In the medium dose range, all compounds except compound III, V, VI, and X increased sleeping time whereas the high doses of all compounds produced a significant increase in sleeping time. CPZ, III, VI, VII, VIII, and IX produced a significant increase in the duration of barbital sleeping time with medium doses. The mean sleeping time of barbital sodium in the saline-treated animals ranged from 65.0 ± 4.8 to 88.3 ± 13.2 min. When the HD_{20} dose of barbital sodium was administered to mice which were pre-treated 30 to 60 min previously with the high dose of either CPZ or one of its metabolites, all but compound X potentiated the sedative action of barbital sodium.

Continuous Lever Pressing Avoidance

This procedure provided measures of the effects of CPZ and the three most potent CPZ metabolites (V, VI, and VII) on the number of shocks and avoidance responses per minute between 0.5 and 1.5 hr following administration. Only CPZ produced a statistically significant increase in shocks and decrease in avoidances in a dose of 2 mg/kg, i.p. 7-Hydroxy-CPZ had similar but much milder effects on both measures, the decrease in avoidances being short of statistical significance. The other two metabolites failed to alter either measure significantly, and contrary to the effects of CPZ, avoidances tended to be increased by this metabolite and 3,7-dihydroxy-CPZ while shocks tended to be increased by 7,8-dihydroxy-CPZ. With the higher dose of 5 mg/kg, all four compounds significantly increased the number of shocks per minute and all except 7,8-dihydroxy-CPZ significantly decreased the number of avoidances per minute. However, CPZ was the most potent of the four compounds investigated.

Pole-Climbing Avoidance

The avoidance responses were made on an average of 75% of the trials in the control condition. Figure 3 summarizes the effects of the four com-

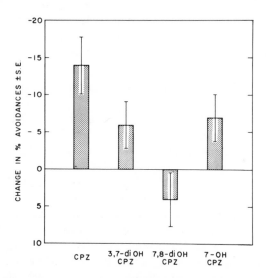

FIG. 3. Effects of chlorpromazine and compounds V, VI, and VII on percentage avoidances in the discriminative pole-climbing avoidance and escape response.

pounds on this measure of performance. A statistically significant decrease in the percentage of avoidances was found with CPZ ($p < 0.01$) and with 7-hydroxy-CPZ ($p < 0.05$). A decrease was also produced by 3,7-dihydroxy-CPZ which was short of statistical significance. A separate measure of average latency of the avoidance response after the onset of the warning signal showed that all four compounds produced an increase in latency. The increase was largest with CPZ and was much smaller with all of the three metabolites.

Discriminative Control by Drug States

Tables 4 and 5 summarize the percentage drug response and percentage approach under various drug conditions by animals trained to make a differential response on the basis of whether they had been treated with

TABLE 4. *Effects of CPZ, three CPZ derivatives, and QCPZ on animals trained to discriminate CPZ (1 mg/kg) from saline*

Drug condition	Dose (mg/kg)	% Drug response	% Approach
Saline	—	23[c]	69
CPZ	1	96[b]	50
CPZ	2	90[b]	44
3,7-diOH-CPZ	2	35[c]	58
	4	0[c]	50
7,8-diOH-CPZ	2	38[c]	31[a]
	4	38	38
7-OH-CPZ	2	77[b]	46
	4	88[a]	62
QCPZ	2	0[c]	50
	4	12	62
	8	38	38

[a] $p < 0.05$ for difference from saline.
[b] $p < 0.01$ for difference from saline.
[c] $p < 0.01$ for difference from CPZ (2 mg/kg).

saline or drug. A drug response means approach (completing five lever presses within 5 min) by one subgroup and avoidance by the other subgroup. The percentage approach combines the same subgroups in a different manner, so that an approach response means a drug response by one subgroup and a saline response by the other subgroup. Many more training sessions were necessary to establish the discriminative response between CPZ (1 mg/kg) and saline (Table 4) than between pentobarbital (10 mg/kg) and saline (Table 5). However, the data for the number of sessions averaged together under these training conditions (Tables 4 and 5) show that a satisfactory discriminative response was obtained between both drugs and the saline condition.

Table 4 shows that 7-hydroxy-CPZ was the only metabolite that elicited

TABLE 5. *Effects of CPZ and three CPZ derivatives on animals trained to discriminate pentobarbital (10 mg/kg) from saline*

Drug condition	Dose (mg/kg)	% Drug response	% Approach
Saline	—	21[a]	45
Pentobarbital	10	97[b]	47
CPZ	2	50	25
3,7-diOH-CPZ	2	17[a]	33
7,8-diOH-CPZ	2	42	8[a]
7-OH-CPZ	2	25	25

[a] $p < 0.05$ for difference from 50%.
[b] $p < 0.01$ for difference from 50%.

the CPZ response whereas the other metabolites elicited predominantly the saline response. The percentage approach was low with 7,8-dihydroxy-CPZ. Quaternary CPZ consistently elicited the saline response except at the very high-dose level of 8 mg/kg. Table 5 summarizes the effects of CPZ and the three metabolites on animals trained to discriminate pentobarbital from saline. None of the four compounds elicited the drug response. Each of these compounds decreased the percentage approach which could possibly be due to CNS depressant or anorexic effects of the compound. This effect was most marked for 7,8-dihydroxy-CPZ, whereas the other two metabolites tended to elicit a preponderantly saline response.

DISCUSSION

Since the LD_{50} of CPZ was higher than most of the metabolites and the safety index 3.8 to 33.2 times greater than the metabolites investigated, it appears that the metabolites were not only less effective in depressing central nervous system (CNS) activity but also more toxic. CPZ was by far the most potent compound in inhibiting spontaneous motor activity (ED_{50} of 2.0 mg/kg, i.p.). Compound VII (7-hydroxy-CPZ) had the highest safety index of the metabolites studied; however, it was slightly less than one-third as effective as CPZ in inhibiting spontaneous motor activity, whereas the LD_{50}'s of the compounds were approximately equal. Although compound VI was extremely toxic, compound II had an LD_{50} in excess of five times that of compound VI. Therefore, the replacement of the 8-hydroxy by an 8-methoxy group markedly decreased the toxicity of the compound; however, it should be noted that it still took a dose of compound II approximately five times greater to equal the depressant effects produced by compound VI. These data suggest that the metabolites are less efficient in depressing CNS activity and more toxic than CPZ.

The compounds potentiated the sleeping time induced by both hexobarbital sodium, which is oxidatively metabolized by the hepatic microsomal enzymes (19), and barbital sodium, which is excreted unmetabolized (20). There were quantitative differences in the effects of each compound on the degree of potentiation of hexobarbital and barbital sleeping time. For example, in comparing the effects of the medium dose of the compounds, CPZ and compounds I and II had a greater effect on hexobarbital sleeping time; compounds III, IV, VI, VIII, IX, and X had a greater effect on barbital sleeping time; compound VII produced equal effects on both barbiturates; and compound V produced a slight decrease in hexobarbital sleeping time without significantly affecting barbital activity. The enhancement of sleeping time induced by barbital, which is not metabolized, suggests that in those instances where the compounds potentiated hexobarbital, the activity was due to a direct depressant effect on the CNS and not to inhibition of hexobarbital metabolism. It is of interest to note that compound V (3,7-dihydroxy-CPZ), the compound which had the lowest ED_{50} of the metabolites investigated (using effects on spontaneous motor activity as the assay procedure), produced minimal effects on barbital sleeping time in both doses used, increasing hexobarbital sleeping time only 6.5% with the low dose of 5 mg/kg, i.p., and 38.6% with the high dose of 20 mg/kg, i.p.

When the behavioral effects of the three most potent metabolites (3,7-dihydroxy-CPZ, 7,8-dihydroxy-CPZ, and 7-hydroxy-CPZ) and CPZ were investigated, all three of the behavioral tests indicated that CPZ was more potent than any of the three metabolites. In both tests of avoidance performance, CPZ was much more potent than the three metabolites tested. Among the metabolites, the detrimental effect of 7-hydroxy-CPZ was greatest and most consistent, whereas the detrimental effect of 7,8-dihydroxy-CPZ was smallest and least consistent. However, the test for discriminative control of behavior by drug states was the only one which effectively differentiated the three metabolites from each other. 7-Hydroxy-CPZ was the only compound eliciting the CPZ response whereas 7,8-dihydroxy-CPZ gave evidence of general CNS depressant effects which could possibly be due to an anorexic action or enhanced avoidance of the shock in this approach-avoidance conflict situation.

The inhibitory effects of 7-hydroxy-CPZ (compound VII) on spontaneous and forced motor activity, its relatively high safety index, its antireserpine activity, and its effects on behavior suggest that this metabolite may have potential utility as a therapeutic agent. Its antagonism of reserpine hypothermia suggests an antidepressant effect which might be combined with the antipsychotic effect of CPZ. The tests for discriminative control of behavior by drug states suggest the same type of central effect. Further evidence for similar effects of CPZ and 7-hydroxy-CPZ have been reported by others (21) who found that both compounds in doses of 10 mg/kg accelerated both accumulation and disappearance of radioactively labeled dopamine in mouse brain following the administration of labeled tyrosine.

SUMMARY

Chlorpromazine and nine of its mono- and disubstituted metabolites were investigated for their effects on the central nervous system of rats and mice. All of the compounds decreased motor activity and rate of respiration and all but two of the compounds decreased heart rate in rats. The most potent metabolite depressing spontaneous motor activity of mice was 3,7-dihydroxy-CPZ having an i.p. ED_{50} of 5.1 mg/kg in comparison to CPZ which had an i.p. ED_{50} of 2.0 mg/kg. However, the metabolite was approximately twice as toxic as CPZ in mice. 7-Hydroxy-CPZ had the highest safety index of all of the metabolites investigated. 7-Hydroxy-CPZ was the only experimental compound that significantly counteracted the decrease in body temperature due to reserpine. Barbiturate sleeping time was potentiated by all of the compounds and appeared to be mainly due to CNS depressant properties rather than inhibition of metabolism. The three most potent metabolites inhibiting spontaneous motor activity in mice (3,7-dihydroxy-CPZ, 7,8-dihydroxy-CPZ, and 7-hydroxy-CPZ) were further investigated for their behavioral effects using the continuous lever pressing, shock-avoidance response (Sidman Schedule), discriminative pole-climbing avoidance and escape response, and discriminative control of behavior by drug states. The 7-hydroxy-CPZ showed a larger and more consistent detrimental effect in the avoidance-response tests than the other two metabolites. 7-Hydroxy-CPZ was the only metabolite which elicited the CPZ response for the discriminative control behavior by drug states.

ACKNOWLEDGMENTS

This study was supported by Research Grant MH 19719 (the National Institute of Mental Health). One of the authors (H.B.) was supported by PHS Research Scientist Development Award K2-MH-5921.

The authors thank Professor J. Cymerman Craig, University of California Medical Center, San Francisco, California, for generously providing the 3,7-dihydroxy-chlorpromazine and Mrs. Ming Shih for her valuable assistance.

REFERENCES

1. Fishman, V., and Goldenberg, H., *J. Pharmacol. Exp. Therap.*, **150**, 122 (1965).
2. Posner, H. S., Hearst, E., Raylor, W. L., and Cosmides, G. J.,*J. Pharmacol. Exp. Therap.*, **137**, 84 (1962).
3. Posner, H. S., and Hearst, E., *Int. J. Neuropharmacol.*, **3**, 635 (1964).
4. Manian, A. A., Efron, D. H., and Goldberg, M. E., *Life Sci.*, **4**, 2425 (1965).
5. Manian, A. A., Watzman, N., Steenberg, M. L., and Buckley, J. P., *Life Sci.*, **7**, 731 (1968).
6. Manian, A. A., Efron, D. H. and Harris, S. R., *Life Sci.*, **10**, 679 (1971).
7. Watzman, N., Manian, A. A., Barry, H., III, and Buckley, J. P., *J. Pharm. Sci.*, **57**, 2089 (1968).

8. Goldstein, J., *Biostatistics,* MacMillan Co., New York, 1964, chap. 11.
9. Watzman, N., and Barry, H., III, *Psychopharmacologia,* 12, 414 (1965).
10. Lapin, I. P., in, *Antidepressant Drugs,* Garattini, S., and Dukes, M. N. G. (eds.), Excerpta Med. Found., Amsterdam, 1967, pp. 266–278.
11. Fujimori, H., *Psychopharmacologia,* 7, 374 (1965).
12. Litchfield, J. T., and Wilcoxon, F. J., *J. Pharmacol. Exp. Therap.,* 96, 99 (1949).
13. Buckley, J. P., Steenberg, M. L., Barry, H., III, and Manian, A. A., *J. Pharm. Sci.,* 62, 715 (1973).
14. Aceto, M. D. G., Kinnard, W. J., and Buckley, J. P., *Arch. Int. Pharmacodyn.,* 144, 214 (1963).
15. Kubena, R. K., and Barry, H., III, *J. Pharm. Sci.,* 58, 99 (1968).
16. Kubena, R. K., and Barry, H., III, *Psychopharmacologia,* 15, 196 (1968).
17. Barry, H., III, and Kubena, R. K., in, *Drug Addiction: Experimental Pharmacology,* Singh, J. M., Miller, L. H., and Lal, H. (eds.), Futura Publishing Co., Mount Kisco, N.Y., 1972, pp. 3–16.
18. Watzman, N., Manian, A. A., Barry, H., III, and Buckley, J. P., *J. Pharm. Sci.,* 57, 2089 (1968).
19. Cooper, J. R., and Brodie, B. B., *J. Pharmacol. Exp. Therap.,* 114, 409 (1955).
20. Burns, J. J., Evans, C., and Trousof, N. J., *J. Biol. Chem.,* 227, 785 (1957).
21. Nyback, H., and Sedvall, G., *Psychopharmacologia,* 26, 155 (1972).

The Phenothiazines and Structurally Related Drugs, edited by I. S.
Forrest, C. J. Carr, and E. Usdin. Raven Press, New York © 1974.

7,8-Dihydroxychlorpromazine: $(Na^+ + K^+)$-ATPase Inhibition and Positive Inotropic Effect

T. Akera, S. I. Baskin, T. Tobin, T. M. Brody, and A. A. Manian*

*Department of Pharmacology, Michigan State University, East Lansing, Michigan 48823,
and * Psychopharmacology Research Branch, National Institute of Mental Health,
Rockville, Maryland 20852*

INTRODUCTION

Chlorpromazine has previously been reported to inhibit $(Na^+ + K^+)$-ATPase activity *in vitro* (1–5). This enzyme system occurs in a wide variety of animal tissues (6) and has been identified as the system responsible for the active transport of Na^+ and K^+ across the cell membrane (7). Subsequently, it was demonstrated that chlorpromazine itself has a rather minimal inhibitory effect on $(Na^+ + K^+)$-ATPase, and the inhibition observed by a number of investigators was possibly due to the formation of a semiquinone free radical of chlorpromazine generated by exposure of the drug-enzyme mixture to light (8–10). The concept that metabolites may be the active forms of phenothiazine tranquilizers is attractive since certain pharmacologic effects of this class of compounds develop rather slowly.

Recently, a highly active metabolite of chlorpromazine, namely 7,8-dihydroxychlorpromazine, has been identified in schizophrenic patients receiving chronic chlorpromazine treatment (11). This metabolite was found to produce a marked efflux of calcium previously accumulated by brain mitochondrial preparations *in vitro* with a concomitant inhibition of respiration (12). It was suggested that interaction of 7,8-dihydroxychlor-promazine with sulfhydryl groups is a possible mechanism of these effects. Since $(Na^+ + K^+)$-ATPase contains essential sulfhydryl groups (13, 14) and the inhibition of this enzyme by chlorpromazine free radical has been attributed to the interaction with these sulfhydryl groups (15), the effect of 7,8-dihydroxychlorpromazine on $(Na^+ + K^+)$-ATPase activity was investigated using partially purified rat-brain enzyme preparations. The results indicated that the 7,8-dihydroxy metabolites of phenothiazine tranquilizers are potent inhibitors of the $(Na^+ + K^+)$-ATPase activity.

This prompted us to undertake a study of cardiac effects of 7,8-dihydroxy-chlorpromazine since most $(Na^+ + K^+)$-ATPase inhibitors produce positive inotropic effects, and it was previously demonstrated that the inhibition of cardiac ($Na^+ + K^+$)-ATPase in the dog parallels the positive inotropic effect produced by cardiac glycosides such as ouabain (16–18). 7,8-Dihydroxychlorpromazine produced a positive inotropic effect in isolated guinea pig hearts and in open-chested anesthetized dogs. Unlike ouabain, however, the effect of 7,8-dihydroxychlorpromazine was abolished by propranolol pretreatment. Whether the cardiac ($Na^+ + K^+$)-ATPase activity was inhibited under these conditions remains to be investigated.

METHODS AND MATERIAL

Brain microsomal fractions from Sprague-Dawley rats were treated with deoxycholic acid and NaI to obtain partially purified ($Na^+ + K^+$)-ATPase preparations according to the method of Akera and Brody (9). ATPase activity was assayed by incubating the enzyme preparation (10 μg of protein) and 5 mM Tris-ATP in the presence of 5 mM $MgCl_2$ and 50 mM Tris-HCl buffer (pH 7.5) in a total volume of 1.0 ml at 37°C for 10 min and assaying the amount of inorganic phosphate released from ATP (9). Before the addition of ATP, enzyme and inhibitor were preincubated for 5 min unless otherwise indicated. Mg^{++}-ATPase activity observed in the absence of added NaCl and KCl was subtracted from the total ATPase activity, assayed in the presence of 100 mM NaCl and 15 mM KCl, to calculate the ($Na^+ + K^+$)-ATPase activity. Mg^{++}-ATPase activity accounted for approximately 5% of the total ATPase activity.

For atrial preparations, guinea pigs of either sex weighing 500 to 700 grams were sacrificed, their left atria removed and placed in aerated (95% O_2 to 5% CO_2) Krebs-Henseleit solution (19) at 35°C. The muscle was stimulated with 5-msec pulses from a 161 Tektronix pulse generator at a frequency of 60 beats/min and a voltage not greater than 10% above threshold. Contractile force was estimated using a Grass FT-03 force-displacement transducer monitored with a recorder.

EFFECTS OF METABOLITES OF PHENOTHIAZINE TRANQUILIZERS ON ($Na^+ + K^+$)-ATPase

When hydroxylated metabolites of phenothiazine tranquilizers were added to the incubation mixture for ATPase assay and the assay was performed in a dark room, the enzyme activities were affected to varying degrees depending on the compound. The inhibition of Mg^{++}-ATPase activity was always significantly less than that of the ($Na^+ + K^+$)-ATPase activity. The concentrations of various derivatives of phenothiazine to produce 50% inhibition of brain ($Na^+ + K^+$)-ATPase activity, calculated from percent inhibition versus log concentration plots, are shown in Table 1. Chlorpromazine and 7-hydroxychlorpromazine failed to inhibit ($Na^+ + K^+$)-ATPase activity significantly without ultraviolet activation, whereas 7,8-dihydroxy derivatives of chlorpromazine, perphenazine, or prochlorperazine produced a significant inhibition of the enzyme activity without such exposure. Three 7,8-dihydroxy derivatives showed similar patterns of inhibition. Ultraviolet exposure of the 7,8-dihydroxychlorpromazine-enzyme mixture enhanced the inhibitory potency of this agent only slightly in contrast to chlorpromazine or 7-hydroxychlorpromazine (Table 1).

TABLE 1. *Concentrations of phenothiazine derivatives to inhibit rat brain $(Na^+ + K^+)$-ATPase activity 50% in vitro*

	Nonexposed[a]	UV-exposed[b]
Chlorpromazine	$> 100 \ \mu M$	$3.5 \ \mu M$
7-hydroxychlorpromazine	> 100	8.5
7,8-dihydroxychlorpromazine	0.80	0.59
7,8-dihydroxyperphenazine	1.6	—[c]
7,8-dihydroxyprochlorperazine	2.2	—[c]
7,8-dioxychlorpromazine	1.1	—[c]

[a] Enzyme activity was assayed in the presence of phenothiazine derivatives in a dark room after a 5-min preincubation during which ATP was absent.

[b] The drug-enzyme mixture was exposed to ultraviolet (UV) light using Mineralight Lamp model R-51 (primary emission wavelength 253.7 nm), with filter removed, in a quartz cuvette with a 1.0-cm light path. The cuvette was placed at a distance of 45 cm from the lamp and exposed for 4 min at room temperature. ATPase activity was subsequently assayed in a dark room and percent inhibition was calculated against enzyme activity observed after ultraviolet exposure of the enzyme in the absence of the drug. The ultraviolet exposure caused a slight decrease (5 to 10%) of enzyme activity.

[c] Not studied.

7,8-Dioxychlorpromazine was also a potent inhibitor of $(Na^+ + K^+)$-ATPase activity without ultraviolet exposure (Table 1). It was noticed that all potent inhibitors of $(Na^+ + K^+)$-ATPase, namely 7,8-dihydroxy and 7,8-dioxy metabolites of phenothiazine tranquilizers, developed a dark red color at pH 7.5 without ultraviolet exposure. The color intensity increased with time even without the exposure to ultraviolet light.

FACTORS WHICH INFLUENCE THE EFFECT OF 7,8-DIHYDROXY-CHLORPROMAZINE ON $(Na^+ + K^+)$-ATPase *IN VITRO*

The addition of dithiothreitol, a potent sulfhydryl-group protecting agent (20), reduced enzyme inhibition by 7,8-dihydroxychlorpromazine (Table 2). However, it is not clear from these experiments whether the effect is due to the reactivation of the essential sulfhydryl groups on the enzyme or due to the chemical interaction between 7,8-dihydroxychlorpromazine and

TABLE 2. *Inhibitions of (Na⁺ + K⁺)-ATPase by 7,8-dihydroxychlorpromazine under various conditions*

Condition	Concentration of 7,8-dihydroxychlor-promazine (μM)	Inhibition
Control	1.0	55.3 ± 3.5[e]%
Presence of 5 μM dithiothreitol[a]	1.0	37.0 ± 3.8[e]
Presence of 50 μM dithiothreitol[a]	1.0	-2.3 ± 1.9[e]
5-min preincubation in the absence of ATP[b]	0.8	50
5-min preincubation in the presence of ATP[c]	1.7	50
1-min preincubation[d]	2.0	7.1 ± 4.0[e]
7-min preincubation[d]	2.0	45.0 ± 3.3[e]
13-min preincubation[d]	2.0	62.4 ± 2.1[e]

[a] Dithiothreitol was present during preincubation and incubation periods for ATPase assay. These concentrations of dithiothreitol did not affect the ATPase activity.

[b] After a 5-min preincubation of the enzyme and 7,8-dihydroxychlorpromazine in the presence of 5 mM $MgCl_2$, 100 mM NaCl, 15 mM KCl, and 50 mM Tris-HCl buffer (pH 7.5), ATP (final concentration; 5 mM) was added to start the reaction.

[c] After a 5-min preincubation of enzyme and 7,8-dihydroxychlorpromazine in the presence of 5 mM Tris-ATP, 5 mM $MgCl_2$, 100 mM NaCl, and 50 mM Tris-HCl buffer (pH 7.5), ATPase reaction was started by the addition of 15 mM KCl. The value observed in the absence of KCl was subtracted to calculate (Na⁺ + K⁺)-ATPase activity.

[d] The enzyme was added to a mixture containing 7,8-dihydroxychlorpromazine and necessary cations at time zero. ATP was added to start the reaction and the ATPase reaction terminated 2 min later by the addition of trichloroacetic acid (final concentration 7.5%).

[e] Mean $\pm$ S.E.M. of five experiments.

dithiothreitol. The addition of dithiothreitol resulted in a fading of the red color of 7,8-dihydroxychlorpromazine, indicating that a chemical interaction occurs between these two compounds.

It has been reported previously that the presence of ATP during the preincubation period partially protected the (Na⁺ + K⁺)-ATPase from sulfhydryl inhibitors such as *n*-ethylmaleimide or *p*-chloromercuribenzoate (13, 14, 21). Similarly, the presence of ATP during the preincubation period doubled the concentrations of 7,8-dihydroxychlorpromazine required for 50% inhibition of (Na⁺ + K⁺)-ATPase (Table 2). This would indicate that essential sulfhydryl groups on (Na⁺ + K⁺)-ATPase are involved in the action of 7,8-dihydroxychlorpromazine, and hence the mechanisms of actions of chlorpromazine free radical and 7,8-dihydroxychlorpromazine would appear to be similar.

An Ackermann-Potter plot (22) of (Na⁺ + K⁺)-ATPase inhibition by various concentrations of 7,8-dihydroxychlorpromazine showed a set of lines passing through the point of origin with different slopes, either after a 5- or 15-min preincubation of the enzyme-inhibitor mixture prior to the assay of the enzyme activity (data not shown). These results may be interpreted as a reversible, equilibrium type interaction between the enzyme and the inhibitor (22). However, the inhibition of (Na⁺ + K⁺)-ATPase activity increased progressively with longer preincubation of the enzyme-inhibitor mixture (Table 2). This would suggest an irreversible, nonequilibrium type of interaction which may be expected from the involvement of sulfhydryl groups. Furthermore, dilution of the inhibited enzyme failed to reduce the magnitude of the inhibition indicating an irreversible or pseudoirreversible nature of the interaction (data not shown). These peculiar kinetics of the interaction should be explored further.

INOTROPIC EFFECT OF 7,8-DIHYDROXYCHLORPROMAZINE

Since $(Na^+ + K^+)$-ATPase inhibitors, such as cardiac glycosides, p-chloromercuribenzoate, n-ethylmaleimide, and fluoride, also produce a positive inotropic response, cardiac effects of 7,8-dihydroxychlorpromazine were studied. 7,8-Dihydroxychlorpromazine produced a sustained positive inotropic response in electrically driven left atrial preparations of guinea pig hearts (Fig. 1). The response developed over a period of several minutes and lasted for several hours, although the inotropic response was readily reversible upon washout of the compound (Fig. 1 *upper tracing*). Addition of cysteine, a known free radical scavenger, partially reversed the inotropic response to 7,8-dihydroxychlorpromazine with a concomitant reduction in the intensity of the red color of 7,8-dihydroxychlorpromazine quinone.

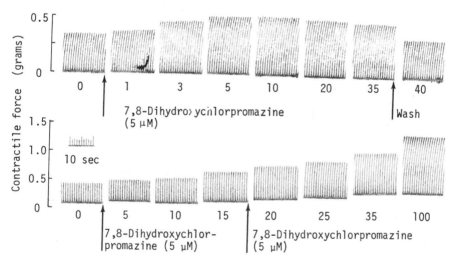

FIG. 1. Inotropic effect of 7,8-dihydroxychlorpromazine in left atrial preparations of guinea pig hearts. These are typical tracings from six experiments. Number below each panel indicates the elapsed time in minutes after the initial addition of 7,8-dihydroxychlorpromazine. Concentrations of 7,8-dihydroxychlorpromazine are the final concentration in 100-ml medium. In the lower tracing, 5 μM dihydroxychlorpromazine was added twice as indicated by arrows. Thus the concentration of the compound after the second addition was 10 μM.

Propranolol pretreatment abolished the inotropic effect of 7,8-dihydroxy-chlorpromazine or isoproterenol. Under these conditions, ouabain was able to produce a positive inotropic response (Fig. 2). These results would indicate that the mechanism by which 7,8-dihydroxychlorpromazine produces a positive inotropic response may be similar to isoproterenol but different from ouabain. It appears that the positive inotropic effect of 7,8-dihydroxychlorpromazine is unrelated to the inhibition of $(Na^+ + K^+)$-ATPase for the following reasons: (a) the inotropic response may be blocked by a β-adrenergic-blocking agent, propranolol; (b) the inotropic effect was readily reversible upon washout of the compound, whereas the inhibition of $(Na^+ + K^+)$-ATPase activity was rather irreversible; (c) arrhythmias, which result from a marked inhibition of $(Na^+ + K^+)$-ATPase (23), were

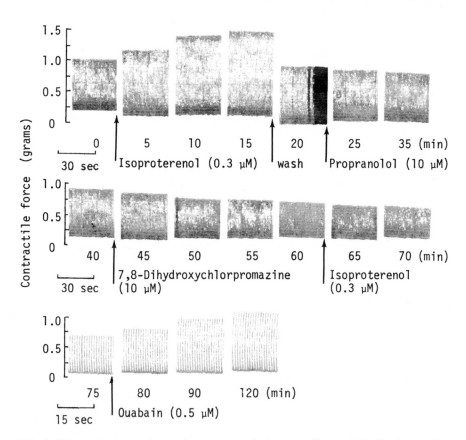

FIG. 2. Effect of propranolol pretreatment on inotropic actions of 7,8-dihydroxychlorpromazine, isoproterenol, and ouabain. These are typical tracings of six electrically driven left atrial preparations of guinea pig hearts. Number below each panel indicates the elapsed time in minutes after the addition of isoproterenol. Isoproterenol was added after 60 min of equilibrium period. Concentrations of the drugs are final concentration in 100-ml medium.

not observed with high concentrations of 7,8-dihydroxychlorpromazine, even after prolonged exposure to the compound. In fact, 7,8-dihydroxychlorpromazine reversed arrhythmias due to toxic concentrations of ouabain or chloroform in Langendorff preparations. It is conceivable that the active site for 7,8-dihydroxychlorpromazine on $(Na^+ + K^+)$-ATPase may not be accessible in intact cells for this polar compound, unless it was formed within the cell, whereas such a site becomes exposed to externally applied compound after homogenization and deoxycholic acid treatment. An alternative explanation may be the differences in animal species or tissues. Whether $(Na^+ + K^+)$-ATPase is inhibited in cardiac tissue *in situ* at a time when the drug elevates contractile force has yet to be determined.

In Langendorff preparations of guinea pig hearts and in anesthetized open-chest dogs, 7,8-dihydroxychlorpromazine produced a positive inotropic effect and a modest increase in heart rate.

CONCLUSION

7,8-Dihydroxylated metabolites of phenothiazine tranquilizers and 7,8-dioxychlorpromazine were potent inhibitors of $(Na^+ + K^+)$-ATPase *in vitro*. 7-Hydroxychlorpromazine was less potent unless activated by ultraviolet light. The inhibition seems to involve sulfhydryl group interactions. 7,8-Dihydroxychlorpromazine possesses positive inotropic properties in the heart although this action does not appear to be related to its ability to inhibit $(Na^+ + K^+)$-ATPase.

ACKNOWLEDGMENT

This work was supported by grant MH-12783–07 (from the National Institute of Mental Health).

REFERENCES

1. Jarnefelt, J., *Biochim. Biophys. Acta,* **59,** 643 (1962).
2. Judah, J. D., and Ahmed, K., *J. Cell Biol.,* **64,** 355 (1964).
3. Squires, R. F., *Biochem. Biophys. Res. Commun.,* **19,** 27 (1965).
4. Davis, P. W., and Brody, T. M., *Biochem. Pharmacol.,* **15,** 703 (1966).
5. Robinson, J. D., Lowinger, J., and Bettinger, B., *Biochem. Pharmacol.,* **17,** 1113 (1968).
6. Bonting, S. L., Simon, K. A., and Hawkins, N. M., *Arch. Biochem. Biophys.,* **95,** 416 (1961).
7. Skou, J. C., *Physiol. Rev.,* **45,** 596 (1965).
8. Akera, T., and Brody, T. M., *Mol. Pharmacol.,* **4,** 600 (1968).
9. Akera, T., and Brody, T. M., *Mol. Pharmacol.,* **5,** 605 (1969).
10. Gubitz, R. H., Akera, T., and Brody, T. M., *Biochem. Pharmacol.,* **22,** 1229 (1973).
11. Turano, P., Turner, W. J., and Manian, A. A., *J. Chromatography,* **75,** 277 (1973).
12. Tjioe, S. A., Manian, A. A., and O'Neill, J. J., *Biochem. Biophys. Res. Commun.,* **48,** 212 (1972).
13. Skou, J. C., *Biochem. Biophys. Res. Commun.,* **10,** 79 (1963).
14. Skou, J. C., *Biochim. Biophys. Acta,* **110,** 359 (1965).

15. Akera, T., and Brody, T. M., *Mol. Pharmacol.*, **6,** 557 (1970).
16. Akera, T., Larsen, F. S., and Brody, T. M., *J. Pharmacol. Exp. Ther.*, **170,** 17 (1969).
17. Besch, H. R., Allen, J. C., Glick, G., and Schwartz, A., *J. Pharmacol. Exp. Ther.*, **171,** 1 (1970).
18. Akera, T., Larsen, F. S., and Brody, T. M., *J. Pharmacol. Exp. Ther.*, **173,** 145 (1970).
19. Winegrad, S., and Shanes, A. M., *J. Gen. Physiol.*, **45,** 371 (1962).
20. Cleland, W. W., *Biochemistry*, **3,** 480 (1964).
21. Akera, T., *Biochim. Biophys. Acta*, **249,** 53 (1971).
22. Ackermann, W. W., and Potter, V. R., *Proc. Soc. Exp. Biol. Med.*, **72,** 1 (1949).
23. Lee, K. S., and Klaus, W., *Pharmacol. Rev.*, **23,** 193 (1971).

The Phenothiazines and Structurally Related Drugs, edited by I. S. Forrest, C. J. Carr, and E. Usdin. Raven Press, New York © 1974.

Session VII: Discussion

Reporter: P. Kaul

1. *F. W. Grant*

Q. Landgraf: Did you look at the decomposition of phenothiazine compounds by using electron spin resonance?
A. No, we have attempted only the most economic experimental methodology, e.g., TLC and absorption spectroscopy.

Q. Curry: I am greatly interested by the observation of Dr. Chignell which has been mentioned concerning covalent reaction between CPZ and a biological protein. Although this is light catalyzed and therefore of less *in vivo* significance, it is, I believe, of great importance as a model to be considered. We have also seen this type of binding, but would it occur in the dark as well?
A. No, but it is very difficult to say.
Shostak: We have seen that CPZ binds to bovine serum albumin in the presence of UV light at position 2.
Potter: Dr. Chignell has not pursued the formation of a CPZ-protein covalent bond, partly because of the low quantity of such binding. In contrast to light activation, microsomal metabolic activation of CPZ to possible alkylating intermediates has also been investigated, using liver microsomal systems. Enzyme-dependent covalent binding was very small, especially in comparison to that seen with a wide variety of other nonphenothiazine compounds that have been investigated in our laboratory. Data on the covalent binding and toxicity of such other compounds, e.g., acetaminophen, show a quantitative correlation of binding with tissue toxicity. On this basis, we are not optimistic about a clear relationship between the covalent binding and toxicity of CPZ being demonstrated.
A. There may be a difference in the antigenicity and the ability of CPZ to bind. For one thing, the binding sites may be differentiated, e.g., side chain versus the ring positions.
Spirtes: Despite the covalent binding shown with serum proteins, the binding of CPZ to biological membranes such as erythrocytes or liver mitochondria is easily reversible with one isotonic saline or sucrose wash. Nevertheless, this low-energy binding changes membrane behavior and may be, at least partially, the important biological effect.
Grant: Yes, this type of binding does exist and I agree, but I am talking about possible toxicological effects in serum. Coupling may occur in the

presence of UV light; you may be surprised but the body appears quite transparent to light.

3. T. A. Grover

Q. Wollemann: Did you also measure tyrosine hydroxylase activity, because CPZ inhibits this enzyme?

A. No, we did not.

Q. Chan: I wonder if you have any data showing the reversibility of the 7-OH-CPZ inhibition, because the competitive inhibition of your results has to be reversible; otherwise your treatment of data is wrong.

Q. Gabay: Yes, it has to be reversible. How pure is your enzyme?

A. It is a crude mixture from mushrooms; about 100 units. It is just a preliminary study.

Q. Conway: Is there a pH-dependence for your thermodynamically reversible reaction of mono- or dihydroxy product?

A. Yes, these reactions are pH-dependent.

Q. Gorrod: In the light of the fact that administration of hydroxy-CPZ to animals produces eye opacities which are not colored, isn't it more likely that the catechol theory is only relevant to skin where pigmentation occurs? If your compounds were produced in the eye, then red pigments might be expected by further oxidation and polymerization.

A. 7,8-dihydroxy-CPZ in rabbits shows opacity.

Q. Grant: If dopaquinone spontaneously polymerizes to melanin, what is the behavior of the quinone of 7,8-dihydroxy-CPZ in this respect?

A. It also polymerizes spontaneously.

Q. Grant: Am I correct in saying that your primary photochemical event is the activation of tyrosinase leading to pigment formation?

A. Yes, and perhaps also some catalysis of the quinone polymerization.

Adams: The confusion about occular changes warrants recognition that in rabbits, corneal opacity occurs, whereas in the human the changes are lenticular and colorless.

Kaufman: Greiner and Nicolson (*Lancet,* 1965) postulated that retinal pigmentation may be due to melanin formation catalyzed by tyrosinase, a copper-containing enzyme. When they gave a Cu^{++} chelating agent to the patient, they obtained Cu^{++} in the urine and arrested the retinal pigmentation.

4. K. S. Rajan

Q. Kaufman: What solvent did you use and how did you carry out the neutralizations? I am also surprised that you mentioned NE interaction with CPZ, because it is DA that is believed to be involved in the neuroleptic effect of these compounds.

A. An equivalent of acid was added to the solutions of the compounds in water, and then back titrated with base. I said that complexes could be formed with biogenic amines of which NE certainly is one.

Gabay: I agree with Dr. Kaufman's remark. This potentiometric work of Dr. Rajan is extremely good work, but we should not apply it to the biological systems.

A. There is evidence that the presence of copper at the presynaptic membranes may facilitate the formation of an ATP-metal-CPZ complex.

Grant: Is there any evidence that these copper-chelating metabolites may be functioning therapeutically by flushing out possible neurotoxic levels of copper? Carl Pfeiffer, for instance, has emphasized the importance of trace metals in this connection.

Breyer: We found no changes in urinary copper before, during, and after a therapeutic chlorpromazine regimen.

Q. Spirtes: Have you looked into the effects of CPZ on calcium in tissues? Some work has been done indicating that CPZ removes this metal from biological membranes.

A. No, but copper was looked at for that very reason.

5. R. P. Maickel

Q. Turner: Is there any evidence for enzyme induction by CPZ and by triflupromazine but not for induction by promazine?

A. There has been a demonstration of induction of liver microsomal hydroxylases by promazine and chlorpromazine, but I have not seen any data for triflupromazine.

Q. Curry: The tolerance and rebound phenomenon is very interesting and similar to that observed with barbiturates. Regarding your brain/plasma ratios, I wonder if your extraction method may not have included the presence of Nor_1CPZ.

A. Yes, it is possible that we are also measuring this metabolite without knowing it.

Q. Lomax: Could some of the effects be explained on the basis of altered neuroendocrine function? For example, CPZ depresses thyroid function in the rat.

A. I did not realize that you could get thyroid effects in 7 to 10 days. We did conduct a few oxygen uptake studies and found slight but not significant changes in O_2 uptake.

Q. Palmer: Do you think that the increased glycogen deposition in the livers of the animals following phenothiazine administration might be due to the hyperglycemia elicited by these drugs, possibly by inhibiting insulin release in the pancreas at the level of adenyl cyclase–cyclic AMP?

A. Yes, it could be.

Q. *Van Woert:* How did you measure rigidity?

A. By using a hard sheet of aluminum, pressing against the animal to see how far the animal would flex.

Q. *Spirtes:* The glycogen effect could also be due to the thyroid effects. I wonder if hypothermia would be responsible for the behavioral changes?

A. Occasional checking showed no significant temperature changes — perhaps 0.2 to 0.3 degree.

6. S. Tjioe

Q. *Gabay:* What method did you use for the purification of your enzyme?

A. We used Ozawa's method.

Q. *Gabay:* Have you used any enzyme markers to ensure that your preparation does not contain any lysosomal enzymes?

Q. *Wollemann:* I did not see any lysosomes in your electron micrographs; so what is the problem about lysosomal enzymes?

A. We did not see any lysosomes, but that does not mean that they are not a problem. If lysosomes are disrupted, then enzymes would be released and might still be present, and could be a problem.

Q. *Chan:* What is the P/O ratio and respiratory quotient of your mitochondria preparation in brain? I observed in your electron micrographs that most of your mitochondria have damaged outer membranes.

A. Respiratory control was 5 with glutamate and 3 with succinate as the substrate. Control mitochondria do not have damaged outer membranes but mitochondria treated with 7,8-dihydroxychlorpromazine during calcium uptake do have altered membranes. The outer membrane as well as the inner membrane may be damaged.

7. J. P. Buckley

Q. *Lomax:* Some of the responses described may be mediated peripherally and some are central actions. Have you related the responses to the partition coefficients of the different compounds?

A. No, we have not.

Q. *Simpson:* How do you explain the split between the ptosis and hypothermia?

A. Possibly different sites of action.

Q. *Conway:* What did you use to calculate the effectiveness in blocking spontaneous motor activity?

A. ED_{50} values.

Q. *Ahtee:* Did any of your compounds cause catalepsy and what were the rates of penetration of these compounds into brain, when compared to CPZ? The toxicity is most probably due to a combination of central and peripheral effects, whereas the effect on spontaneous motor activity results from an action on the CNS.

A. Yes, monohydroxy compound did seem to enter the brain.

Q. Potter: These compounds must pass through the liver before entering the main blood stream, since you used i.p. administration. Have you, or has anybody else, measured the relative plasma and tissue levels of CPZ and 7-OH-CPZ after i.p. administration?

A. No, we did not.

Q. Curry: Following injections of ^{35}S-CPZ in rats, at 24 hr, the activity remaining is largely due to the metabolites. Has anyone measured the solubilities and partition coefficients of these metabolites? This data is urgently needed.

Conway: 7-OH-CPZ is nearly as soluble as CPZ in aqueous medium at pH 1.5.

A. Partition coefficient is important, but the drug activity is far more complex.

Q. I. Forrest: How much time had elapsed between the avoidance training under CPZ and your testing with the hydroxylated metabolites?

A. None.

Q. Kaul: What was your basis for saying that your compounds did not inhibit the hexobarbital metabolism?

A. Only indirect evidence; since we saw prolongation of sleeping time of both the barbital and hexobarbital and we know that barbital does not get metabolized.

8. *T. Akera*

Q. Kaul: Your 7-8-dihydroxy-CPZ is a potent inhibitor of (NA^+, K^+)-ATPase and at the same time also a positive inotropic agent. You have concluded that this compound acts by a mechanism by which norepinephrine and isoproterenol act. Have you studied the effect of these catecholamines on the (Na^+, K^+)-ATPase?

A. Yes, but they show no effect on the enzyme.

Q. Conway: In your figure showing the kinetic curves of inhibition, I believe that interpolation of these curves, with two apparent slopes, to zero can be misleading. A lot more and possibly different things may be happening in the reaction, than what the interpolated straight line tells us.

A. Yes, but the parachloromercuric benzoate curve was parallel.

Wolleman: CPZ activates adrenyl cyclase. If your compound also did it, that would perhaps explain the inotropic activity you see.

I. Forrest: Tris buffer seems to hydroxylate CPZ, but I do not know what it does to phenolic metabolites.

A. We used 50 mM of Tris buffer. I do not know if this would effect 7,8-dihydroxy-CPZ in any way.

Session VIII

Clinical Session:
Pharmacological Effects of Phenothiazines and Related Drugs

Chairmen: Samuel C. Kaim and Pavel Stern

The Phenothiazines and Structurally Related Drugs, edited by I. S. Forrest, C. J. Carr, and E. Usdin. Raven Press, New York © 1974.

Antipsychotic Efficacy of Clozapine in Correlation to Changes in Catecholamine Metabolism in Man

M. Ackenheil, H. Beckmann, W. Greil, G. Hoffmann, E. Markianos, and J. Raese

Psychiatrische Klinik der Universität München, München, Germany

INTRODUCTION

Until now, the antipsychotic activity of classic neuroleptic drugs (e.g., haloperidol and chlorpromazine) has been assumed to be correlated with major disturbances of extrapyramidal functions in man. Simultaneously, the pharmacological characteristics of these drugs have been the cataleptic effect and the ability to inhibit pharmacogenic stereotyped behavior in animals. These effects are also thought to be due to a blockade of the dopamine receptor in the brain, leading to an enhanced turnover of dopamine measurable by an increased level of homovanillic acid (HVA), the major metabolite of dopamine. This increased level of HVA has been found in the brains of animals as well as in the cerebrospinal fluid (CSF) of patients treated with neuroleptic drugs (8, 9).

In addition to these changes in HVA, changes in 5-hydroxyindoleacetic acid (5-HIAA), the major metabolite of serotonin, and 3-methoxy-4-hydroxyphenylglycol (MHPG), the major metabolite of norepinephrine (NA), can also be assumed.

Recently, the tricyclic drug 8-chloro-11-(4-methyl-1-piperazinyl)-5-H-dibenzo (b,c) (1,4) diazepine (Clozapine®) was found in different clinical studies to possess antipsychotic efficacy in schizophrenia without producing major disturbances in extrapyramidal functions in man (2–4, 7). It also has no cataleptogenic effect in animals (26). On the other hand, an enhanced dopamine and NA turnover has been reported (6).

It was our intention to investigate whether these changes could be found in patients also, and whether there was any correlation between the antipsychotic action and the level of amine metabolites in CSF. Furthermore, we were interested in the excretion of these metabolites in urine in relation to the CSF levels, and the plasma content of the drug in relation to the onset of the antipsychotic efficacy.

Finally, we were interested in finding out whether there were any changes in serum dopamine-β-hydroxylase (DBH) activity after Clozapine® treatment, according to the theory that an increased or decreased activity of this enzyme influences the ratio of HVA/MHPG.

METHODS

Patients and Drug Treatments

Studies were made on a group of nine male patients on a ward at the Psychiatric Clinic of the University of München. All patients (mean age 28 ± 10) in this study had been free of drugs for at least 4 weeks prior to admission to the hospital. They suffered from an acute exacerbation of mania (three patients) or schizophrenia (six patients), and hospitalization was necessary for therapy. The diagnoses were made by consensus of two of the authors. Emphasis was placed on behavioral and phenomenological criteria. At days 0, 5, 10, 20, and 30, each patient was rated independently by two raters (always the same) using the AMP rating system (1). By means of a screening program (laboratory data, EEG, X-ray), a check was made for signs of any organic illness. In case of pathological findings, the patients were excluded from the study.

The first day after admission, no drugs were provided with the exception of chloralhydrate. The patient was kept in bed from 7 P.M. until the next morning (usually 8 A.M.), when the first lumbar puncture was carried out in a sitting position. Before the patient had breakfast, 13.5 ml of CSF was collected in four portions (0.5, 3, 3, and 7 ml). The first two portions were used for routine diagnosis. The other two portions were immediately frozen and stored at $-40°C$ until analysis. A second lumbar puncture was done after 10 (or in two cases, 20) days of treatment with Clozapine, and CSF was stored in the same way.

On the same days, 24-hr urine was collected with Na-metabisulfite (50 mg/100 ml) and stored at $-40°C$. On days 0, 5, 10, 20, and 30, 10 ml of blood was taken before the first medication of Clozapine. After cooling, the blood was centrifuged, the plasma decanted and immediately frozen. This plasma was used to estimate the Clozapine level and to assay the DBH activity. Clozapine was given at fixed dosage of 100 mg, three times per day, with one exception, 3×200 mg/day.

Chemical Estimations

Clozapine in blood plasma was estimated by gas chromatography using a nitrogen detector. The Clozapine estimations were made in the laboratories of the Sandoz Company, Basle, by W. Pacha. MHPG in urine was estimated gas chromatographically, using a slightly modified method of Dekirmenjian (11). MHPG in CSF was estimated by use of a slightly modified method of E. Gordon (14). HVA in urine and CSF was measured fluorimetrically by using the methods of Sato (23), and Ashcroft and Sharman (5), also with slight modifications. For the measurement of 5-HIAA, Gerbode's method (13) was used. The serum DBH activity was determined by a method developed in our laboratory, which is based on a thin-layer chromatographic separation of ^{14}C-tyramine from the β-hydroxylated product, ^{14}C-octopamine. The chromatograms were then scanned on a thin-layer chromatographic scanner. The amounts of tyramine and octopamine were estimated by using the scanner integrator or a planimeter. The percentage of hydroxylated tyramine was calculated. The DBH activity is expressed in nmoles of tyramine hydroxylated per milliliter of serum and hour *(to be published)*.

RESULTS

Plasma Level of Clozapine and Clinical Status during Treatment

Nine male patients suffering from an acute episode of either mania [3] or schizophrenia [6] had been treated with Clozapine. The plasma level of Clozapine was estimated for four patients (Fig. 1). An increase of plasma level was found up to the 10th day of treatment, at which time a steady state was reached. The concentration of Clozapine in plasma was between 0.2 and 0.6 μg/ml plasma.

The mean value of the sum of the rating scores of all patients was remarkably reduced after 10 days of treatment, indicating a good response to the treatment (Fig. 2). Considering each patient separately (Table 1), a very good improvement of psychiatric status was found in seven patients;

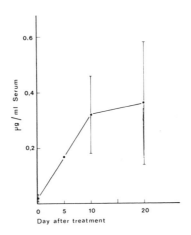

FIG. 1. Clozapine® serum level during 20 days of treatment; means ± SEM (*n* = 4), at day 5, *n* = 2.

Table 1: Changes in MHPG, HVA and 5-HIAA concentration with respect to changes in clinical state after clozapine treatment

Pat.	Age	diagn.	Clozapine treatment	MHPG CSF ng/ml	MHPG URINE ng/mg CREAT.	HVA CSF ng/ml	HVA URINE ng/mg CREAT.	5-HIAA CSF ng/ml	AMP-score
1	22	M	before	112	551	30.1	630	21.7	56
			after	52.5	158	21.5	1030	< 5	16
2	22	M	before	47	826	63.0	1790	15.5	39
			after	32	1267	90.1	1210	21.7	16
3	44	M	before	55	304	17.2	2190	< 5	29
			after	39	688	24.3	1800	21.7	14.5
4	51	S	before	11	369	2.9	–	< 5	41
			after	15	106	61.5	–	31.0	18
5	25	S	before	22	144	18.6	1000	6.2	28
			after	1	242	71.6	1430	34.1	22.5
6	27	S	before	38	828	15.8	4180	< 5	43
			after	35	291	54.4	3040	6.2	7.5
7	24	S	before	34	253	118.8	2242	43.4	78
			after	24	195	131.6	1550	27.9	33
8	21	S	before	14	255	15.8	–	12.4	23
			after	9	–	61.5	–	24.8	7
9	24	S	before	50	412	40.1	1940	9.2	– [+]
			after	31	781	70.1	2610	15.5	33

+) Patient was stuporous

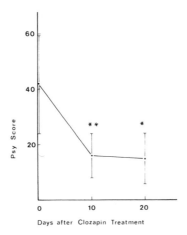

FIG. 2. Psychiatric status of patients before and during Clozapine® treatment; scores of the AMP rating system, means ± SEM ($n = 9$). *$p < 0.001$; **$p < 0.005$.

two of them did not respond well. In no case were major disturbances in the extrapyramidal system observed. Occasionally, other somatic side effects appeared, such as tiredness, hypersalivation, elevation of body temperature and pulse rate, accompanied by a tendency to orthostatic disregulations probably caused by lowered blood pressure.

MHPG, HVA, and 5-HIAA in CSF (Fig. 3)

The basic levels of MHPG, HVA, and 5-HIAA in the CSF were estimated. We compared the levels on the first day of admission with the levels

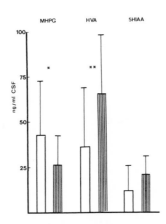

FIG. 3. Lumbar CSF MHPG, HVA, and 5-HIAA before and during Clozapine treatment; unshaded bars—before treatment, shaded bars—after 10 days of treatment, means ± SEM ($n = 9$). *$p < 0.05$, **$p < 0.005$: paired Student's t-test.

after 10 (in two cases, after 20) days of treatment with Clozapine. There was a decrease of 38% in MHPG, which was found to be significant in the paired Student's-t-test ($p < 0.005$). The 5-HIAA level was increased, but this increase was not statistically significant.

MHPG and HVA Excretion in Urine (Fig. 4)

On the same days that the lumbar punctures were carried out, 24-hr urines were collected and the excretion of HVA and MHPG was measured and calculated per mg creatinine. There was no difference between the values for the first day of admission and those for the 10th day. No correlation was found between CSF levels and excretion of MHPG and HVA in urine.

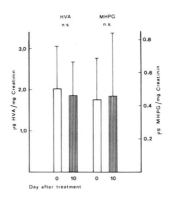

FIG. 4. HVA and MHPG excretion in urine before and during Clozapine treatment; unshaded bars — before treatment, shaded bars — after 10 days of treatment, means ± SEM ($n = 9$), n.s. — not significant.

DBH Activity in Serum (Fig. 5)

The DBH activity in the serum of six patients before and during treatment with Clozapine was measured. After treatment, a 20 to 30% decrease was generally observed. This reduction was seen during the entire period of treatment. It was independent of the plasma level of Clozapine.

Comparison of MHPG, HVA, and 5-HIAA Levels in CSF between Mania and Schizophrenia (Fig. 6)

In manics, we found a higher MHPG level in CSF (71 ± 35 ng/ml) than in schizophrenics (28 ± 15 ng/ml). The decrease after Clozapine treatment

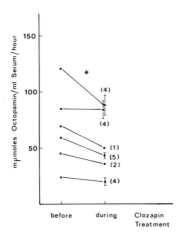

FIG. 5. Serum DBH activity before and during Clozapine treatment. Samples taken within 4 weeks in parentheses; *$p < 0.05$ paired Student's t-test.

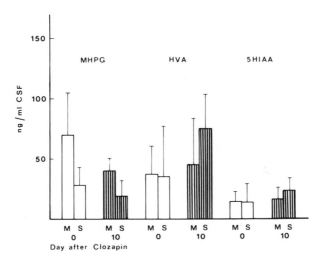

FIG. 6. Lumbar CSF MHPG, HVA, and 5-HIAA in manic (M) ($n = 3$) and schizophrenic (S) ($n = 6$) patients before and during treatment with Clozapine; unshaded bars—before treatment, shaded bars—after 10 days of treatment, means ± SEM.

was even greater in manics (33%) than in the group of schizophrenics (23%). The basic levels of HVA and 5-HIAA did not differ in both groups, but the HVA increase after treatment was higher in schizophrenics (114%) than in manics (25%). Because of the small number of patients studied (three manics and six schizophrenics), the results did not lend themselves to statistical analysis.

DISCUSSION

Our results confirm the findings of other authors who reported good antipsychotic effects of Clozapine in a great number of patients (about 120) without observing major disturbances in extrapyramidal functions (3, 4, 7). From the clinical point of view, there was no correlation between antipsychotic efficacy and extrapyramidal side effects, although such a correlation has been assumed for some time (16). However, we cannot exclude the possible occurrence of very slight disturbances in the extrapyramidal system which could be observed with special techniques only. It is probable that other properties of Clozapine, e.g., anticholinergic or, peripherally, α-adrenolytic, are able to block these extrapyramidal side effects (26).

The plasma level of Clozapine was not found to correlate with antipsychotic efficacy or biochemical data. This could be due to the small number of patients examined for plasma levels of Clozapine.

Surprisingly, the biochemical data are very similar to those obtained after use of other neuroleptic drugs, with regard to dopamine turnover, but differ with regard to the clinical effects. Like other authors (8, 9) who have investigated the influence of neuroleptics (e.g., chlorpromazine and haloperidol), we also found a significant increase of HVA in CSF during Clozapine treatment. This increase was even greater than that found during treatment with haloperidol *(unpublished results)*. These findings agree with the results of Bartholini et al. (6), who found Clozapine to have the same effects on dopamine turnover as other neuroleptics, without producing catalepsy. The lack of cataleptogenic properties has also been reported by Stille (26), who investigated the pharmacology of this drug. Furthermore, Clozapine does not inhibit the pharmacologic stereotypes and conditioned avoidance response. Therefore, it is doubtful that a blockade of dopamine receptors alone is important for these effects of the drug. This blockade would lead to an enhanced dopamine turnover, which should be indicated by an increased HVA level. Perhaps anatomical differences in striatal and limbic dopamine systems (1) are more important. On the other hand, it is not clear whether higher HVA levels always indicate a blockade of dopamine receptors. Keller et al. (18) recently showed that "spreading depression" also leads to higher HVA levels. In addition, it should be remembered that noradrenergic systems in spinal cord or in brain are certainly also affected by neuroleptic drugs. Assuming MHPG to be the main metabolite of brain NA, our results show a decrease of central NA turnover. There are relatively few reports (25) on CSF MHPG levels in man after treatment with neuroleptics. A remarkably reduced content of NA was found in the brains of animals. This decrease was even more pronounced after blockade of NA synthesis by α-methylparatyrosine, indicating an enhanced NA turnover. This increased turnover must be due to a blockade of NA receptors, leading to an increased impulse flow as a consequence of a feedback mechanism (6). The authors assumed that the synthesis of NA was not sufficient to compensate for the increased consumption of NA. They also could not find an inhibition of DBH in the brains of these animals.

In our study, it was important to determine if there were any changes in the serum DBH activity after Clozapine treatment. Since the development of a sensitive assay for DBH (22), this enzyme has been the focus of much brain research. Nevertheless, the influence of neuroleptics on this enzyme has not yet been investigated. We determined the serum DBH activity before and during treatment with Clozapine by a new method. After 10 days of treatment, we found a significant decrease of serum DBH activity. This effect persisted throughout the entire treatment period. If the serum DBH activity reflects the DBH activity in the brain, this effect could account for the decreased CSF MHPG level after Clozapine treatment. On the other hand, no differences in CSF MHPG levels or serum DBH activity have been observed after treatment with haloperidol *(unpublished results)*. Nevertheless, other factors which probably affect the CSF MHPG level, such as mood and activity of the patient (20, 21, 24), or sedative effects of the drug (19), should be considered. Changes in urinary MHPG execretions were observed in depressive and manic patients. In our Clozapine-treated patients, we did not find significant differences in urinary MHPG and HVA excretions. Furthermore, the excretion in urine did not correlate with the CSF levels of these two metabolites. Therefore, we must assume that the CSF HVA and MHPG levels reflect the activity of the central nervous system due to Clozapine administration. In contrast to the significantly increased CSF HVA level and to the decreased MHPG level in CSF, the CSF 5-HIAA level was not notably different before and after treatment. Nonetheless, there is a slight but not significant increase of 5-HIAA during treatment with Clozapine. Assuming that CSF 5-HIAA reflects, at least to some extent, the turnover of serotonin in brain (a not universally accepted theory) (10), the changes observed may be related either to the drowsiness or to the elevated body temperature of the patient. In both of these states, which sometimes occurred during treatment, serotonin is believed to be involved (17, 12). Furthermore, a specific drug effect cannot be excluded, because other neuroleptics (e.g., chlorpromazine) (15) elevate the 5-HIAA concentration in the brains of animals. Tentatively, we tried to compare the data for manics and schizophrenics. In mania, we found a higher CSF level and a more accentuated decrease of MHPG than in schizophrenia. The basic values of CSF HVA in schizophrenia and mania were not different. However, the increase after Clozapine treatment was higher in schizophrenia. Further investigations are necessary to confirm these findings.

CONCLUSIONS

In summary, we found Clozapine to have a good antipsychotic action without signs of extrapyramidal dysfunctions. As with other neuroleptics, the CSF HVA level was increased during treatment. In the case of these other neuroleptics, the receptor blockade and the resulting increase in HVA was thought to be related to extrapyramidal dysfunctions and anti-psychotic action. The effects of Clozapine make this hypothesis doubtful. In this instance, the effects are probably related not only to the dopamine system, but also to the noradrenergic system, which is markedly influenced by this drug.

SUMMARY

Clozapine in a dosage of 300 mg/day markedly improves acute psychotic patients, without producing disturbances in extrapyramidal functions.

The plasma level of Clozapine increases up to the 10th day, when it reaches a steady-state level.

CSF HVA is significantly increased and CSF MHPG is significantly decreased after treatment with Clozapine. Only a slight increase in CSF 5-HIAA was found.

In urine, no changes in HVA and MHPG excretion were observed before and after treatment.

The serum DBH activity after treatment with Clozapine is significantly reduced.

In mania, the CSF MHPG was higher than in schizophrenia. The decrease after treatment in mania was more accentuated than in schizophrenia. The increase of CSF HVA after treatment was higher in schizophrenia than in mania.

ACKNOWLEDGMENTS

The authors wish to thank Dr. W. Pacha for the estimations of Clozapine plasma level and Miss I. Nystrom, Mrs. C. Lampart, and Miss E. Schmitt for skillful assistance.

REFERENCES

1. Andén, N. E., Butcher, S. G., Corrodi, H., Fuxe, K., and Ungerstedt, U., *Europ. J. Pharmacol.*, **11**, 303 (1970).
2. Angst, J., Battegay, R., Bente, D., Berner, P., Broeren, W., Corny, F., Dick, P., Engelmeier, M. P., Heimann, H., Heinrich, K., Helmchen, H., Hippius, H., Poeldinger, W., Schmidlin, P., Schmitt, W., and Weis, P., *Arzneim.-Forsch.*, **19**, 399 (1969).
3. Angst, J., Bente, D., Berner, P., Heimann, H., Helmchen, H., and Hippius, H., *Pharmakopsychiat.*, **4**, 201 (1971).
4 Angst, J., Jaenicke, U., Padrutt, A., and Scharfetter, Ch., *Pharmakopsychiat.*, **4**, 192 (1971).
5. Ashcroft, G. W., and Sharman, D. F., *Brit. J. Pharmacol.*, **19**, 153 (1962).
6. Bartholini, G., Haefely, W., Jalfre, M., Keller, H. H., and Pletscher, A., *Brit. J. Pharmacol.*, **46**, 736 (1972).
7. Berzewski, H., Helmchen, H., Hippius, H., Hoffman, H., and Kanowski, S., *Arzneim.-Forsch.*, **19**, 495 (1969).

8. Bowers, M. B., Jr., Heninger, G. R., and Gerbode, F., *Internat. J. Neuropharmacol.,* **8,** 255 (1969).
9. Bowers, M. B., Jr., *Psychopharmacologia (Berlin),* **28,** 309 (1973).
10. Bulat, M., and Zivković, B., *Science,* **173,** 738 (1971).
11. Dekirmenjian, H., and Maas, J. W., *Analyt. Biochem.,* **35,** 113 (1970).
12. Feldberg, W., and Myers, R. D., *J. Physiol. (London),* **173,** 226 (1964).
13. Gerbode, F. A., and Bowers, M. B., Jr., *J. Neurochem.,* **15,** 1053 (1968).
14. Gordon, E. K., and Oliver, J., *Clin. Chim. Acta,* **35,** 145 (1971).
15. Gumulka, W., Samanin, R., and Valzelli, L., *Europ. J. Pharmacol.,* **12,** 276 (1970).
16. Haase, H. J., *Fortschr. Neurol. Psychiat.,* **29,** 245 (1961).
17. Jouvet, M., in *Speaker Abstracts, Frontiers in Catecholamine Research, III International Catecholamine Symposium,* Strasbourg, May, 1973.
18. Keller, H. H., Bartholini, G., Pieri, L., and Pletscher, A., *Europ. J. Pharmacol.,* **20,** 287 (1972).
19. Lidbrink, P., Corrodi, H., Fuxe, K., and Olson, L., *Brain Res.,* **45,** 507 (1972).
20. Maas, J. W., and Fawcett, J. A., *Gen. Psych.,* **26,** 252 (1972).
21. Mendels, J., Frazer, A., Fitzgerald, R. G., Ramsey, T. A., and Stokes, J. W., *Science,* **175,** 1380 (1972).
22. Molinoff, P. B., Brimijoin, S., Weinshilboun, R., and Axelrod, J., *Proc. Nat. Acad. Sci. (U.S.A.),* **66,** 453 (1970).
23. Sato, T. L., *J. Lab. and Clin. Med.,* **66,** 517 (1965).
24. Schildkraut, J. J., in *Speaker Abstracts, Frontiers in Catecholamine Research, III International Catecholamine Symposium,* Strasbourg, May, 1973.
25. Shopsin, B., Wilk, S., Gershon, S., Davis, K., and Suhl, M., *Arch. Gen. Psychiat.,* **28,** 230 (1973).
26. Stille, G., Hippius, H., *Pharmakopsychiat.,* **4,** 182 (1971).

The Phenothiazines and Structurally Related Drugs, edited by I. S. Forrest, C. J. Carr, and E. Usdin. Raven Press, New York © 1974.

The Effect of Phenothiazines on Botulinus Intoxication

P. Stern and K. Valjevac

Department of Pharmacology, Medical Faculty, University of Sarajevo, 71001 Sarajevo, Yugoslavia

INTRODUCTION

Having been concerned with the problem of Botulinus (Bt) intoxication for 15 yr, and particularly with its therapeutic aspects, we have tested the therapeutic value of about 1,000 substances all of which could, in theory, favorably affect Botulinus intoxication (1–3).

Among them were some phenothiazine (Ph) substances. The theoretic reasons for their study were based on the following facts. It is well known that some of them cause extrapyramidal symptoms, which results in rigor and in an increased activity of ACh because of the decreased level of dopamine after the application of Ph (4). Considering that essentially the mechanism of Bt toxine activity is the irreversible blocking of ACh release from its vesicles at the motor-nerve endings (5), it is quite clear that this prompted our attempt to treat this intoxication with Ph.

Since fluphenazine produced the optimum and chlorpromazine the weakest effect, the Phs were classified into three groups according to their mode of action and to some characteristics of their structure (6): (a) Phs that cause strong extrapyramidal symptoms and contain fluorine in their molecule (fluphenazine, trifluoperazine); (b) Phs that also cause strong extrapyramidal symptoms but have no fluorine (F) in their molecule (perazine, thioproperazine, butaperazine); (c) Phs that do not cause extrapyramidal symptoms or to a very minor extent only and contain halogens in their molecule (trifluopromazine or chlorpromazine).

In order to determine whether the presence of F in the molecule of Ph is important, or whether it can be replaced by some other halogen, perphenazine was tested since it contains Cl (7). Furthermore, the butyrophenone drugs, which cause extrapyramidal symptoms, were tested. Some of the compounds of this group contain F in the molecule and some do not (1).

Substances which had an effect and prolonged the life of intoxicated mice were tested again, combined now with antitoxic serum. We have recently shown that *Lathrodectus tredecimguttatus* (LT) toxin is a specific antidote for Bt intoxication, and we therefore examined the effect of Phs combined with LT toxin. It was expected that these two substances would act as synergists, and that the therapeutic effect would be more than additive, and hence better than the effect of each substance alone.

METHOD

White mice of both sexes (Pasteur Institute, Novi Sad) weighing 20 to 25 g were used in the experiments. The mice were divided into experimental and control groups, each consisting of 10 animals. Both the experimental and control groups received 250 mld/kg[1] of Bt[2] subcutaneously. This dose of Bt toxin is lethal within 48 ± 6 hr. In another series of experiments, the dose was much higher and was administered intraperitoneally, which caused death within 2 to 3 hr (10). The test substances were administered 15 to 20 min prior to Bt toxin. They were administered each day up to the death of the animals. Dose and route of application are presented in Table 1. Antitoxic serum was injected i.m. at the rate of 0.05 ml of the original dilution, and was applied 17 hr after Bt intoxication. We had found previously that application of antitoxic serum will protect only 20 to 30% of the mice from intoxication (8).

TABLE 1. *Dose and route of application of test substances*

Substance	Dose (mg/kg, i.p.)	BT + substance X (±SE)	BT control X (±SE)	p
Fluphenazine	10	78.20 (±1.46)	45.60 (±1.09)	<0.001
Fluphenazine	10 24 hr prior to BT	57.60 (±3.91)	50.40 (±2.40)	N.S.
Fluphenazine	10 (2 × daily)	74.40 (±4.30)	45.60 (±2.40)	<0.001
Perphenazine	10	72.00 (±3.50)	43.20 (±3.20)	<0.001
Perphenazine	5	60.00 (±4.00)	45.60 (±2.40)	<0.05
Trifluoperazine	20	62.40 (±3.91)	43.20 (±3.20)	<0.05
Perazine	25	52.80 (±3.20)	48.00 (±3.57)	N.S.
Thioproperazine	20	50.40 (±2.40)	48.00 (±3.57)	N.S.
Butaperazine	10	52.80 (±4.71)	48.00 (±3.57)	N.S.
Trifluopromazine	20	52.80 (±3.20)	48.00 (±6.19)	N.S.
Chlorpromazine	10	48.00 (±3.56)	45.60 (±5.60)	N.S.
Butyrophenone (Haloperidol)	10	62.40 (±5.30)	43.20 (±3.20)	<0.05
Butyrophenone without F (Compound R-1532)	10	50.40 (±2.40)	48.00 (±3.57)	N.S.

X—mean value for survival time from application of BT until death of the animals (in hours).
SE—standard error of the value.
p—statistical significance.
N.S.—not significant.

---

[1] mld—medial lethal dose.
[2] Bt was kindly supplied by Boehringer Werke AG, Marburg a/L.

LT toxin was obtained by the extraction of the venomous glands. The glands were ground in a mortar and the toxin was extracted by 10 ml of physiologic NaCl solution (9). This preparation of toxin was administered subcutaneously, 0.1 ml per mouse. We used solutions of LT toxin which cause rigor within 5 to 6 hr, but did not kill the animals.

Mice were fed with "Kalinovica" (stock diet) cakes. They had water *ad libitum* and were kept in an air-conditioned room with an air temperature of 22°C. The time of death of every mouse of the experimental and control groups was recorded, and the results were elaborated statistically by the Student *t*-test.

RESULTS

The effects of fluphenazine and of two substances of the butyrophenone group on the survival time of intoxicated mice is presented in Table 1. These mice were intoxicated with 250 mld/kg Bt. Table 2 represents the influence of fluphenazine and of perphenazine upon the life span of mice intoxicated with large doses of Bt.

It can be clearly seen from Table 1 that the best effect was achieved with fluphenazine and perphenazine. Fluphenazine application 24 hr prior to Bt intoxication had no protecting effect. When the dose was doubled, the therapeutic effect was no better than that of the single dose. Decrease of the perphenazine dose to 5 mg/kg daily weakened the protecting effect.

A significant increase in survival time was achieved with trifluoperazine and with haloperidol, while haloperidol without F (Compound 1532) and other substances had no effect.

It can be seen from Table 2 that the increase of life span was highly significant after the application of fluphenazine and perphenazine. These mice were intoxicated with enormous doses of Bt (10) and each animal was given more than 10,000 mld intraperitoneally.

Since fluphenazine proved most effective, it was subsequently applied together with antitoxic serum (8) and LT. Table 3 shows the percentage of

TABLE 2. *Influence of fluphenazine and perphenazine*

Substance	Dose (mg/kg i.p.)	BT + substance X (±SE–n)	BT control X (±SE–n)	p
Fluphenazine	10	351.50 (±8.50–10)	163.00 (±4.95–10)	<0.001
Perphenazine	10	330.00 (±2.98–10)	163.00 (±4.95–10)	<0.001

X—mean value for survival time from the application of BT until death of the animals (in minutes).
SE—standard error of the value.
n—number of animals in the group.
p—statistical significance.

TABLE 3. *Percentage of survival*

BT + antitox. serum	BT + antitox. serum + fluph.	BT control
30%	10%	0%

survival of mice which were only given antitoxic serum and of mice which received serum + fluphenazine. The experiments were repeated several times, but the results of the combined antitoxic serum + fluphenazine treatment were never better than the ones with antitoxic serum alone. Actually, the effect of the combined treatment was weaker.

Table 4 shows the results of the treatment with fluphenazine + LT. The effect of this combination did not prove superior to separate application of the individual compounds.

TABLE 4. *Results of the treatment with fluphenazine and LT*

Substance	Dose and route of administration	BT + substance X (±SE–n)	BT control X (±SE–n)	p
Fluphenazine	10 mg/kg i.p.	351.50 (±8.50–10)	163.00 (±4.95–10)	<0.001
LT	0.1 ml 1:10 s.c.	388.75 (±8.48–10)	192.50 (±2.83–10)	<0.001
Fluphenazine +	10 mg/kg i.p.			
		379.20 (±2.09–10)	163.00 (±4.95–10)	<0.001
LT	0.1 ml 1:10 s.c.			

X — mean value from application of BT until death of the animals (in minutes).
SE — standard error of the value.
n — number of animals in the group.
p — statistical significance.

DISCUSSION

If the results of these experiments are examined carefully, several important facts are obvious. First of all, we may conclude that some compounds of the Ph group had a beneficial effect on the survival of the mice intoxicated with Bt. This is particularly true for fluphenazine and perphenazine, while trifluoperazine had a somewhat weaker, but nevertheless obvious effect. Haloperidol exerted a similar effect, while the other neuroleptics examined had no effect. Fluphenazine proved to be the best, and we therefore suggest that fluphenazine therapy be tentatively applied in intoxicated humans as well.

It is also evident that the Ph compounds that cause extrapyramidal symptoms, and have F in position 2 of the nucleus (fluphenazine and trifluoperazine) had an effect on Bt intoxication. Since perphenazine also exerted a good effect, it may be concluded that F does not have to be present in the Ph molecule in order to achieve a good effect, but that Cl and perhaps some other halogen might be suitable substituents. It was, however, important that suitable drugs produce extrapyramidal symptoms as well as have a halogen substituent at position 2 of the nucleus.

Thus trifluopromazine, which contains F in its molecule but causes weak extrapyramidal symptoms, had no effect on Bt intoxication. Similarly, perazine, which has no F in its molecule but causes strong extrapyramidal symptoms, had no effect.

Similar considerations apply to the butyrophenone group. Haloperidol, which causes strong extrapyramidal symptoms, protected animals from intoxication, whereas "compound 1532" had no effect.

The correlation between the structural formula, the extrapyramidal effects, and the effect on Bt intoxication is shown in Table 5.

TABLE 5. *Correlation between structural formula, extrapyramidal effects, and Bt intoxication*

Substance	Structural formula	Extra-pyramidal symptoms	Effect on BT intoxication
Fluphenazine		+ + + +	+ + + +
Perphenazine		+ + + +	+ + + +
Trifluoperazine		+ + + +	+ + +
Trifluopromazine		+ − − −	− − − −

TABLE 5 *(Continued)*

Substance	Structural formula	Extra-pyramidal symptoms	Effect on BT intoxication
Chlorpromazine		+ − − −	− − − −
Perazine		+ + + +	− − − −
Thioproperazine		+ + + +	− − − −
Butaperazine		+ + + +	− − − −
Butyrophenone (Haloperidol)		+ + + +	+ + +
Butyrophenone without F (Compound R-1532)		+ + + +	− − − −

The good effects of fluphenazine, perphenazine, trifluoperazine, and haloperidol on Bt intoxication are due to the increased activity of ACh and the decreased level of dopamine (11), at the motor-nerve end plates and in CNS, which may, for a certain period of time, prolong the function of neuromuscular transmission blocked by Bt toxin (4).

But our results clearly showed that the extrapyramidal effects as such are not sufficient for the good effect on Bt intoxication and that the simultaneous presence of a halogen is necessary (1, 12). Hence, the substances that cause very strong extrapyramidal effects have no effect on Bt intoxication, unless they contain halogen. We had previously shown that F alone had no effect on Bt intoxication. We have examined dexamethazone and DFP, and neither of these compounds had any effect (4, 12). Therefore, the importance of the halogen in the nucleus could partly be explained by the well-known phenomenon that introduction of a halogen potentiates the activity of many drugs. It is, however, clear that this explanation is not adequate, and the role of halogen in Bt intoxication remains unclear. We are also unable to explain why fluphenazine did not exert a superior effect when combined with LT, i.e., why the therapeutic effects were not synergistic, and why fluphenazine in fact decreased the protective activity of the antitoxic serum.

SUMMARY

The protective effect of some phenothiazine drugs on Bt intoxication was examined. A significant increase of the life span of the intoxicated animals was observed only when substances which cause strong extrapyramidal symptoms and contain halogen in position 2 of the nucleus were applied. The correlation between the chemical structure of the compounds studied, their extrapyramidal effects and their antibotulinus effects were tentatively defined.

REFERENCES

1. Stern, P., Boras, J. (1968): Proc. of the European Society for the Study of Drug Toxicity Ics, **9**, 189.
2. Stern, P., Boras, J. (1968): Toxicon **5**, 187.
3. Boras, J., Stern, P. (1969): Arhiv za higijenu rada i toksikologiju **20**, 161.
4. Boras, J., Stern, P. (1967): Iug. Physiol. et Pharmacol. Acta **3**, 225.
5. Wright, G. P. (1955): **7**, 413.
6. Bohaček, N., Hajnsek, F., Sartorius, N. (1963). Fortschr. Neurol. Psychiat. **31**, 565.
7. Valjevac, K., Stern, P. (1970): Arhiv za higijenu rada i toksikologiju **21**, 143.
8. Stern, P., Valjevac, K. (1973): RADOVI Akademije nauka i umjetnosti BiH **17**, 13.
9. Stern, P., Valjevac, K.: In preparation for publication.
10. Boroff, D. A., Fleck, U. (1967): J. Pharm. exper. Therapeut. **157**, 427.
11. Stern, P. (1968): Wien. klin. Wschr. **80**, 181.
12. Stern, P., Valjevac, K., Boras, J. (1971): Subsidia medica **23**, 3.

The Phenothiazines and Structurally Related Drugs, edited by I. S. Forrest, C. J. Carr, and E. Usdin. Raven Press, New York © 1974.

Clinical Differences Among Phenothiazines in Schizophrenics

Leo E. Hollister

Veterans Administration Hospital, Palo Alto, California 94304

INTRODUCTION – SPECIFIC INDICATIONS FOR ANTIPSYCHOTICS: ELUSIVE END OF THE RAINBOW

Beginning of the Idea

As soon as there was more than one antipsychotic drug, clinicians made the observation that patients who did not respond to one might respond to another. Such individual differences in response to drugs persisted even after most phenothiazine drugs had been repeatedly found to be equally efficacious when the responses of groups of patients were compared (1, 2). The more sedative phenothiazines, such as chlorpromazine (Thorazine®) or thioridazine (Mellaril®), were thought initially to be preferable for patients with agitation, less sedative drugs, such as trifluoperazine (Stelazine®) and perphenazine (Trilafon®), being considered as drugs best for patients with symptoms of withdrawal and retardation. Such a differential action was based more on armchair reasoning than on experimental evidence.

To complicate matters, the notion of target symptoms, originally proposed simply to provide a guide to setting goals and evaluating results of drug therapy in individual patients, became confused with differences between drugs. Depending upon which clinician you consulted, drug A was particularly good for hallucinations, drug B, for social withdrawal, and drug C preferable for hostile or belligerent behavior. Based on such unproved assumptions, it was easy to justify the use of combined drug therapy, giving a pinch of each drug for the symptom or sign it was thought especially to benefit. Combinations of several antipsychotic drugs were used in the same patient, and in addition, antidepressant, stimulant, or sedative drugs were thrown into the mill. Today it is rare to find a schizophrenic patient being treated with a single antipsychotic drug.

The original phenomenon still holds. Patients do respond in individual ways to drugs. Is there any way to predict in advance which patients will do best with which drug?

Our Past Attempts with This Problem

For over a decade, my collaborators and I have studied a variety of antipsychotic drugs, both in controlled and uncontrolled studies, not only to compare their efficacy, but also to distinguish differing patterns of clinical indications. We have used increasingly sophisticated techniques for looking into the matter and have never failed to find some promising leads. As will soon become evident, it is one thing to find leads and another to prove them.

A controlled comparison of the new antipsychotic drug, haloperidol (Haldol®) and the phenothiazine, thiopropazate (Dartal®), not surprisingly revealed no difference between the two drugs in terms of total efficacy (3). It did suggest that in patients classified as "nonparanoid," halperidol was somewhat more effective. A study of the phenylpiperazine derivative, oxypertine, again suggested a special spectrum of activity (4). This drug had little apparent effect on "paranoid" symptoms and considerable effect on a small group of patients classified as "depressed" schizophrenics. An uncontrolled study of the benzoquinolizine derivative, benzquinamide, placed it among active antipsychotic drugs (5). Response to benzquinamide was significantly correlated with pretreatment ratings in five items from the Brief Psychiatric Rating Scale (BPRS). Benzquinamide appeared to be specifically indicated for patients having high BPRS ratings on hallucinatory behavior and unusual thought content relative to ratings on emotional withdrawal, mannerisms, and posturing and depressive mood. Summed scores on the first pair of ratings minus those on emotional withdrawal, mannerisms, and posturing provided a simple "prediction index" that, at least retrospectively, correlated highly with the observed improvement. A new butyrophenone derivative, trifluperidol, also fell within the range of efficacy of most antipsychotic drugs we had studied (6). What was most intriguing was that the mean BPRS change scores in a small group of patients classified as "paranoid" were the highest we had ever observed in this group. Other toxicity removed this drug from further study, so it was impossible to check this interesting but distressing finding. Distressing it was, for it was quite the opposite from what we had found with haloperidol, a closely related compound.

Our first attempt at a replicative study was a controlled comparison of acetophenazine (Tindal®), perphenazine, and benzquinamide (7). Once again, we could find no overall difference between the drugs. In this instance, too, we could find no significant difference in the patterns of symptoms which responded. Patients classified as "paranoid" tended to do generally better with drugs than those in the "nonparanoid" category. A study which simultaneously evaluated thiothixene (Navane®) in both schizophrenic and depressed patients provided some apparent differences in responses among the schizophrenic patients (8). These were classified, according to computer profiles of BPRS ratings, into five empirical types: primary; hallucinatory-thinking disturbance; anxious-depressed; paranoid hostile-suspicious; and nonhallucinatory-thinking disturbance. The latter two categories represented the extremes, the paranoid group being the most severely ill and the nonhallucinatory group showing the lowest total pathology scores. The degree of improvement was highest in the paranoid and hallucinatory-thinking groups (which comprised 50% of the sample) and least in the non-hallucinatory group. It was disappointing that clinical division of patients into paranoid and nonparanoid groups failed to distinguish between them. A controlled comparison of the acridane derivative, SKF 14336, with chlorpromazine revealed the former drug to be somewhat less effective (9). It was conspicuously so in patients classified as having "florid thinking disorders" where specific antipsychotic effects of a drug might be most likely to show. A replicative study comparing thiothixene with oxypertine provided somewhat more encouragement (10). Thiothixene was once again found to be somewhat better in "paranoid" patients, whereas oxypertine was better in "nonparanoid" patients, especially those categorized as "depressed." The results of some studies in which patients were classified into "paranoid," "core," and "depressed" types are shown in Table 1.

TABLE 1. Change scores BPRS total pathology in various schizophrenic subtypes

Drug	Paranoid	Core schiz.	Depressed
Thioridazine	24.3	22.4	25.9
Acetophenazine	32.5	27.6	24.5
Acetophenazine	30.8	28.5	24.8
Perphenazine	30.0	25.8	14.2
Benzquinamide	35.9	28.7	
Benzquinamide[a]	36.6	23.2	10.7
Trifluperidol[a]	46.3	23.9	21.2
Oxypertine[a]	13.5	29.5	35.7
Thiothixene[a]	31.7	21.7	25.4
Oxypertine	7.7	24.3	34.6
Thiothixene	34.5	23.4	26.2

The higher the change score, the greater the improvement.
[a] Uncontrolled study.

Looking back, it is difficult to see why we continued on this search. One can only argue that new leads kept appearing and that sometimes, rather infrequently to be sure, they were confirmed. At the same time, a search for specific indications for antidepressant drugs, which was proceeding concurrently, was producing definite and reproducible indications for these drugs.

Attempts Made by Others

We were not alone in our folly. Another group in the Veterans Administration (VA) analyzed data from a VA Cooperative Study to develop regression equations which might predict responses to chlorpromazine and fluphenazine (Prolixin®) (11). In the area of excitement versus retardation, chlorpromazine produced best results in patients with high scores on the Inpatient Multidimensional Psychiatric Scale (IMPS) factors of excitement, disorientation, and hostility, and fluphenazine did better in patients with high scores on paranoid projection and conceptual disorganization and low scores on perceptual distortion, retardation, and grandiosity. Similar approaches were taken to predicting improvement in "schizophrenic disorganization" and "paranoid process." When these equations were applied to data from a N.I.M.H. study, the interactions between the actual and predicted results were significant. Such an elegant approach is something of a statistical tour de force, for it is difficult, if not impossible, to translate these factors to a specific patient. An attempt to cross-validate this approach using data from a new VA Cooperative study failed to support the hypothesis that those patients who received the putative drug of choice would respond more favorably than those randomly assigned to the other drug (12). This same group explored the predictive value of dividing patients into the older categories of "hypodynamic" and "hyperdynamic," based on the degree of activity and socialization (13). No differential response was found between carphenazine (Proketazine®), trifluoperazine, and chlorpromazine, despite the fact that the first two drugs were reputed to be better for the "hypodymanic" type.

An N.I.M.H. group also looked into this question (14). Schizophrenics were divided into four types, "core," "paranoid," "bizarre," and "depressive," and the actions of four phenothiazines were compared in each. Evidence was suggestive that chlorpromazine was the most efficacious for core, acetophenazine was the most efficacious for bizarre and depressive, acetophenazine and chlorpromazine were more effective than fluphenazine in paranoid, and fluphenazine was the most suitable for depressives. A later attempt by the principal members of the same group failed to replicate these findings of specificity of action of antipsychotic drugs (15).

ANOTHER LOOK AT THE QUESTION

Our most recent attempt to examine this question will probably be our last. In this study, we assigned 320 newly admitted schizophrenic men randomly to three types of phenothiazines, aliphatic, piperidine, and piperazine derivatives (16). Physicians were free, once the assignment had been made, to choose drugs within the class assigned and were encouraged to use them to the maximal clinical advantage. Thus, except for the random assignment to type of drug, conditions of treatment mimicked the usual clinical situation. As it turned out, almost all the patients assigned to piperidines were treated with thioridazine, most assigned to aliphatics received chlorpromazine, and most assigned to piperazines received either acetophenazine, fluphenazine, or perphenazine.

As might now be readily expected, we found no main differences in clinical effects among the three classes of drugs, that is, they were equals in terms of therapeutic potential in large groups of patients. Looking at individual characteristics of patients, we found that piperazine derivatives were superior in the treatment of older schizophrenic patients, as well as those diagnosed as "nonparanoid;" the reverse situation applied to the piperidine series, and to a lesser extent, the aliphatics (Table 2). On the whole, nonparanoid patients tended to respond somewhat better to any phenothiazine.

Considering more specific symptoms, we found that piperazines tended to improve thinking disturbance in contrast to withdrawal-retardation, the piperidines showed the least differences in response, and the aliphatics were somewhere in between (see Table 3). The piperazines were also superior in the poor premorbid history, process types of schizophrenia. Based on global ratings, the piperazine derivatives looked to be somewhat more superior overall than the other two classes, but these differences were not significant.

Such differences as were found in this study were internally consistent and largely consonant with prevailing clinical beliefs. That is, piperazine derivatives were more effective than the other two types in treating older schizophrenic patients, a group that tended also to include patients classified as nonparanoid, core schizophrenics with primary disturbances of thinking. The idea that piperazine derivatives have more specific antipsychotic activity was given some support.

TABLE 2. *BPRS schizophrenia syndrome change scores following three types of phenothiazines*

Drug/Age group	<30	30–39	40 +
Aliphatic	7.7 (40)[a]	7.8 (22)	6.3 (42)
Piperazine	6.0 (41)	8.8 (18)	8.4 (44)[a]
Piperidine	7.8 (47)[a]	7.8 (23)	6.6 (43)

Drug/Schiz. subtype	Paranoid	Nonparanoid
Aliphatic	7.0 (34)	7.9 (70)
Piperazine	6.7 (29)	8.8 (74)[a]
Piperidine	8.4 (38)[a]	7.0 (75)

[a] Significantly different from others, complex analysis of covariance.
( ) N, size of sample.

TABLE 3. *BPRS change scores for thinking disturbances (TD) and withdrawal-retardation (WR) responses to three types of phenothiazines*

Drug/Symptom	TD	WR	TD-WR
Aliphatic	4.6	2.3	2.2
Piperazine	5.1	2.2	2.9[a]
Piperidine	4.5	2.7	1.8

[a] Difference in change significantly greater for piperazine treatment group ($p < 0.05$).

Satisfying as these results might be, they are rather meager. Further, in contrast to the present study, one of our past studies had suggested a better overall response among paranoid, rather than nonparanoid, patients (7). Thus the record of the past remains unblemished; no study completely replicates any which preceded it.

SOME GENERAL CONCLUSIONS ABOUT SPECIFICITY OF ACTION

The notion that different antipsychotic drugs affect target symptoms selectively, a still prevalent belief, has failed to find experimental support in all of these studies. It has been essentially impossible to sort out any pattern of symptoms and signs, or demographic variables, or any combinations of these, which can be used to predict responses of an individual patient. Many of the differences found retrospectively have been based on contrast functions, that is, patients relatively high in one set of symptoms and low in another respond better to one drug than another. Such studies, even should they be valid, would be useless for clinical purposes, for it would be rare to find in advance patients who fitted so neatly into such artificial categories. As a corollary to the failure to delineate specific antipsychotic effects of drugs, the hope that subtypes of schizophrenia might be defined on the basis of their specific responses to drugs also seems rather remote, at least if one considers responses among various phenothiazines.

It may very well be the case that differences between various phenothiazines in individual patients may be more due to idiosyncratic kinetics and metabolism of these drugs than to any important pharmacological differences between them. Evidence is accumulating that chlorpromazine, the most widely studied of these drugs in this regard, may be variably absorbed and metabolized in different patients (17, 18). Until we know more about the fate of these drugs in the body, and what this may mean in regard to clinical outcome, clinicians must continue to choose these drugs largely on an *empirical basis*.

ACKNOWLEDGMENTS

Work cited in this paper was supported in part by grants MH 03030 and 05144, from the U.S. Public Health Service.

REFERENCES

1. Casey, J. F., Lasky, J. J., Klett, C. J., and Hollister, L. E., *Am. J. Psychiat.* **117,** 97 (1960).
2. National Institute of Mental Health-Psychopharmacology Service Center Collaborative Study Group, *Arch. Gen. Psychiat.,* **10,** 246 (1964).
3. Hollister, L. E., Overall, L. E., Caffey, E., Jr., Bennett, J. L., Meyer, F., Kimbell, I., Jr., and Honigfeld, G., *J. Nerv. Ment. Dis.,* **135,** 544 (1962).
4. Hollister, L. E., Overall, J. E., Kimbell, I., Jr., Bennett, J. L., Meyer, F., and Caffey, E., Jr., *J. New Drugs,* **3,** 26 (1963).
5. Overall, J. E., Hollister, L. E., Bennett, J. L., Shelton, J., and Caffey, E. M., Jr., *Current Therap. Research,* **5,** 335 (1963).
6. Hollister, L. E., Overall, J. E., Bennett, J. L., Kimbell, I., Jr., and Shelton, J., *J. New Drugs,* **5,** 34 (1965).
7. Hollister, L. E., Overall, J. E., Bennett, J. L., Kimbell, I., Jr., and Shelton, J., *Clin. Pharmacol. Therap.,* **8,** 249 (1967).
8. Overall, J. E., Hollister, L. E., Shelton, J., Kimbell, I., Jr., and Pennington, V., *Clin. Pharmacol. Therap.,* **10,** 36 (1969).
9. Overall, J. E., Hollister, L. E., Prusmack, J. J., Shelton, J., and Pokorny, A. D., *J. Clin. Pharmacol.,* **9,** 328 (1969).
10. Hollister, L. E., Overall, J. E., Katz, G., Higginbotham, W. E., and Kimbell, I., Jr., *Clin. Pharmacol. Therap.,* **12,** 531 (1971).
11. Klett, C. J., and Mosely, E. C., *J. Consult. Psychol.,* **29,** 546 (1965).
12. Galbrecht, C. R., and Klett, C. J., *J. Nerv. Ment. Dis.,* **147,** 173 (1960).
13. Platz, A. R., Klett, C. J., and Caffey, E. M., Jr., *Dis. Nerv. Syst.,* **28,** 601 (1967).
14. National Institute of Mental Health and PRB Collaborative Study Group, *Dis. Nerv. Syst.,* **28,** 369 (1967).
15. Goldberg, S. C., Frisch, W. A., Drossman, A. K., Schooler, N. R., and Johnson, G. F. S., *Arch. Gen. Psychiat.,* **26,** 367 (1972).
16. Hollister, L. E., Overall, J. E., Kimbell, I., Jr., and Pokorny, A. D. (*In press,* 1974).
17. Sakalis, G., Curry, S. H., Mould, G. P., and Lader, M. H., *Clin. Pharmacol. Therap.,* **13,** 931 (1972).
18. Usdin, E., CRC Critical Reviews in Clin. Lab. Sciences, **2** (3), 347 (1971).

The Phenothiazines and Structurally Related Drugs, edited by I. S. Forrest, C. J. Carr, and E. Usdin. Raven Press, New York © 1974.

Prediction of Neuroleptic Effects from Animal Data

O. Vinař and M. Kršiak

Institute of Psychiatry, Prague, Czechoslovakia, and Institute of Pharmacology, Academy of Sciences, Prague, Czechoslovakia

INTRODUCTION

There is widespread disagreement on the value of the results of pharmacological tests in animals in predicting therapeutic efficacy of a psychotropic drug. There are optimists and pessimists in this respect and Irwin (1) showed that their attitudes might influence their findings.

The test conditions in animals differ greatly from conditions in which psychotropic drugs are administered to patients. The comparability of a so-called average experimental animal or of homogeneous groups of such animals with heterogeneous groups of mentally ill human individuals is really very low. Usually, acute animal experiments are compared with observations following chronic application in patients. In addition, the clinical findings are based on optimal dosage which varies from individual to individual, from hospital to hospital, and even from one country to another, whereas the pharmacological findings are based on the effective doses that are relatively stable. These might be reasons for the fact that animal models of psychotropic drug action generally have little relevance to the clinical use of these compounds, and extrapolation of drug effects from animals to psychiatric patients is still an inexact procedure.

Nevertheless, an empirical approach has enabled us to screen pharmacologically thousands of compounds from which a few hundred have been proposed for clinical investigation in psychiatry. Many of them were shown to be of therapeutic value and were produced by the pharmaceutical industry with satisfactory results for both patients and pharmaceutical companies.

There have been many attempts to correlate animal data with clinical findings (2–5). However, these studies did not usually formalize the correlation statistically. Moreover, correlations were usually sought between a certain animal test and the global therapeutic efficacy in schizophrenic psychoses, depressions, anxiety neuroses, etc., and little attention was paid to the fact that various drugs have different effects on various symptoms of schizophrenia or of endogenous depression.

The present study attempted to elaborate the correlation between various

675

pharmacological tests and the therapeutic efficacy in various psychotic symptoms in a mathematically formalized manner for 11 neuroleptic drugs. Its aim was to find out whether and which pharmacological tests could predict the effects on specific psychotic symptoms.

METHOD

Clinical data were obtained from observation of patients treated on the wards of the Department of Psychopharmacology of the Institute of Psychiatry in Prague. During the last 8 yr, a system of continuous controlled trial has been in operation on these wards (6).

The main characteristics are that the double-blind procedure is not reinstated for each subsequent trial of a new drug, but that it is a general policy on these wards which is applied without exception to all patients admitted. The criteria for selection of patients are strictly stipulated, allowing only patients with functional psychoses to be admitted. Drugs are allocated to individual patients at random according to a design whereby about three neuroleptic drugs and two or three antidepressants are tested at any one time. Short placebo wash-out periods precede each investigational trial in the individual patient. Their purpose is exclusion of placebo reactors: drugs to be tested are not assigned to patients who ameliorate on placebo. Placebo periods last 7 to 10 days on the average depending on whether and when the condition of the patient deteriorates. The duration of the trial with neuroleptics is 6 weeks, but it is prolonged in many patients when an amelioration occurs indicating that the particular drug helps the patient to the extent that his discharge appears likely. For the purpose of most of our studies—and also for the purpose of this study, data on the therapeutic response after 6 weeks of treatment are used. The clinical condition of the patients is evaluated by a number of standardized tests for the assessment of the current state of the patients and observed changes. Data obtained by the FKP rating scale (7) were used in this study. This rating scale was developed in our Institute to evaluate drug effects on 18 psychotic target symptoms; its reliability has been checked by repeated studies of inter-rater agreement; and several factor analyses were performed with its scores comparing them with the scores of the Brief Psychiatric Rating Scale of Overall and Gorham (8).

We believe that this system facilitates comparison of the effects of various drugs tested during the last 8 yr (9–14), providing that we control for the comparability of the patient samples in parameters relevant for the prognosis of the short-term treatment (age, sex, duration of illness, pretreatment symptomatic profiles, etc.).

In addition, data were used, obtained in a controlled multiclinical trial performed in 17 psychiatric hospitals where identical evaluation instruments and a similar study design were used (15).

Five hundred and sixty-one patients with a diagnosis of schizophrenia in its broad meaning yielded data for the study. A group treated by one of the trial drugs contained 38 to 120 patients. The effects of the drugs on each item of the rating scale FKP were the basis for producing a scale according to the average relative decrease of the score. The differences in the effects of the trial drugs were statistically significant only in about 20% of the comparisons. Accordingly, we obtained 18 rankings of 11 drugs, one for each item, where the first one had the least and the last one the highest effect on the symptom described by the item.

Similar rankings were produced in 19 various pharmacological animal tests as reported (16–21). Only those animal tests were selected which yielded reliable data obtained by one author — or one group of authors working in a laboratory which published the test results for a number of neuroleptic drugs, the efficacy of which was compared in a quantified manner.

We suppose that rankings of drugs for efficacy in a certain test are sufficiently reliable only if the work was done in the same laboratory. We wanted to avoid the risk of comparing the ED_{50} if the data were obtained in different laboratories by different workers. Thus, the papers by Irwin (3), Julou et al. (19), Janssen et al. (17, 18), and Tedeschi et al. (20, 21) were relevant for the present study.

To increase the comparability between the animal and human data, the rankings of drugs in animal tests were modified using a ratio of the average therapeutic daily dose and ED_{50}.

$$y = \frac{\text{average daily therapeutic dose}}{ED_{50}}$$

The ratio shows to what extent a given drug is effective in a particular test, in relation to the optimal therapeutic dosage in patients. Table 1 shows the drugs that were compared and the average daily doses used in the trials. These doses cannot necessarily be considered optimal according to various clinicians: the views differ in this respect and there is a discrepancy between

TABLE 1. *Drugs and their average therapeutic daily dose*

Thioridazine	450 mg
Chlorprothixene	400 mg
Levopromazine	350 mg
Chlorpromazine	300 mg
Clopenthixol	175 mg
Carphenazine	120 mg
Prochlorperazine	80 mg
Perphenazine	48 mg
Trifluoperazine	40 mg
Methylperidol	35 mg
Propericiazine	25 mg

somewhat lower doses used in Europe and higher doses used in the United States. The figures in Table 1 represent averages of doses actually used in the trials permitting flexibility according to the therapeutic response.

RESULTS

First, we were interested in the correlations between the optimal therapeutic doses in patients and the ED_{50} in animals. As shown in Tables 2–4, the tests for catalepsia, ptosis (according to Tedeschi), inhibition of amphetamine and apomorphine effects, and the inhibition of exploratory activity and of conditioned avoidance response were found to have a certain predictive value for therapeutic response, on the basis of comparison of dosage only. No statistically significant correlations were found in tests using mice, which might suggest that the mouse is not a good model for man. However, this finding can be explained simply by the fact that tests where a correlation for rats and dogs was observed, were not repeated in mice (with the exception of catalepsia).

TABLE 2. *Rank correlations between optimum therapeutic doses in man and ED_{50} in animals*

Effect	Mice	Rats
LD_{50} per os	+0.08	+0.19
LD_{50} i.v.	+0.35	+0.21
Loss of righting reflex	−0.39	
Fall off rota-rod	+0.36	
Ptosis		+0.70*
Catalepsia	+0.40	+0.74*
Analgesia (hot-plate)	−0.18	

Figures are Spearman's coefficients; *statistically significant ($p = 0.05$).

TABLE 3. *Rank correlations between optimum therapeutic doses in man and ED_{50} in animals*

Antagonism of	Rats	Dogs
Epinephrine − pressor effect	−0.60	
− lethal effect	−0.57	
Norepinephrine − lethal effect	−0.57	
Tryptamine convulsions	+0.02	
Amphetamine–gnawing	+0.95*	
Apomorphine–gnawing	+0.95*	
− vomiting		+0.70*

Figures are Spearman's coefficients; *statistically significant ($p + 0.05$).

TABLE 4. *Rank correlations between optimum therapeutic doses in man and ED_{50} in animals*

Inhibition of	Mice	Rats	Dogs
Foot-shock fighting	−0.68		
Exploration − horizontal		+0.83*	
− vertical		+0.79*	
Conditioned avoidance response		+0.76*	+0.75*

Figures are Spearman's coefficients; *statistically significant ($p = 0.05$).

The absence of a significant correlation between the LD_{50} and the therapeutic doses can have important theoretical implications: it could support the optimistic view that catalepsia, ptosis, inhibition of exploratory activity, etc., are indicative of some specific action of neuroleptics, related to their therapeutic effects, and not only a nonspecific consequence of the intoxication of the experimental animals.

Secondly, we wanted to compare the efficacy in 19 selected animal tests with the therapeutic responses in 18 items of the psychiatric rating scale. Tables 5 and 6 show the values of the Spearman's correlation coefficients. From the total number of 342 correlations, 27 are statistically significant (14 of the coefficients with the $p < 0.01$, 4 with $p < 0.02$, and 9 with $p < 0.05$). Thus, the number of significant correlations exceeds the number that would be obtained by chance only.

The test of catalepsia was correlated with the highest number of psychotic symptoms, the second most successful test was the inhibition of the apomorphine emesis. From these two tests it was obvious that the animal data can predict the clinical effects for different symptoms.

There are clinical symptoms that do not correlate with any animal test: this lack of correlation is surprising, especially in the symptoms connected with the impairment of motor activity. We expected that it would not be difficult to find an animal model for motor activity in man. On the other hand, it could be anticipated that such symptoms as disorders of sociability, appearance, orientation, and insight would not be correlated with animal tests. Anxiety was a symptom where we expected to find some correlations.

Our negative findings were due, perhaps, to the fact that anxiety in psychotic patients is different from neurotic anxiety, for which most of the anxiolytics are used. Also, anxiety is usually not considered to be among the most important target symptoms with regard to neuroleptic drugs.

The pathology of affectivity is correlated with the greatest number of animal tests. This might not be too surprising, taking into consideration the fact that the brain structures involved in the regulation of affectivity in man do not differ much from those that control the instincts in animals. Very probably, it is not by chance that psychotic aggressivity responds to drugs in relation to their capacity to antagonize some effects of epinephrine. The

TABLE 5. Correlations between the efficacy in animal tests and in target symptoms/
Spearman's coefficients

RATS	INHIBITION OF						ANTAGONIZATION OF					
	CAR	EXPLORATION		SELF STIMULATION	CATALEPSIA	PTOSIS	GNAWING		TRYPTAMINE CONVULSIONS	LETHALITY		BLOOD PRESSURE EPINEPHRINE
		VERTICAL	HORIZONTAL				AMPHETAMINE	APOMORPHINE		NE	EPINEPHRINE	
SLEEP	0	-16	-14	-80	-23	-72	+10	+24	-26	-50	-64	-80
EATING	-7	-23	-31	-40	-14	-56	-11	+17	-42	-45	-59	-100
MOOD	-21	-40	-35	-20	-42	-35	0	+2	+5	-19	-33	-60
SELF-EVALUATION	+16	-14	-19	-20	-19	+20	+7	-29	+69	+63	+28	+20
AFFECT	-52	-83	-71	-40	-50	+30	-91	-81	-7	+17	+4	-30
MOTOR ACTIVITY	-7	-9	-35	-20	-21	-31	+33	+31	-31	-7	-5	0
SPEECH	-28	-42	-7	-60	-19	-30	-73	+2	-29	-48	-57	-100
INCOOPERAT	-19	-23	-50	-20	-28	-59	+6	+17	-48	-38	-48	-90
SOCIABILITY	-45	-61	-38	-40	-35	+42	-62	-57	+26	+26	+23	-20
APPEARANCE	+8	+4	+40	+40	0	-17	+12	-2	-7	+9	0	-10
ORIENTATION	-45	-47	-64	+20	-40	+27	-31	-45	+6	+31	+34	+10
ANXIETY	-2	-4	-12	+20	+12	+40	-5	+2	+31	+31	+44	+10
AGGRESSIVITY	-33	-38	-19	-80	-40	-71	-12	+19	-48	-71	-81	-90
HALLUCINATIONS	-21	-45	-42	-20	-50	-21	+5	0	+19	0	-12	-30
DELUSIONS	-23	-67	-36	-20	-45	+28	-48	-45	+35	+21	+16	-30
THINKING	-14	-45	-26	-20	-28	+49	-48	-66	+62	+65	+36	+20
DISSIMULATION	-59	-74	-71	-20	-64	+51	-54	-80	+29	+48	+52	+40
INSIGHT	-19	-28	+6	-20	-19	+43	-10	-14	+50	+33	+36	+30

Figures in thick squares are significant on 0.01 level.
Figures in thin squares are significant on a 0.02 or 0.05 probability level.
Circled figures are on 0.1 probability level.

TABLE 6. *Correlations between the efficacy in animal tests and in target symptoms/Spearman's coefficients*

	MICE					DOGS	
	INHIBITION OF FOOT-SHOCK AGGRESSION	HOT PLATE	ROTA ROD	LOSS OF RIGHTING REFLEX	CATALEPSIA	INHIBITION OF APOMORPHINE EMESIS	CAR
SLEEP	-50	-71	-57	-12	-60	0	-8
EATING	-39	-43	-32	-32	-80	+69	+31
MOOD	0	-14	-7	-7	-100	-22	-13
SELF-EVALUATION	+57	+29	+43	+43	-100	-30	-3
AFFECT	-7	-36	+14	+14	-20	-88	-86
MOTOR ACTIVITY	-7	-4	-43	-43	+20	-33	-22
SPEECH	-50	(-68)	-14	-14	-80	-8	-20
INCOOPERAT	-32	-11	-46	-46	-100	-3	-4
SOCIABILITY	+14	0	+43	+43	-60	-48	-40
APPEARANCE	+11	+39	-11	-11	-80	-11	+9
ORIENTATION	-25	+46	+18	+18	0	-28	-16
ANXIETY	+35	+29	+50	+50	0	+17	+3
AGGRESSIVITY	(-71)	-79	-57	-57	-40	-3	-15
HALLUCINATIONS	+11	-11	-4	-4	-100	-31	-18
DELUSIONS	+21	-21	+36	+36	-100	(-60)	(-55)
THINKING	+42	+7	+57	+57	-100	-40	-24
DISSIMULATION	+42	+32	+54	+36	+40	-84	-91
INSIGHT	+39	+7	+46	+46	0	-51	-46

See Table 5 for explanation of symbols.

number of significant correlations found between dissimulation and the animal tests was surprising.

DISCUSSION

There are limitations for drawing far-reaching conclusions from our study: most important seem to be the methodological ones.

(a) Not all of the correlation coefficients are based on comparison of the effects of all 11 drugs. Sometimes there were simply not enough comparative pharmacological data available for all drugs used in the clinic.

(b) We still are improving the interpretation of the effect of standardization on the results. Here, first of all, the great number of negative correlation coefficients is perplexing. Just to demonstrate the complexity of the problem, let me try to express the possible meaning of such a negative correlation: the greater the effect of a drug in inducing catalepsia, the lower its effect against hallucinations. Or, in other words: we determined the ratio of the efficacy of neuroleptics in a certain animal test to its daily therapeutical dose in man and correlated it with the therapeutic response in various psychopathological symptoms. At best, the results are difficult to interpret at present, especially in the case of negative correlations, despite our attempts to standardize the results. On the other hand, we are sure that some relationship exists between the efficacy in animal tests and psychotic symptoms, if a statistically significant correlation is found. We just do not understand the relationship at present. For this reason, we intend to repeat the whole procedure with nonstandardized raw input data.

(c) When we performed a factor analysis of the scores of the rating scale, important correlations between the items were found. The same might be true for correlations between the results within the pharmacological tests. In such a situation, multivariate statistical techniques such as canonical correlation analysis or a factor analysis, could reduce the complexity of the findings and facilitate interpretation. The present study is a starting point for further work in this direction.

CONCLUSIONS

In an attempt to correlate the efficacy of 11 neuroleptic drugs in 19 pharmacological animal tests to their action as measured by the therapeutical response in 18 psychotic symptoms in 561 schizophrenic patients, 27 rank correlations were found to be statistically significant.

The test of catalepsia in mice predicts the effects in the greatest number of psychotic symptoms. Disorders of affect were correlated to the highest number of pharmacological animal tests.

REFERENCES

1. Irwin, S., *Amer. J. Psychiat.*, **124**, 1–19 (1968).
2. Pöldinger, W., and Stille, G., in *The present status of psychotropic drugs*, Cerletti, A., Bové, F. J., (eds.), Excerpta Medica, Amsterdam, 1969, pp. 529–531.
3. Irwin, S., *Arch. Int. Pharmacodyn*, **132**, 279 (1961).
4. Benešová, O., and Náhunek, K., *Psychopharmacologia* **20**, 337 (1971).
5. Káto, L., Gözsy, B., Lehmann, H. E., and Ban, T. A., *J. Clin. Exper. Psychopathol. Quart. Rev. Psychiat. Neurol.*, **23**, 75 (1962).
6. Vinař, O., in the *VII. Internat. Congr. of the Collegium Internationale Neuro-Psychopharmacologicum*, Prague, August 11–15, 1970.
7. Vinař, O., Váňa, J., and Grof, S., *Activ. Nerv. Super. (Prague)* **8**, 405 (1966).
8. Overall, J. E., and Gorham, D. R., *Psychol. Rep.*, **10**, 799 (1962).
9. Vinař, O., and Baštecký, J., *Activ. Nerv. Super. (Prague)*, **6**, 225 (1964).
10. Vinař, O., Baštecký, J., and Formánková, M., *Activ. Nerv. Super. (Prague)*, **8**, 453 (1966).
11. Vinař, O., Formánková, M., Taussigová, D., and Růžička, S., *Activ. Nerv. Super. (Prague)*, **9**, 353 (1967).

12. Vinař, O., Baštecky, J., Taussigová, D., Formánková, M., and Růžička, S., *Activ. Nerv. Super. (Prague)*, **9,** 401 (1967).
13. Vinař, O., and Taussigová, D., *Activ. Nerv. Super. (Prague)*, **7,** 250 (1965).
14. Vinař, O., and Taussigová, D., *Activ. Nerv. Super. (Prague)*, **8,** 447 (1966).
15. Vinař, O., *Agressologie* **IX,** 315 (1968).
16. Janssen, P. A. J., Documentation about Luvatrene ® (methylperidol) to be registered at the Ministry of Health, Prague, Czechoslovakia, 1972.
17. Janssen, P. A. J., Niemegeers, A. J. E., and Schellekens, K. H. L., *Arzneimittel-Forschung,* **15,** 104 (1965).
18. Janssen, P. A. J., Niemegeers, C. J. E., and Schellekens, K. H. L., *Arzenimittel-Forschung,* **15,** 1196 (1965).
19. Julou, L., Bardone, M. C., Ducroft, R., Laffargue, B., and Loiseau, G., in *Neuro-Psycho-Pharmacology,* ICS 129, Brill, H., Cole, J. O., Deniker, P., Hippius, H., and Bradley, P. B. (eds.), Excerpta Medica, Amsterdam, 1967, pp. 293–303.
20. Tedeschi, D. H., in *Neuro-Psycho-Pharmacology,* ICS 129, Brill, H., Cole, J. O., Deniker, P., Hippius, H., and Bradley, P. B. (eds.), Excerpta Medica, Amsterdam, 1967, pp. 314–320.
21. Tedeschi, D. H., Tedeschi, R. E., and Fellows, J., *Arch. Int. Pharmacodyn.,* **132,** 172 (1961).

The Phenothiazines and Structurally Related Drugs, edited by I. S.
Forrest, C. J. Carr, and E. Usdin. Raven Press, New York © 1974.

Prevention of Delirium Tremens: Use of Phenothiazines Versus Drugs Cross-Dependent with Alcohol

Samuel C. Kaim

Friends of Medical Science Research, Baltimore, Maryland 21228

INTRODUCTION

Sedatives, and more recently tranquilizers, have been used symptomatically for many years in the treatment of alcohol withdrawal states. But it has been only in the past few years that we have come to understand that some of the sedatives or tranquilizers employed have more than symptomatic value. In fact, some are specific remedies in that they suppress, or even prevent, the usual abstinence symptoms when given in a systematic detoxication program.

RESULTS OF VA COOPERATIVE STUDIES

Two large-scale cooperative studies have been conducted by the VA to compare the safety and efficacy of commonly employed drugs in the treatment of "incipient" and full-fledged delirium tremens.

The first study (1) was a double-blind comparative evaluation of chlordiazepoxide, chlorpromazine, hydroxyzine, thiamine, and placebo in the (predelirium tremens) alcohol withdrawal syndrome. It was conducted on 537 patients in 23 VA hospitals employing an identical protocol. Symptoms were rated three times per day on a Nurses' Rating Scale and once per day on Lorr's Mood Scale. Symptoms improved rapidly in all treatment groups, paradoxically most rapidly in the placebo and thiamine groups. Strangely, the chlorpromazine group actually fared worst (of the five groups) in the "hallucinating-confused" cluster of symptoms; and the chlordiazepoxide group reported more anger and tension than the others. As judged by the two rating instruments employed, the study drugs had little or no effect on the natural tendency toward remission of alcohol withdrawal symptoms.

This study (2), however, demonstrated one clinically important result: delirium tremens and/or convulsions developed in only 2% of the chlordiazepoxide group, compared to 10% or more in each of the other groups.

As chlordiazepoxide was the only agent in this study that is cross-dependent with alcohol, the result would appear to support the thesis that to prevent delirium and convulsions, alcohol withdrawal is best treated with pharmacologic substitutes for alcohol.

Just as in subjects physiologically dependent on barbiturates or opiates, chronically alcohol-intoxicated individuals can be withdrawn abruptly. However, in all three cases it has been found safer to withdraw addicts (including alcoholics) with the aid of drugs showing cross-dependence with the abused substance. By substituting such pharmacologic equivalents, it is possible to ameliorate the distressing symptoms of abstinence and to prevent convulsions, delirium, and, in the case of barbiturates and alcohol, even death.

The second cooperative study (3) was undertaken in 17 VA hospitals to determine whether drugs cross-dependent with alcohol influence the course of delirium tremens more favorably than drugs without this characteristic. Chlordiazepoxide, paraldehyde, and pentobarbital were chosen for this study as representative of agents cross-dependent with alcohol. Perphenazine was selected to represent drugs not showing this quality. Two hundred and two patients were admitted to this study on the basis of exhibiting the three cardinal symptoms of delirium tremens: disorientation, tremors, and hallucinations. All four drugs were effective in safely controlling the syndrome, with no significant differences in outcome among the four groups. However, in considering a combination of the three chief outcome factors, duration and severity of the delirium, and incidence of treatment failures, paraldehyde and chlordiazepoxide appeared to hold an advantage over pentobarbital and perphenazine.

The failure of the drugs cross-dependent with alcohol to effect a significantly better outcome than the phenothiazine used in this study may indicate that uncomplicated delirium tremens has a time-limited course relatively uninfluenced by the type of drug treatment employed. One quality shared by the four agents in the study is the ability to produce sedation. The overall favorable outcome of these 202 patients may have been due to the effective sedation achieved in all four groups, as well as to the quality of supportive care, which was prescribed in detail in the research protocol.

DISCUSSION

In the second VA Cooperative Study (3), the mean duration of the delirium ranged from 74 hr in the chlordiazepoxide group to 80 hr in the pentobarbital group. The same duration, about 3 days, was reported in 1841 by Ware (4), who observed: "This disease is not capable of being arrested in its course of treatment . . . but will continue a certain time and then arrive at a spontaneous termination either in death or recovery."

Although the results of this VA study tend to corroborate Ware's statement of 132 years ago that the course of delirium tremens cannot be halted, the findings of the first VA study (2) lend support to the notion that delirium tremens may be prevented by use of a pharmacologic agent during treatment of the alcohol withdrawal syndrome.

PREVENTION OF DELIRIUM TREMENS BY DRUG THERAPY

Before the first VA cooperative study Victor (5) voiced the opinion that there were no adequate data to show that any of the newer psychoactive drugs were effective in preventing delirium tremens. The VA study (2) was the first well-controlled trial to find that the use of one of these newer agents, chlordiazepoxide, did result in a significant reduction in the development of delirium among patients undergoing withdrawal from alcohol. In that study only one of 103 patients who received chlordiazepoxide developed delirium, a significantly lower incidence than the 7% in the chlorpromazine group of 98, and the 6% in the placebo group of 130.

What about the older drugs which have been used in the treatment of acute withdrawal from alcohol? Hart (6) compared the use of promazine and paraldehyde in patients in alcohol withdrawal. Twenty-three percent of the promazine group of 57 developed delirium, versus 16% of the paraldehyde group of 56.

In a similar study of 67 patients in alcohol withdrawal, Thomas and Freedman (7) reported that 12% of the group receiving promazine developed delirium, versus none in the paraldehyde group. Another study (8) reported delirium tremens developed in one of 12 subjects on a combination of paraldehyde and chloral hydrate versus 18 of 37 on other regimens.

THEORIES CONCERNING DEVELOPMENT OF DELIRIUM TREMENS

Gross et al. (9) monitored the EEG of four adult males suffering from acute alcoholic psychoses. Two of these four patients slept during the first recording day, much of the period in REM-type EEG activity, with no Stage IV delta-sleep activity. The other two patients did not appear to sleep, but showed REM activity when their eyes were closed. During several of these episodes they reported hallucinations.

On the basis of their behavioral and EEG observations, the authors speculated that very high concentrations of alcohol may block the discharge of REM, perhaps by preventing the raising of consciousness to the level at which adequate REM discharge is possible. When that level is reached, nightmares are experienced, the patient awakens, drinks, and repeats this series of events. Repetitive cycles of this nature could lead to great increases in the propensity for REM, which, when alcohol is withdrawn, results in a massive eruption of REM of such magnitude that it may appear also in the wake state, manifested with hallucinations.

Greenberg and Pearlman (10) studied 14 subjects, three of whom were given increasing amounts of alcohol and then withdrawn; the other 11 were admitted in a state of alcohol withdrawal. The initial effect of alcohol was suppression of REM sleep. With increasing doses of alcohol, REM activity usually remained suppressed, although on some nights REM increased markedly.

During withdrawal from alcohol, REM activity increased greatly, often appearing also during long waking periods preceding sleep. The major EEG difference between the patients who developed delirium tremens and those who did not, was the higher percentage of REM sleep in the former. One subject studied before delirium developed had continuous REM activity the night before his delirium started. Another patient had 100% REM before a nightmare of hallucinatory intensity (the second night after alcohol was discontinued).

EFFECTS OF BRAIN AMINES ON STAGES OF SLEEP

Jouvet (11) has reported that increased cerebral serotonin leads to a state which resembles Stage IV sleep (suppression of REM activity, followed by a rebound of REM). During REM rebound (after its selective deprivation in rats) there is increased turnover of cerebral norepinephrine. Acetylcholine triggers REM (in cats). Pujol (12) reported decreased NE turnover during REM deprivation; increased NE turnover during REM.

Jouvet (11) suggests that the REM mechanism may require three "keys" for its operation—serotonin, acetylcholine, and norepinephrine. He feels that this may constitute a fail-safe mechanism which ordinarily prevents the intrusion into the waking state of the hallucinatory processes involved in dreaming.

EFFECTS OF SEDATIVE-HYPNOTICS ON EEG SLEEP PATTERNS

Although not all reports coincide, the majority (10, 13–16) tend to show the following effects of sedative-hypnotic agents on REM and Stage IV Sleep.

Alcohol depresses REM and Stage IV. REM rebounds above baseline levels during withdrawal from alcohol. Stage IV remains depressed during withdrawal.

The barbiturates also depress REM and Stage IV. During withdrawal, REM rebounds above baseline levels, and Stage IV returns to baseline.

The phenothiazines also depress REM, but increase Stage IV. REM rebounds above baseline during withdrawal.

Some of the benzodiazepines are reported to depress REM, others apparently do not alter REM time. Most report a decrease in Stage IV sleep. During withdrawal, REM returns to (or stays at) baseline levels, while Stage IV remains depressed.

Chloral hydrate has little effect on REM, which remains near baseline levels also during withdrawal. Paraldehyde is reported to increase Stage IV sleep.

EFFECTS OF SEDATIVE-HYPNOTICS ON BRAIN AMINES

Bradley (17) has reported that chlorpromazine decreases the activity of neurons which respond to norepinephrine, apparently acting as a specific antagonist to NE in those sites in the brainstem at which NE has excitatory effects. Pletscher (18) reported that the phenothiazines block the actions of serotonin, decreasing its tissue uptake.

Mendelson (19) has reported increased excretion of catecholamines in subjects with high blood-alcohol levels. When alcohol ingestion was discontinued and severe withdrawal symptoms ensued, catecholamine levels remained elevated until symptoms remitted, at which time they returned to baseline.

Stein et al. (20) reported that the barbiturates and the benzodiazepines decrease the turnover of norepinephrine, dopamine, and serotonin in the brain. These authors injected rats daily for 6 days with oxazepam, a benzodiazepine. Significant increases were observed in the serotonin levels of the rats treated with single and repeated doses of oxazepam. However, only the rats treated with a single dose of the benzodiazepine had an increase of norepinephrine. A decrease in NE turnover was no longer seen after six consecutive daily doses of oxazepam.

Essman (21) reported that benzodiazepines significantly increase synaptosomal levels of acetylcholine.

ATTEMPT AT SYNTHESIS

Although our knowledge is still quite limited—most of the pertinent experiments have not yet been performed, or, at least, reported—some suggestive clues have been uncovered.

1. Admittedly based on a very small series of cases, one factor in the development of delirium tremens may be the intrusion into wakefulness of the hallucinatory-dream activity associated with the REM state, during periods of massive REM rebound encountered after cessation of excessive ingestion of alcohol.

2. Two of the three drugs reported to prevent the development of delirium (when used during the alcohol withdrawal syndrome) do not show the phenomenon of REM rebound when their use is discontinued: the benzodiazepines and chloral hydrate. The pertinent sleep studies have not been reported in the case of the third effective drug, paraldehyde.

3. The REM phenomenon may be mediated by a sequence of brain-amine effects. Imbalances brought about by excessive alcohol intake and then withdrawal may account for the massive REM rebound phenomenon.

The lack of REM rebound during withdrawal from benzodiazepines and chloral hydrate may indicate a different sequence of brain amine changes than is obtained for alcohol. Could this account for the prophylactic action of the benzodiazepines and chloral hydrate in preventing delirium tremens?

Some of the answers to these outstanding questions might further clarify the role of the brain amines, and of the stages of sleep in the development of delirium tremens. They might also help explain why certain drugs, and not others, used in the treatment of the alcohol withdrawal syndrome, can prevent the development of delirium.

To secure some of these answers, much work remains to be done. A most important study would be of the brain amines and EEG stages of sleep during administration of paraldehyde, chloral hydrate, a barbiturate, a benzodiazepine, and a phenothiazine, while patients are being treated for the (predelirium) alcohol withdrawal syndrome. Because of technical problems, some of the amine work may have be to conducted in mice rather than men.

REFERENCES

1. Klett, C. J., Hollister, L. E., Caffey, E. M., Jr., and Kaim, S. C., *Arch. Gen. Psychiat.*, **24**, 174 (1971).
2. Kaim, S. C., Klett, C. J., and Rothfeld, B., *Amer. J. Psychiat.*, **125**, 1640 (1969).
3. Kaim, S. C., and Klett, C. J., *Quart. J. Stud. Alcohol*, **33**, 1065 (1972).
4. Ware, J., *Med. Commun. Mass. Med. Soc.*, **6**, 175 (1841) [cited in *Alc. Treat. Dig.*, **23**, 14 (May, 1973)].
5. Victor, M., *Psychosom. Med.*, **28**, 636 (1966).
6. Hart, W. T., *Amer. J. Psychiat.*, **118**, 323 (1961).
7. Thomas, D. W., and Freedman, D. X., *JAMA*, **188**, 244 (1964).
8. Golbert, T. M., Sanz, C. J., Rose, H. D., and Leitschuh, T. H., *JAMA*, **188**, 99 (1967).
9. Gross, M. M., Goodenough, D., Tobin, M., Halpert, E., Lepore, D., Perlstein, A., Sirota, M., Dibianco, J., Fuller, R., and Kisher, I., *J. Nerv. Ment. Dis.*, **142**, 493 (1966).
10. Greenberg, R., and Pearlman, C., *Amer. J. Psychiat.*, **124**, 133 (1967).
11. Jouvet, M., *Science*, **163**, 32 (1969).
12. Pujol, J. F., Mouret, J., Jouvet, M., and Glowinski, J., *Science*, **159**, 112 (1968).
13. Feinberg, I., Wender, P. H., Koresko, R. L., Gottlieb, F., and Piehut, J. A., *J. Psychiat. Res.*, **7**, 101 (1969).
14. Kales, A., Malmstrom, E. J., Scharf, M. B., and Rubin, R. T., in *Sleep: Physiology and Pathology*, Kales, A. (ed.), Lippincott, Philadelphia, 1969.
15. Johnson, L. C., Burdick, J. A., and Smith, J., *Arch. Gen. Psychiat.*, **22**, 406 (1970).
16. Gross, M. M., *Quart. J. Stud. Alcohol*, **28**, 655 (1967).
17. Bradley, P. B., in *Biochemical and Pharmacologic Mechanisms Underlying Behavior*, Bradley, P. B., and Brimblecombe, R. W. (eds.), Elsevier, Amsterdam, 1972.
18. Pletscher, A., Kunz, E., Staebler, H., and Gey, K. F., *Biochem. Pharmacol.*, **12**, 1065 (1963).
19. Mendelson, J. H., *New Engl. J. of Med.*, **283**, 71 (1970).
20. Stein, L., Wise, C. D., and Berger, B. D., in *The Benzodiazepines*, Garattini, S., Mussini, E., and Randall, L. O. (eds.), Raven Press, New York, 1973.
21. Essman, W. B., in *The Benzodiazepines*, Garattini, S., Mussini, E., and Randall, L. O. (eds.), Raven Press, New York, 1973.

The Phenothiazines and Structurally Related Drugs, edited by I. S.
Forrest, C. J. Carr, and E. Usdin. Raven Press, New York © 1974.

Clinical Effectiveness of Piperacetazine Injection in Schizophrenic Patients: A Controlled Study

A. S. Kulkarni *

*Medical Department, Dow Pharmaceuticals, The Dow Chemical Company, Indianapolis,
Indiana 46077*

INTRODUCTION

The primary objective of the study was to determine the effectiveness of
piperacetazine (Quide ®) injection therapy in control of agitated, aggressive,
schizophrenic patients. Chlorpromazine injection was used as a positive
control so that the comparative efficacy and safety of the two drugs could be
evaluated.

Piperacetazine is a phenothiazine derivative with a piperidine moiety
(Fig. 1). Animal studies have shown that piperacetazine is many times more
potent than chlorpromazine in a variety of tests. Clinical trials in man have
shown that piperacetazine, used in the tablet form, is an effective antipsychotic.

Schizophrenic patients of both sexes were admitted to the study. These
patients were uncooperative, aggressive, agitated, hyperactive, and unmanageable. Patients whose condition was a result of acute alcoholism or
drug addiction were excluded. Patients showing evidence or a history of
kidney or liver dysfunctions were also excluded.

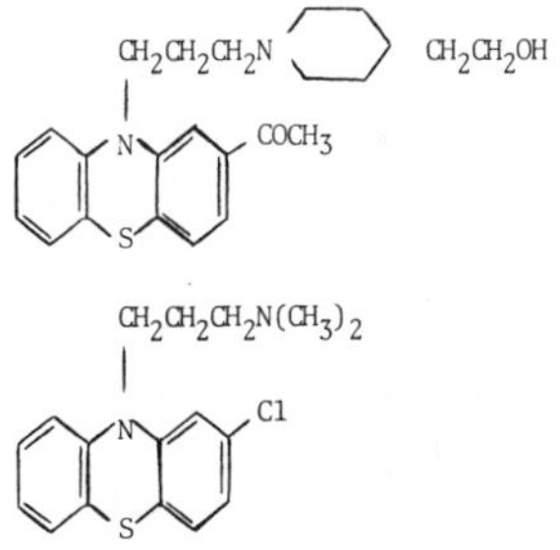

FIG. 1. Structural formulas.

---

* At present Associate Director Clinical Research, Section Head Neuropsychiatry, Abbott
Laboratory, N. Chicago, Illinois 60064.

DESIGN

After enrollment, each patient in the study was identified by a sequential number and was assigned to a medication, piperacetazine or chlorpromazine, using a randomization scheme. The two drugs cannot be physically altered to disguise the identity of the solution; however, all other measures were taken to maintain a double-blind status. The rating physicians and the nurses were blinded from the identity of the assigned medication. This was done using medication nurses who did no rating and who were instructed not to divulge any information concerning the physical characteristics. Therapy was begun after initial evaluation and was continued in conjunction with repeated observations of the patient. The first injection was 1 ml (2 mg/ml of piperacetazine or 25 mg/ml of chlorpromazine). One hr later the patient was evaluated again and another injection of 1 to 2 ml could be administered if needed. Later 1 to 4 ml of the drug was allowed at approximately four intervals thereafter, until the patient became manageable and capable of receiving oral medication. The maximum period of treatment and observation was 72 hr. The treatment and observation was discontinued when the patient became manageable or when the physician in charge judged the therapy to be ineffective or unsatisfactory.

EVALUATION PROCEDURES

Therapy was rated as successful when in the opinion of the investigator, an agitated, aggressive patient became manageable and the oral medication was initiated. If at the end of 72 hr the patient had not improved sufficiently, he was judged as a failure. Any time during the treatment period, if the patient was not showing a satisfactory improvement, in the opinion of the investigator, and treatment was discontinued, the patient again was judged to be a failure.

The Target Symptom Rating Scale, consisting of 10 items usually presented by an agitated, aggressive patient, was utilized. The patient was rated on this scale before each injection. Each item was rated on a four-point scale (0 — not present; 1 — mild; 2 — moderate; 3 — severe). The decrease in the score after the therapy indicated the degree of improvement in the patient.

Evaluations were also conducted using Brief Psychiatric Rating Scale (N.I.M.H. Form 9–6) before and after the treatment. This evaluation was used in our studies as supportive to the clinical improvement and the Target Symptom Rating Scale described above.

As an additional measure, patients were also evaluated before and after the therapy using Clinical Global Impressions (N.I.M.H. Form 9–12). Although the injection therapy may not result in the global improvement of the mental disease of the patient because of its short duration of treatment, it was employed again as a secondary evaluation of the therapy in our studies.

The improvement, measured by the difference in pre- and posttreatment scores, was statistically analyzed using a nonparametric test (Wilcoxon Rank-Sum).

Side effects observed in these patients were noted on Treatment Emergent Symptoms Scale (N.I.M.H. Form 9–3). Medical and psychiatric history was obtained and physical examination conducted on these patients, before admission to the study.

The drugs were packaged in 10-cc multiple-dose vials and had double-blind labels. In most cases, amber color syringes were employed.

RESULTS

Seven investigators provided the data on which this summary is based. A total of 182 acutely agitated, aggressive, uncooperative schizophrenics were admitted to the studies, as shown in Table 1.

TABLE 1. *Investigators and locations*

Investigator		Location	Number of patients
Ulett	A[a]	St. Louis, Mo.	26
McLaughlin	B	Fort Worth, Tex.	26
Leonard	C	Terrell, Tex.	26
Kiev	D	New York, N.Y.	26
Kiev		New York, N.Y.	12
Johnson	E	Imola, Calif.	26
Holden		St. Louis, Mo.	10
Merlis		Central Islip, N.Y.	30

[a] The studies with assigned code letters are the only ones used for statistical analysis.

Ninety patients received piperacetazine injection and 92 received chlorpromazine. Demographic information on the two groups is given in Table 2. The diagnostic categories are also shown. There was a preponderance of paranoid schizophrenia followed by chronic undifferentiated type and catatonics.

Clinical Effectiveness

As seen in Table 3, of 90 patients on piperacetazine, 80 showed a successful response, nine were failures, and one patient dropped out because of side effects. In the chlorpromazine group, of the 92 patients enrolled in the group, 78 showed a successful response, 13 were considered failures, and one dropped out due to side effects. As one can see, a very large majority of the patients responded successfully to both drugs. To give you some idea as

TABLE 2. *Demographic and diagnostic data*

	Number of patients	
	Piperacetazine	Chlorpromazine
Sex: male	49	56
female	41	36
Race: Caucasian	77	79
Negro	13	13
Schizophrenia, paranoid	39	33
Schizophrenia, catatonic	10	13
Schizophrenia, hebephrenic	5	4
Schizophrenia, chronic undifferentiated	21	20
Miscellaneous:	15	22
Acute episode		
Schizo-affective		
Simple type		
Unspecified		

Patients receiving piperacetazine ranged in age from 16 to 76 years, patients receiving chlorpromazine from 14 to 69 years.

to how fast the response was achieved, Table 3 describes this information according to the number of injections the patients received. Out of the 80 patients that successfully responded to piperacetazine, 52 responded after one injection, 14 after two injections, and another 14 after three injections. This means that in approximately 9 to 10 hr after the treatment was initiated, a successful response was achieved and further injections were discontinued in all the patients on piperacetazine. In the chlorpromazine group, out of the 78 patients responding to the treatment, 47 responded successfully after the first injection, 14 after two injections, and another 12 after three injections.

TABLE 3. *Clinical effectiveness*

	Number of patients	
	Piperacetazine	Chlorpromazine
Successful response	80	78
Failures	9	13
Dropouts due to side effects	1	1
Responded after 1 injection	52	47
Responded after 2 injections	14	14
Responded after 3 injections	14	12
Responded after 4 injections	0	3
Responded after 9 injections	0	1
Responded after 12 injections	0	1

Successful response—patient cooperative and capable of receiving oral medication.

Failure—patient not responding to the treatment according to the judgment of the investigator.

There were three patients who needed four injections, one patient needed nine injections, and another one needed 12 injections of chlorpromazine.

Target Symptom Rating Scale (Table 4)

When the total scores were examined, the improvement observed in both the groups was statistically significant ($p < 0.01$). The improvement for piperacetazine was from a score of 17 to 5 or approximately 71%. The improvement in the chlorpromazine group was from 17 to 6 or approximately 65%. All the individual 10 items of the scale also showed a statistically significant improvement ($p < 0.01$). This was true when all the data from five studies were pooled together. When the total scores for each of the five studies were examined separately for the two drugs (Table 6), they again showed a statistically significant improvement after the therapy with both the drugs.

TABLE 4. *Target symptom rating scale*

	Pre–Post improvement	
	Piperacetazine (65 patients)	Chlorpromazine (65 patients)
Pacing	1.5	1.6
Combative	1.1	0.9
Uncooperative	1.6	1.6
Tense	1.5	1.5
Hostile	1.3	1.3
Cursing	1.1	0.9
Disabled	0.5	0.6
Destructive	0.8	0.5
Yelling	1.0	0.9
Angry	1.5	1.4
Total	11.8	10.9

Each item was scored on a four-point scale: $0 =$ absent, $1 =$ mild, $2 =$ moderate, $3 =$ severe.

All improvements were significant ($p < 0.01$, Wilcoxon Test)

Brief Psychiatric Rating Scale

When the data from all the studies were pooled and the changes for each item on the Brief Psychiatric Rating Scale were examined, significant improvements were noted with both drugs on all of the items (Table 5). This is also true when the individual studies were examined separately and the improvement in the total score for each item was evaluated (Table 6). The total improvement noted in the piperacetazine group was from 65 to 50 — an improvement greater than 23%. The improvement noted in the chlorpromazine group was from 63 to 47 — an improvement of approximately 25%.

TABLE 5. *Brief psychiatric rating scale*

	Pre–Post improvement	
	Piperacetazine (65 patients)	Chlorpromazine (65 patients)
Somatic concern	0.5	0.5
Anxiety	1.6	1.6
Emotional withdrawal	0.8	0.6
Conceptual disorganization	0.8	0.9
Guilt feelings	0.3	0.3
Tension	2.0	2.2
Mannerisms and posturing	0.6	0.4
Grandiosity	0.1[a]	0.2
Depressive mood	0.5	0.4
Hostility	1.6	1.8
Suspiciousness	0.9	1.0
Hallucinatory behavior	0.6	0.6
Motor retardation	(worse 0.1)	No change
Uncooperativeness	1.8	1.8
Unusual thought	0.4	0.4
Blunted affect	0.2	0.1[a]
Excitement	2.0	2.4
Disorientation	0.3	0.4
Total	15.0	15.6

[a] Not significant, all other values significant ($p < 0.05$, Wilcoxon Test)
N.I.M.H. (MH–9–6) forms were used. A seven-point rating scale was employed: 1 — not present, 2 — very mild, 3 — mild, 4 — moderate, 5 — moderately severe, 6 — severe, 7 — extremely severe.

TABLE 6. *Changes in the mean total scores of target symptom rating scale and brief psychiatric rating scale*

Study	Patients in each drug group	Piperacetazine		Chlorpromazine	
		Pre	Post	Pre	Post
Target symptom rating scale					
A	13	12	4	11	2
B	13	17	8	18	8
C	13	20	1	20	6
D	13	17	5	15	4
E	13	19	10	20	9
Brief psychiatric rating scale					
A	13	52	41	51	39
B	13	68	51	68	51
C	13	80	53	73	52
D	13	60	49	61	48
E	13	69	59	62	46

Each pre-post change is significant ($p < 0.05$).

Clinical Global Impressions

A total score for the combined studies improved from 5.5 to 4.6 in the piperacetazine group and from 5.4 to 4.7 in the chlorpromazine group ($p < 0.05$). This presents an approximate improvement of about 20% in the severity of the mental illness (Item 1 of the Clinical Global Impressions). In terms of therapeutic effect, again the two groups were rated very closely (Table 7). In the piperacetazine group there were nine patients showing marked improvement, 40 moderate, 33 minimal, six were unchanged, and two became worse. In the chlorpromazine group, nine patients showed marked improvement, 31 moderate, 35 minimal, and four became worse.

TABLE 7. *Therapeutic effect*

	Number of patients	
	Piperacetazine	Chlorpromazine
Marked improvement	9	9
Moderate improvement	40	31
Minimal improvement	33	35
Unchanged	6	13
Worse	2	4
Total	90	92

N.I.M.H. (MH-9–12) forms—Clinical Global Impressions were used.

Side Effects

Twenty patients in the piperacetazine group complained of one or more side effects. There were nine patients in the chlorpromazine group. When only the patients with two or more side effects were considered, there were nine such patients in the piperacetazine group and six in the chlorpromazine group. It may be worthwhile to point out that there is only one patient who dropped out because of side effects from each of the two drug groups. Table 8 gives a breakdown of the various symptoms reported.

DISCUSSION

As noted above piperacetazine injection appears to be approximately equal to chlorpromazine injection in effectiveness and in the incidence of side effects. As shown in Table 3, 80 patients out of 90 successfully responded to piperacetazine therapy and 78 out of 92 patients successfully responded to chlorpromazine. The total number of failures and dropouts was 10 in piperacetazine and 14 in chlorpromazine. The average dose (mg)

TABLE 8. *Side effects: number of reports*

	Piperacetazine		Chlorpromazine	
	Total reports	Severe or needed action	Total reports	Severe or needed action
Akathisia	1	None	1	None
Dizziness	4	3	4	1
Drowsiness	14	3	5	1
Dry mouth	–	–	2	1
Dystonic symptoms	1	1	2	1
Excitement	1	1	1	1
Faintness	4	2	5	2
Headache	1	1	–	–
Hypotension	6	3	2	2
Nausea	1	1	2	2
Rigidity	–	–	1	None
Syncope	2	2	1	1
Tachycardia	2	1	–	–
Toxic confusional state	1	None	–	–
Tremor	2	1	2	None
Vomiting	2	1	2	2
Weakness	4	2	5	2
Local reaction	6	None	9	None
Total	52	22	44	16

of chlorpromazine used in these studies was approximately 10 to 30 times that of piperacetazine depending on the study. Overall average dose of piperacetazine was approximately 4.4 mg while that for chlorpromazine was approximately 66 mg. The amounts for patients who were failures or dropouts was 6.6 mg for piperacetazine and 85 mg for chlorpromazine. In these studies dealing with acutely agitated, aggressive, and uncooperative schizophrenics the total clinical response in terms of the manageability of the patient after treatment was the most important one. The effectiveness of the two drugs in this respect was similar. Target Symptom Rating Scale may also be meaningful in the evaluation of the effectiveness of the drugs. In most of the individual studies, significant improvement was shown by both drug treatments, and the degree of improvement was similar. The Brief Psychiatric Rating Scale and Clinical Global Impressions were used in these studies essentially as additional supportive measures. Evaluation on both the scales has shown significant improvement with both the drugs.

It appears that there is some variation in the investigator's evaluation of the degree of manageability needed for the patient in order to stop the injection therapy. For example in some studies only one injection was needed to control the patient, in others several injections were required. Such evaluation, however, was approximately the same for both the drugs in a given study. It is worth noting that, in general, patients were rated between mild to moderately ill on target symptoms and BPRS before the treatment. On the clinical global, they were rated as moderately severe.

CONCLUSION

The data reported in these studies indicate that piperacetazine injection is effective in immediate management of agitation and aggression of the schizophrenic patients. A vast majority of patients on either of the drugs responded within approximately 10 hr of the beginning of the treatment, and were manageable so that the oral treatment could be started. Statistically significant pre- to postimprovement in various ratings was observed in these patients after therapy with piperacetazine or chlorpromazine. This was apparent in the total scores and the individual items of TSRS, BPRS, and CGI either in individual studies or in all the studies combined. Side effects and local reactions associated with piperacetazine or chlorpromazine injection were also similar. In terms of mg of drug used, piperacetazine is approximately 15 times more potent than chlorpromazine.

The Phenothiazines and Structurally Related Drugs, edited by I. S.
Forrest, C. J. Carr, and E. Usdin. Raven Press, New York © 1974.

Session VIII: Discussion

Reporter: W. Turner

1. *M. Ackenheil*

Q. Vinar: You studied nine patients; was the response always a good
one? Did you observe any relation between the plasma levels or the metabolic parameters and the therapeutic response?

A. No, there was no relation between plasma levels and therapeutic
responses. We now have six patients on Clozapine and there was no relationship.

Q. Denber: I understand that Clozapine is strongly sedative.

A. Yes, at the beginning of treatment but after about 5 days there no
longer is such a strong sedative effect.

Q. Denber: You mentioned that the extrapyramidal effects could be
demonstrated by using special techniques?

A. Yes. We have not applied such special techniques, but Angst and
Hippius did in 120 patients and have not seen extrapyramidal side effects.

Q. Shostak: How did you measure the plasma levels? Would you comment on the cis- and transisomers with respect to their clinical effects?

A. The levels were determined at the Sandoz Company using G. C.
with a nitrogen detector. We have not tried to determine differences between
the two isomers.

Q. Kulkarni: Would you tell us a little bit about its animal pharmacology?
Does it inhibit the conditioned avoidance response?

A. There was no catalepsy; no stereotyped behavior, and there was no
CAR inhibition.

2. *P. Stern*

Q. F. Forrest: Your observation that phenothiazine and Latrodectus
do not act more effectively together than either one alone may be explained
by interaction of two substances: Fluphenazine being an electron donor
and Latrodectus being an electron acceptor, they may interact.

A. This theory does not appear plausible. Latrodectus acts on the
presynaptic membrane. Fluphenazine acts on the spinal neurons. I don't
know enough physical chemistry to advance a plausible theory.

3. *L. E. Hollister*

Q. Vinar: Clinicians know many patients who respond therapeutically to a drug. These patients may even resemble patients who do not respond to the same drug with regard to symptomatology. Until now, we have not been able to tell these responders from nonresponders. In this respect, I agree with Dr. Hollister's conclusion that only studies of drug metabolism and studies of the interaction of the drug with neurotransmitters in individual patients could explain some of the causes of this variability.

It is true also that much of the efforts to find clinical clues for selecting the right drug for the right patients were not too successful. Usually, studies which used predictive formulas for selecting different neuroleptics for specific patient populations failed in attempts to cross-validate these formulas. Nevertheless, this unfortunate state of affairs should not prevent us from pursuing work in this direction. We must face the reality that there are 10 to 15 neuroleptics used in routine practice, and the clinicians wish to know what their differential indications in psychotic patients are. It is a common experience that a patient who did not respond to one drug, did respond to another. I do not think that we have done enough to be able to state that a neuroleptic drug can be chosen at random and then changed on a trial-and-error basis. I am optimistic with respect to the ultimate development of sophisticated statistical techniques for routine practice. If we succeed in developing, e.g., differential multiple regression equations where the scores of a simple rating scale would be predictors of the drug response to be cross-validated, then it might be a very easy arithmetic procedure for the clinician to choose the optimum drug for the individual patient. We just have to look for the clinical parameters most relevant for such a prediction. However, I do not wish to say that in the process of selecting the right drug for the individual patient, metabolic studies could not be of great help. But I am afraid that such metabolic studies cannot be expected to have practical relevance in the near future.

A. I take it that you believe the end of the rainbow can still be found. I would only remark that people generally select a prototypic drug from one of the drug families. We have only three major families of drugs and three subtypes of phenothiazines, which limits you to about five. You can exploit the differences between these drugs; if one fails, another might work. But if you put a patient before me I'd be hard put to tell you which drug would be most useful to him at that moment.

Q. Clark: Your last figure showed that piperazines were better in older people (> 40) and nonparanoids (usually older). Do you have any data on dose, that might be used to confirm the observation of Puiew and Cole that indicated interaction between dose and age in which younger people (< 40), hospitalized less than 10 years responded best to high doses of chlorpromazine?

A. That figure had to do with paranoid patients and age groups: piperazine derivatives seemed to be more effective in older age groups, whereas the piperidines were more effective in the younger age groups. Paranoid patients largely were present in the younger age group, and piperidines were most useful there.

Q. Clark: Did you have any information on doses?
A. The instructions were to use the drugs to the maximum advantage, as they would be used clinically, so no attempt to standardize the dose was made. In previous studies, we had attempted to standardize the dose, but we thought the time had come to do what is done in real life, in newly admitted patients. I suspect you get better results in a real life situation than in trying to outguess the needs of different patients by a single protocol.

4. O. Vinar

Stern: As a pharmacologist I consider it most difficult to find a relation between psychotic disease and animal experiments.

Q. Goodwin: In a matrix of 300 correlations you might expect 10 to 20 correlations at the $p < 0.05$ level by chance alone. In light of this, could you tell us if the theoretically important correlations between affect and animal tests were stronger than the $p < 0.05$ level?
A. Yes. Those figures enclosed in thick squares were at the 0.01 level, and those in circles were at the 0.05 level. We have not yet performed multivariate statistical analysis.

Q. Goodwin: Do you recall whether the significant relationship between affect in animals and clinical efficacy was strong?
A. Yes. That was strong.

Q. I. Forrest: Do you plan to use other than rats and mice and, if so, by what criteria would you choose your animal models?
A. Until now we used data from the literature; we did not do any ourselves. We used only those papers which compared at least eight to 10 neuroleptic drugs which were compared in the same laboratory. This limited work to mice, rats, dogs, and cats. We were surprised to learn that the mouse is not a good animal model, except for the test of catalepsia. The dog is a better animal for other tests.

Q. Stern: Did you find a model simulating schizophrenia? The method by Stein, which uses 6-hydroxydopamine to induce catalepsy, is not adequate to establish a model for schizophrenia.
A. About 8 years ago I thought that a good model would be the LSD state in humans, but that turned out to be a disappointment when reserpine, which has some antipsychotic action, was found to aggravate the LSD reaction.

5. *S. C. Kaim*

Q. F. Forrest: Are you the first to describe these phenomena of REM and Stage IV sleep in alcoholics?

A. No, Grosz described this in 1966.

Q. F. Forrest: Re REM sleep. I would like to refer to a paper a year ago in which I presented evidence that the REM phenomena are derived from CNS activity of bottom-feeding reptiles, now seen also in sea mammals. Three dangers face the alcoholic: B-vitamin deficiencies, brain edema, and inflammation of the gut. The first is treated by large doses of B vitamins, the second by Benadryl, and the third by i.m. chlorpromazine. In view of this, your study did not have too much significance. You can't treat alcoholic psychoses with just one drug.

A. Jaffe has aptly said (in his chapter in Goodman and Gilman) that such supportive treatment is desirable, but cannot substitute for the specific effects of the drugs which are pharmacologic equivalents of alcohol and suppress the abstinence symptoms.

Q. Hollister: I'm going to please Dr. Forrest by recommending multiple pharmacy for DT.

A. Again, vitamin and other supportive treatment are desirable adjuncts to the specific drugs which are cross-dependent with alcohol, but cannot by themselves effectively suppress the withdrawal symptoms.

6. *A. S. Kulkarni*

Q. Shostak: Do you know of anyone who has done a control with sodium amytal or Librium ®? I am curious how you got this kind of control in 15 hr, and I wonder if this is a nonspecific type of effect.

A. No, that is possible but I doubt it. The patients were selected on the basis of their uncooperativeness and unmanageability when acutely admitted to hospital or clinic, or from already hospitalized patients who suddenly took a turn for the worse. This therapy is given to achieve temporary control, rather than to relieve the basic illness.

Q. Turner: There are still a number of us here with grey hair who remember how things were before 1950. We then encountered many agitated, terrified patients who entered the hospital after prolonged periods of sleeplessness. They suffered not only from schizophrenia, if at all, but also from oneirophrenia, a waking sleep, dream state. If one then administered sufficient hypnotic drugs to induce sound sleep, they would be tremendously improved. I am not sure that chlorpromazine or any of these drugs do more in this period than to assure patients sufficient sleep.

A. This is quite possible and I would venture to say that inclusion of a placebo group would have enhanced the value of the study quite a bit.

Q. Denber: I think we should look again at the figures. It appears that more than half of the patients were brought under control by a single injection. This suggests that the patients were not terribly agitated.

A. Yes. I could show you in one study we used a psychiatrist in private practice and he found more than half of his "uncontrolled, unmanageable" patients were controlled after one injection. Thus we take it to indicate that "uncontrolled, unmanageable" varies with the definition of the investigator. We were hoping that by a double-blind comparison with CPZ, we would not be biasing the results in favor of our drug or the other.

Q. Denber: My experience with CPZ goes back to 1954. I do not recall achieving control of an acutely agitated depression by one single injection.

A. This is quite possible. Milder patients were admitted, but four of the studies were conducted in a hospital setting. Perhaps physicians today try to use these drugs more often on milder conditions than they used to.

Session IX

Phenothiazine Effects on Macromolecules and Neurotransmitters

Chairmen: Albert A. Manian and Maria Wollemann

The Phenothiazines and Structurally Related Drugs, edited by I. S. Forrest, C. J. Carr, and E. Usdin. Raven Press, New York © 1974.

Effect of Phenothiazines on Central Cholinergic Activity

Melvin H. Van Woert, Vimala H. Sethy, and Lalit M. Ambani

Departments of Internal Medicine and Pharmacology, Yale University School of Medicine, New Haven, Connecticut 06510

INTRODUCTION

Both cholinergic and dopaminergic neurons, located in the basal ganglia, participate in the regulation of extrapyramidal function. This conclusion is based on biochemical and pharmacological investigations in Parkinson's disease and in animal models of parkinsonism. The concentration of dopamine is decreased in the basal ganglia in Parkinson's disease (1). L-DOPA, which increases brain dopamine (2), and apomorphine, which stimulates dopamine receptors (3), improve the neurological status of parkinsonian patients (4, 5).

On the other hand, physostigmine, which increases brain acetylcholine levels by cholinesterase inhibition, consistently aggravates the neurological manifestations (6, 7), while anticholinergic drugs improve parkinsonism. This hypersensitivity to cholinergic stimulation by physostigmine in Parkinson's disease is probably secondary to low brain-dopamine concentration, since the physostigmine effect is inhibited by L-DOPA (7). Furthermore, choline-acetylase and cholinesterase activities are normal in the parkinsonian brain (8). A similar hypersensitivity to physostigmine was observed in an animal model of Parkinson's disease produced by serial intracisternal injections of 6-hydroxydopamine, a chemical which selectively destroys dopaminergic and noradrenergic neurons in the brain (9). 6-Hydroxydopamine-treated dogs developed hypokinesia, tremor, and rigidity, which were aggravated by an injection of physostigmine (10). As observed in parkinsonian patients, L-DOPA suppressed the neurological effects of physostigmine in 6-hydroxydopamine-treated dogs, presumably by repleting brain dopamine.

Phenothiazine drugs also can produce parkinsonian symptoms, presumably by blocking striatal dopamine receptor sites (11). In the present chapter we shall describe (a) the effects of physostigmine on extrapyramidal signs in psychiatric patients being treated with phenothiazine drugs and (b) the effect of phenothiazine drugs on physostigmine-induced tremor and the concentration of acetylcholine, choline, and cholinesterase activity in the brain of the rat. The purpose of these studies was to determine if central cholinergic hyperactivity or hypersensitivity, like that observed in idiopathic Parkinson's disease, also occurs in drug-induced parkinsonism.

EFFECT OF PHYSOSTIGMINE ON PHENOTHIAZINE-INDUCED EXTRAPYRAMIDAL REACTIONS

In 10 psychiatric patients (nine schizophrenics, one drug addict) admitted to the hospital, the effect of an intravenous injection of 1 mg of physostigmine salicylate (Eserine) on their neurological status was investigated prior to and during treatment with either chlorpromazine or trifluoperazine (Table 1). Methscopolamine bromide (0.25 mg), which blocks the peripheral muscarinic effects of physostigmine but has no effect on the central nervous system, was administered intravenously immediately after the physostigmine injection. Prior to phenothiazine therapy, all 10 patients had normal neurological examinations and none developed any neurological signs after the intravenous injection of physostigmine salicylate (1 mg) and methscopolamine bromide (0.25 mg). As seen in Table 1, cases 1 to 7 were treated with trifluoperazine (10 to 40 mg/day) and cases 8 to 10 with chlorpromazine (300 to 1200 mg/day). After 12 to 16 days of therapy, the physostigmine test was repeated. Patients 1 through 5 and 8, who had developed minimal rigidity and/or tremor during phenothiazine therapy, exhibited a worsening of these signs after the physostigmine injection (Table 1). These six patients (cases 1 to 5 and 8) later were administered anticholinergic medication (benztropine) with good relief of the extrapyramidal side effects. Akathisia was present in cases 1 and 6 but this side effect was not aggravated by the injection of physostigmine. Physostigmine did not induce any dyskinetic or dystonic reactions during phenothiazine therapy.

In order to investigate the mechanism of this phenothiazine-induced hypersensitivity to cholinergic stimulation, we measured the effect of various phenothiazine drugs on physostigmine-induced tremor, brain acetylcholine and choline concentration, and cholinesterase activity in the rat.

EFFECT OF PHENOTHIAZINE DRUGS ON THE TREMORIGENIC ACTION OF PHYSOSTIGMINE IN RATS

One-hundred-fifty-two Sprague-Dawley rats weighing 180 to 220 g were used in the experiments. Tremor was recorded on a Lafayette 501 activity platform (Lafayette Instruments, Lafayette, Indiana) set at a sensitivity adjustment of 10 which minimized counts due to exploratory movements but still recorded tremor. After a 3-min period to permit the rats to familiarize themselves with the new environment, activity was recorded for 15 min. Measurements were obtained before and after the intraperitoneal

TABLE 1. *Effect of intravenous physostigmine (1 mg) on neurological side effects of phenothiazine therapy in psychiatric patients*

Case no.	Sex	Age (yr)	Drug[c]	Dose (mg/day)	Neurological signs				Benztropine[b] (mg/day)
					Before physostigmine		After physostigmine		
					Rigidity[a]	Tremor[a]	Rigidity[a]	Tremor[a]	
1	M	28	TFP	10	+	0	++	++	6
2	F	19	TFP	20	+++	0	+++	0	4
3	M	20	TFP	20	+++	0	+++	0	4
4	M	22	TFP	20	+	0	++	0	2
5	F	35	TFP	40	0	+	0	++	2
6	F	20	TFP	15	0	0	0	0	—
7	F	37	TFP	40	0	0	0	0	—
8	M	25	CPZ	1200	+	0	++	0	2
9	M	25	CPZ	300	0	0	0	0	—
10	F	22	CPZ	300	0	0	0	0	—

[a] Rigidity and tremor were graded as 0 = none, + = minimal, ++ = moderate, +++ = marked, ++++ = severe.
[b] Benztropine (cogentin) therapy was started after the physostigmine tests were completed.
[c] TFP = trifluoperazine; CPZ = chlorpromazine.

injection of 0.25 mg/kg physostigmine salicylate. The ratio of the post-physostigmine activity to prephysostigmine activity was called the activity index which proved to be a quantitative measurement of the tremorigenic effect of physostigmine in these animals. Physostigmine (0.25 mg/kg) produced minimal tremor in about 50% of the rats. The ratio of postphysostigmine activity to prephysostigmine activity (activity index) was less than one in the control rats because 0.25-mg physostigmine has minimal tremorigenic action and reduces exploratory movements due to its sedative effect (Fig. 1). The activity index was also less than one when the various neuroleptic drugs were administered without physostigmine. One hr after the intraperitoneal injection of chlorpromazine HCl (15 mg/kg), physostigmine produced moderate to severe tremor in all four extremities of the treated rats. This was reflected by a 26-fold increase in the activity index compared to control rats (Fig. 1). Physostigmine-induced tremor was increased 23-fold by reserpine (10 mg/kg) administered 1 hr prior to the

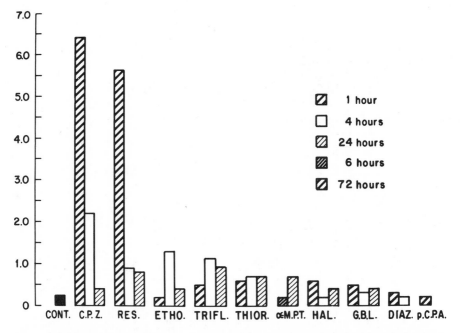

FIG. 1. Effect of various drugs on physostigmine-induced tremor. The activity index (ratio of postphysostigmine counts to prephysostigmine counts) indicates the tremorigenic action of physostigmine (0.25 mg/kg) as affected by different compounds. The hours indicated are the time intervals between the neuroleptic drug administration and the physostigmine injection. Two rats were placed on the activity platform at one time, and each value is the mean of five groups of rats. The abbreviations are: CONT, control; CPZ, chlorpromazine; RES, reserpine; ETHO, ethopropazine; TRIFL, trifluoperazine; THIOR, thioridazine; α-MPT, α-methyl-p-tyrosine; HAL, haloperidol; GBL, γ-butyrolactone; DIAZ, diazepam; pCPA, p-chlorophenylalanine.

physostigmine injection. L-DOPA (500 mg/kg) injected 1 hr before physostigmine reduced the tremorigenic effect of physostigmine in rats pretreated with reserpine but had no effect on tremors produced by physostigmine in rats pretreated with chlorpromazine. Benztropine (4 mg/kg), administered 0.5 hr prior to physostigmine, decreased the tremorigenic activity of physostigmine induced by both reserpine and chlorpromazine. Other drugs, which alter catecholamine metabolism, ethopropazine (30 mg/kg), trifluoperazine HCl (1 mg/kg), thioridazine (0.5 mg/kg), alpha-methyl-p-tyrosine (200 mg/kg), haloperidol (10 mg/kg), and gamma-butyrolactone (250 mg/kg) enhanced physostigmine-induced tremor, but to a lesser degree. Diazepam (3 mg/kg) and p-chlorophenylalanine (316 mg/kg) had no effect on the tremorigenic activity of physostigmine.

EFFECT OF PHENOTHIAZINE DRUGS ON PHYSOSTIGMINE-INDUCED INCREASE IN RAT-BRAIN ACETYLCHOLINE AND INHIBITION OF CHOLINESTERASE

Several studies have demonstrated that there is a causal relationship between drug-induced increase in brain acetylcholine and tremor (12–14). Therefore, we measured the concentration of brain acetylcholine as well as choline and cholinesterase activity before and after the injection of physostigmine (0.25 mg/kg) in rats pretreated with some of the phenothiazine drugs that potentiated the tremor in Fig. 1. Acetylcholine and choline were assayed by the gas-chromatographic procedure of Jenden et al. (15) and Hanin et al. (16) with the previously described modifications (17). Cholinesterase was determined by the method of McCaman et al. (18). Sixty min after the intraperitoneal injection of chlorpromazine (15 mg/kg), thioridazine (10 mg/kg), ethopropazine (30 mg/kg), and trifluoperazine (1 mg/kg) there was no significant change in brain acetylcholine concentration or brain cholinesterase activity (Table 2). Twenty min after the intraperitoneal injection of 0.25 mg/kg of physostigmine, there was a 25% increase in brain-acetylcholine concentration and a 44% inhibition of cholinesterase activity. However, the administration of thioridazine or chlorpromazine 40 min prior to the physostigmine injection, significantly potentiated the increase in acetylcholine concentration produced by physostigmine. The combination of thioridazine or chlorpromazine with physostigmine produced approximately 20% greater inhibition of cholinesterase than observed with physostigmine alone. This potentiation of physostigmine-induced inhibition of cholinesterase also was seen when the rats were placed in an incubator to prevent the hypothermia produced by chlorpromazine. Pretreatment with either ethopropazine or trifluoperazine did not enhance the increase in acetylcholine produced by physostigmine. None of the phenothiazines, either alone or in combination with physostigmine, altered brain choline concentration.

TABLE 2. *Effect of phenothiazines alone or in combination with physostigmine on rat brain acetylcholine (ACh) and choline concentration and cholinesterase activity*

	Dose (mg/kg)	Acetylcholine (n moles/g)	% Increase	Cholinesterase (μ moles ACh hydrolyzed/g/h)	% Inhibition	Choline (n moles/g)
Control	—	18.3 ± 0.4 (27)		580 ± 22 (12)		59 ± 8 (27)
Chlorpromazine	15	18.6 ± 0.8 (9)	2	583 ± 23 (6)	0	65 ± 2 (9)
Thioridazine	10	19.2 ± 0.7 (7)	5	619 ± 31 (6)	0	67 ± 4 (7)
Ethopropazine	30	18.7 ± 0.7 (5)	2	—		62 ± 3 (5)
Trifluoperazine	1	19.6 ± 1.0 (5)	7	—		64 ± 4 (5)
Physostigmine	0.25	22.9 ± 0.7^a (27)	25	323 ± 16^a (13)	44	64 ± 2 (27)
Chlorpromazine + physostigmine	15, 0.25	25.9 ± 0.9^{a,b} (10)	42	223 ± 11^{a,c} (8)	62	69 ± 2 (10)
Thioridazine + physostigmine	10, 0.25	28.0 ± 0.9^{a,c} (8)	53	215 ± 11^{a,c} (8)	63	66 ± 4 (8)
Ethopropazine + physostigmine	30, 0.25	23.4 ± 1.5^a (5)	28	—		59 ± 5 (8)
Trifluoperazine + physostigmine	1, 0.25	22.7 ± 0.7^a (5)	24	—		55 ± 2 (5)

Acetylcholine, choline, and cholinesterase were measured 20 min after physostigmine and 60 min after the phenothiazine injection. The values are the mean ± SE and the numbers in parenthesis are the number of animals used in each experiment.

^{a} p < 0.001, compared to control.
^{b} p < 0.02, compared to physostigmine.
^{c} p < 0.001, compared to physostigmine.

DISCUSSION

The data presented in this chapter suggest that phenothiazine drugs can induce a hypersensitivity to central cholinergic stimulation by physostigmine in humans and rats similar to that observed in Parkinson's disease (6, 7). This phenothiazine-induced hypersensitivity to physostigmine results in a potentiation of the tremorigenic action of physostigmine in the rat and increased rigidity and/or tremor in humans.

Physostigmine is a tertiary amine which crosses the blood–brain barrier, inhibits the enzyme cholinesterase, and thereby stimulates central cholinergic pathways by increasing brain acetylcholine levels (19). Previous studies in our laboratory demonstrated a correlation between the rise in rat-brain acetylcholine concentration and tremor induced by physostigmine (14). The potentiation by chlorpromazine of both the increase in brain acetylcholine and the rigidity and tremor produced by physostigmine suggest a causal relationship between the biochemical and neurological effects of the interaction of these two drugs. The potentiation of the physostigmine-induced increase in brain acetylcholine by chlorpromazine and thioridazine may be due to their enhancement of cholinesterase inhibition. Dasgupta and Mukherjie (20) and Maickel (21) had shown by *in vitro* studies that high concentrations of chlorpromazine can inhibit brain cholinesterase. However, chlorpromazine and thioridazine might also alter acetylcholine metabolism by their blocking action on the dopamine receptor site. Dopamine may act as a presynaptic inhibitor of certain central cholinergic neurons (22). A depressant action of dopamine on the neuronal discharge frequency of the caudate (23, 24), lateral geniculate nucleus (25), thalamus (26), hypothalamus (27), and hippocampus (28) has been demonstrated. Phenothiazine drugs, by blocking dopamine receptors, could increase the discharge frequency of some central cholinergic neurons and enhance acetylcholine release and turnover in these neurons. The inhibition of cholinesterase by physostigmine may increase further the quantity of acetylcholine released and the neuronal concentration of acetylcholine. Hyperactivity of striatal cholinergic neurons could produce the parkinsonian side effects of phenothiazine therapy such as rigidity and tremor. By decreasing brain dopamine levels, reserpine might produce similar changes in the same cholinergic neurons. The effects of striatal cholinergic hyperactivity would be blocked by anticholinergic drugs which are the most effective therapeutic agents in drug-induced parkinsonism.

Despite the high incidence of extrapyramidal side effects associated with trifluoperazine therapy in patients, this phenothiazine had little effect on the action of physostigmine in the rat. Multiple factors such as dosage, duration of therapy, and species sensitivity to each phenothiazine drug might be important in determining its interaction with physostigmine.

SUMMARY

The intravenous injection of 1 mg of physostigmine induced and/or aggravated rigidity and tremor in six out of 10 psychiatric patients treated with chlorpromazine and trifluoperazine. Prior to phenothiazine therapy, physostigmine produced no neurological effects. A similar effect was demonstrated in rats. The tremorigenic activity of physostigmine was increased 26- and 23-fold 1 hr after the injection of chlorpromazine and reserpine respectively. Other phenothiazine drugs also potentiated the tremorigenic effect of physostigmine to a lesser extent. The increase in rat brain acetylcholine concentration produced by physostigmine was enhanced significantly by chlorpromazine and thioridazine but not by ethopropazine or trifluoperazine, although these phenothiazines had no effect on brain acetylcholine or choline when administered alone. The combination of thioridazine or chlorpromazine with physostigmine produced approximately 20% greater inhibition of brain cholinesterase than observed after the injection of physostigmine alone.

The mechanism of phenothiazine-induced extrapyramidal reactions may include direct effects on central cholinergic as well as catecholamine metabolism.

ACKNOWLEDGMENTS

This work was supported by grant NS07542 (from the U.S. Public Health Service). V. H. Sethy is the recipient of special NIH Fellowship, Grant No. 1-F-10-NSO 2597–01. The authors thank the following for their generous donations of compounds used in these studies: Smith Kline and French Laboratories (chlorpromazine and trifluoperazine), Warner-Chilcott Laboratories (ethopropazine), and Pfizer, Inc. (*p*-chlorophenylalanine).

REFERENCES

1. Hornykiewicz, O., *Wien. Klin. Wschr.,* **75,** 309 (1963).
2. Everett, G. M., and Borcherding, J. W., *Science,* **168,** 849 (1970).
3. Anden, N. E., Rubenson, A., Fuxe, K., and Hokfelt, T., *J. Pharm. Pharmacol.,* **19,** 627 (1967).
4. Cotzias, G. C., Van Woert, M. H., and Schiffer, L. M., *New Eng. J. Med.,* **276,** 374 (1967).
5. Schwab, R. S., Amador, L. V., and Lettvin, J. Y., *Trans. Amer. Neurol. Assoc.,* **76,** 251 (1951).
6. Duvoisin, R. C., *Arch. Neurol.,* **17,** 124 (1967).
7. Weintraub, M. I., and Van Woert, M. H., *New Eng. J. Med.,* **284,** 412 (1971).
8. McGeer, P. L., and McGeer, E. G., *Arch. Neurol.,* **25,** 265 (1971).
9. Breese, G. R., and Traylor, T. D., *J. Pharmacol. Exp. Ther.,* **174,** 413 (1970).
10. Van Woert, M. H., Ambani, L. M., and Bowers, M. B., Jr., *Neurology,* **22,** 86 (1972).
11. Van Rossum, J. M., in *Proceedings of the Vth International Congress of the Collegium Internationale. Neuropsychopharm,* Wash. 28–31, March 1968. Excerpta Med. Int. Congress, Series no. 129.

12. Holmstedt, B., and Lundgren, G., in *Mechanisms of Release of Biogenic Amines,* von Euler, U. C., Rosell, S., and Urnas, B. (eds.) Pergamon Press, New York, 1966, p. 439.
13. Slater, P., and Rogers, K. J., *Europ. J. Pharmacol.,* **4,** 390 (1968).
14. Sethy, V. H., and Van Woert, M. H., *Biochem. Pharmacol.,* **22,** 2685 (1973).
15. Jenden, D. J., Hanin, I., and Lamb, S. I., *Analyt. Chem.,* **40,** 125 (1968).
16. Hanin, I., Massarelli, R., and Costa, E., *J. Pharmacol. Exp. Ther.,* **151,** 10 (1972).
17. Sethy, V. H., and Van Woert, M. H., *Neuropharm.,* **12,** 27 (1973).
18. McCaman, M. W., Tomey, L. R., and McCaman, R. E., *Life Sci.,* **7,** 233 (1968).
19. Rosecrans, J. A., Dren, A. T., and Domino, E. F., *Int. J. Pharmac.,* **7,** 127 (1968).
20. Dasgupta, S. R., and Mukherjie, K. L., *Bull. Calcutta Sch. trop. Med. Hyg.,* **4,** 123 (1956).
21. Maickel, R. P., *Int. J. Neuropharmac.,* **7,** 23 (1968).
22. Wooley, D. F., *Physiologist,* **12,** 399 (1970).
23. Bloom, F. E., Costa, E., and Salmoiraghi, G. C., *J. Pharmacol. Exp. Ther.,* **150,** 244 (1965).
24. McLennan, H., and York, D. H., *J. Physiol. (London),* **189,** 393 (1967).
25. Phillis, J. W., Tebecis, A. K., and York, D. H., *J. Physiol. (London),* **190,** 563 (1967).
26. Anderson, P., and Curtis, D. R., *Acta Physiol. Scand.,* **61,** 100 (1964).
27. Bloom, F. E., Oliver, A. P., and Salmoiraghi, G. C., *Int. J. Neuropharmac.,* **2,** 181 (1963).
28. Biscol, T. J., and Straughan, D. W., *J. Physiol. (London),* **183,** 341 (1966).

The Phenothiazines and Structurally Related Drugs, edited by I. S.
Forrest, C. J. Carr, and E. Usdin. Raven Press, New York © 1974.

Induction of Increased Aryl Hydrocarbon Hydroxylase Activity by Phenothiazines

Lee W. Wattenberg

Department of Pathology, University of Minnesota, Minneapolis, Minnesota 55433

A number of phenothiazines have been studied for their inducing effect
on microsomal aryl hydrocarbon hydroxylase activity of the small intestine
and liver of the rat (1). Phenothiazine has a strong inducing activity, and, in
most instances, its derivatives show either a comparable or a lesser activity.
Certain of its derivatives, i.e., those with side chains substituted onto the
nitrogen, induce approximately twice as much activity in the mucosa of
the small intestine as phenothiazine. These compounds are chlorpromazine
HCl, chlorpromazine (free base), chlorpromazine sulfoxide HCl, and
pyrathiazine HCl. The relative inducing capacity of various phenothiazines
toward the liver and the mucosa of the small intestine differs, i.e., phenothiazine has a much greater effect on the liver than the small intestine,
whereas thioridazine had a greater effect on the small intestine.

The results of several chemical modifications of the phenothiazines on
their inducing capacity have been determined (1). Oxidation of the sulfur
of the phenothiazine ring of chlorpromazine HCl does not significantly alter
its inducing capacity. Administration of chlorpromazine as the free base
dissolved in sesame oil or as the hydrochloride in aqueous solution results
in similar inducing activities. Some substitutions markedly reduce inducing
activity. Thus, phenothiazine propionic acid and its methyl ester are devoid
of significant inducing activity. Likewise, the quaternary salt of chlorpromazine, chlorpromazine methyliodide, is devoid of activity. Alteration of
the phenothiazine ring structure results in a profound loss of inducing
capacity. If the sulfur atom remains in the ring, some activity persists, e.g.,
thianthrene and chlorprothixene. Replacement of the sulfur atom results
in virtually complete loss of inducing capacity, e.g., acridan, phenoxazine,
and phenazine.

The effect of administration of phenothiazine on the aryl hydrocarbon
hydroxylase activity of several tissues other than the liver and small intestine were also studied in the rat (1). Phenothiazine induced a marked
increase in activity in the kidney and lung. The activities in the spleen and
thymus were enhanced, but to a lesser extent. In addition to *in vivo* experiments, induction of increased aryl hydrocarbon hydroxylase activity by
phenothiazines has also been carried out *in vitro* (2).

Experiments were carried out to determine biological implications of induction of aryl hydrocarbon hydroxylase activity by phenothiazines. In this work, adrenal necrosis and mammary tumor formation in the rat resulting from DMBA administration were employed as test systems. In both of these test systems, rats receiving phenothiazine were protected (1, 3, 4). In addition, phenothiazine inhibits intestinal and urinary bladder tumors induced in rats fed Bracken Fern (5). The possibility that phenothiazines might alter drug metabolism and/or the response to toxic environmental agents in patients receiving these compounds for therapeutic purposes merits evaluation.

REFERENCES

1. Wattenberg, L. W., and Leong, J. L., *Cancer Res.,* **25,** 365 (1965).
2. Wattenberg, L. W., Leong, J. L., and Galbraith, A. R., *Proc. Soc. Exp. Biol. and Med.,* **127,** 467 (1968).
3. Wattenberg, L. W., and Leong, J. L., *Fed. Proc.,* **26,** 692 (1967).
4. Wattenberg, L. W., *Toxicology and Applied Pharmacology,* **23,** 741 (1972).
5. Pamukcu, A. M., Wattenberg, L. W., Price, J. M., and Bryan, G. T., *J. National Cancer Institute,* **47,** 155 (1971).

The Phenothiazines and Structurally Related Drugs, edited by I. S. Forrest, C. J. Carr, and E. Usdin. Raven Press, New York © 1974.

Interactions of Chlorpromazine with Monoamines in the Hypothalamic Thermoregulatory Centers

Peter Lomax and W. E. Kirkpatrick

Department of Pharmacology, School of Medicine, and Brain Research Institute, University of California, Los Angeles, California 90024

INTRODUCTION

Chlorpromazine has been in clinical use since 1952 but its mode of action has yet to be established. In an early study of the pharmacological properties of the drug, Courvoisier and his associates (1) characterized its anticholinergic, adrenolytic, antihistaminic, and local anesthetic activity. Since acetylcholine, norepinephrine, and histamine may serve as neurotransmitters in the central nervous system, it has been suggested that chlorpromazine's central pharmacological effects are a consequence of some interaction between the drug and these putative transmitters (2).

Although it can be shown that chlorpromazine can reverse or block a variety of adrenergic and cholinergic effects at peripheral receptor sites, such actions in the central nervous system have not been convincingly demonstrated. Indeed, the rigid criteria for establishing that norepinephrine and acetylcholine act as central neurotransmitters have not been completely met, although the evidence for such a role appears to be overwhelming. Part of the difficulty in making such determinations and in investigating the effects of centrally active compounds on these neurotransmitter functions has stemmed from the lack of a suitable model central-neuronal test system.

One such system on which the effects of a variety of drugs have been extensively studied in recent years is that in the rostral hypothalamic thermoregulatory centers (3). Since it has long been known that chlorpromazine may modify body temperature, it seemed likely that an investigation of the effects of the drug on temperature regulation might prove fruitful in elucidating its general mode of action in the central nervous system.

THE ROLE OF MONOAMINES IN CENTRAL TEMPERATURE REGULATION

Norepinephrine

The brainstem, particularly the hypothalamus, contains high concentrations of monoamines, including norepinephrine (4). Brodie and Shore

(5) and von Euler (6) suggested that these endogenous monoamines may be involved in the central regulation of body temperature. Injection of norepinephrine into the cerebral ventricles of cats caused a fall in temperature (7) but in other species variable responses were seen (8). In the rat, intracerebral injection of norepinephrine may cause a rise or fall in core temperature (9). Lomax et al. (10) studied the interactions of norepinephrine and cholinomimetics on the thermoregulatory centers of the rat and suggested that norepinephrine may exert a modulating influence on ongoing cholinergic activity analogous to the interactions of these amines on peripheral autonomic ganglia. This view is consistent with the data of Beckman and Eisenman (11) who showed that rostral hypothalamic thermosensitive neurons, which increased their firing rates when acetylcholine was applied iontophoretically, decreased their frequency in response to norepinephrine. However, in spite of the considerable volume of research that has been carried out, the role of norepinephrine in central temperature regulation is at present unresolved.

Acetylcholine

There is a growing body of evidence to support the concept that acetylcholine plays a role in central thermoregulatory mechanisms (12). Iontophoretic injection of acetylcholine into the rostral hypothalamic thermoregulatory centers causes a fall in body temperature in the rat (13) and this response is abolished by prior systemic injection of atropine indicating a specific effect at cholinergic receptor sites. Direct injection of atropine into the rostral hypothalamus of the rat produces hyperthermia, presumably due to blockade of central cholinergic activity (14). Knox et al. have investigated the effect of acetylcholine on unit activity in the thermoregulatory centers of rats (15). Units that increased their firing frequency in response to heating the skin showed a similar response to direct application of acetylcholine. Since raising the environmental temperature would be expected to lower the set point of the hypothalamic thermostat, it was suggested that the pathways involved contained a cholinergic link and that the hypothermic effect of cholinomimetics is due to a lowering of the set temperature. As a corollary to this interpretation, the hyperthermic effect of cholinolytics is due to a raising of the set point.

THE EFFECTS OF CHLORPROMAZINE ON BODY TEMPERATURE

Systemic Administration

Administration of chlorpromazine (2 mg/kg i.p.) to rats causes a fall in core temperature within a few minutes with the lowest level being attained in 90 to 120 min. The mean fall in a group of eight animals was $2.8 \pm 0.29°C$

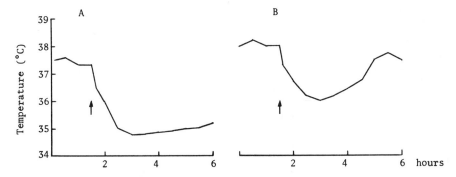

FIG. 1. Temperature records from 2 rats. The fall in temperature following systemic injection of chlorpromazine (2 mg/kg i.p.) (A) was more rapid and of longer duration than that seen after N-methyl chlorpromazine (5 mg/kg i.p.) (B).

($\pm$ SEM). A typical response is seen in Fig. 1A. The quaternary analogue, N-methyl chlorpromazine (5 mg/kg i.p.) led to a similar fall in temperature but of lesser degree ($1.5 \pm 0.20°C$ in eight animals) and shorter duration (Fig. 1B). Since it is unlikely that the highly charged N-methyl chlorpromazine is able to penetrate into the central nervous system in appreciable amounts (16), these results indicate that the hypothermic action of chlorpromazine is probably mediated at peripheral sites. Increased heat loss from the skin is most likely the major factor contributing to the fall in temperature (17).

Intracerebral Microinjection

Six rats were injected with chlorpromazine (2 μg i.c.) at the same sites in the rostral hypothalamus: in each case this resulted in a rise in temperature with a mean increase for the group of $1.5 \pm 0.19°C$. The hyperthermia persisted for 3 to 4 hr before slowly subsiding. A record from one of these animals is seen in Fig. 2A.

The effect of injection of the quaternary derivative into the thermoregulatory centers was also investigated. Since N-methyl chlorpromazine had proved to be less potent when administered systemically the intracerebral dose used was 5 μg. Here again a gradual rise in temperature occurred in six rats to give a mean of $1.9 \pm 0.04°C$ which was not significantly different ($0.05 < p < 0.1$) from that seen after chlorpromazine. The hyperthermia was less prolonged after N-methyl chlorpromazine with the temperature recovering to control values in under 4 hr (Fig. 2B).

Histological examination of the brains of these 12 animals revealed that the injection sites lay in the preoptic/anterior hypothalamic nuclei, within 1 mm of the midline. Injection of chlorpromazine (2 μg i.c.) into various sites in the middle and caudal hypothalamus failed to produce any significant changes in core temperature.

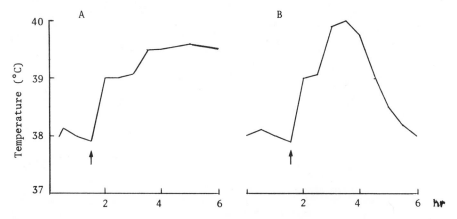

FIG. 2. Hyperthermia following injection of chlorpromazine (2 μg) (A) and N-methyl chlorpromazine (5 μg) (B) into the rostral hypothalamic thermoregulatory centers of 2 rats. The duration of action of the tertiary drug was much longer than that of the quaternary derivative.

Conclusions

Although it is generally considered to be a hypothermic agent, these studies suggest that this action of chlorpromazine is mediated at peripheral sites and that the effect of the drug on the rostral hypothalamic thermoregulatory centers is to cause a rise in body temperature. These data do not, however, rule out the possibility that the hypothermic effect could be due, in part, to an action at other sites in the central nervous system.

On the basis of the studies of the effects on temperature regulation of norepinephrine and acetylcholine, discussed above, it might be postulated that chlorpromazine raises the core temperature by modifying the function of these amines in the rostral hypothalamus. In order to test these possibilities, the effects of chlorpromazine and its N-methyl derivative on peripheral noradrenergic and cholinergic receptors were compared.

THE EFFECTS OF CHLORPROMAZINE ON PERIPHERAL RECEPTORS

Cholinergic Sites

(i) *Guinea pig ileum* Both chlorpromazine and N-methyl chlorpromazine antagonize cholinergic stimulation of the isolated guinea pig ileum. The apparent affinity constants of the antagonists were estimated by plotting the intercept of each curve at 50% of its maximum against the agonist concentration at which it was obtained. As seen in Fig. 3, a plot of this type made from data obtained with tertiary and quaternary chlorpromazine is

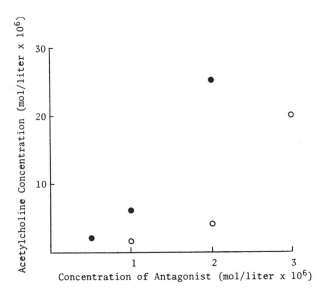

FIG. 3. Isoboles obtained by plotting concentration of acetylcholine required to produce 50% of the maximum contraction of the isolated guinea-pig ileum in the presence of varying concentrations of chlorpromazine (open circles) or N-methyl chlorpromazine (solid circles).

nonlinear; the curves do not pass through the origin. These data are indicative of noncompetitive antagonism. Also, the quaternary compound proved to be more active.

(ii) *Superior cervical ganglion* Contractions of the ipsilateral nictitating membrane of the cat were recorded following intra-arterial injection of muscarinic (McN A343, 10 μg) or nicotinic (DMPP, 10 μg) agents into the superior cervical ganglion. Systemic injection of chlorpromazine or N-methyl chlorpromazine antagonized the response to McN A343 while leaving the response to DMPP unaltered. In Fig. 4, the inhibition of the responses to McN A343 is seen compared to that produced by atropine. The doses of each agonist (expressed as moles/kg body weight) producing 50% inhibition were: atropine sulfate, 5×10^{-9}; N-methyl chlorpromazine iodide, 2×10^{-6}; and chlorpromazine hydrochloride, 2×10^{-5}.

Noradrenergic Sites

(i) *Rabbit aorta* Both tertiary and quaternary chlorpromazine antagonized the norepinephrine-induced contractions of rabbit aortic strips *in vitro*. The tertiary drug was about 100 times more potent than the quaternary derivative (Fig. 5). The concentration producing complete blockade was about 10 times the minimum effective dose for each drug.

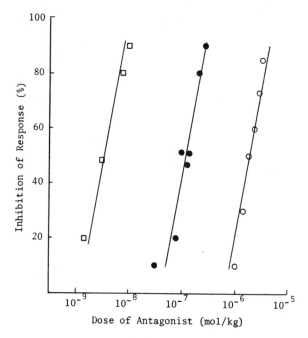

FIG. 4. Inhibition of the maximum contraction of the cat nictitating membrane, induced by injection of Mc A343 (10 μg) into the ipsilateral superior cervical ganglion, by varying concentrations of atropine (open squares), chlorpromazine (open circles), or N-methyl chlorpromazine (solid circles) injected systemically.

Conclusions

The noncompetitive nature of the cholinergic blocking effect of the phenothiazines (Fig. 3) on the ileum, coupled with the much greater potency of atropine on the muscarinic receptors in the superior cervical ganglion, does not encourage the view that the central thermoregulatory effects of the drugs are due to direct antagonism of endogenous acetylcholine in the rostral hypothalamus. Earlier studies (14) showed that the hyperthermic effect of atropine, when injected into the thermoregulatory centers, was comparable in degree and duration to that produced by the same dose of chlorpromazine (2 μg). At the peripheral cholinergic sites investigated, the N-methyl derivative was consistently more potent than the parent tertiary compound, whereas the reverse was the case in respect to their action on the thermoregulatory centers (Fig. 2).

On comparing the peripheral noradrenergic blocking effects, the relative potencies of the two phenothiazines are in the right direction but the magnitude of the difference (tertiary:quaternary—100:1, Fig. 5) is much greater than that seen centrally (Fig. 2). However, the major objection to assigning such a role to explain the central thermoregulatory actions resides

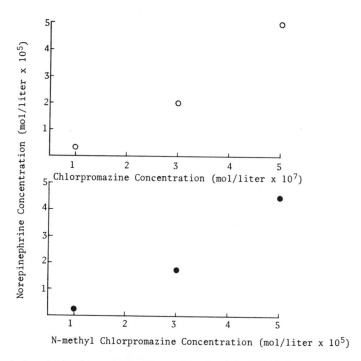

FIG. 5. Isoboles obtained by plotting concentration of norepinephrine required to produce 50% of the maximum contraction of rabbit aortic strips in the presence of varying concentrations of chlorpromazine (open circles) or N-methyl chlorpromazine (solid circles).

in the uncertainty regarding the importance of hypothalamic noradrenergic activity in temperature regulation. The α-adrenergic blocking agent, tolazoline, when injected into the rostral hypothalamus, has no significant effect on body temperature by itself (10) but enhances the effect of subsequently injected cholinomimetics (10). By analogy to the interaction of cholinomimetics and norepinephrine on peripheral autonomic neurons (18), it has been postulated that norepinephrine hyperpolarizes the thermoregulatory neurons causing an upward setting of the thermostat (10). Thus, depending on the degree of ongoing cholinergic activity, which tends to lower the set point, noradrenergic blockade might be expected to lower, rather than raise, the core temperature.

Thus, the effects at peripheral cholinergic and noradrenergic receptors lend scant support to the hypothesis that the actions of the phenothiazines on central neuronal systems can be explained on the basis of inhibiting the actions of acetylcholine or norepinephrine at specific receptor sites.

THE EFFECT OF CHLORPROMAZINE ON NEURONAL CONDUCTION

In common with the phenothiazine derivatives, chlorpromazine has been described as exhibiting local anesthetic activity (1), being more potent and having a longer duration of action *in vivo* than cocaine or procaine.

The isolated frog sciatic nerve preparation has been used to compare the ability of procaine, chlorpromazine, and their quaternary derivatives to block neuronal conduction (19). Typical results are illustrated in Fig. 6: procaine (6 mM) caused a 50% reduction of the height of the action potential in 28 min; chlorpromazine (0.6 mM) achieved this in 15 min. N-methyl procaine (12 mM) was without effect on the propagated action potentials whereas N-methyl chlorpromazine (0.6 mM) had about the same activity as the tertiary analogue. No recovery of conduction occurred in spite of prolonged washing (24 hr or longer) of the nerves treated with the phenothiazines.

These data indicate that although both phenothiazines and local anesthetics are able to stabilize neuronal membranes, their mechanisms of action are fundamentally different. In order to exert a local anesthetic effect, procaine and related drugs must penetrate the nerve membrane to reach receptor sites on the inner surface (20, 21). Since N-methyl chlorpromazine is as effective as the tertiary compound, the blockade appears to be due to an action on the external surface of the nerve membrane. The mechanism by which the membrane is stabilized seems to be fundamentally different than that of the clinically useful local anesthetics. Nevertheless, the end result on neuronal conduction is the same.

Like chlorpromazine, procaine causes a rise in core temperature when injected directly into the thermoregulatory centers of the rat (22). This hyperthermic effect could be due to stabilization of the neurons controlling the set point with a consequent upward setting similar to that postulated to occur when norepinephrine is applied to the thermoregulatory centers (10).

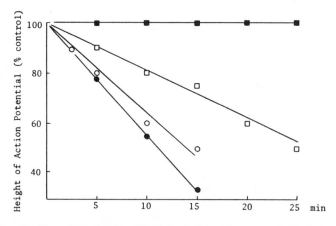

FIG. 6. The kinetics of conduction block in isolated frog sciatic nerves for procaine (6 mM) (open squares), N-methyl procaine (12 mM) (solid squares), chlorpromazine (0.6 mM) (open circles), and N-methyl chlorpromazine (0.6 mM) (solid circles).

Thus, the phenothiazines may act on neurons to cause a nonspecific stabilization of the membranes and, in the case of the rostral hypothalamic thermoregulatory centers, so mimic the effect of norepinephrine.

This stabilization could, alternatively, reduce the activity of cholinergic neurons directly. Studies of unit activity in the thermoregulatory centers indicate that the setting of the thermostat is under tonic cholinergic control (15). Such ongoing cholinergic activity, mediated from cutaneous thermoreceptors, seems to be necessary to prevent the set temperature from rising. Increased cholinergic stimulation appears to lower the set point and, hence, the body temperature (23).

The effect of chlorpromazine (2 mg/kg or 10 mg/kg) on whole brain acetylcholine levels of the rat was measured using the gas chromatographic method developed by Hanin and Jenden (24). The levels were unchanged 20 min after injection of the drug (Table 1). It is possible that localized hypothalamic changes are masked when whole brain levels are measured; of greater interest, however, would be the effect of phenothiazines on acetylcholine turnover in the rostral hypothalamus.

At the present stage it is clear that current data allow the precise mechanism of action of chlorpromazine on the thermoregulatory centers to be determined.

TABLE 1. *The effect of chlorpromazine on whole brain acetylcholine levels in the rat*

Treatment	Number of animals	Acetylcholine concentration (nanomoles/g $\pm$ S.E.M.)
0.9% NaCl	8	17.42 $\pm$ 0.54
Chlorpromazine (2 mg/kg i.p.)	4	17.25 $\pm$ 0.61[a]
Chlorpromazine (10 mg/kg i.p.)	4	18.17 $\pm$ 0.65[a]

[a] p > 0.50

SUMMARY

The mechanism of action of chlorpromazine on the central nervous system is unknown. It is possible that the central pharmacological effects of the drug are a consequence of some interaction between it and neurochemical transmitters in the central nervous system. Chlorpromazine antagonizes acetylcholine at peripheral cholinergic receptor sites and some of its central effects may be due to anticholinergic activity. Investigation of the inhibitory action of chlorpromazine and chlorpromazine methyl iodide at peripheral cholinergic sites indicates that both drugs are noncompetitive antagonists of acetylcholine at muscarinic and nicotinic receptor sites. This suggests the possibility that chlorpromazine inhibits cholinergic transmission within the central nervous system. Both drugs also exert a noncompetitive inhibitory action at peripheral adrenergic receptor sites.

There is evidence that acetylcholine serves as a neurotransmitter in the hypothalamic thermoregulatory centers. Iontophoretic application of acetylcholine to the thermoregulatory centers of the rat caused a fall in core temperature. In light of the fact that intracerebral microinjection of other cholinomimetic agents also produced hypothermia it seems likely that central cholinergic neurones are involved in activation of heat loss mechanisms. Since chlorpromazine possesses considerable anticholinergic activity, chlorpromazine might antagonize acetylcholine in the hypothalamic thermoregulatory centers.

Investigation of the effects of chlorpromazine on thermoregulation involved two general approaches: one centered around the response to quaternary chlorpromazine and the other based on the use of intracerebral microinjection. Both chlorpromazine and methyl chlorpromazine caused a fall in temperature following systemic injection in the rat. Since the polar quaternary derivative does not cross the blood–brain barrier, this response must be mediated at sites outside the central nervous system.

Chlorpromazine and methyl chlorpromazine caused an increase in core temperature following intracerebral microinjection into the hypothalamic thermoregulatory centers of the rat. Hyperthermia was also seen following intracerebral microinjection of anticholinergic drugs. These responses are probably due to inhibition of endogenous acetylcholine in the hypothalamic thermoregulatory centers. The specificity of the blockade induced by chlorpromazine could not be established, however, since the drug also produced a generalized neuronal blockade.

REFERENCES

1. Courvoisier, S., Fournel, J., Ducrat, R., Kolsky, M., and Koetschet, P., *Arch. Int. Pharmacodyn. Thér.*, **92**, 305 (1953).
2. Brodie, B. B., Sulser, F., and Costa, E., *Ann. Rev. Med.*, **12**, 349 (1961).
3. Schönbaum, E., and Lomax, P., *The Pharmacology of Thermoregulation*, Karger, Basel, 1973.
4. Vogt, M., *J. Physiol. (London)*, **123**, 451 (1954).
5. Brodie, B. B., and Shore, P. A., *Ann. N.Y. Acad. Sci.*, **66**, 631 (1957).
6. von Euler, C., *Pharmacol. Rev.*, **13**, 361 (1961).
7. Feldberg, W., and Myers, R. D., *Nature*, **200**, 1325 (1963).
8. Veale, W. L., and Cooper, K. E., in *The Pharmacology of Thermoregulation*, Schönbaum, E., and Lomax, P. (eds.), Karger, Basel, 1973, p. 289.
9. Feldberg, W., and Lotti, V. J., *Brit. J. Pharmacol.*, **31**, 152 (1967).
10. Lomax, P., Foster, R. S., and Kirkpatrick, W. E., *Brain Research*, **15**, 431 (1969).
11. Beckman, A. L., and Eisenman, J. S., *Science*, **170**, 334 (1970).
12. Brimblecombe, R. W., in *The Pharmacology of Thermoregulation*, Schönbaum, E., and Lomax, P., (eds.), Karger, Basel, 1973, p. 182.
13. Kirkpatrick, W. E., and Lomax, P., *Neuropharmacology*, **9**, 195 (1970).
14. Kirkpatrick, W. E., and Lomax, P., *Life Sci.*, **6**, 2273 (1967).

15. Knox, G. V., Campbell, C., and Lomax, P., *Brain Research*, **51**, 215 (1973).
16. Hansson, E., and Schmiterlöw, C. G., *Arch. Int. Pharmacodyn. Thér.*, **131**, 309 (1961).
17. Chevillard, L., Giorno, H., and Laury, M.-Cl., *C. R. Séanc. Soc. Biol.*, **152**, 1074 (1958).
18. de Groat, W. C., and Volle, R. L., *J. Pharmacol.*, **154**, 200 (1966).
19. Kirkpatrick, W. E., and Lomax, P., *Res. Comm. Chem. Path. Pharmacol.*, **1**, 149 (1970).
20. Ritchie, J. M., and Greengard, P., *Ann. Rev. Pharmacol.*, **6**, 405 (1966).
21. Narahashi, T., Anderson, N. C., and Moore, J. W., *Gen. Physiol.*, **50**, 1413 (1967).
22. Kirkpatrick, W. E., *M. A. dissertation*, University of California, Los Angeles, 1968, pp. 63–74.
23. Lomax, P., and Knox, G. V., in *The Pharmacology of Thermoregulation*, Schönbaum, E., and Lomax, P., (eds.), Karger, Basel, 1973, p. 146.
24. Hanin, I., and Jenden, D. J., *Biochem. Pharmacol.*, **18**, 837 (1969).

The Phenothiazines and Structurally Related Drugs, edited by I. S. Forrest, C. J. Carr, and E. Usdin. Raven Press, New York © 1974.

The Action of Chlorpromazine on the Metabolism of Cyclic Adenosine 3′,5′-Monophosphate

Maria Wollemann

Institute of Biochemistry, Biological Research Center, Hungarian Academy of Sciences, Szeged, Hungary

INTRODUCTION

The difficulties of explaining the effects of chlorpromazine (CPZ) on the molecular level are due primarily to the multiplicity of effects. The problem is how to select the specific ones from among all these effects.

Many of the phenothiazine actions are interpreted as membrane effects. The most varied types of membranes are used as models, such as artificial lipid-bilayer membranes (1), mitochondria (2), lysosomes (3), synaptosomes (4), thyroid-plasma membranes (5), muscle membranes (6), and erythrocytes (7). The phenothiazine binding to the proteins and lipids is generally explained by the cationic properties of the molecule. Enzymatic effects on soluble crystalline dehydrogenases (8–11) and membrane-bound ATPase (12) are attributed to the formation of free radicals from CPZ.

Effects of CPZ on the metabolism of cyclic adenosine 3′,5′-monophosphate (cAMP) are also reported but inconsistent. Kakiuchi and Rall (13, 14), using rabbit brain cortex and cerebellum, found a decreased cAMP level after histamine and norepinephrine stimulation of cerebellar slices with 5 and 50 μM CPZ. Injecting 15 mg/kg CPZ into rabbits 80 min prior to sacrifice, cAMP levels in brain cortex were diminished. Palmer et al. (15) reported a decrease of norepinephrine-stimulated cAMP levels without decrease of base levels of cAMP in chopped rat brain hypothalamus after treatment with 50 μM CPZ. Similar results were obtained by Uzunov and Weiss (16).

In contrast Ferendelli et al. (17) treated mice with 10 mg/kg CPZ and found no changes after 4 hr in the cAMP level of cerebellum, but a reduction in the cyclic guanosine 3′,5′-monophosphate (cGMP) level.

The metabolism of cAMP is regulated by the synthesizing enzyme, adenylate cyclase (18), and by the hydrolyzing enzyme, cyclic 3′,5′-nucleotide phosphodiesterase (19). The effect of CPZ on the membrane-bound adenylate-cyclase activity in thyroid, adrenal, and liver tissue, was investigated by Wolff and Jones (20). Base level activity was unaffected but hormone stimulation (thyrotropin, prostaglandin E_1, adrenocorticotropin, and epinephrine) was inhibited at 50 μM CPZ concentration. In contrast, fluoride-stimulated adenylate-cyclase activity was increased at similar CPZ concentrations (5, 20).

The effect of phenothiazines on the soluble phosphodiesterase activity was studied in rabbit brain and beef heart (21). The enzyme in brain was more sensitive to CPZ inhibition than the one in heart.

In view of these data, it seemed of interest to investigate the effect of CPZ on the cAMP level regulating enzymes in the same tissue. Rabbit and rat heart tissues were selected for this purpose and ventricles and atria were also compared.

EXPERIMENTAL PROCEDURE

Methods

Adult white inbred Wistar rats and young gray rabbits (1 to 1.2 kg body weight) were used for the experiments. Hearts were quickly excised in ether anesthesia and washed free from blood in Ringer solution. One gram of heart tissue was homogenized with 9 vol of 0.05 M Tris-HCl pH 7.4 buffer. The homogenate was centrifuged at 10,000 g at 0°C and washed twice with the same volume of buffer solution. The final precipitate was dissolved in 9 vol of Tris buffer and used immediately for measurements of adenylate-cyclase activity. Lubrol-PX® (Sigma Chemicals) solubilization was performed according to Levey (22). When no ATP-regenerating system was used, Tris buffer was supplemented with a final concentration of 0.25 M sucrose.

The reaction mixture for assay of adenylate cyclase activity contained 2 mM ATP (0.2 μCi ^{14}C-ATP); 3mM $MgCl_2$; 50 μg bovine serum albumin; 2 mM cAMP and 1 mM tetrahydroperparine were added to inhibit enzymatic destruction of labeled cAMP; 0.1 ml enzyme solution and 0.1 mg pyruvate kinase and 2 mM phosphoenolpyruvate were used for ATP regeneration. Hormones were added in a concentration of 50 μM if not otherwise indicated. The final volume was 0.3 ml. The incubation was carried out at 34°C for 10 min, if not otherwise indicated, and before boiling the samples at 100°C for 3 min, 0.1 ml recovery mixture (10 mM ATP and 1 mM cAMP) was added. After cooling, the samples were centrifuged and 0.05 ml of the supernatants were used in parallel assays for paper chromatography on Whatman 3-MM with the appropriate standard solutions. As solvents n-butanol, acetone, ammonia (5%), acetic acid, and water were used in a ratio 9:3:2:2:4. Four passes by ascending paper chromatography were performed. After complete separation of the adenine nucleotides, the appropriate spots were detected in ultraviolet light, excised, and the radioactivity of the samples was counted in a Packard Liquid Scintillation Spectrometer using Bray's solution.

Phosphodiesterase activity was measured in the following reaction mixture: 2mM 3',5'cAMP (5 μCi ^{3}H-cAMP), 2 mM MgCl$_2$, 0.1-ml enzyme. The supernatant from the first centrifugation was used for phosphodiesterase purification according to Drummond (19). The incubation and determination of ^{3}H-AMP was carried out essentially in the same way as described for the adenylate-cyclase assay, except that finally ^{3}H-AMP was determined. In order to follow ^{3}H-AMP degradation, labeled adenosine was also measured in some cases with and without addition of 5'nucleotidase (0.1-mg Crotalus adamanteus venom). Protein was measured with the biuret method.

Materials

All fine chemicals were purchased from Sigma, St. Louis, Missouri; radioactive chemicals were from New England Nuclear, Boston. CPZ was a gift from Specia, Paris. Irradiated CPZ was prepared as published previously (8, 9).

RESULTS

Membrane-Bound Adenylate-Cyclase Activity

In Table 1, the action of CPZ on the particulate adenylate-cyclase activity of rabbit atria and ventricles is demonstrated. The base level activity of adenylate cyclase was higher in the atrium than in the ventricle, but it was not affected by CPZ. Irradiated CPZ stimulated the base level adenylate-cyclase activity. The stimulating actions of isoproterenol, norepinephrine, and histamine were inhibited by CPZ. Glucagon stimulation was not inhibited. Stimulators of alpha-receptor such as phenylephrine and methoxa-

TABLE 1. *The effect of CPZ on the adenylate-cyclase activity from rabbit heart*

Addition	Picomoles cAMP accumulated/10 min/mg protein			
	Ventricle		Atrium	
	Control	CPZ 100 μM	Control	100 μM CPZ
—	958 ± 42	920 ± 36	1330 ± 52	1280 ± 63
Isoproterenol 50 μM	1528 ± 72	963 ± 28	1950 ± 43	1250 ± 30
Norepinephrine 50 μM	1475 ± 64	942 ± 47	2000 ± 75	1260 ± 44
Histamine 50 μM	1640 ± 85	1016 ± 30	2420 ± 61	1340 ± 54
Glucagon 10 μM	1720 ± 52	1684 ± 48	2385 ± 78	2290 ± 57
Phenylephrine 50 μM	1030 ± 45	1090 ± 62	1410 ± 54	1470 ± 43
Methoxamine 50 μM	1100 ± 24	1042 ± 45	1460 ± 38	1480 ± 37
Ca^{++} 1 mM	450 ± 28	500 ± 30	845 ± 46	912 ± 39

Each value represents the mean ± S.E. of four samples.

mine had no effect on base levels of adenylate-cyclase activity. The action of fluoride on the adenylate-cyclase activity was potentiated by CPZ. Ca^{++} inhibition of adenylate-cyclase activity was not significantly influenced by CPZ.

Solubilized Adenylate-Cyclase Activity

After solubilization of the membrane-bound adenylate-cyclase, activity with the anionic detergent Lubrol-PX®, hormonal stimulation is lost but fluoride stimulation is retained (22). In Table 2, data are demonstrated for the effect of CPZ on the solubilized adenylate cyclase activity. The inhibitory as well as stimulatory actions of CPZ on the adenylate-cyclase activity ceased completely after solubilization of the enzyme. The stimulating effect of irradiated CPZ on the base level of cyclase activity was lost after solubilization. Stimulatory actions of CPZ on the solubilized enzyme could not be restored by the addition of phospholipids (phosphatidylserine and phosphatidylinositol) (23).

TABLE 2. *The effect of CPZ and fluoride on the base level and solubilized adenylate-cyclase activity from rabbit heart*

	Picomoles cAMP accumulated/10 min/mg protein			
	Ventricle		Atrium	
Addition	Base level	NaF 8 mM	Base level	NaF 8 mM
—	945 ± 27	1980 ± 74	1420 ± 32	2570 ± 53
CPZ 50 μM	959 ± 33	2310 ± 56	1385 ± 43	2780 ± 48
CPZ 100 μM	930 ± 42	3650 ± 63	1390 ± 37	3980 ± 57
CPZ 250 μM	918 ± 29	4140 ± 49	1348 ± 52	4890 ± 65
CPZ 500 μM	910 ± 48	2540 ± 38	1363 ± 34	3250 ± 42
CPZ+ 100 μM	1440 ± 29	—	1890 ± 51	—
Lubrol-PX® 20 mM	1090 ± 45	1870 ± 57	1610 ± 44	2750 ± 53
CPZ 100 μM+LUBROL-PX®	1045 ± 39	1848 ± 28	1660 ± 36	2800 ± 61
CPZ 250 μM+LUBROL-PX®	1067 ± 44	1833 ± 42	1597 ± 57	2772 ± 53
CPZ+ 100 μM+LUBROL-PX®	1120 ± 28	—	1635 ± 37	—

Each value represents the mean ± S.E. of four samples.
CPZ+ = irradiated chlorpromazine.

Cyclic 3',5'-Nucleotide Phosphodiesterase Activity

The inhibitory action of CPZ on the phosphodiesterase activity of rabbit heart ventricles and atria were noncompetitive as determined from the double reciprocal plots according to Lineweaver and Burk (Figs. 1 and 2) (24). K_i Values were obtained graphically by the Dixon method (Figs. 3 and 4) (25). The K_i values were different for atria and ventricles; atria were more sensitive to CPZ inhibition. Base levels of phosphodiesterase activity differed insignificantly in atria and ventricles (Table 3).

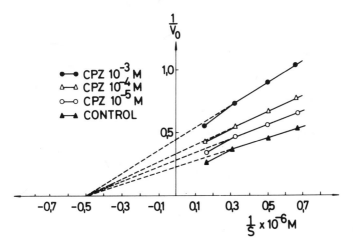

FIG. 1. Lineweaver-Burk plots of phosphodiesterase inhibition by chlorpromazine in rabbit-heart ventricle.

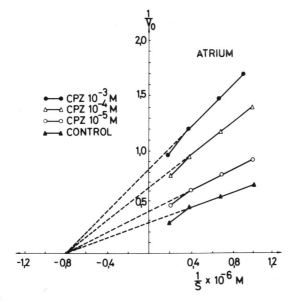

FIG. 2. Lineweaver-Burk plots of phosphodiesterase inhibition by chlorpromazine in rabbit-heart atrium.

DISCUSSION

According to the reported results the base level of adenylate-cyclase activity is not influenced by CPZ, whereas hormone stimulation of the enzyme is inhibited by CPZ. This effect of CPZ is most probably exerted

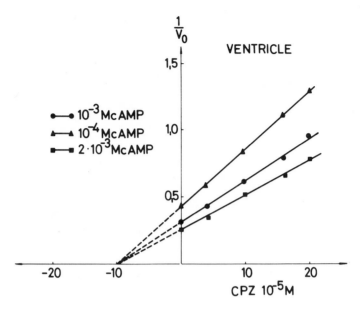

FIG. 3. Dixon plots of the effect of chlorpromazine on the phosphodiesterase activity in rabbit-heart ventricle.

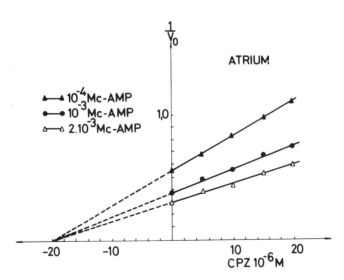

FIG. 4. Dixon plots of the effect of chlorpromazine on the phosphodiesterase activity in rabbit-heart atrium.

through the hormone receptor, rather than through direct action on the enzyme itself. The stimulatory effect of CPZ on fluoride activation of the thyroid adenylate-cyclase activity has been explained by Wolff and Jones (5, 20) as a membrane-expanding detergent action. This is further confirmed in our experiments by the fact that after Lubrol® solubilization, this action

TABLE 3. *Apparent K_m and K_i values for phosphodiesterase activity in rabbit heart*

	Atrium	Ventricle
cAMP K_m	1.2×10^{-5} M	2×10^{-5} M
CPZ K_i	2.1×10^{-5} M	1×10^{-4} M

of CPZ is also abolished, and it could not be restored even after addition of phospholipids (23).

The phosphodiesterase activity was inhibited in a noncompetitive manner both in atria and ventricles, but atria were more sensitive to CPZ inhibition. The differences in inhibition can be explained either by the different iso-enzyme composition of phosphodiesterase (26) or by the different quantities of phosphodiesterase activators (27, 28).

In the generally used CPZ concentrations (50 to 100 μM), Mg^{++}-stimulated ATPase activity was not influenced in our preparations, but the Ca^{++}-stimulated ATPase was inhibited by CPZ. At the same time CPZ did not influence Ca^{++} inhibition of adenylate cyclase (29), thus no competition occurred between Ca^{++}- and CPZ-binding sites on the enzyme (30).

The higher adenylate-cyclase activity of atria is inconsistent with previous data obtained on tissue slices (31). However, the adenylate-cyclase activity in slices depended also on the rate of ATP synthesis from labeled adenosine or adenine. We observed differences in activity between atria and ventricles after *in vivo* reserpine treatment of rabbits (0.5 mg/kg) injected 24 hr before sacrifice and after solubilization with Lubrol-PX®.

CONCLUSIONS

In conclusion, the double effect of CPZ consisting partly of the inhibition of hormonal activation of adenylate-cyclase activity and partly of the inhibition of the phosphodiesterase activity, might result in a regulatory action on the level of *c*AMP. Which of the two effects will dominate *in vivo* depends on the actual hormone and CPZ concentrations in the investigated tissue.

ACKNOWLEDGMENT

The author wishes to thank Aniko Nagy and Katalin Adam for technical assistance in these studies.

REFERENCES

1. Mueller, P., and Rudin, D. O., *Nature,* **213,** 603 (1967).
2. Spirtes, M. A., and Guth, P. S., *Nature,* **190,** 274 (1961).
3. Koenig, H., and Jirbel, A., *Biochim. Biophys. Acta,* **65,** 543 (1962).
4. Guth, P. S., *Fed. Proc.,* **21,** 6, 1100 (1962).

5. Wolff, J., and Jones, A. B., *J. Biol. Chem.*, **246**, 3939 (1971).
6. Balzer, H., Makinose, M., Fiehn, W., and Hasselbach, W., *Arch. Pharmakol. Exp. Pathol.*, **260**, 456 (1968).
7. Seeman, P., and Weinstein, J., *Biochem. Pharmacol.*, **15**, 1737 (1966).
8. Wollemann, M., and Elodi, P., *Biochem. Pharmacol.*, **6**, 228 (1961).
9. Wollemann, M., *Biochem. Pharmacol.*, **12**, 757 (1963).
10. Nagy, A., and Wollemann, M., *Biochem. Pharmacol.*, **20**, 3331 (1971).
11. Levey, L., and Burbridge, T. N., *Biochem. Pharmacol.*, **16**, 1249 (1967).
12. Akera, T., and Brody, T. M., *Mol. Pharmacol.*, **4**, 600 (1968).
13. Kakiuchi, S., and Rall, T. W., *Mol. Pharmacol.*, **4**, 367 (1968).
14. Kakiuchi, S., and Rall, T. W., *Mol. Pharmacol.*, **4**, 379 (1968).
15. Palmer, G. C., Robison, G. A., and Sulser, F., *Biochem. Pharmacol.*, **20**, 236 (1971).
16. Uzunov, P., and Weiss, B., *Neuropharmacology*, **10**, 697 (1971).
17. Ferrendelli, J. A., Kinscherf, D. A., and Kipnis, D. M., *Biochem. Biophys. Res. Commun.*, **46**, 2114 (1972).
18. Sutherland, E. W., Rall, T. W., and Menon, T., *J. Biol. Chem.*, **237**, 1220 (1962).
19. Drummond, G. I., and Perrot-Yee, S., *J. Biol. Chem.*, **236**, 1126 (1961).
20. Wolff, J., and Jones, A. B., *Proc. Nat. Acad. Sci. U.S.A.*, **65**, 454 (1970).
21. Honda, F., and Imamura, H., *Biochim. Biophys. Acta*, **161**, 267 (1968).
22. Levey, G. S., *Biochem. Biophys. Res. Commun.*, **38**, 86 (1970).
23. Levey, G. S., *Ann. N.Y. Acad. Sci.*, **185**, 449 (1971).
24. Lineweaver, H., and Burk, D., *J. Am. Chem. Soc.*, **56**, 658 (1934).
25. Dixon, M., *Biochem. J.*, **55**, 170 (1953).
26. Monn, E., and Christiansen, R. O., *Science*, **173**, 540 (1971).
27. Cheung, W. Y., *J. Biol. Chem.*, **246**, 2859 (1971).
28. Teo, T. S., Wang, T. H., and Wang, J. H., *J. Biol. Chem.*, **248**, 588 (1973).
29. Bradham, L. S., Holt, D. A., and Sims, M., *Biochim. Biophys. Acta*, **201**, 250 (1970).
30. Kwant, W. O., and Seeman, P., *Biochim. Biophys. Acta*, **183**, 338 (1969).
31. Lee, T. P., Kuo, J. F., and Greengard, P., *Biochem. Biophys. Res. Commun.*, **45**, 991 (1971).

The Phenothiazines and Structurally Related Drugs, edited by I. S. Forrest, C. J. Carr, and E. Usdin. Raven Press, New York © 1974.

Inhibition by Phenothiazines of Adenylate Cyclase in Adrenal and Brain Tissue

Charles A. Free, Velma S. Paik, and J. Dennis Shada

Department of Biochemical Pharmacology, Squibb Institute for Medical Research, Princeton, New Jersey 08540

INTRODUCTION

The observation was made by Wolff and Jones (1) that phenothiazines inhibit the hormonally stimulated activity of adenylate cyclase preparations from thyroid, adrenal, and liver tissue. In a more recent study (2), five phenothiazines were found to inhibit the isoproterenol-activated adenylate cyclase activity of guinea pig lung; the same compounds also acted as potent inhibitors of ACTH-activated steroidogenesis in the rat adrenal cell and of epinephrine-activated lipolysis in the rat epididymal fat cell, a pair of metabolic processes considered to be regulated by adenosine 3',5'-cyclic monophosphate (cyclic AMP) (3). The present study was conducted to explore the mechanisms of inhibition by phenothiazines and related compounds in cyclic AMP-mediated biological systems at the cellular level.

EXPERIMENTAL PROCEDURE

Materials

The experimental compounds and drugs employed in the study were generously provided by the following sources: thioridazine, Sandoz Pharmaceuticals; imipramine, Geigy Pharmaceuticals; amitriptyline, Merck, Sharp, and Dohme; promethazine, Wyeth Laboratories; chlorpromazine, Smith, Kline, and French Laboratories; triflupromazine, 3-chloro-10-(3-dimethylaminopropyl) phenothiazine, 2-trifluoromethyl-10-(3-chloropropyl) phenothiazine, and 3-chloro-10-phenothiazinepropionitrile, E. R. Squibb and Sons; pyrvinium pamoate, Parke-Davis and Co.; haloperidol, McNeil Laboratories; aminoglutethimide, Ciba Pharmaceutical Co. Puromycin hydrochloride and cyclic AMP were purchased from Nutritional Biochemicals Corp. and Jem Research Products, respectively. Tritium-labeled adenine (15.8 C/mmole) was purchased from Schwarz-Mann and purified according to the procedure of Humes et al. (4) prior to use. ^{32}P-Cyclic AMP was purchased from New England Nuclear.

Methods

The preparation and incubation of isolated rat adrenal cells were according to established procedures (5, 6). In brief, decapsulated rat adrenals were digested with collagenase; the resulting cells were washed and resuspended in Krebs-Ringer bicarbonate buffer containing 3% albumin and 0.2% glucose. Of the experimental compounds employed in the study, 2-trifluoro-methyl-10-(3-chloropropyl) phenothiazine, 3-chloro-10-phenothiazinepropionitrile, pyrvinium pamoate, and haloperidol were dissolved in dimethyl sulfoxide and added to incubation mixtures in volumes of 10 μl or less; the remaining compounds were added as aqueous solutions in volumes of 100 μl or less. Individual incubation mixtures, each containing cells equivalent to one adrenal gland, experimental compound, and Krebs-Ringer buffer to a final volume of 2.5 ml, were incubated at 35°C, under 95% O_2:5% CO_2, for 2 hr. After incubation, the corticosterone concentrations in the mixtures were measured by a fluorimetric procedure (6, 7).

The accumulation of ^{3}H-cyclic AMP in hippocampal slices from male, Hartley strain guinea pigs, was measured by the procedure of Chasin and colleagues (8). In brief, slices approximately 0.2 mm in height, width, and depth were prepared with a McIlwain tissue chopper, and then suspended (35 to 40 mg of tissue/ml) in Krebs-Ringer bicarbonate buffer containing 0.2% glucose and ^{3}H-adenine (10 to 25 μC/ml). The slices were incubated initially for 10 min, then were redistributed in 2-ml aliquots to individual flasks and incubated again for 40 min. Finally, 1 ml of buffer containing appropriate hormone and/or test substance, was added to each flask; this addition was followed by a third incubation for 15 min. All incubations were at 37°C under 95% O_2:5% CO_2. After termination of the third incubation by the addition of trichloroacetic acid containing ^{32}P-cyclic AMP (>5 nC), the cyclic AMP in the incubation mixtures was purified and quantitated by liquid-scintillation spectrometry. Accumulations of ^{3}H-cyclic AMP are expressed in disintegrations per min (dpm) per mg of protein, after correction for recovery of ^{32}P-cyclic AMP.

RESULTS

Inhibition of Steroidogenesis in Isolated Adrenal Cells

Previous studies (5) have shown that cyclic AMP and ACTH activate adrenal cells to the same maximum rate of corticosterone formation; the concentrations required for half-maximal activation are approximately 0.1 to 0.2 nM for ACTH and 3 mM for cyclic AMP, respectively. Thirteen compounds, including previously known inhibitors of steroidogenesis as well as phenothiazines and related tricyclic agents, were examined for relative potency as inhibitors in adrenal cells half-maximally activated by ACTH and cyclic AMP. The inhibition of steroidogenesis at various concentrations of two representative phenothiazines, promethazine and chlorpromazine, is shown in Fig. 1. Each compound generated a pair of inhibition curves that varied with the activator of the adrenal cells; each inhibitor was considerably more effective in cells activated by ACTH than in those activated by cyclic AMP. Two other inhibitors (puromycin and aminoglutethimide) each generated a pair of virtually superimposable curves (Fig. 2) in the presence of ACTH and cyclic AMP, respectively.

By interpolation from their inhibition curves, the concentrations (I_{50} values) required to inhibit steroidogenesis by 50% were determined for the agents shown in Figs. 1 and 2, and for the nine other compounds. These I_{50} values are summarized in Table 1. On the basis of the ratios of their I_{50} values in cyclic AMP- versus ACTH-activated cells, the inhibitors tend to divide into two groups. The initial seven compounds in the table, including phenothiazines and related tricyclic agents, constitute a group characterized by inhibitory potencies ranging from three- to 10-fold greater against ACTH-activated than against cyclic AMP-activated steroidogenesis. Two additional phenothiazines failed to inhibit steroidogenesis in the presence of ACTH or of cyclic AMP. The last four compounds in Table 1 comprise a second group characterized by inhibitory potencies against ACTH-activated cells that are similar to those against cyclic AMP-activated cells.

The inhibition of steroidogenesis by chlorpromazine at various concentrations of ACTH is illustrated in Fig. 3. With increasing concentrations of hormone, the degree of inhibition successively decreased. Chlorpromazine at 50 μM, for example, inhibited the effects of 0.05, 0.1, 0.2, and 2.0 nM

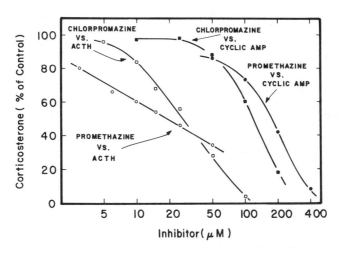

FIG. 1. Effects of inhibitors on ACTH(0.1 nM)—versus cyclic AMP(3 mM)—activated steroidogenesis in rat adrenal cells. Each point represents the mean from duplicate incubation mixtures.

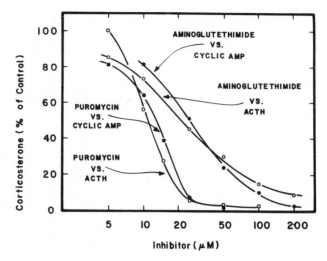

FIG. 2. Effects of inhibitors on ACTH(0.1 nM)−versus cyclic AMP(3 mM)−activated steroidogenesis in rat adrenal cells. Each point represents the mean from duplicate incubation mixtures.

TABLE 1. Inhibitors of steroidogenesis in rat adrenal cells

	Activator		
	ACTH (0.1 nM)	Cyclic AMP (3mM)	
Compound	I_{50} (μM)		I_{50} Ratio[a]
Thioridazine	7	65	9.3
Imipramine	16	140	8.8
Amitriptyline	18	175	9.7
3-Chloro-10-(3-dimethylamino-propyl) phenothiazine	18	75	4.2
Promethazine	19	175	9.2
Chlorpromazine	26	120	4.6
Triflupromazine	50	160	3.2
2-Trifluoromethyl-10-(3-chloropropyl) phenothiazine	Inactive[b]	Inactive	—
3-Chloro-10-phenothiazine-propionitrile	Inactive	Inactive	—
Pyrvinium pamoate	0.18	0.15	0.8
Puromycin	11	13	1.2
Haloperidol	13	28	2.2
Aminoglutethimide	21	25	1.2

[a] Cyclic AMP I_{50}/ACTH I_{50}.
[b] No inhibition at 200 μM.

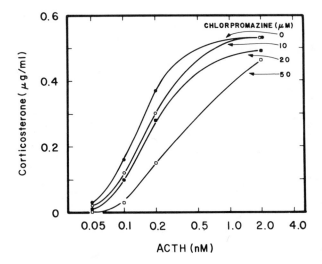

FIG. 3. Inhibition by chlorpromazine of steroidogenesis in rat adrenal cells as a function of ACTH concentration. Each point represents the mean from duplicate incubation mixtures.

ACTH by 100, 81, 59, and 13%, respectively, indicating that high concentrations of hormone can reverse the inhibitory action of the phenothiazine.

Inhibition of Accumulation of Cyclic AMP in Guinea Pig Hippocampus

The neurohormones epinephrine and histamine stimulate the accumulation of ^{3}H-cyclic AMP in slices from the hippocampus of guinea pig brain, following prelabeling of the slices with ^{3}H-adenine (9). Typical stimulations achieved with 100 μM concentrations of epinephrine or histamine are two- and eightfold, respectively. Figure 4 illustrates the effects of chlorpromazine, at various concentrations, on the histamine-stimulated tissue. Inhibition of accumulation of cyclic AMP is evident at chlorpromazine concentrations of 1 μM or lower; 10 μM chlorpromazine inhibited the histamine-stimulated increase by 55%. In contrast, basal levels of ^{3}H-cyclic AMP were not affected by chlorpromazine at 100 μM. Table 2 summarizes the effects of chlorpromazine on both histamine- and epinephrine-stimulated activities. Chlorpromazine also reversed the stimulation by epinephrine; at concentrations of 1, 10, and 100 μM, chlorpromazine blocked the increase of ^{3}H-cyclic AMP by 31, 49, and 77%, respectively.

Table 3 shows the effects of the dibenzazepine imipramine on the accumulation of ^{3}H-cyclic AMP. Like chlorpromazine, the compound had little effect on the accumulation of cyclic AMP in the absence of hormone. Imipramine was comparable in potency to chlorpromazine as an inhibitor of histamine-stimulated activity, but appeared relatively weaker as an inhibitor

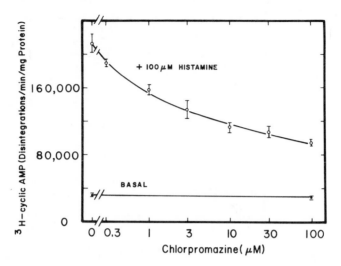

FIG. 4. Inhibition by chlorpromazine of the histamine-stimulated accumulation of ³H-cyclic AMP in slices from guinea pig hippocampus. Each point represents the mean ± standard error from triplicate incubation mixtures.

TABLE 2. *Inhibition by chlorpromazine of accumulation of ³H-cyclic AMP in slices of guinea pig hippocampus*

	Percent of basal ³H-cyclic AMP ± SEM[a]			
	Chlorpromazine (μM)			
Stimulator	0	1	10	100
None	100 ± 5[b]	—	—	92 ± 6
Histamine (100 μM)	663 ± 34	490 ± 19	350 ± 18	296 ± 12
None	100 ± 8[c]	—	—	89 ± 10
Epinephrine (100 μM)	171 ± 12	149 ± 8	136 ± 5	116 ± 1

[a] Each value is the mean from triplicate incubation mixtures.
[b,c] The mean basal accumulations of ³H-cyclic AMP are 32,100[b] and 62,900[c] dpm per mg of protein, corresponding to conversions of 0.51 and 0.35% from total ³H-adenine, respectively.

of epinephrine-stimulated cyclic AMP accumulation as indicated by the lack of significant effect at an imipramine concentration of 10 μM.

DISCUSSION

Phenothiazines such as chlorpromazine, at concentrations of 2 to 20 μM, bind to cell membranes with consequent alterations in properties of the membranes (10). In the case of the plasma membrane of the human erythrocyte, these alterations include an increase in surface area and an increased resistance to osmotic lysis. The activity of a membrane-associated enzyme,

TABLE 3. *Inhibition by imipramine of accumulation of ^{3}H-cyclic AMP in slices of guinea pig hippocampus*

	Percent of basal ^{3}H-cyclic AMP ± SEM[a]			
	Imipramine (μM)			
Stimulator	0	1	10	100
None	100 ± 4[b]	—	—	78 ± 5
Histamine (100 μM)	478 ± 17	381 ± 27	275 ± 21	201 ± 7
None	100 ± 9[c]	—	—	90 ± 5
Epinephrine (100 μM)	186 ± 7	197 ± 4	184 ± 12	135 ± 6

[a] Each value is the mean from triplicate incubation mixtures.

[b,c] The mean basal accumulations of ^{3}H-cyclic AMP are 33,400[b] and 26,600[c] dpm per mg of protein, corresponding to conversions of 0.42 and 0.36% from total ^{3}H-adenine, respectively.

ATPase, is inhibited by various phenothiazines at concentrations of 50 μM or less (11). A second membrane-associated enzyme, adenylate cyclase, is likewise inhibited by chlorpromazine and trifluoperazine (1). The latter study, employing cyclases of rat adrenal, rat liver, and bovine thyroid membranes, as well as more recent investigations with the adenylate cyclase of guinea pig lung (2), indicated that the phenothiazines interfere with activation of the cyclase by various hormones, with little effect on the basal activity of the enzyme.

In a study of the effects of 158 therapeutic agents on cyclic AMP metabolism (2), the phenothiazines and related compounds were found to be particularly effective inhibitors of ACTH-activated steroidogenesis in the isolated adrenal cell. This observation suggested that phenothiazines might act as inhibitors of adenylate cyclase in intact cells or tissues as well as at the subcellular level. Current theory holds that the steroidogenic effects of ACTH are mediated through cyclic AMP synthesized by ACTH-activated adenylate cyclase in the adrenal cell membrane. Because it appeared reasonable that agents inhibiting steroidogenesis specifically through inhibition of adenylate cyclase would be effective primarily against stimulation of steroidogenesis by ACTH, but not by exogenous cyclic AMP, the inhibitory effects of a series of phenothiazines were measured in the presence of half-maximally activating concentrations of ACTH versus cyclic AMP. The first seven phenothiazines and tricyclic compounds in Table 1, all potent inhibitors of ACTH-activated steroidogenesis, were only one-10th to one-third as potent as inhibitors of steroidogenesis produced by exogenous cyclic AMP. The cellular inhibitory actions of these agents thus appeared to result from their inhibition of ACTH-activated adenylate cyclase. Interestingly, 2-trifluoromethyl-10-(3-chloropropyl) phenothiazine and 3-chloro-10-phenothiazinepropionitrile, each lacking a side-chain amino group, were totally inactive.

For comparative purposes, a group of inhibitors with structures differing from those of the phenothiazines was tested for relative inhibition of ACTH-versus cyclic-AMP-activated steroidogenesis. Those agents inhibiting events in the steroidogenic pathway distal to the site of action of cyclic AMP, or those acting as general metabolic inhibitors or cytotoxic agents might be expected to inhibit equally the actions of ACTH or exogenous cyclic AMP. Both puromycin, a probable inhibitor of the synthesis of protein required for corticosteroidogenesis (12), and aminoglutethimide, an inhibitor of cholesterol desmolase (13), were, in fact, equally effective as inhibitors of the actions of ACTH or of cyclic AMP. Pyrvinium pamoate, an agent with an unknown inhibitory mechanism in the adrenal cell, was likewise equally effective against ACTH- or cyclic AMP-activated steroidogenesis. Haloperidol, an agent with properties characteristic of an inhibitor of adenylate cyclase in rat brainstem (14) and rat cerebellum (15), displayed an I_{50} of 13 μM against ACTH-activated steroidogenesis. Because of its relatively potent I_{50} of 28 μM in the presence of cyclic AMP, however, haloperidol was not grouped with the tricyclic compounds.

Competition experiments with ACTH and chlorpromazine in the isolated adrenal cell demonstrated that high concentrations of ACTH reverse the inhibitory action of chlorpromazine. This finding lends further support to an inhibition mechanism wherein phenothiazines interfere with the activation of adenylate cyclase by ACTH. A related observation has been made with canine thyroid slices (16), in which the inhibitory effects of chlorpromazine on thyrotropin-stimulated cyclic AMP levels were partially reversed by increased concentrations of thyrotropin. The inhibition of corticosterone formation by chlorpromazine has been previously reported by Haksar and Peron (17), who utilized a preparation of quartered rat adrenals. These authors, however, observed that chlorpromazine, at concentrations of 50 to 500 μM, produced similar inhibitions regardless of whether ACTH ($>$500 nM) or cyclic AMP (5 to 12 mM) had been used to activate the tissue. The results of the latter study are not necessarily at variance with ours, in that we have also observed similar inhibitions of about 12% (Figs. 1 and 3) with 50 μM chlorpromazine in the presence of 2 nM ACTH or 3 mM cyclic AMP; the more potent and selective inhibition of steroidogenesis by chlorpromazine was observed only during activation of adrenal cells by concentrations of ACTH $<$ 2 nM.

The accumulation of ^{3}H-cyclic AMP in brain slices prelabeled with ^{3}H-adenine was employed as a second test system for assessing the effects of inhibitors of adenylate cyclase in an intact tissue. The hippocampus of guinea pig brain was selected because of its dual sensitivity to histamine or epinephrine (9). Experiments with chlorpromazine revealed a very potent inhibition of the accumulation of ^{3}H-cyclic AMP resulting from stimulation by either histamine or epinephrine. Imipramine, although similar in potency to chlorpromazine as an inhibitor of the effects of histamine, was a weaker inhibitor of the accumulation of ^{3}H-cyclic AMP resulting from stimulation by epinephrine.

The preceding results are consistent with the reported actions of phenothiazines on cyclic AMP in other brain preparations. For example, chlorpromazine has been shown to inhibit the accumulation of cyclic AMP produced by norepinephrine or histamine in rabbit cerebellum (18), or by norepinephrine in rat brainstem and hypothalamus (14, 19). Chlorpromazine also appeared to inhibit the postdecapitation increase of cyclic AMP in the rabbit cerebral cortex (20), as well as in the rat cerebellum (19). More recently, Huang and Daly (21), employing prelabeling with ^{3}H-adenine, have observed that histamine- and epinephrine-stimulated accumulations of ^{3}H-cyclic AMP in cerebral cortex of guinea pig are inhibited by chlorpromazine and imipramine at 100 μM; at 500 μM, however, both chlorpromazine and imipramine acted to increase levels of ^{3}H-cyclic AMP.

SUMMARY

Seven phenothiazines and related tricyclic amines inhibited the ACTH-activated formation of corticosterone in isolated adrenal cells at I_{50} concentrations ranging from 7 to 50 μM. The same compounds were only one-10th to one-third as potent as inhibitors of cyclic AMP-activated steroidogenesis, suggesting a primary inhibition at the level of adenylate cyclase in the cells. High concentrations (2 nM) of ACTH reversed the inhibitory effect of chlorpromazine, lending further support to the concept of an inhibitory mechanism involving interference by the phenothiazines in activation of adenylate cyclase by ACTH.

Chlorpromazine and imipramine (1 to 100 μM) also inhibited the histamine- or epinephrine-stimulated accumulation of ^{3}H-cyclic AMP in ^{3}H-adenine-prelabeled slices of guinea pig hippocampus, a system designed to measure direct effects of the compounds on synthesis of cyclic AMP in a hormone-sensitive tissue.

These studies provide evidence that phenothiazines and related compounds that act as potent inhibitors of hormonally activated adenylate cyclase at the subcellular level can demonstrate effects that are consistent with this locus of inhibition in the cyclic AMP-mediated systems of intact cells.

REFERENCES

1. Wolff, J., and Jones, A. B., *Proc. Nat. Acad. Sci. U.S.A.*, **65**, 454 (1970).
2. Weinryb, I., Chasin, M., Free, C. A., Harris, D. N., Goldenberg, H., Michel, I. M., Paik, V. S., Phillips, M., Samaniego, S., and Hess, S. M., *J. Pharm. Sci.*, **61**, 1556 (1972).
3. Robison, G. A., Butcher, R. W., and Sutherland, E. W., *Cyclic AMP*, Academic Press, New York, 1971.
4. Humes, J. L., Rounbehler, M., and Kuehl, F. A., *Anal. Biochem.*, **32**, 210 (1969).
5. Free, C. A., Chasin, M., Paik, V. S., and Hess, S. M., *Biochemistry*, **10**, 3785 (1971).

6. Free, C. A., in *Methods in Cyclic Nucleotide Research*, Chasin, M. (ed.), Marcel Dekker, New York, 1972, pp. 223–254.
7. Mattingly, D., *J. Clin. Pathol.*, **15**, 374 (1962).
8. Chasin, M., Rivkin, I., Mamrak, F., Samaniego, S. G., and Hess, S. M., *J. Biol. Chem.*, **246**, 3037 (1971).
9. Chasin, M., Mamrak, F., Samaniego, S. G., and Hess, S. M., *Fed. Proc.*, **31**, 440 Abs (1972).
10. Kwant, W. O., and Seeman, P., *Biochim. Biophys. Acta*, **183**, 530 (1969).
11. Davis, P. W., and Brody, T. M., *Biochem. Pharmacol.*, **15**, 703 (1966).
12. Garren, L. D., Davis, W. W., Crocco, R. M., and Ney, R. L., *Science*, **152**, 1386 (1966).
13. Cohen, M. P., *Proc. Soc. Exp. Biol. Med.*, **127**, 1086 (1968).
14. Palmer, G. C., Robison, G. A., and Sulser, F., *Biochem. Pharmacol.*, **20**, 236 (1971).
15. Uzunov, P., and Weiss, B., in *Advances in Cyclic Nucleotide Research, Vol. 1*, Greengard, P., Robison, G. A., and Paoletti, R. (eds.), Raven Press, New York, 1972, pp. 435–453.
16. Yamashita, K., Bloom, G., Rainard, B., Zor, U., and Field, J. B., *Metabolism*, **19**, 1109 (1970).
17. Haksar, A., and Peron, F. G., *Biochem. Biophys. Res. Commun.*, **44**, 1376 (1971).
18. Kakiuchi, S., and Rall, T. W., *Mol. Pharmacol.*, **4**, 367 (1968).
19. Uzunov, P., and Weiss, B., *Neuropharmacology*, **10**, 697 (1971).
20. Kakiuchi, S., and Rall, T. W., *Mol. Pharmacol.*, **4**, 379 (1968).
21. Huang, M., and Daly, J. W., *J. Med. Chem.*, **15**, 458 (1972).

The Phenothiazines and Structurally Related Drugs, edited by I. S.
Forrest, C. J. Carr, and E. Usdin. Raven Press, New York © 1974.

Effects of Phenothiazines and Phenothiazine Metabolites on Adenyl Cyclase and the Cyclic AMP Response in the Rat Brain

Gene C. Palmer and Albert A. Manian*

*Department of Pharmacology, University of New Mexico School of Medicine, 915 Stanford N.E., Albuquerque, New Mexico 87106, and *National Institute of Mental Health, Rockville, Maryland 20852*

INTRODUCTION

The brain contains one of the highest adenyl cyclase activities (1) and brain slices incubated in the presence of neurohumoral agents readily accumulate cyclic 3',5'-adenosine monophosphate (cyclic AMP) (2–5). Likewise, neurohumoral agents activate the enzyme in both neuronal and glial elements (6–8). However, it has been shown that synaptosomes contain the highest adenyl cyclase activity of any central subcellular fraction (9). Subsequent investigations have indicated an active role for cyclic AMP in certain types of synaptic transmission (10, 11).

Several lines of evidence suggest that a correlation exists between the psychotropic potency of certain drugs and their ability to modify central adenyl cyclase activity (2, 4, 12–16). In this regard pharmacologically active phenothiazines are indeed potent inhibitors of brain adenyl cyclase activity as well as antagonizing the neurohumoral-induced accumulation of cyclic AMP in brain slices *in vitro* (2, 12, 13, 17–19). Perhaps the central antiadrenergic effects of phenothiazines are exerted at the level of the adenyl cyclase-receptor complex.

The present experiments were initiated in order to study, in a more extensive and precise way, the manner in which several phenothiazines and their derivatives modify the adenyl cyclase cyclic AMP system in the rat brain. To provide a means to demonstrate an effect of phenothiazines upon the catalytic component of the enzyme, broken cell preparations were utilized. In this regard preparations were isolated from either the high-speed particulate fraction of the hypothalamus and cerebral cortex or disrupted neuronal and glial-enriched fractions from the cerebral cortex. In an attempt to demonstrate the action of phenothiazines on the receptor component of adenyl cyclase, the drugs were added to incubated tissue slices (cerebral cortex and medial and lateral hypothalamus) in the presence of norepinephrine (NE) and the resultant levels of cyclic AMP were determined.

EXPERIMENTAL PROCEDURE

Broken Cell Preparations

Male rats (Sprague-Dawley-Holtzman) weighing 100 to 140 gm were decapitated and the cerebral cortex and hypothalamus were dissected free, weighed, and homogenized in 10 vol of cold glycyl glycine buffer (2 mM + 1 mM $MgSO_4$, pH 7.4). The samples were then centrifuged at $100,000 \times g$ for 30 min, the supernatant removed and the pellet resuspended in glycyl glycine buffer and recentrifuged. Following the centrifugation, the supernatant was again discarded, the pellet resuspended, frozen in liquid nitrogen, and stored at $-40°C$. Within 1 week the samples were thawed and diluted with glycyl glycine buffer to a volume equal to 10 times the weight of the individual pooled brain areas and assayed for adenyl cyclase activity according to the method of Klainer et al. (1). The washed particles were incubated for 12 min at 37°C in the presence or absence of phenothiazines and 5 mM sodium fluoride. The reaction was terminated by boiling the sample for 5 min followed by centrifugation. Cyclic AMP was measured in the supernatant by the protein-binding assay of Gilman (20) and adenyl cyclase activity was expressed as pmoles of cyclic AMP formed per mg of protein during 12-min incubation.

Preparation of Disrupted-Neuronal and Glial-Enriched Fractions

The procedure for isolation of neuronal perikarya and glial-enriched fractions was identical to that developed by Sellinger et al. (21). Briefly, the cerebral cortices were placed into a cold solution of 7.5% (w/v) polyvinyl-pyrrolidone, 1% bovine serum albumin and 10 mM $CaCl_2$. The tissue was minced and poured into a truncated disposable syringe and eased through successive passes of different pore sizes of nylon bolting cloth (333, 110, and 73 μ, three times each). The suspension was layered onto a discontinuous gradient of 1.75 and 1.0 M sucrose and centrifuged at 20,000 rpm in an SW 25.1 swinging bucket rotor. This first density-gradient centrifugation yielded a pellet of relatively pure neuronal perikarya, while the band containing the crude glial fraction was subjected to one additional density-gradient centrifugation (1.65 M sucrose, 1.2 M sucrose, and 30% Ficoll). The cells from the isolated neuronal and glial-enriched fractions were disrupted by agitation in cold glycyl glycine buffer (2 mM + 1 mM $MgSO_4$, pH 7.4) and centrifuged at $1,000 \times g$ for 10 min. The resultant pellets containing membrane fragments were resuspended in glycyl glycine buffer, vigorously shaken, and aliquots were removed for protein determinations (22). Phenothiazines were added to the isolated fractions in the presence or absence of sodium fluoride and adenyl cyclase activity was determined as described (1, 8).

Incubation of Tissue Slices

Tissue slices from the cerebral cortex and medial and lateral hypothalamus were prepared according to previously reported methods (2, 17). The tissues were preincubated at 37°C in Krebs-Ringer bicarbonate buffer for 30 min while O_2 containing 5% CO_2 was bubbled into the individual samples. The buffer was changed and at this time either phenothiazines or control solutions were added. The incubations were continued for 14 min at which time d,1NE (5×10^{-5} M) was pipetted into the samples. The reaction was terminated 6 min later by adding the contents of the reaction mixture to an operating Waring blender containing 2 ml of 1 N HCl. An aliquot was removed for protein determination (22), the remainder was centrifuged at $12,000 \times g$. and the cyclic AMP was isolated from the supernatant using Dowex 50 according to Butcher et al. (23), assayed (20), and expressed as pmoles per mg protein.

Materials

Prochlorperazine (Ppz), chlorpromazine (CPZ), CPZ-SO, and 3-hydroxyphenothiazine (3-OH-Ph) were gifts from Smith, Kline and French Laboratories. Promethazine and promazine (PZ) were donated by Wyeth Laboratories. Haloperidol and 3-OH-CPZ were kindly supplied by McNeil Laboratories and Rhone-Poulenc respectively. The generous donations of fluphenazine (Fz) and perphenazine (Pz) from the Schering Corporation are also appreciated. 7-OH-Fz and 8-OH-Fz were generously supplied by the Squibb Institute for Medical Research. The Psychopharmacology Research Branch, N.I.M.H., provided the following phenothiazine derivatives: 7-OH-CPZ; 8-OH-CPZ; 7,8-diOH-CPZ; 7,8-dioxo-CPZ; 8-OH-7-MeO-CPZ; 7-OH-8-MeO-CPZ; 7-MeO-CPZ; 7,8-diMeO-CPZ; 3,7-diMeO-CPZ; 7-OH-Ppz; 7,8-diOH-Ppz; 2-OH-PZ; 3-OH-PZ; 2,3-diOH-PZ; 7-OH-Pz; 7,8-diOH-Pz; phenothiazine (Ph); and 2-Cl-7,8-dioxo-Ph. Many of the compounds were obtained in the hydrochloride form and were dissolved in 0.1% ascorbic acid. The following compounds were initially dissolved in 0.1 N HCl and diluted to the appropriate volumes in distilled water: 3-OH-CPZ; 7-OH-CPZ; 7-OH-8-MeO-CPZ; 8-OH-7-MeO-CPZ; 7-OH-Ppz; 2-OH-PZ; and 3-OH-PZ. Ethanol (100%) was used to solubilize Ph; 2-Cl-7,8-dioxo-Ph; 3-OH-Ph; and haloperidol. All solutions were prepared immediately before use.

RESULTS

Effects of Phenothiazines on Adenyl Cyclase Prepared from the High-Speed Particulate Fraction

Several different preparations of the enzyme were made. In the first group, four separate preparations were utilized in order to test the ability of the CPZ-related compounds to modify enzyme activity. Three individual preparations were similarly used in the second group in which the remainder of the compounds were studied. The amounts of enzyme protein per sample were as follows: Group I, cerebral cortex 2.4 mg; hypothalamus, 3.0 mg; Group II, cerebral cortex 1.9 mg and hypothalamus 1.76 mg. The mean values ($\pm$ SEM) for the basal and fluoride activation of adenyl cyclase in these preparations were: Group I, cerebral cortex 5 ± 2 to 78 ± 3; hypothalamus 7 ± 2 to 49 ± 7; Group II, cerebral cortex 30 ± 3 to 83 ± 3, and hypothalamus 25 ± 6 to 91 ± 11 pmoles of cyclic AMP per mg sample protein in 12 min.

The phenothiazine compounds that exhibited an antagonism of either basal- or fluoride-stimulated adenyl cyclase are listed in Tables 1 and 2 in

TABLE 1. *Modification by phenothiazines of adenyl cyclase using the 100,000 $\times$ g particulate fraction from the rat cerebral cortex*

Treatment	Drug concentrations			
	10^{-3}	10^{-3} + F	10^{-4} + F	10^{-5} + F
7,8-dioxo-CPZ	81 ± 2	95 ± 5	86 ± 4	22 ± 6
7,8-diOH-Ppz	81 ± 0	93 ± 0	52 ± 7	18 ± 13
7,8-diOH-CPZ	25 ± 1	95 ± 5	85 ± 1	16 ± 3
7,8-diOH-Pz	81 ± 2	94 ± 1	72 ± 5	—
2,3-diOH-PZ	49 ± 25	62 ± 5	68 ± 9	24 ± 12
7-OH-8-MeO-CPZ	—	78 ± 9	28 ± 17	6 ± 3
8-OH-7-MeO-CPZ	—	72 ± 12	23 ± 12	12 ± 6
7-OH-Pz	43 ± 8	27 ± 12	23 ± 18	17 ± 10
8-OH-CPZ	—	30 ± 10	—	—
7-OH-Ppz	67 ± 9	28 ± 11	—	—
CPZ	—	24 ± 13	—	—
8-OH-Fz	52 ± 7	20 ± 9	—	—
Ppz	51 ± 20	17 ± 6	—	—
7-OH-CPZ	—	15 ± 8	17 ± 12	16 ± 9
Fz	54 ± 2	14 ± 3	—	—
3,7-diMeO-CPZ	39 ± 16	—	—	—
3-OH-PZ	36 ± 10	—	—	—
PZ	34 ± 6	—	—	—
Pz	30 ± 8	—	—	—
Promethazine	25 ± 6	—	—	—

Different concentrations of phenothiazines were added to the crude enzyme in either the presence or absence of sodium fluoride (5 mM) and incubated for 12 min at 37°C. The values represent the percent inhibition ($\pm$ SEM of 3 to 4 experiments) of either basal activity or the stimulation of adenyl cyclase by fluoride.

TABLE 2. *Modification by phenothiazines of adenyl cyclase using the 100,000 × g particulate fraction from the rat hypothalamus*

Treatment	Drug concentrations			
	10^{-3}	10^{-3} + F	10^{-4} + F	10^{-5} + F
7,8-diOH-CPZ	45 ± 6	94 ± 1	78 ± 5	15 ± 6
7,8-diOH-Pz	69 ± 4	94 ± 1	67 ± 1	25 ± 10
7,8-dioxo-CPZ	73 ± 3	90 ± 4	63 ± 16	33 ± 10
7,8-diOH-Ppz	65 ± 6	89 ± 2	40 ± 7	17 ± 11
2,3-diOH-PZ	44 ± 4	77 ± 8	57 ± 6	25 ± 10
8-OH-7-MeO-CPZ	—	48 ± 5	11 ± 5	—
8-OH-Fz	37 ± 4	44 ± 9	—	—
7-OH-Pz	65 ± 2	43 ± 9	—	—
Pz	42 ± 11	43 ± 13	—	—
7-OH-8-MeO-CPZ	—	41 ± 11	—	—
Ppz	55 ± 1	39 ± 8	—	—
3-OH-PZ	—	14 ± 9	30 ± 9	—
3,7-diMeO-CPZ	—	28 ± 7	—	—
7-OH-Pz	—	24 ± 12	—	—
Fz	—	23 ± 11	—	—
Promethazine	—	22 ± 10	—	—
PZ	—	20 ± 9	—	—
CPZ	—	10 ± 1	—	—

Different concentrations of phenothiazines were added to the crude enzyme in either the presence or absence of sodium fluoride (5 mM) and incubated for 12 min at 37°C. The values represent the percent inhibition (± SEM of 3 to 4 experiments) of either basal activity or the stimulation of adenyl cyclase by fluoride.

approximate order of potency. The dihydroxylated and dioxo derivatives of CPZ, Pz, Ppz, and PZ exerted the greatest antagonism of the enzyme. The monohydroxylated derivatives and the parent compounds demonstrated a weaker effect on adenyl cyclase. 3,7-diMeO-CPZ was the only methoxylated derivative that inhibited the enzyme. No effect on adenyl cyclase was observed with 7,8-diMeO-CPZ, 7-MeO-CPZ, CPZ-SO, PZ, 2-OH-PZ, Ph, 3-OH-Ph, 2-Cl-7,8-dioxo-Ph, and haloperidol.

Effects of Phenothiazines on Brain Slices

Tissue slices were prepared from the lateral and medial hypothalamus (24) and the cerebral cortex. Basal levels as well as the NE-induced accumulation of the cyclic nucleotide were highest in the medial hypothalamic area followed by the lateral hypothalamus and the cerebral cortex in that order (Tables 3–6). When various concentrations of phenothiazines (10^{-4} to 10^{-6} M) were added to the incubations, the greatest antagonism of the cyclic AMP response was observed with the pharmacologically active compounds and their respective monohydroxylated metabolites (CPZ, PZ, promethazine, Fz, Ppz, Pz, 7-OH-CPZ, 8-OH-7-MeO-CPZ, 3-OH-CPZ, 2-OH-PZ, 3-OH-PZ, 7-OH-Fz, 8-OH-Fz, 7-OH-Ppz, and 7-OH-Pz) (Tables 3–6). The

TABLE 3. *Antagonism by chlorpromazines (CPZ) of the NE-induced accumulation of cyclic AMP in tissue slices of the rat brain*

Treatment and concentration (molar)		Brain region		
		Lateral hypothalamus	Medial hypothalamus	Cerebral cortex
Control		34 ± 4	46 ± 4	24 ± 3
NE		90 ± 6	150 ± 20	68 ± 5
CPZ	10^{-4}	35 ± 4	51 ± 5	20 ± 3
	10^{-4} + NE	41 ± 1 (56)	58 ± 4 (61)	23 ± 3 (66)
	10^{-5} + NE	81 ± 12 (10)	97 ± 9 (35)	46 ± 7 (32)
	10^{-6} + NE	87 ± 4 (3)	98 ± 6 (35)	85 ± 3
7-OH-CPZ	10^{-4}	35 ± 11	40 ± 5	27 ± 4
	10^{-4} + NE	35 ± 6 (61)	50 ± 12 (67)	38 ± 5 (44)
	10^{-5} + NE	48 ± 8 (47)	68 ± 15 (55)	48 ± 4 (29)
	10^{-6} + NE	96 ± 15	107 ± 24 (29)	80 ± 11
3-OH-CPZ	10^{-4}	23 ± 1	31 ± 2	18 ± 3
	10^{-4} + NE	67 ± 2 (26)	46 ± 2	33 ± 4 (51)
	10^{-5} + NE	—	—	45 ± 6 (34)
	10^{-6} + NE	—	—	48 ± 4 (29)
8-OH-7-MeO-CPZ	10^{-4}	38 ± 10	44 ± 11	37 ± 3
	10^{-4} + NE	35 ± 11 (61)	33 ± 4 (78)	54 ± 6 (21)
	10^{-5} + NE	100 ± 29	98 ± 13 (35)	51 ± 12 (25)
	10^{-6} + NE	173 ± 13	157 ± 19	68 ± 5
7,8-diOH-CPZ	10^{-4}	35 ± 3	40 ± 6	38 ± 3
	10^{-4} + NE	63 ± 10	125 ± 23	65 ± 7
	10^{-5} + NE	106 ± 8	164 ± 20	67 ± 12
	10^{-6} + NE	106 ± 12	118 ± 14	77 ± 16
3,7-diMeO-CPZ	10^{-4}	—	—	29 ± 3
	10^{-4} + NE	—	—	30 ± 1 (56)
	10^{-5} + NE	—	—	83 ± 12
	10^{-6} + NE	—	—	90 ± 6

Tissue slices were preincubated for 30 min, the buffer changed, and the various chlorpromazines added. Fourteen min later, NE (5×10^{-5} M) was introduced and after 6 min the samples were homogenized and cyclic AMP isolated and determined. Values are expressed as pmoles of cyclic AMP/mg sample protein ± SEM of four separate experiments. The values in parentheses are the mean percent inhibition of the total NE response.

TABLE 4. Antagonism by promazines (PZ) haloperidol and promethazine of the NE-induced accumulation of cyclic AMP in tissue slices of the rat brain

Treatment and concentration (molar)		Brain region		
		Lateral hypothalamus	Medial hypothalamus	Cerebral cortex
Control		35 ± 5	43 ± 3	23 ± 3
NE		86 ± 6	134 ± 15	68 ± 6
PZ	10^{-4}	33 ± 1	29 ± 4	17 ± 1
	10^{-4} + NE	52 ± 4 (40)	51 ± 14 (62)	22 ± 2 (68)
	10^{-5} + NE	47 ± 4 (45)	49 ± 5 (63)	23 ± 2 (66)
	10^{-6} + NE	47 ± 4 (45)	129 ± 9	40 ± 15 (41)
2-OH-PZ	10^{-4}	25 ± 3	38 ± 2	28 ± 2
	10^{-4} + NE	42 ± 6 (51)	67 ± 10 (50)	47 ± 3 (31)
	10^{-5} + NE	54 ± 5 (37)	97 ± 14 (28)	64 ± 10
	10^{-6} + NE	59 ± 8 (31)	106 ± 23 (21)	94 ± 9
3-OH-PZ	10^{-4}	—	—	30 ± 2
	10^{-4} + NE	—	—	38 ± 3 (56)
	10^{-5} + NE	—	—	61 ± 4 (10)
	10^{-6} + NE	—	—	64 ± 4
2,3-diOH-PZ	10^{-4}	36 ± 3	47 ± 4	21 ± 4
	10^{-4} + NE	53 ± 2 (40)	108 ± 5 (19)	64 ± 6
	10^{-5} + NE	66 ± 9 (23)	101 ± 13 (25)	70 ± 3
	10^{-6} + NE	70 ± 8 (13)	86 ± 10 (36)	50 ± 6 (26)
Haloperidol	10^{-4}	48 ± 7	47 ± 8	27 ± 4
	10^{-4} + NE	101 ± 18	104 ± 13 (22)	38 ± 3 (44)
	10^{-5} + NE	147 ± 20	185 ± 28	51 ± 7 (25)
	10^{-6} + NE	156 ± 18	171 ± 14	52 ± 2 (24)
Promethazine	10^{-4}	28 ± 5	38 ± 2	—
	10^{-4} + NE	25 ± 3 (71)	39 ± 11 (72)	—
	10^{-5} + NE	58 ± 8 (33)	73 ± 11 (46)	—
	10^{-6} + NE	134 ± 12	116 ± 13 (13)	—

Tissue slices were preincubated for 30 min, the buffer changed, and the various phenothiazines added. Fourteen min later, NE (5×10^{-5} M) was introduced and after 6 min the samples were homogenized and cyclic AMP isolated and determined. Values are expressed as pmoles of cyclic AMP/mg sample protein ± SEM of four separate experiments. The values in parentheses are the mean percent inhibition of the total NE response.

TABLE 5. *Antagonism by prochlorperazines (Ppz) and perphenazines (Pz) of the NE-induced accumulation of cyclic AMP in tissue slices of the rat brain*

Treatment and concentration (molar)	Brain region		
	Lateral hypothalamus	Medial hypothalamus	Cerebral cortex
Control	28 ± 1	50 ± 4	20 ± 1
NE	96 ± 9	137 ± 9	69 ± 6
Ppz 10^{-4}	35 ± 4	46 ± 7	29 ± 4
10^{-4} + NE	54 ± 6 (44)	54 ± 9 (61)	40 ± 2 (42)
10^{-5} + NE	45 ± 7 (53)	75 ± 8 (45)	59 ± 7 (14)
10^{-6} + NE	74 ± 1 (23)	76 ± 8 (45)	62 ± 6 (10)
7-OH-Ppz 10^{-4}	24 ± 2	52 ± 4	17 ± 2
10^{-4} + NE	59 ± 6 (39)	69 ± 4 (50)	32 ± 4 (54)
10^{-5} + NE	71 ± 4 (26)	106 ± 6 (23)	41 ± 5 (41)
10^{-6} + NE	94 ± 14	149 ± 15	66 ± 8
7,8-diOH-Ppz 10^{-4}	33 ± 1	54 ± 8	22 ± 1
10^{-4} + NE	51 ± 9 (47)	86 ± 10 (37)	47 ± 5 (32)
10^{-5} + NE	72 ± 15 (25)	102 ± 13 (26)	45 ± 7 (35)
10^{-6} + NE	78 ± 17 (19)	105 ± 7 (23)	54 ± 2 (22)
Pz 10^{-4}	30 ± 3	35 ± 2	30 ± 3
10^{-4} + NE	57 ± 3 (41)	47 ± 10 (66)	26 ± 3 (62)
10^{-5} + NE	51 ± 3 (47)	67 ± 10 (51)	48 ± 9 (30)
10^{-6} + NE	77 ± 8 (20)	113 ± 18 (18)	49 ± 5 (29)
7-OH-Pz 10^{-4}	24 ± 5	39 ± 6	22 ± 2
10^{-4} + NE	57 ± 8 (41)	65 ± 11 (53)	55 ± 6 (20)
10^{-5} + NE	93 ± 3	114 ± 7 (17)	64 ± 2 (7)
10^{-6} + NE	93 ± 14	139 ± 5	89 ± 14
7,8-diOH-Pz 10^{-4}	22 ± 3	38 ± 3	28 ± 5
10^{-4} + NE	44 ± 4 (54)	81 ± 12 (41)	81 ± 8
10^{-5} + NE	64 ± 10 (33)	66 ± 8 (52)	101 ± 11
10^{-6} + NE	67 ± 5 (30)	82 ± 8 (40)	99 ± 11

Tissue slices were preincubated for 30 min, the buffer changed, and the various phenothiazines added. Fourteen min later, NE (5×10^{-5} M) was introduced and after 6 min the samples were homogenized and cyclic AMP isolated and determined. Values are expressed as pmoles of cyclic AMP/mg sample protein ± SEM of four separate experiments. The values in parentheses are the mean percent inhibition of the total response.

TABLE 6. Antagonism by fluphenazines (Fz) and 7,8-dioxo-CPZ of the NE-induced accumulation of cyclic AMP in tissue slices of the rat brain

Treatment and concentration (molar)		Brain region		
		Lateral hypothalamus	Medial hypothalamus	Cerebral cortex
Control		32 ± 8	48 ± 6	26 ± 6
NE		91 ± 7	125 ± 14	72 ± 7
Fz	10^{-4}	18 ± 1	22 ± 2	16 ± 3
	10^{-4} + NE	27 ± 3 (70)	39 ± 4 (69)	35 ± 2 (51)
	10^{-5} + NE	37 ± 1 (59)	58 ± 3 (54)	48 ± 6 (33)
	10^{-6} + NE	75 ± 7 (18)	98 ± 10 (22)	51 ± 7 (29)
7-OH-Fz	10^{-4}	18 ± 1	25 ± 2	33 ± 5
	10^{-4} + NE	40 ± 2 (56)	46 ± 3 (63)	63 ± 9
	10^{-5} + NE	35 ± 3 (62)	55 ± 4 (56)	60 ± 6
	10^{-6} + NE	48 ± 5 (47)	105 ± 16 (16)	88 ± 10
8-OH-Fz	10^{-4}	26 ± 6	27 ± 2	29 ± 6
	10^{-4} + NE	49 ± 14 (46)	53 ± 4 (58)	35 ± 7 (51)
	10^{-5} + NE	57 ± 6 (37)	78 ± 15 (38)	27 ± 5 (63)
	10^{-6} + NE	91 ± 11	102 ± 14 (10)	80 ± 14
7,8-dioxo-CPZ	10^{-4}	27 ± 9	39 ± 5	39 ± 5
	10^{-4} + NE	66 ± 3 (27)	88 ± 5 (30)	67 ± 7
	10^{-5} + NE	175 ± 18	243 ± 54	87 ± 5
	10^{-6} + NE	95 ± 15	171 ± 19	103 ± 7

Tissue slices were preincubated for 30 min, the buffer changed, and the various phenothiazines added. Fourteen min later, NE (5×10^{-5} M) was introduced and after 6 min, the samples were homogenized and cyclic AMP isolated and determined. Values are expressed as pmoles of cyclic AMP/mg sample protein ± SEM of four separate experiments. The values in parentheses are the mean percent inhibition of the total NE response.

dihydroxylated metabolites of the pharmacologically active phenothiazines were usually less effective on the tissue slices; however, the hypothalamic areas were sometimes inhibited with the higher drug concentrations. The medial hypothalamus appeared to be more susceptible to inhibition by the pharmacologically active compounds. Haloperidol antagonized the NE-induced cyclic AMP response only in the cerebral cortex (Table 4). The remainder of the compounds investigated were ineffective, namely: CPZ-SO, Ph, 3-OH-Ph, and 2-Cl-7,8-dioxo-Ph. In some preliminary studies using tissue slices from the cerebral cortex, 3-OH-PZ and 3,7-diMeO-CPZ were effective at the highest concentrations in antagonizing the cyclic AMP response to NE while 7-MeO-CPZ was without effect (Tables 3 and 4). As a rule, basal levels of the cyclic nucleotide were unchanged by the highest concentration of the drug (10^{-4} M). The compounds that exhibited inhibition on basal levels of cyclic AMP in some or all brain regions were PZ, 2-OH-PZ, Fz, 7-OH-Fz, 8-OH-Fz, and 3-OH-CPZ. Compounds that enhanced basal levels of cyclic AMP in certain brain regions were 7,8-diOH-CPZ, 7,8-dioxo-CPZ, 8-OH-7-MeO-CPZ, 3-OH-Ph, and 2-Cl-7,8-dioxo-Ph.

Antagonism of Adenyl Cyclase by Phenothiazines in Disrupted Neuronal and Glial-Enriched Fractions

Phase microscopy of the neuronal and glial fractions revealed a relatively pure neuronal fraction consisting mainly of perikarya, while the glial fraction was contaminated with small neuronal cells, broken-cell debris, and capillaries. For the most part, the glial-enriched fraction contained clumps of astrocytes. Adenyl cyclase activity varied from preparation to preparation in that basal activity of the enzyme might be as low as 30 pmoles cyclic AMP/mg protein after 12-min incubation or as high as 100. Fluoride (5 mM) consistently activated the enzyme by 80 to 120%. This twofold stimulation was somewhat less than that observed for the enzyme in the high-speed particulate fraction. Likewise this purification process resulted in higher basal activities of the enzyme in either the neuronal or the glial-enriched fractions. Basal- and fluoride-activated adenyl cyclase activities were somewhat higher (20 to 80%) in the neuronal when compared to the corresponding glial-enriched fraction. Since enzyme activities were inconsistent, three separate preparations were used for each drug. Therefore the data plotted in Figs. 1–5 represent the percent inhibition of either basal or fluoride stimulation of adenyl cyclase at three to five different drug concentrations.

At the highest drug concentrations (10^{-3} M), almost all phenothiazine drugs inhibited either basal- or fluoride-activation of adenyl cyclase. The exceptions were: CPZ-SO, Ph, 2-Cl-7-8-dioxo-Ph, and haloperidol (Figs. 1–5). The most potent inhibitors of the enzyme were the dihydroxylated

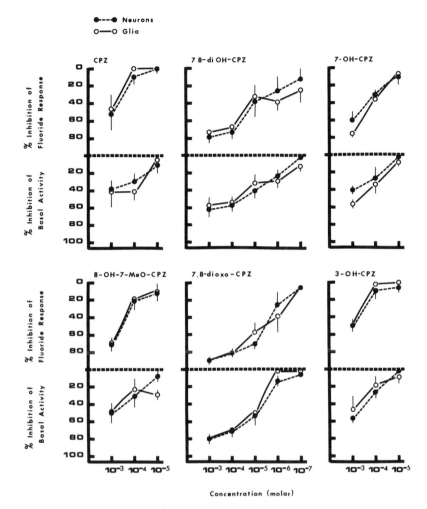

FIGS. 1–5. Adenyl cyclase activity was determined in disrupted neuronal and glial-enriched fractions isolated from the rat cerebral cortex. Various concentrations of phenothiazines were added to the crude enzyme and the activity of either basal or fluoride (5 mM) activation of adenyl cyclase was determined. The values represent the mean percent inhibition of either basal- or fluoride-stimulated adenyl cyclase ± SEM of at least three separate experiments.

derivatives of CPZ, Ppz, Pz, PZ, and 7,8-dioxo-CPZ. An intermediate antagonism of the enzyme was seen with the parent compounds and mono-hydroxylated derivatives of Ppz, Pz, Fz, and, to a lesser extent, CPZ. The methylated derivatives of CPZ (7-MeO and 3,7-diMeO-CPZ) were as potent as CPZ while 7,8-DiMeO-CPZ, 3-OH-CPZ, PZ, 2-OH-PZ, 3-OH-Pz, promethazine, and 3-OH-Ph exhibited lesser potency. No remarkable differences were noted between drug effects on either the neuronal or glial-enriched fractions.

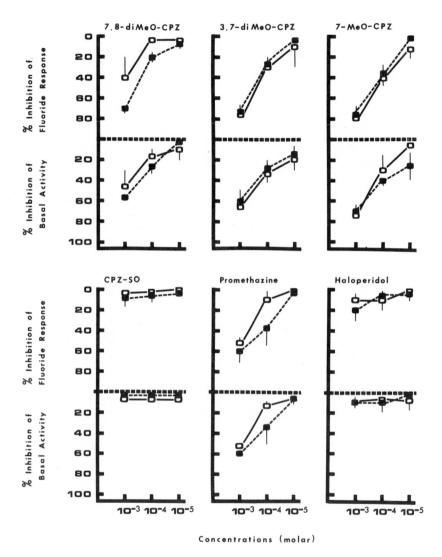

FIG. 2.

DISCUSSION

Biogenic amines in the central nervous system, particularly the cate-cholamines, have been implicated in the mechanism of action of psycho-tropic drugs (25). Carlsson and Lindquist (26) proposed that CPZ acts to antagonize adrenergic receptors within the brain. Subsequent investigations

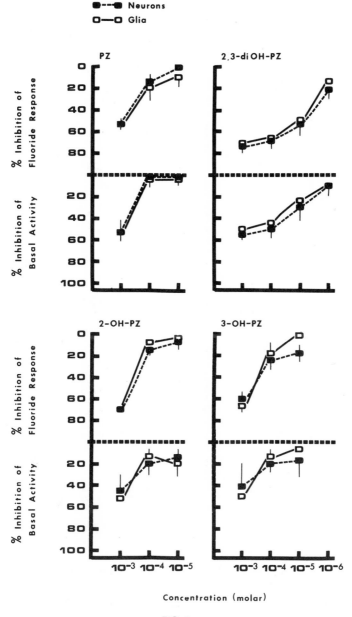

FIG. 3.

have supported this hypothesis (27, 28). Many of the peripheral actions of the catecholamines, especially those involving adrenergic *beta* receptors appear to be mediated by cyclic AMP (29). Based on the receptor model of Robison et al. (29) adenyl cyclase is thought to exist in at least two com-

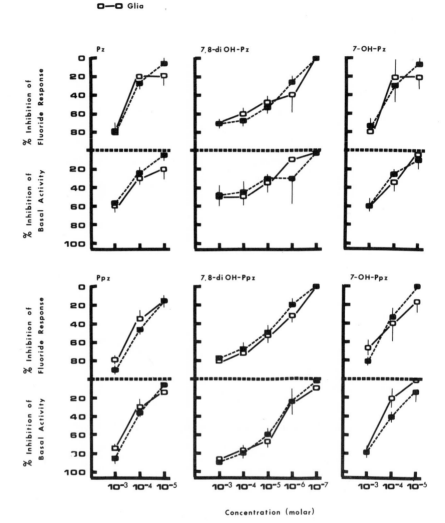

FIG. 4.

partments within the cell. One, the receptor component, faces the external milieu of the cell and is subjected to activation by specific hormones. The other component, the catalytic site, is thought to be accessible to the interior of the cell and is subject to, by an unknown mechanism, stimulation by fluoride. A series of recent investigations with the brain and peripheral tissues indicate that the antiadrenergic actions of pharmacologically active phenothiazines and monohydroxylated metabolites are manifested at the level of adenyl cyclase–cyclic AMP (2, 12, 13, 17–19, 30–32). This action occurred in either broken-cell preparations or tissue slices that were in-

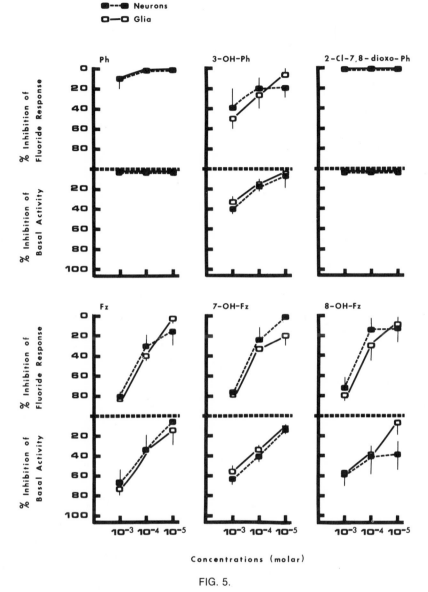

FIG. 5.

cubated in the presence of catecholamines. The former effect (broken cells) is presumably a drug action exerted on the catalytic moiety of adenyl cyclase, while the latter represents an effect on the receptor component of the enzyme. Furthermore, in an *in vivo* study, it was reported that pharmacologically active phenothiazines, but not the sulfoxide analogues, blocked the postdecapitation rise in cyclic AMP in rats (13).

The availability of various metabolites and derivatives of several pheno-thiazines allowed us the opportunity to test the relative potencies of these compounds toward adenyl cyclase–cyclic AMP under three experimental conditions. At first, a crude enzyme was prepared from the high-speed particulate fraction taken from the rat cerebral cortex and hypothalamus. In an attempt to localize the action of the phenothiazines at more precise loci within the cerebral cortex, disrupted neuronal and glial-enriched fractions were utilized in the second study. The dihydroxylated and dioxo de-rivatives of the pharmacologically active phenothiazines were the most potent inhibitors of adenyl cyclase in these broken-cell preparations. To a lesser extent, the parent compounds and the monohydroxylated metabolites exhibited anti-adenyl cyclase actions. Methoxylated and sulfoxide deriva-tives of CPZ, along with haloperidol, Ph and its analogues, were ineffective. The one exception was observed with 3,7-diMeO-CPZ. The enzyme pre-pared from the neuronal and glial-enriched fractions was more sensitive to the highest concentrations of almost all the compounds. No salient differ-ences were noted between the actions of the phenothiazines on either the neurons or glia.

As a means to determine the actions of phenothiazines on the adrenergic receptor, the third experiment consisted of incubating tissue slices in the presence of drugs and measuring the antagonism of the cyclic AMP ac-cumulation induced by NE. In this study, the greatest antagonism was exerted by pharmacologically active compounds (including promethazine) and their monohydroxylated derivatives. The dihydroxylated analogues were of lesser effect. Analogues of phenothiazine and methoxylated and sulfoxide derivatives of CPZ were ineffective. The one exception was seen with 3,7-diMeO-CPZ. Haloperidol, a structurally unrelated butyro-phenone, exerted an inhibitory action in only the cerebral cortex. This lack of effect by haloperidol on the hypothalamus has been previously noted (17). A few active compounds inhibited basal levels of the cyclic nucleotide. An elevation of basal levels of cyclic AMP by some of the dihydroxylated and dioxo derivatives is difficult to interpret. A possible explanation might be that the catechol configuration of the dihydroxylated derivatives re-sembles NE and acts as a weak hormone. A recent study, however, has shown that pharmacologically active phenothiazines enhance the turnover of labeled adenine into cyclic AMP in guinea pig brain slices (14). The medial and lateral areas of the hypothalamus were investigated individually because Grossman (33) reported that microinjections of CPZ and mono-hydroxylated metabolites caused differential effects in these two brain areas while using diverse conditioned avoidance behavioral responses. 7-OH-CPZ and 3-OH-CPZ were effective in the lateral hypothalamus in suppression of a double-grill shock-avoidance effect, while CPZ, 8-OH-CPZ, and 3-OH-CPZ were more effective in the medial hypothalamus in suppression of a one-way sound-avoidance paradigm. If any compound was injected into either the septal area, the amygdala, or the midbrain reticular formation, no suppression of any conditioned avoidance response was noted. In our study, many of the active phenothiazines and monohydroxylated derivatives were more potent in the medial hypothalamus in their ability to antagonize the cyclic AMP response elicited by NE.

From the present experiments, a comparison of the structure-activity relationships can be made concerning the actions of phenothiazines on central adenyl cyclase–cyclic AMP. In the broken-cell preparations, the dihydroxylated compounds were the most potent inhibitors at the catalytic site of the enzyme. This action might result from the rapid formation of free radicals (Zwitter ions), which could affect the enzyme. In this regard, 7,8-dioxo-CPZ was as potent in antagonizing adenyl cyclase activity. The side chain on the phenothiazine basic structure is also important for this activity because 2-Cl-7,8-dioxo-Ph did not possess any anti-adenyl cyclase activity. It has been established that the rabbit liver can form 7,8-diOH-CPZ (34) but from the effects observed on tissue slices, it is doubtful whether the compound can enter the brain. Again, it is possible that 7,8-diOH-CPZ is formed within the brain cells themselves and, along with other metabolites, exerts additional effects, namely, inhibition of sodium, potassium-activated ATPase (30, 35, 36), prevention of calcium accumulation by mitochondria (37), chelation of metals (38), and inhibition of protein kinase and phosphodiesterase (13, 39, and Petzold, G., and Greengard, P., *personal communication*). Likewise, recent reports suggest that this diOH analogue of CPZ exerts powerful peripheral toxic effects (40) including ophthalmopathies (41). The pharmacologically active parent compounds and monohydroxylated derivatives were considerably less effective in broken cells, but exerted the most potent actions in their ability to modify the cyclic AMP response to NE in tissue slices. Monohydroxylated metabolites of CPZ (7-OH and 8-OH) are readily accumulated in brain tissue (42) and are almost as potent as the parent compound in several pharmacologic and behavioral investigations *in vivo*. In these studies, methylated metabolites were less effective (40, 43, 44). Some dimethoxy metabolites of CPZ did, however, influence these behavior tests (44) as well as antagonize adenyl cyclase–cyclic AMP in the study discussed in this chapter.

From the present experiments it is assumed that parent compounds of pharmacologically active phenothiazines and their corresponding monohydroxylated derivatives first antagonize the receptor component of the enzyme and then penetrate the cell and affect the catalytic moiety of adenyl cyclase. The action exerted inside the cell might be due to a formation of free radicals. Holmes and Piette (45), using the electron spin-resonance technique, have demonstrated a binding effect of only the active phenothiazines to isolated red blood cell ghost membranes. Moreover, Mercier and Dumont (46) have shown that phenothiazines display high electron-donating properties and postulated that an essential role in the mechanisms of psychotropic activity of these drugs is played by a positive radical ion.

In conclusion, we would like to postulate that in addition to antiadrenergic actions exerted at the level of adenyl cyclase, the phenothiazines by their chemical nature are responsible for a host of effects on other central processes. The psychotropic activity of any parent compound might also be realized through one or a combination of its hydroxylated metabolites and the accumulation of these analogues might account for some of the side effects in patients undergoing phenothiazine therapy.

SUMMARY

The actions of several derivatives of phenothiazines were evaluated in the rat brain with respect to the enzyme receptor, adenyl cyclase. In order to evaluate the action of the compounds at the catalytic site of the enzyme, the drugs were added to broken-cell preparations consisting of either a high-speed particulate fraction from the cortex and the hypothalamus or disrupted neuronal and glial-enriched fractions from the cortex. The dihydroxylated analogues of chlorpromazine, promazine, prochlorperazine, and perphenazine along with 7,8-dioxochlorpromazine exerted the most profound inhibition of either basal or fluoride activation of adenyl cyclase. To a lesser extent these parent compounds including fluphenazine and promethazine and respective monohydroxylated and methoxylated derivatives were effective. No actions were observed with any analogue of phenothiazine, haloperidol, or chlorpromazine sulfoxide. Tissue slices were used to examine at the receptor level the effects of these compounds on the norepinephrine-induced accumulation of cyclic AMP. In these studies the parent compounds and the monohydroxylated analogues were the most potent inhibitors at the receptor site of adenyl cyclase. The results suggest that cellular actions of phenothiazines may in addition be reflected through a combination of one or more active metabolites.

ACKNOWLEDGMENTS

The authors are especially grateful to Mr. Halbert Scott, Mr. Rufus Putnam, and Mrs. Jo Palmer for technical assistance. This work was supported by grant MH–21584 (from the National Institute of Mental Health).

REFERENCES

1. Klainer, L. M., Chi, Y. M., Freidberg, S. L., Rall, T. W., and Sutherland, E. W., *J. Biol. Chem.*, **237**, 1239 (1962).
2. Kakiuchi, S., and Rall, T. W., *Molec. Pharmacol.*, **4**, 367 (1968).
3. Kakiuchi, S., and Rall, T. W., *Molec. Pharmacol.*, **4**, 379 (1968).
4. Palmer, G. C., Sulser, F., and Robison, G. A., *Neuropharmacol.*, **12**, 327 (1973).
5. Daly, J. W., Huang, M., and Shimizu, H., *Adv. Cyclic Nucleotide Res.*, **1**, 375 (1972).
6. Clark, R. B., and Perkins, J. P., *Proc. Nat. Acad. Sci. U.S.A.*, **68**, 2757 (1971).

7. Gilman, A. G., and Nirenberg, M., *Proc. Nat. Acad. Sci. U.S.A.,* **68,** 2165 (1971).
8. Palmer, G. C., *Res. Commun. Chem. Path. Pharmacol.,* **5,** 603 (1973).
9. DeRobertis, E., Delores Arnaiz, G. A., Alberici, M., Butcher, R. W., and Sutherland, E. W., *J. Biol. Chem.,* **242,** 3487 (1967).
10. Johnson, E. M., Ueda, T., Maeno, H., and Greengard, P., *J. Biol. Chem.,* **247,** 5650 (1972).
11. Siggins, G. R., Hoffer, B. J., and Bloom, F. E., *Science,* **165,** 1018 (1969).
12. Palmer, G. C., Robison, G. A., Manian, A. A., and Sulser, F., *Psychopharmacologia Berl.,* **23,** 201 (1972).
13. Uzunov, P., and Weiss, B., *Neuropharmacol.,* **10,** 697 (1971).
14. Huang, M., Shimizu, H., and Daly, J., *J. Med. Chem.,* **15,** 458 (1972).
15. Huang, M., Shimizu, H., and Daly, J., *J. Med. Chem.,* **15,** 462 (1972).
16. Forn, J., and Valdecasas, F. G., *Biochem. Pharmacol.,* **20,** 2773 (1971).
17. Palmer, G. C., Robison, G. A., and Sulser, F., *Biochem. Pharmacol.,* **20,** 236 (1971).
18. Palmer, G. C., and Manian, A. A., *Trans. Amer. Soc. Neurochem.,* **4,** 86 (1973).
19. Weinryb, I., Chasin, M., Free, C. A., Harris, D. N., Goldenberg, H., Michel, I. M., Paik, V. S., Phillips, M., Samaniego, S., and Hess, S. M., *J. Pharm. Sci.,* **61,** 1556 (1972).
20. Gilman, A. G., *Proc. Nat. Acad. Sci. U.S.A.,* **67,** 305 (1970).
21. Sellinger, O. Z., Azcurra, J. M., Johnson, D. E., Ohlsson, W. G., and Lodin, Z., *Nature (New Biol.),* **230,** 253 (1971).
22. Lowry, O. H., Rosebrough, N. J., Farr, A. L., and Randall, R. J., *J. Biol. Chem.,* **193,** 265 (1951).
23. Butcher, R. W., Ho, R. J., Meng, H. C., and Sutherland, E. W., *J. Biol. Chem.,* **240,** 4515 (1965).
24. DeGroot, J., *Verh. Kon. Ned. Acad. Wet. B. Naturkunde,* **52,** 1 (1959).
25. Sulser, F., and Sanders-Bush, E., *Ann. Rev. Pharmacol.,* **11,** 209 (1971).
26. Carlsson, A., and Lindquist, M., *Acta Pharmacol.,* **20,** 140 (1963).
27. Bradley, P. B., Wolstencroft, J. H., Hosli, L., and Avanzino, G. L., *Nature,* **212,** 1425 (1966).
28. Gordon, M., in *Psychopharmacological Agents,* XI, Gordon, M., (ed.), Academic Press, New York, 1967, pp. 1–198.
29. Robison, G. A., Butcher, R. W., and Sutherland, E. W., in *Fundamental Concepts in Drug-Receptor Interactions,* Danielli, J. F., Moran, J. F., and Triggle, D. J., (eds.) Academic Press, New York, 1969, p. 59.
30. Wolff, J., and Jones, A. B., *Proc. Nat. Acad. Sci. U.S.A.,* **65,** 454 (1970).
31. Kakiuchi, S., Rall, T. W., and McIlwain, H., *J. Neurochem.,* **16,** 485 (1969).
32. Palmer, G. C., *Biochim. Biophys. Acta,* **252,** 561 (1971).
33. Grossman, S. P., *Commun. Behavl. Biol.,* **1,** 9 (1968).
34. Daly, J. W., and Manian, A. A., *Biochem. Pharmacol.,* **16,** 2131 (1967).
35. Akera, T., Baskin, S. I., Tobin, T., Brody, T. M., and Manian, A. A. *(these proceedings, 1973).*
36. Hackenberg, H., and Krieglstein, J., *Naunyn-Schmiedeberg's Arch. Pharmacol.,* **274,** 63 (1972).
37. Tjioe, S., and O'Neill, J. J. *(these proceedings, 1973).*
38. Rajan, K. S., Manian, A. A., and Davis, J. M. *(these proceedings, 1974).*
39. Honda, F., and Imamura, H., *Biochim. Biophys. Acta,* **161,** 267 (1968).
40. Buckley, J. P., Steenberg, M. L., Barry, H., III, and Manian, A. A., *J. Pharm. Sci.,* **62,** 715 (1973).
41. Adams, H. R. *(these proceedings, 1973).*
42. Manian, A. A., Efron, D. H., and Harris, S. R., *Life Sciences,* **10,** 679 (1971).
43. Manian, A. A., Efron, D. H., and Goldberg, M. E., *Life Sciences,* **4,** 2425 (1965).
44. Manian, A. A., Watzman, N., Steenberg, M. L., and Buckley, J. P., *Life Sciences,* **7,** 731 (1968).
45. Holmes, D. E., and Piette, L. H., *J. Pharmacol. Exp. Ther.,* **173,** 78 (1970).
46. Mercier, M. J., and Dumont, P. A., *J. Pharm. Pharmacol.,* **24,** 706 (1972).

The Phenothiazines and Structurally Related Drugs, edited by I. S.
Forrest, C. J. Carr, and E. Usdin. Raven Press, New York © 1974.

Effects of Chlorpromazine on Acetylcholine Turnover *In Vivo*

Donald J. Jenden

*Department of Pharmacology, School of Medicine, and Brain Research Institute,
University of California, Los Angeles, California 90024*

While drug effects on the levels of biogenic amines may provide some
clues as to their mechanism of action, it is now increasingly recognized
that neurotransmitter metabolism must be studied dynamically to derive a
valid assessment of the roles played by neurotransmitters in normal function or the alterations induced by drugs. A variety of techniques have been
described to measure the turnover of catecholamines and serotonin (1), but
until recently the approaches available to study acetylcholine have been
limited because of a lack of analytical methods of sufficient sensitivity and
specificity. Several new methods have recently been described (2, 3), of
which the one used in the present study is based on integrated gas chroma-
tography/mass spectrometry. The results indicate that chlorpromazine
produces a significant reduction in the turnover rate of acetylcholine in
mouse brain *in vivo*, although it leaves mean levels of acetylcholine unaltered.

ANALYTICAL METHODS

The gas chromatographic analysis of acetylcholine requires preliminary
conversion to a volatile derivative. Although several derivatives have been
employed (2), the N-demethylation product has the advantage of uniqueness,
and is now most commonly used. N-Demethylation can be accomplished
by pyrolysis (4–7) or by reaction with sodium benzenethiolate, the procedure used in the work reported here. Details of the sample preparation
and analytical procedure have been described elsewhere (8–10). Choline is
estimated simultaneously following acylation with propionyl chloride and
subsequent N-demethylation (11). This procedure has a sensitivity limit
of about 50 pmoles using a conventional flame-ionization detector.

Mass-spectrometric detection offers three major advantages for the work
to be described: an increase in sensitivity of approximately 1,000-fold,
greatly enhanced specificity, and the capability of using stable isotopic
labels for purposes of internal standardization and as tracers. When using
an isotopic internal standard, the procedure is in effect an isotope dilution

769

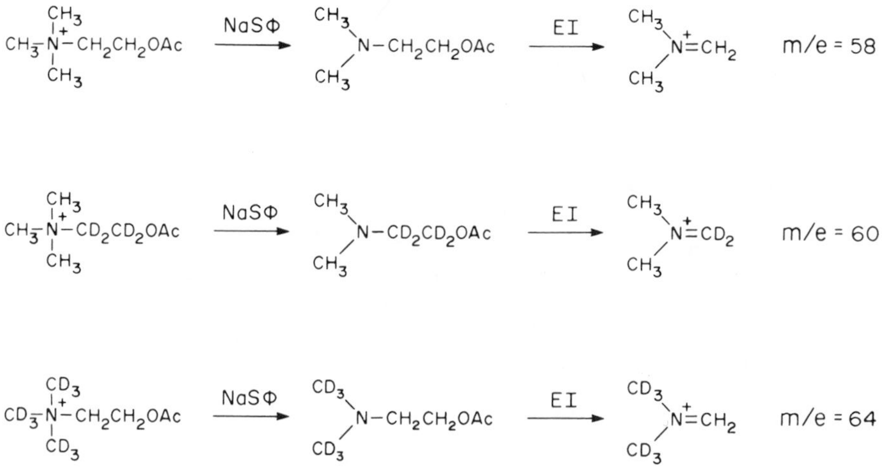

FIG. 1. Scheme showing derivatization of acetylcholine variants by N-demethylation with sodium benzenethiolate, followed by electron-impact ionization to yield dimethyleneimmonium ions which are the base peaks, with m/e 58, 60, and 64.

analysis and is capable of great precision [~1%; (12)]. Two isotopic variants of choline and acetylcholine were used in this work, with deuterium substitution as shown in Fig. 1. Following N-demethylation and electron impact ionization, they generate base peaks at m/e 60 (for d_4-choline and d_4-acetylcholine) and 64 (for d_9 compounds), whereas the endogenous unlabeled compounds have base peaks at m/e 58.

An EAI Quad 300 quadrupole mass spectrometer was multiplexed to focus continuously on m/e 58, 60, and 64. The mass spectrometer was used to monitor the output from a Varian 1400 gas chromatograph to which it was coupled by a Carle 2800 valve and glass frit separator (13). A 2 m × 2 mm (ID) silanized glass column was packed with 5% OV 101 and 5% DDTS (14) on Gas Chrom Q. The demultiplexed output from the mass spectrometer was recorded on a four-channel Rikadenki potentiometric recorder. Figure 2 shows a typical gas chromatogram of a mouse brain extract, with specific ion detection at m/e 58, 60, and 64. The channel responding at m/e 58 represents predominantly the unlabeled endogenous variants; the m/e 60 channel responds primarily to the d_4-variants used as tracers, and the channel recording at m/e 64 responds predominantly to the d_9-labeled internal standards. Calculation of the precise quantities of each variant requires the solution of three simultaneous linear equations, since all six variants give some response (<5% of base peak) at the three masses monitored (12).

ESTIMATION OF ACETYLCHOLINE TURNOVER

The procedure described above allows the simultaneous absolute estimation of endogenous and tracer variants of choline and acetylcholine. It

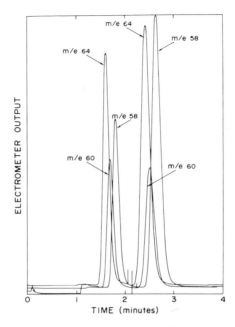

FIG. 2. Gas chromatograms of mouse brain extract with specific ion detection at m/e 58, 60, and 64 as indicated. Mouse was sacrificed 20 sec after intravenous injection of d_4-choline, 20 μmol kg^{-1}. There is a time offset in the recorder corresponding to a delay of 0.1 min for m/e 60 and 0.2 min for m/e 58 relative to m/e 64. The first set of peaks corresponds to acetylcholine, converted to dimethylaminoethyl acetate, with sensitivities of 120, 6, and 30 nA full scale for m/e 58, 60, and 64 respectively. Gain settings were changed at 2.1 min. The second set of peaks represents choline, converted to dimethylaminoethyl propionate, with sensitivities of 240, 60, and 60 nA full scale for m/e 58, 60, and 64 respectively. The quantities of d_9-choline and acetylcholine used as internal standards were 5 nmol and 2.5 nmol respectively. The quantities of derivatized d_0- and d_4-acetylcholine injected were calculated as 167 and 3.96 pmols, corresponding to 20.9 and 0.495 nmol gm^{-1} of brain; quantities of d_0- and d_4-choline injected were 293 and 25.1 pmols, corresponding to 36.6 and 3.13 nmol gm^{-1} of brain. Specific activities of acetylcholine and choline were 2.31 and 7.90 moles percent respectively.

was used to implement an experimental design originally used by Schuberth, Sundwall, and Sparf (15) with radioisotopically labeled choline. Groups of 11 to 16 mice each were given d_4-choline (20 μmol kg^{-1}) by a pulse intravenous injection, and were subsequently sacrificed at time intervals from 20 sec to 30 min. The brain was rapidly (<25 sec) removed, frozen in liquid nitrogen, and analyzed as described above. Although the injection undoubtedly causes a transient change in the plasma choline level, the total levels of choline and acetylcholine in the brain are unaltered at all time points from 20 sec to 30 min (Fig. 3). In the sense that the brain choline pool is labeled without any detectable change in the steady-state levels, the dose of d_4-choline employed is a tracer amount as far as brain metabolism is concerned. The specific activity of choline falls rapidly from the 20-sec value of 0.08 to 0.10 (mole ratio), while the specific activity of acetylcholine

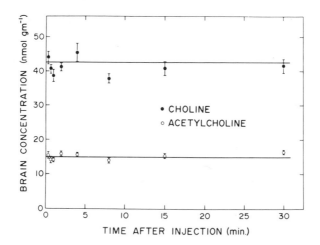

FIG. 3. Mean total brain levels of choline and acetylcholine following pulse intravenous injection of d_4-choline (20 μmol kg^{-1}). Each point represents the average of 11 to 15 mice.

rises to a peak of about 0.03 at 2 to 4 min and declines thereafter. Several approaches have been proposed for the further analysis of these data (16), of which one is considered in greater detail below.

EFFECTS OF CHLORPROMAZINE

Groups of at least 40 mice each were given chlorpromazine intraperitoneally at doses of 3, 10, 30, and 100 μmol kg^{-1} ($\sim$1 to 30 mg kg^{-1}), 40 min prior to a pulse intravenous injection of d_4-choline. They were sacri-

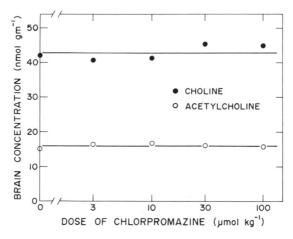

FIG. 4. Mean brain levels of choline and acetylcholine 40 to 70 min after chlorpromazine (100 μmol kg^{-1}). Each point represents the average of at least 40 mice. Values at different time intervals were not significantly different.

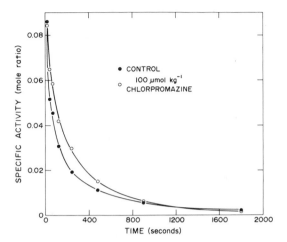

FIG. 5. Specific activity of d_4-choline in brain as a function of time after the pulse intravenous injection of d_4-choline (20 μmol kg^{-1}), in control mice and after chlorpromazine (100 μmol kg^{-1}).

ficed in subgroups of five at time intervals of 20 sec to 30 min and the brains were analyzed as described above.

Figure 4 presents the mean brain levels of choline and acetylcholine as a function of dose of chlorpromazine. There is no significant change following any dose, which is in agreement with previously reported data (17–19).

The specific activity of choline in brain following the pulse injection is unaltered after chlorpromazine initially, but declines somewhat more

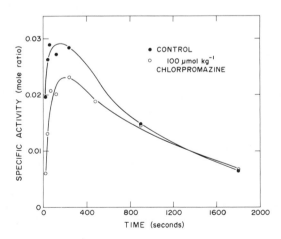

FIG. 6. Specific activity of d_4-acetylcholine in brain as a function of time after the pulse intravenous injection of d_4-choline (20 μmol kg^{-1}), in control mice and after chlorpromazine (100 μmol kg^{-1}).

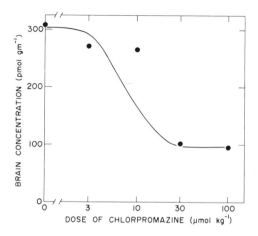

FIG. 7. Mean concentration of d_4-acetylcholine in brain 20 sec following an intravenous pulse injection of d_4-choline (20 μmol kg^{-1}) as a function of the dose of chlorpromazine given 40 min earlier.

slowly during the ensuing 10 to 15 min (Fig. 5). The specific activity of acetylcholine is depressed by chlorpromazine at the early time points following the pulse injection of choline, but is unchanged at 15 and 30 min (Fig. 6). Many agents have been found to exert significant effects only on the early part of this curve (Jenden, D. J., *unpublished observation*), and it is possible that the kinetics of the later part of it are determined by factors other than the functional activity of cholinergic neurons (16). The most pronounced effect of chlorpromazine is seen at the first time point, and Fig. 7 shows the mean concentration of d_4-acetylcholine in the brain 20 sec after the pulse intravenous injection of d_4-choline (20 μmol kg^{-1}), as a function of the dose of chlorpromazine. A highly significant effect appears at a dose between 10 and 30 μmol kg^{-1} ($\sim$3 to 10 mg kg^{-1}), i.e., well within the therapeutic dose range.

Since there is essentially no d_4-choline in the brain until after it is injected (natural abundance of deuterium would provide a mole ratio of $< 10^{-7}$), the 300 pmol gm^{-1} d_4-acetylcholine found 20 sec after the d_4-choline injection must have been synthesized in less time than this, i.e., the rate of synthesis must be at least 0.9 nmol gm^{-1} min^{-1} in animals untreated with chlorpromazine. But it is most unlikely that the choline pool from which acetylcholine is synthesized is completely replaced by the labeled choline injected; synthesis is also proceeding from unlabeled choline, for which some correction should be made. A reasonable correction has been derived, albeit with a number of assumptions that remain to be validated, which probably provides a better turnover estimate than the uncorrected figure (16).

Let x and y represent the total concentrations of choline and acetylcholine respectively, and an asterisk* be used to indicate the labeled tracer variants. Then if V_S is the total rate of synthesis of acetylcholine, and the synthesis occurs exclusively from choline, the rate of synthesis of labeled acetylcholine is $V_S x^*/x$; similarly, the rate of degradation of labeled acetylcholine is $V_D y^*/y$, where V_D is the total rate of degradation of acetylcholine. Hence the rate of accumulation of labeled acetylcholine per unit weight is given by the expression

But in a steady state, the total concentration of acetylcholine is constant, and hence $V_S = V_D \equiv V$, the turnover rate. Therefore

$$\frac{dy^*}{dt} = V\left(\frac{x^*}{x} - \frac{y^*}{y}\right). \tag{2}$$

In the experiments described, x, x^*, y, and y^* have all been measured at every time point; dy^*/dt may be estimated graphically at each time point or by fitting a semiempirical equation and differentiating (16). If dy^*/dt is plotted against $x^*/x - y^*/y$, a straight line should be obtained which passes through the origin and has a slope equal to the turnover rate. Figure 8 shows the data for control animals and the largest dose of chlorpromazine analyzed in this way. The theoretical model clearly provides a satisfactory fit for the data, and the turnover rates calculated from regression lines passing through the origin are 7.5 and 3.6 nmol gm^{-1} min^{-1}. It seems reasonable to conclude that chlorpromazine at this dose (100 μmol kg^{-1}) produces a twofold re-

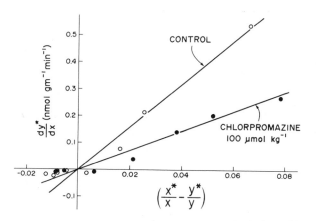

FIG. 8. Acetylcholine turnover estimation by differential method described in text [see Eq. (2)], in control mice and after chlorpromazine (100 μmol kg^{-1}).

duction in the turnover rate of acetylcholine without affecting the steady-state levels of either acetylcholine or choline.

The significance of these results in relation to the psychotropic actions of chlorpromazine will require additional work to establish. It cannot yet be stated whether the decreased turnover reflects an essential part of the mechanism by which the neuroleptic properties of the drug are exerted, a secondary response to the manifestation of these properties, or an entirely unrelated phenomenon. It is unlikely that the decreased turnover of acetylcholine is secondary to nonspecific sedative effects, since these are generally associated with a rise in acetylcholine levels (17, 20–22). Both this and earlier studies have failed to demonstrate a rise following chlorpromazine (17–19). The decreased turnover is apparently not due to a hypothermic action of chlorpromazine, since it occurs also in mice which are housed at an environmental temperature (32°C) in which no fall in body temperature occurs (Jenden, D. J., *unpublished observations*).

A possible explanation lies in the blockade of a dopaminergic system and increased turnover of striatal dopamine for which evidence has been presented (23, 24). There is substantial evidence of mutually antagonistic cholinergic and dopaminergic systems in the striatum (24, 25). Blockade of a dopaminergic pathway might therefore be expected to lead to an adaptive inhibition of the cholinergic system, and a resulting decrease in acetylcholine turnover, as a result of the operation of a negative-feedback loop. In this context it may be significant that a central cholinergic agonist, oxotremorine, profoundly decreases brain-acetylcholine turnover (15) and increases the turnover of dopamine (26).

A great deal of additional work will be required to assess the functional significance of the effects described. We believe that comparative studies on chemically and pharmacologically related compounds, measurements of turnover in individual brain regions, and identification of the subcellular basis for the changes in acetylcholine turnover are likely to help in finding a neurochemical basis for some of the actions of chlorpromazine.

ACKNOWLEDGMENTS

The author wishes to thank Margareth Roch and Ruth A. Booth for their advice and assistance. This study was supported by U.S. Public Health Service grant MH 17691.

REFERENCES

1. Costa, E., and Neff, N. H., in *Handbook of Neurochemistry*, Vol IV, Plenum Press, New York, chap. 3, pp. 45–90.
2. Jenden, D. J., in *Drugs and Cholinergic Mechanisms in the CNS* Heilbronn, E., and Winter, A., (eds.), Research Institute of National Defence, Stockholm, 1970, p. 374.

3. Hanin, I., *Handbook of Chemical Methods for the Assay of Acetylcholine and Choline*, Raven Press, New York, 1973.

4. Szilagyi, P. I. A., Schmidt, D. E., and Green, J. P., *Anal. Chem.*, **40**, 2009 (1968).

5. Schmidt, D. E., Szilagyi, P. I. A., Alkon, D. L., and Green, J. P., *Science*, **165**, 1370 (1969).

6. Schmidt, D. E., Szilagyi, P. I. A., Alkon, D. L., and Green, J. P., *J. Pharmacol.*, **174**, 337 (1970).

7. Szilagyi, P. I. A., Green, J. P., Brown, O. M., and Margolis, S., *J. Neurochem.*, **19**, 2555 (1972).

8. Jenden, D. J., Hanin, I., and Lamb, S. I., *Anal. Chem.*, **40**, 125 (1968).

9. Hanin, I., and Jenden, D. J., *Biochem. Pharmacol.*, **18**, 837 (1969).

10. Jenden, D. J., Campbell, L. B., and Roch, M., *Anal. Biochem.*, **35**, 209 (1970).

11. Jenden, D. J., Booth, R. A., and Roch, M., *Anal. Chem.*, **44**, 1879 (1972).

12. Jenden, D. J., Roch, M., and Booth, R. A., *Anal. Biochem.*, **55**, 438 (1973).

13. Jenden, D. J., Cho, A. K., and Silverman, R. W., in Proceedings of First International Symposium on Stable Isotopes in Chemistry, Biology and Medicine (Klein, P. D., ed) USAEC CONF 730525, National Technical Information Center, Argonne, Ill., May 9–11, 1973.

14. Jenden, D. J., Roch, M., and Booth, R. A., *J. Chromatogr. Sci.*, **10**, 151 (1972).

15. Schuberth, J., Sundwall, A., and Sparf, B., *J. Neurochem.*, **16**, 695 (1969).

16. Jenden, D. J., Choi, L., Silverman, R. W., Steinborn, J. A., Roch, M., and Booth, R. A., *Life Sci.*, **14**, 55 (1974).

17. Consolo, S., Ladinsky, H., Peri, G., and Garattini, S., *Eur. J. Pharmacol.*, **18**, 251 (1972).

18. Rogers, K. J., and Slater, P., *J. Pharm. Pharmacol.*, **23**, 135 (1971).

19. Van Woert, M. H., Sethy, V. H., and Ambani, L. M., in *Effects of Phenothiazine on Central Cholinergic Activity, 3rd International Symposium on Phenothiazines and Structurally Related Drugs*, N.I.M.H., Washington, D.C., June 25–28, 1973.

20. Crossland, J., and Merrick, A. J., *J. Physiol.*, **125**, 56 (1954).

21. Tobias, J. M., Lipton, M. A., and Lepinat, A. A., *Proc. Soc. Exp. Biol. Med.*, **61**, 51 (1948).

22. Richter, J. A., and Goldstein, A., *J. Pharmacol.*, **175**, 685 (1970).

23. Anden, N. E., Butcher, S. G., Corrodi, H., Fuxe, K., and Ungerstedt, V., *Europ. J. Pharmacol.*, **11**, 303 (1970).

24. Corrodi, H., Fuxe, K., and Lidbrink, P., *Brain Research*, **43**, 397 (1972).

25. Janowski, D. S., Davis, J. M., El-Yousef, M. K., and Sekerke, H. J., *Lancet*, **7778**, 632 (1972).

26. Perez-Cruet, J., Gessa, G. L., Tagliamonte, A., and Tagliamonte, P., *Fed. Proc.*, **30**, 216 (1971).

The Phenothiazines and Structurally Related Drugs, edited by I. S.
Forrest, C. J. Carr, and E. Usdin. Raven Press, New York © 1974.

Session IX: Discussion

Reporter: S. Gabay

1. M. H. Van Woert

Q. Lomax: Do you feel that the neuronal model consisting of a dopaminergic neuron inhibiting an activating cholinergic neuron is a more useful one than one in which the dopaminergic and cholinergic neurons inhibit and activate respectively a common effector neuron?

A. Both models were possible, but I thought the data we have would be more compatible with what I proposed in my report.

Q. Kaufman: There was no change in the steady-state concentration of ACh upon administration of CPZ. What were the changes in the rate of synthesis, release, and turnover of ACh?

A. We do not have the data, but I believe Dr. Jenden has some data on that.

Q. Usdin: Years ago we observed that levels of CPZ comparable to those reported by you did inhibit AcChE *in vitro*. Have others found *in vivo* the same result you did—i.e., no inhibition of AcChE by CPZ (at your levels)?

A. Nobody has reported any inhibition *in vivo*. *In vitro* levels are much higher.

2. L. W. Wattenberg

Q. Carr: Is the increased induction of aryl hydrocarbon hydroxylase enzyme a protective mechanism on the part of the animal organism? Have these studies with the phenothiazines been published? Where?

A. Yes. These studies have been documented extensively in the following papers: *J. Natl. Cancer Inst.,* **47,** 155 (1971) and *Toxicol. Appl. Pharmacol.,* **23,** 741 (1972).

Q. Gorrod: How do you quantitate this fluorescent histochemical technique and also how long does it take to "induce" in your tissue culture experiments? If, as your experiments show, you can protect turnover induction with phenothiazines, this suggests that at least two processes are induced as the former toxicity is due to methyl oxidation, and the latter to ring epoxidation. It is also worth noting that British workers at the British Industrial Biological Research Association have also been able to demonstrate another microsomal mixed function oxidase-aniline hydroxylase by histochemical techniques.

A. Tissue culture experiments were carried out primarily with lung specimens and some with liver. The histochemical technique used, although modified, has been essentially that which we described in a paper entitled "Anti-hydroxylase activity in the small intestine," published in 1961 by Wattenberg and Leong in *Cancer Research*.

F. Forrest: I was especially interested in your statement that phenothiazines increase the activity of the kidney as much as 30%. This inducing effect could be the reason for the often observed fact that CPZ drug-treated patients develop enormous thirst—drinking as much as 10 liters of water per day. Also, their weight gain may be correlated to this induction.

A. Possible!

Curry: I am most interested in these observations concerning the existence of an enzyme system capable of metabolizing CPZ in the intestinal villi. Some years ago, we reported that metabolism of CPZ during absorption, but not in the hepatic portal system, is a major factor affecting CPZ plasma levels *in vivo*, shown by differences in concentrations following injected and oral doses. There is a major difference in the degree of metabolism in different communities. For example, plasma levels *per mg of dose* are higher in the U.K. compared with those in the U.S.A. We have always suspected that this is a diet-dependent phenomenon.

3. P. Lomax

Q. Kaufman: The guinea pig ileum is used extensively in studying narcotics, especially by Kosterlitz at Aberdeen. Narcotics inhibit the release of ACh from the presynapse. What effect does CPZ have on ACh release under the same conditions?

A. CPZ blocks the receptors of ACh. As far as CPZ effect on the release of ACh is concerned, to our knowledge no experiments have been reported.

Q. Gutmann: Why would acetylcholine turnover reduction *in vivo* be compatible with the complexation of ACh with CPZ on a membrane surface? The CPZ bulk concentration would be far below the surface concentration or absorbed CPZ.

A. The data we have show a presynaptic phenothiazine blocking the release of ACh rather than the release at the postsynaptic site. Since CPZ and atropine were used, the kinetics did not show any competitive inhibition.

Davis: It is important to keep in mind that the phenothiazines have anticholinergic properties. Recently Dr. Janowski, myself, and our colleagues observed that several patients treated by a cocktail of drugs, instead of becoming better, became markedly worse on chlorpromazine, tricyclic antiparkinsonian drugs, and anticholinergic antiparkinsonian agents. They manifested florid visual hallucination, a severe deficit in immediate (30 sec) memory and disorientation. When a central cholinomimetic (physostigmine) was given, this syndrome was dramatically reversed. This evidence was interpreted to suggest that this behavioral toxicity was a central anticholinergic syndrome consequent to the combined anticholinergic properties of all the patients' drugs. Although the phenothiazine derivatives are less potent on a mg/kg basis than the atropine-like drugs in this respect, they are administered to man in substantially higher doses (e.g., 100 to 200 times for chlorpromazine).

4. M. Wollemann

Gabay: Dr. Wollemann is to be congratulated for her very elegant experiments. One wishes to see these experiments on the brain tissue rather than on rat and rabbit heart, for all the parameters studied in brain tissue will be more relevant to the antipsychotic action of CPZ. In this connection I wish to state that to my knowledge the gray matter of the CNS has the highest activities of adenyl cyclase and phosphodiesterase of any mammalian tissue studied to date (1972). This is also to some extent a function of the age of the animal. I am sure that Dr. Wollemann will agree that this kind of data is badly needed.

5. C. A. Free

Q. Lomax: It is most interesting that CPZ and ACTH appear to be competitive on the adrenal cells since CPZ inhibits endocrine function, and the fact that administration of the trophic hormone overcomes the inhibition has been taken to indicate an effect of CPZ on the hypothalamus or pituitary gland. These views need to be reconsidered in the light of the present findings. Do the *in vitro* drug levels reflect *in vivo* concentrations of CPZ?

A. Inhibition of hormonally stimulated adenylate cyclase activity in adrenal cells or hippocampal slices was generally at I_{50} concentrations in the range of 5 to 50 μM for the active phenothiazines employed in our studies. CPZ displayed some inhibition at 1 μM in the hippocampal slice and at 5 μM in the adrenal cell, concentrations that might be attained *in vivo*.

F. Forrest: I was especially interested in this antagonism of CPZ and ACTH. My clinical experience confirms this antagonism. Quite a few CPZ-treated patients developed moderate to severe leukopenia, down to a dangerous level (4,000, 3,000, 2,000 leukocytes). *I could promptly reverse this leukopenia* in all cases by injections of ACTH of 80 units at 3-day intervals. ACTH could perhaps be tried to treat other side effects.

Curry: In any comparison between concentrations occurring *in vivo* and those used *in vitro,* it is most important to consider the significance of protein binding, and this is very difficult with tissues.

A. The ability of phenothiazines to bind to tissue proteins may affect the concentrations of phenothiazines in biological fluids, *in vivo,* perhaps reducing them to levels insufficient for activity *in vitro*. On the other hand, such binding might increase the effective phenothiazine concentration in the vicinity of membrane-associated adenylate-cyclase, and indeed, may well be related to the mechanism by which phenothiazines modify the activity of membrane-associated adenylate cyclase.

Gabay: Dr. Free's data, secured from all of his studies, were subjected to an analysis employing dose-effect curves. Prior to the examination of these curves, I should like to point out that comparisons of potency of drugs of all kinds are difficult and often misleading. *In vitro* and *in vivo* potencies can be different. One point overlooked in *in vitro* work is the establishment of parallelism of the dose-effect curve. Unless a parallelism of these curves is established, it is of questionable validity to say that a certain inhibitor is several times more potent than another. Since a near parallelism was shown to exist between promethazine and CPZ, it is apparent that the phenothiazines used exhibit a common mode of action. However, I would like to point out that the system does not discriminate between promethazine (an antihistaminic agent) and CPZ (an antipsychotic agent). These two compounds, at least on the basis of dose-response curves, seem to have a similar effect on the adenyl-cyclase receptor and thus show a certain lack of specificity.

Palmer: In answer to Dr. Gabay's comment about the action of promethazine on the adenyl-cyclase receptor, we are going to present some data that this drug is as potent as CPZ in blocking the norepinephrine-induced accumulation of cyclic AMP in rat-brain slices. Perhaps the close similarity in the structure of this compound to CPZ accounts for these antiadrenergic actions.

Buckley: Your data is most interesting in light of previous data that we obtained in our stress studies. Chronic stress exposure increases corticosterone secretion threefold and theoretically CPZ should protect the experimental animals from the lethal effects of stress exposure. However, CPZ increased mortality twofold and reserpine threefold; our data suggested increased ACTH secretion leading to adrenal insufficiency with necrosis of the zona fasiculata. In light of your data perhaps we should reconsider our previous conclusion.

6. *G. C. Palmer*

Q. I. Forrest: Could the differential effects of the (OH) CPZ metabolites observed on glia and neurons have something to do with the endogenous metabolism of these structures, e.g., pentose pathway in glia and Krebs cycle in cortex, as assumed by Laborit?

A. I believe that the next step in understanding the role of cyclic AMP in the brain is studying the possible differential responses that this molecule elicits in either neurons or glia, especially with respect to metabolism of sugars.

F. Forrest: This difference of CPZ action on adenyl cyclase within cortical and subcortical neurons could possibly be explained by the difference of neuromelanin contents in cortical and subcortical (including hypothalamic) nerve cells. The strong affinity of CPZ, especially the 7, 8-dihydroxy-CPZ-metabolite to neuromelanin may decrease a metabolic activity of neuromelanin (so far not well-defined), which in turn may inhibit adenylcyclase turnover within the pigmented neurons. I suggest that the "melanostatic" activity of CPZ (well established by recent research) should be further investigated in this connection.

Turner: I've been using propranolol for the severe anxieties in deeply depressed patients, for example with tremulous or "butterfly" feelings in epigastrium. These are quite distressing. With 40-mg propranolol daily one has excellent relief which improves depression, too.

7. D. Jenden

Q. Usdin: Have you tried other phenothiazines or CPZ metabolites?

A. No, we have not tried other phenothiazines, but we have tried other drugs.

Q. Usdin: Would you care to speculate as to what you would observe with such compounds?

A. Speculation at this stage is premature — we would have to experiment to find out.

Q. Van Woert: What effect would acetylcholine release by CPZ have on your turnover data? And secondly, why is the decrease in acetylcholine turnover induced by CPZ only seen during the initial measurement and not throughout the entire curve?

A. Compounds which release ACh, in general, produce an increase because the synthesis keeps up with the release.

Q. Kaul: Dr. Jenden, thank you for a very lucid and excellent presentation. I wonder if your demethylating reagent is capable of removing methyl groups from a tertiary or quatenary nitrogen as well as it does from the quatenary carbon? If so, what is the relative ease of dealkylation among mixed alkyl functions on the nitrogen?

A. The demethylating reagent does not react with the tertiary amines.

Q. Curry: Wouldn't it be more appropriate to hypothesize that CPZ complexes with choline, thereby making it less available for acetylation?

A. Complex formation between CPZ and ACh might account for the data. I could not, at this moment, imagine a mechanism that might be responsible for this.

Q. Ahtee: Have you tried any drugs which stimulate the dopaminergic system such as apomorphine together with CPZ?

A. No.

Session X

Round Table Conference

Chairmen: Jerome Levine and Oldrich Vinař

The Phenothiazines and Structurally Related Drugs, edited by I. S. Forrest, C. J. Carr, and E. Usdin. Raven Press, New York © 1974.

Roundtable Conference on Relevance of New Basic Data to Clinical Parameters

O. Vinař

We now come to the main question of this round table: what was the impact of the new findings of chemistry and pharmacology for clinical practice in the last five years? If I had to answer this question, I would say that the psychiatrists began to think not only in terms of target symptoms when initiating a drug treatment but also in terms of how the drug is metabolized, how it interacts with other drugs given simultaneously or subsequently; they are more concerned with the proper dosage, etc. And in many instances (e.g., in maintenance treatment with long-acting injections with fluphenazine decanoate, with tricyclic antidepressants, with the exception of lithium) they become seriously interested in the blood levels of the drug. Unfortunately, they did not usually go beyond a theoretical interest: they could not begin to measure plasma levels of chlorpromazine and its metabolites.

Psychopharmacology is an interdisciplinary branch of science. A psychiatrist is confronted with this fact daily: if there is a surprising change in the clinical state of the patient, it might be due to the fact that the right metabolite of the drug he is taking was formed. But other causes could be relevant as well: he might have started to take the drug because he liked the nurse who distributed the drugs that night and stopped intake thereafter; he might get the news that his mother-in-law decided to move out of his house or that his father was dying. It is not easy to control all levels in clinical research beginning with the molecular ones and finishing with the interpersonal or social ones.

One strategy could help to solve some of the problems: to select matched pairs of patients who are comparable in all respects known to be relevant for programs from the clinical point of view, but who respond differently to the same drug in the same doses and to investigate their plasma levels, metabolic pathways, and interaction with their central neurotransmitters. This way, we might find out what really is relevant for the therapeutic response.

S. Curry

Comments: I suppose the question at issue is: "Is it or is it not a metabolite or the unchanged drug that matters in schizophrenia?" and "When we know, will it be worth measuring the appropriate compound in blood and relating therapy to it?"

The answer to the first question is still unknown but it is nearer. To the second question, the answer must be "yes," but the relationship is and will be complex, and there is a huge communication problem involved in investigating it.

John M. Davis

Comments: The dose-response relationship of amount of drug which reaches the site of action of a therapeutic effect or a given side effect of a psychotropic drug can be represented as in Fig. 1 for a typical patient. How much drug reaches these sites of action may be a function of the dose administered and such clinical pharmacologic parameters as plasma level and plasma binding. The dose administered could be thought of as the coarse adjustment and the amount of free plasma drugs as the fine adjustment of the control mechanism that determines the amount of drug which reaches these sites. One level of discourse which relates plasma level to effectiveness would involve the patient who fails to manifest clinical improvement because he had a low plasma level and too little drug reached the critical site of action. Conversely, another patient may do poorly because he may have excessively high plasma levels and suffer from excess toxicity (e.g., excess sedation). Thus there may not necessarily be a direct linear relationship between blood level and clinical efficacy. Indeed the relationship may be a U-shaped function or more precisely a bridge-shaped relationship (see Fig. 2). At the optimal plasma level, the relationship between drug level and response may be a straight line. At low or high levels it drops to zero. The reason it drops to zero (the clinical response being nil) is that behavioral toxicity supersedes the beneficial clinical effects (e.g., by excessive sedation). In other words, within the therapeutic window the patient does well. Above or below this therapeutic window the patient does poorly. The patient may do just as well just above the lower window sill as near the top of the therapeutic window. Generally, clinicians will not push the dose above the therapeutic window because the patients show overt toxicity.

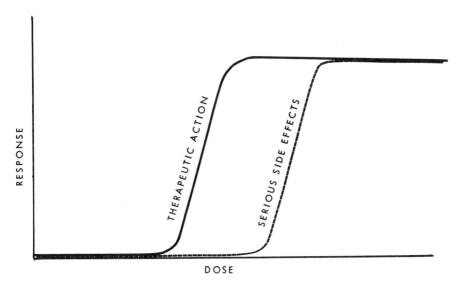

FIG. 1. Dose-response relationship.

Let us raise the question whether a given drug produces covert toxicity. For example, this might occur in the upper one-half of the therapeutic window (see Fig. 2). This would be clinically silent toxicity. If a given drug does not produce clinically silent toxicity with blood levels corresponding to the lower end of the therapeutic window, he may derive the same benefits from the drug, as if he were treated with drugs which produce higher levels. However, if he were treated with drugs producing higher blood levels which did not cause overt toxicity but cause silent toxicity, the patient may in fact pay for this later. This is not an unlikely situation in psychiatric patients exposed to long-term toxicity. Tardive dyskinesia or cardiac problems would be examples. In the first instance, tardive dyskinesia might be related to the total dose administered over the years. If a patient were administered an excess of dose over the minimum to achieve maximum improvement, he may be more likely because of the therapeutically silent toxicity to develop tardive dyskinesia. In the second example, it may be that cardiac toxicity is virtually unknown at levels close to the bottom of the therapeutic window. However, cardiac toxicity may occur in the predisposed patient near the top of the therapeutic window. Since this is a rare side effect, it may be due to silent toxicity. By assaying plasma levels for fine adjustment, one might be able to treat patients at the maximum of the dose-therapeutic response curve, before the toxicity reaches appreciable levels with respect to overt and covert manifestations.

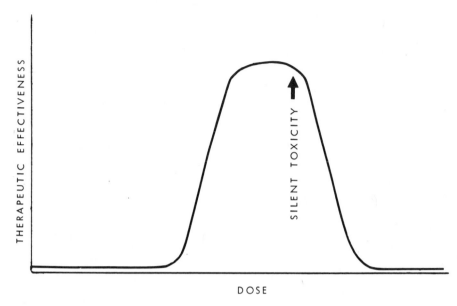

FIG. 2. Therapeutic effectiveness — therapeutic actions — side effects.

In considering the therapeutic window, it is relevant to note that in order to define how many patients need to be studied, we must know how many patients fall below or above the therapeutic window for a given drug. One cannot accurately estimate how many subjects need to be studied from the variance of two linearly related variables, since this is not relevant to a bridge-shaped curve.

C. J. Carr

Comments: Clinicians still neglect proof of who is actually taking their drug in their reports today even though we know that many do not receive their drug. There are methods to measure absorption and excretion and these are as important as the assessment of behavioral changes. We need proof of drug absorption.

There is need for collaborative studies by clinicians that also include some biochemical measures.

A group has now been formed to collaborate with each other to test reproducibility of their analytical methods and to test analytical methods between laboratories using different methods. This is one result of this meeting.

Evidence has now been brought forward by the physical chemists that shows profound changes in the geometry of the protein mosaic of cell membranes. These alone may account for changes in cell function, release of neurogenic amines, cell metabolism, and ionic exchanges of the cell.

George Simpson

Comments: I would first like to respond to Dr. Carr's comment that we should at least be able to determine that the patient got the drug. Unfortunately, to do this we take blood or urine from a patient and give it to you to get the answer. I sometimes think the pharmacologists now are where we clinicians were 12 years ago, with much promising methodology to be validated.

To return to the program, I think in agreement with Dr. Crane that CPZ might be the greatest disaster since the Plantation of Ulster. For this reason I was pleased to hear that Dr. Davis is working with butaperazine. I would add that although the method is simpler, we seem to have encountered enzyme induction and this might be a variable to look at.

Obviously, blood levels are of tremendous help to the clinician as witness lithium and even our ability to predict the therapeutic range. The least we should do is to predict toxicity.

The situation with imipramine is technically more simple and already we have learned that toxicity is related to this and that the practice of administering the total dose at bedtime will change. The problem of binding is also important and I would like to know if this may change the course of the illness. Do other drugs change this?

If we turn to the MAOI drugs, it is only in the last year that they were demonstrated to be effective in two studies using two different blood-level techniques. I am referring to the study in Vermont where they actually tested platelet MAO and dose and showed it to be active. Another recent study giving phenelzine in depression showed that if the patients were divided into slow and rapid acetylators, the latter did not show any difference from placebo, whereas the slow acetylators did.

All of this and the more precise diagnosis that already has resulted leads me to be optimistic, although I feel that the work on CPZ metabolism has probably contributed more to basic research and less to psychiatry.

George Crane

Comments: I recommend that more research be done in the area of current practices in clinical psychopharmacology. Emphasis should be placed on determining safe and effective doses of neuroleptics, particularly in long-term drug therapy.

Donald J. Jenden

Comments: The problem of correlating the total pharmacokinetics of CPZ with its clinical pharmacology and toxicology may well be outside the boundary of practical feasibility. Nevertheless, there are some approaches to it which may help to achieve a practical solution. First, it is essential to define which metabolites may contribute to the antipsychotic activity of CPZ — not just those that have some resemblance to CPZ in a behavioral screen in animals. Secondly, some metabolites of CPZ such as the sulfoxide may be converted back to the parent compound and thus serve as reservoirs. These must be documented and the conditions of reversibility defined. Finally, consideration should be given to correlating the rates of the six or so metabolic reactions with individual response or toxicity rather than the concentrations of the 200 or so possible metabolites. This could be accomplished clinically using stable-isotope-labeled compounds to measure the rates.

G. Gardos

Comments: The panelists focused on the "dose" side of the dose-response problem. The "response" side also deserves close attention. Clinical efficacy is not a unitary phenomenon and consists of a multitude of clinical actions. This is analogous to the profile of actions which the pharmacologist presents us with. Each action has its own dose-response relationship. We should put a prism to the white light of "clinical response" to examine its constituents. For example, the sedative-hypnotic effects of chlorpromazine appear quicker and at a lower dose than those associated with antipsychotic effect. Clinical dose-response studies are needed to determine these relationships for each important action for each commonly used effective antipsychotic. Clinically, this approach implies a target-symptom approach. In view of the enormous difficulties in carrying out adequate dose-response studies, collaborative efforts in this direction would be very helpful.

J. W. Gorrod

Comments: I would like to think that one of the most significant findings which should be further considered is that of Beckett and Essien [*J. Pharm. Pharmacol.*, **25**, 188 (1973)], who reported the finding of CPZ-hydroxylamines as metabolites. From our knowledge of N-hydroxylation of other "drug" molecules we know that in every case the parent drug is converted into a potent toxicant, for example, aniline yields phenylhydroxylamine, in methemoglobin formation, urethane yields N-hydroxy urethane, in carcinogenesis, and many other examples.

The hydroxylamines from chlorpromazine are lipid soluble persistent metabolites which are among the most chemically reactive compounds metabolically formed and should be considered as possible intermediates in the etiology of both the pharmacological and toxicological effects.

I would argue for the continued study of plasma levels not only of the drug, but of its metabolites: low plasma does not always mean enzyme induction. I have just learned that patients on CPZ often pass as much as 8 liters of urine daily and become fluid loaded; these are all phenomena which can produce low plasma levels.

I would like to interpolate a word of caution in the use of pure physical-chemical data for drug-metabolism studies. If one considers any molecules with a choice of oxidative site, then electron-distribution studies may give very good correlation providing that certain factors are incorporated into the calculation. However when you consider the metabolism of this same group of drugs in another species, no correlation can be observed, yet the electron-distribution remains the same.

I would also like to recommend that "classical pharmacologists" when carrying out experiments purported to elucidate the mechanisms of action of drugs *in vitro,* spend a little time putting some metabolites through the same system, rather than those structurally similar but differing in pharmacological activity. This may produce some more relevant data, particularly on small structural changes after producing remarkable changes in metabolism which are usually not produced in their systems, but may be of prime importance in drug action.

Alexander Glassman

Comments: In this symposium there has been an emphasis on the use of plasma levels to predict or explain clinical outcome. There is no question that these levels will be useful in explaining some clinical failures or preventing certain kinds of toxicity. However, it would be naive to expect all of the variability in human drug response to be on the side of the drug. In the long run it will be what drug levels do *not* explain that will be their most useful contribution. In recent years there have been many instances in which pharmacology has been used as a tool to explore both disease entities and normal biological functioning. Solomon Snyder's work using D- and L-amphetamine to explore the role of dopamine in a model psychosis is a recent example. This use of a drug is obviously limited by the degree of uncertainty as to the amount of the drug available. As in any system, it is only when you can fix one variable that you can examine others. As our technical ability improves in the measurement of blood or tissue levels, we will be better able to discriminate among these other variables.

I don't think that knowing blood levels will mean we can get a drug response from every depressive or every schizophrenic; rather, we will recognize different subtypes of these diseases. In some cases we undoubtedly will improve our therapeutic capability but more significantly the clarification of these variables in the long run will be an important source of new knowledge.

J. J. Kaufman

Comments: Perhaps one could enlarge the focus of the study of metabolites to include the question of whether it is possible to prepare substituted chlorpromazines which would not be as subject to metabolism. In particular, substitution of F in the positions which are normally hydroxylated and testing the neuroleptic effects and the length of time for which the drug is effective, could shed some light on the metabolic problem.

In the next 5 years, the use of the animal data on the rate of synthesis, release, and turnover (1) of DA in the presence of neuroleptics could indicate the neuroleptic efficacy of these drugs, (2) of NE in the presence of neuroleptics could indicate the sedative side effect of these drugs, (3) of ACh in the presence of neuroleptic drugs could indicate the possible parkinsonian effects (due to too little ACh).

It seems to be fairly general that if a drug blocks a receptor site of a normal neurotransmitter, it increases the rate of synthesis and release of the normal neurotransmitter whose receptor site is blocked, whereas if the release of a normal neurotransmitter is blocked from the presynapse, the synthesis and release of the normal neurotransmitter is decreased.

It is important for clinicians to understand the biochemical effects these drugs cause since multiple-drug therapy is used and sometimes, as Dr. Davis pointed out, it can have unfortunate effects.

In reply to Dr. Gorrod I would like to say that pure physical chemistry and theoretical chemistry do have positive contributions to make to the field of psychoactive drugs, especially when the results are viewed in the perspective of the biochemical mechanisms of drug actions. For the preliminary studies it was important to establish that quantum chemical calculations could be carried out successfully on these isolated compounds. Obviously, species difference must take into account the milieu in which the molecules react—and this is a further step which must be taken. However, the book edited by D. Efron in 1967 mentioned that there had been 10,000 papers written on CPZ from 1954 to 1967 and there have been several more thousand papers written since. We have had the opportunity to initiate our theoretical studies recently, and it would be appropriate to give physical and theoretical chemical studies a fair chance.

P. Lomax

Comments: Several speakers have raised the point that qualitative and quantitative assays are needed. Immunoassay methods for a number of drugs are now available (digoxin, opium alkaloids, THC and its metabolites, etc.). These are available because there has been sufficient demand, for a variety of reasons, to render the commercial development of these assays viable. The phenothiazines and their metabolites are not technically difficult molecules for the development of highly specific immunoassays. If these assays are needed, it is up to the scientific community to advertise such a demand so that the kits will be produced and the clinical laboratories will institute the tests.

S. Curry

Comments (reply to Lomax): Our experience with plasma chlorpromazine measurements is as follows:

(1) Regardless of whether the activity is mediated by a metabolite, a measurement can be of value in special cases, such as: (a) nonresponse to

CPZ caused by zero plasma levels (try another drug), (b) poor response to CPZ caused by levels over 300 ng/ml (reduce dose).

(2) Screening of whole hospital populations is inappropriate.

(3) There is a need for specialist collaboration between an *interested* psychiatrist and an *interested* pharmacologist. We are not yet ready to recommend to psychiatrists and pharmacologists to make measurements on an ad hoc basis.

I firmly believe that we need an improvement in methods of psychopharmacological evaluation before we can make specific recommendations for achievement of a concentration within a review range. This is the exact opposite of an earlier comment that the pharmacologists are 10 years behind the psychiatrists, in regard to methods. The pharmacologists are 10 years ahead.

Leonor Rivera-Calimlim

Comments: As a clinical pharmacologist, I can't get away from terms like "controlled study" and "double-blind clinical investigation." I have a strong belief that a well-designed clinical investigation on plasma levels of drug and clinical response must take the following important factors into consideration: (1) a reliable, accurate method of determination of plasma level of chlorpromazine; (2) a reliable and conscientious psychiatrist to work hand in hand with the pharmacologist.

We conducted a preliminary study in the correlation of plasma levels of chlorpromazine and clinical response in psychiatric patients in a double-blind fashion. Data showed that patients who did not improve clinically (assessed by Brief Psychiatric Rating Score) showed very low plasma levels (less than 30 ng/ml). Those who showed some improvements showed plasma levels ranging from 150 to 300 ng/ml.

We looked into the patients who had very low plasma levels and one common factor noted was the presence of trihexyphenidyl (Artane®). We conducted an intrapatient investigation of the effect of Artane on CPZ levels. One group of patients received Artane plus CPZ on the 1st to 3rd week, discontinuing Artane after the 3rd week. Another group of patients was started on CPZ alone during the 1st and 2nd week and during the 3rd week Artane was added up to the 6th week. Plasma levels were assayed at 0, 2, 3, and 4 hr after medication once a week. The investigation was again carried out by a double-blind technique. Assay of plasma CPZ was done by gas chromatography with an electron-capture detector. Results suggested that trihexyphenidyl diminished plasma levels of CPZ. I am quite optimistic on the future meaningful collaboration between pharmacologists and clinicians and I see a glimpse of hope in the realization of the goal of this meeting, that is, to apply the vast information of basic and clinical studies to the solution of problems in the therapy of psychiatric patients.

Another important point for consideration is to stratify the items of the global crude clinical scoring assessment and determine which of the groups of symptoms, i.e., thinking disorders, paranoid delusions, depression, withdrawal, and retardation, are more responsive to chlorpromazine. With our own few patients, the data suggested that thinking disorders and paranoid delusions are more sensitive to chlorpromazine than depression, withdrawal, and retardation.

W. J. Turner

Comments: We should address ourselves to a question of Dr. Levine's, namely, what do we wish to happen and what may we hope to bring about?

We are here because CPZ has a beneficial effect in schizophrenia. Schizophrenics have a wholly different way of being than the healthy minded. No matter how bizarre or weird the delusions or hallucinations, each has a real personal history. It is not the content which is to be treated by CPZ; it is the way of thinking and feeling about that history.

In treating schizophrenia we deal with a mixed bag. It is to be hoped and possibly expected that the geneticists and enzymologists will help us in the next 5 yr to know *who* is being treated, and what biological systems are involved. CPZ then may help us to treat more specifically "the proper schizophrenia." This may well leave the patient still in trouble, because he has years of unrewarding and damaging experiences. Yet at that point social or psychiatric therapy may enable the patient to live as a whole human being.

James M. Perel

Comments: Two points were made:

(1) I dispute the use of purely clinical drug studies in psychiatry without pharmacodynamic considerations. They will lead to nothing but more of the confusion reigning today. On the other hand, the utilization of pharmacological animal studies with dosages such as 90 mg/kg of phenobarbital for enzyme induction is erroneous and irrelevant with regard to clinical

applications. The solution is a closer collaboration between the psychiatrist and the clinical pharmacologist, without intermediate disciplines.

(2) In confirmation of the data on the interaction of chlorpromazine and Artane® in man, we found that a patient taking a huge dose of imipramine (estimated 5.0 g) together with an unspecified amount of Artane®, survived an otherwise lethal dose. The blood level of antidepressant did not exceed 600 ng/ml. This is because the anticholinergic effects of Artane® prevented most of the gastrointestinal absorption of imipramine. This work was done in collaboration with Dr. Nathan Carliner, Emory University School of Medicine, Atlanta, Georgia.

F. M. Forrest

Comments: Some new biological parameters should be introduced into this field of research, especially the effect of CPZ on tissue cultures of glia. CPZ might have a regenerating effect on the pentose metabolism of *glia* which in turn reactivates neurons, dormant in the CNS, for example, in catatonia. Glia cells should be investigated with regard to their capacity to grow, nourish neurons, and activate the growth of dendrites and axon cylinders in formerly "hibernating" cortical nerve centers.

Also, the hidden function of neuromelanin and its relationship to phenothiazines should be more intensively investigated. This could elucidate many so far little-understood cell functions and their behavioral consequences.

J. P. Buckley

Comments: The correlation of blood levels of CPZ with therapeutic efficacy is extremely complex. One question that can be asked is: "Is CPZ the molecule that should be monitored or should it be one of the metabolites?" The time course is also of utmost importance.

Dr. Piette presented a paper on the incubation of RBC's with phenothiazines and demonstrated marked activity. We have repeated these experiments and find that CPZ, 7-OH-CPZ and imipramine can be incubated with RBC's, reinjected into the animal and produce marked pharmacological effects. On the other hand, 7,8-$(OH)_2$-CPZ was not effective. Therefore, another question is: "How much of CPZ and its active metabolites carried by RBC's would *not* be reflected in serum levels?"

Irene Forrest

Comments: For doing pharmacokinetic studies of individual CPZ metabolites, as was suggested, you had to have a qualitative and quantitative idea on what these were.

Blood-level methods for CPZ are very new and are only beginning to be reliable. Accumulation of a significant body of data for a representative number of patients of various diagnostic categories is needed before clinical correlations can be made with some degree of confidence.

The *Phenothiazines and Structurally Related Drugs,* edited by I. S.
Forrest, C. J. Carr, and E. Usdin. Raven Press, New York © 1974.

Summary

Frederick K. Goodwin

Section on Psychiatry, National Institute of Mental Health, Bethesda, Maryland 20014

I would like to preface my summary of this rich and varied series of papers
with some overall impressions that were brought into focus during the
stimulating panel discussions. First is the enormous complexity and individual variability in dealing with the problem of the mechanism of action of
the phenothiazine drugs in schizophrenia. Second is the marked *intrade-
pendence* between the various areas of work in this field which may be illustrated with an example: if one is to evaluate meaningfully the efficacy of a
phenothiazine neuroleptic, one cannot ignore knowledge concerning its
metabolism and distribution, since in order to decide that a patient is a treatment failure, one must be sure that this particular patient has a sufficient
blood level of the drug or its active metabolites to qualify as a "therapeutic
level." On the other hand, with regard to the mechanism of action of
phenothiazines, one must attend to the data concerning clinical efficacy in
order to identify which of the multiple biological actions are meaningful in
terms of correlating with clinical effectiveness. A final overall impression
relates to the increasing convergence of the data around several critical
hypotheses—a convergence which has not heretofore been characteristic of
research in this most difficult area. This convergence point focuses on those
central neuronal systems which involve the amine neurotransmitters, particularly the catecholamines dopamine and norepinephrine.

In undertaking a summary, one is challenged by the wide variety of inter-
locking subjects presented in this volume. Although many chapters overlap,
there are basically five broad areas of focus:

(1) the biological effects of the phenothiazines and related drugs on
various *in vitro* and *in vivo* systems;

(2) the methods for the measurement of these drugs and their metabolites
in tissues and body fluids;

(3) the metabolism of these drugs in animal systems and in man, including a consideration of those metabolites with biological activity and/or
clinical effects;

(4) studies in man of uptake, distribution, and elimination of these drugs,
including studies of blood levels, half life, and binding to plasma and
tissue constituents;

(5) the clinical efficacy and side effects of the neuroleptic drugs, including the question of predictor variables.

Now, a few of the individual highlights of the meeting. Dr. Carr set the stage for the entire meeting when he pointed out that, even today in the 20th year since the discovery of the phenothiazines, the fate of chlorpromazine in the body is still an open question.

(1) Appropriately, the volume begins with papers focused on the molecular level; Dr. Fenner reports that very small structural changes in the tricyclic phenothiazine molecule can result in very large steric conformational changes, and points out the biological significance in these steric changes, particularly in regard to drug-membrane interactions. In a series of papers relating to the correlation between physicochemical properties of these drugs and their biological activity, there are discussions of charge transfer interactions, quantum chemical calculations, X-ray crystallography, and spectroscopic characteristics of the phenothiazine drugs. Each of these approaches reveals some correlation between chemical properties and biological activity, but no clear pattern emerges.

In other sections on the mode of action of the phenothiazine drugs, evidence concerning the direct effect of chlorpromazine on biological membranes is reviewed, particularly the effects on membrane proteins and the mechanism by which chlorpromazine might produce membrane swelling. The possible involvement of calcium in this process is of special interest since it is critically involved in the mechanism of release of neurotransmitters at the synaptic membrane.

The work on the effects of phenothiazine derivatives on the uptake of monoamines by blood platelets is of considerable interest, since the blood platelet can be shown to be a reasonable model in many respects for the central aminergic nerve ending. Considerable work with the blood platelet system is being done in the field of manic-depressive illness; it has been found that the major psychoactive drugs, which are thought to exert some of their effects on transport of biogenic amines at the nerve ending membrane, can be shown to have the expected effect on the platelet when used in standard doses in patients.

In a section dealing with specific metabolites and studies of the mechanism of action, data are presented concerning the effects of chlorpromazine and its metabolites on tyrosinase, on metal chelation, and on ATPase. Since all of these biochemical processes are involved in neurotransmitter function, they are of particular interest.

In Session VIII, recent clinical data are reported on Clozapine, a drug of considerable theoretical importance since it is an effective antipsychotic and yet has little or no extrapyramidal side effects in doses with clear antipsychotic effect. The animal data reviewed indicate this drug has an effect on both dopamine and norepinephrine neurons. Some of the most important current questions concerning the role of dopamine in the mechanism of action of phenothiazines are clarified. Noteworthy is the recent debate concerning the proper interpretation of the amphetamine psychosis model for schizophrenia as it regards dopamine involvement. The earlier formulation of Snyder and his co-workers suggesting that the ratio of effects of the D and L isomers of amphetamine indicated that the amphetamine psychosis was produced by alterations in dopamine metabolism, has now been called into some question. In addition, the recent provocative data of Stein and Weiss indicating a 50% reduction in the activity of dopamine-beta-hydroxylase in brains from chronic schizophrenics compared to controls (*Science, 181,* 344, 1973) is of particular interest in light of the bits of evidence suggesting some disturbance in the ratio of dopaminergic to noradrenergic function in schizophrenia.

Of further relevance to the question of the mechanism of action of these drugs are a group of papers dealing with the interrelationship between dopaminergic and cholinergic systems, an interrelationship which has also been demonstrated at the clinical level in both schizophrenia and affective disorders. The paper on the very elegant technique for measuring turnover of acetylcholine in the central nervous system is especially encouraging since it is applicable to man. This is made possible by the use of deuterium labeling with subsequent quantification of the label by mass spectroscopy; since deuterium is a stable, nonradioactive isotope, very large amounts of label can safely be given to man. These techniques, using nonradioactive isotopes as tracers, are now being applied in other laboratories to the study of catecholamine turnover and function and to the mechanism of action of a variety of drugs.

The papers concerning cyclic AMP suggest that some final common pathway probably mediates the effects of a variety of neurotransmitters, and that this final common pathway might be an important focus for the effects of phenothiazines. These studies have assumed a new clinical relevance since cyclic AMP can now be measured in cerebrospinal fluid and can be shown to accumulate following probenecid, suggesting perhaps a methodology for indirectly assessing cyclic AMP turnover in the central nervous system of patients.

(2) A number of papers in several sessions deal specifically with the critical area of assay procedures for the phenothiazines and their metabolites. The two basic problems of separation versus detection are brought into focus. It cannot be overemphasized that the solvent extraction steps that are a prerequisite for further purification and final detection are often the "Achilles heel" of an otherwise elegant method: unless prior separation has been quantitative, the detection method remains limited in its interpretability.

Many of the problems inherent in chromatographic methodologies are discussed. For example, small variations in the thickness of thin-layer plates can cause considerable variation in results, whereas the elegant gas chromatographic methods for the measurement of chlorpromazine in plasma do not suffer from these problems. However, in this field one is faced with the question of how heavily the results might depend on the skill of an individual investigator in the application of gas chromatographic methods — particularly those requiring the use of the electron-capture detector. Clearly, in some skillful hands the methods are quite reproducible, but the question of reproducibility in more routine clinical settings still remains. The chapters reporting progress in the development of a radioimmunoassay for chlorpromazine perhaps point the way to a new era in the detection of these compounds in which methods can be set up that are simple, reproducible, and sensitive. If these immunoassay procedures can be made more specific, they will certainly represent a major breakthrough in this field, particularly since they are less dependent upon the skill of the individual doing the assay.

There are several papers concerned with measurements of very small amounts of phenothiazines and their metabolites using mass spectroscopy and mass fragmentography. These techniques which can provide absolute detection and quantification of very small amounts of drugs should prove particularly useful in research settings and should, in the next few years, add substantially to our understanding in these areas.

(3) A number of chapters report the problems of the metabolism of phenothiazines and related drugs in animals and in man. Of special interest is the consensus concerning the existence of several metabolites which possess considerable biological activity — particularly the 7-hydroxy metabolite of chlorpromazine.

(4) The chapters in this session which stimulated perhaps the most debate are those dealing with the distribution, binding, and elimination of phenothiazines in man. The chapter on red cell binding of chlorpromazine presents a system that might provide for the study of actual tissue binding of these compounds in patients. The relative importance of tissue binding versus the binding of these drugs by plasma proteins is extensively discussed. The possibility that binding by the red cell might be more analogous to tissue binding at the site of action deserves consideration. In addition, it is pointed out that in the case of a drug with rapid uptake and binding in the tissues, and with a very high volume of distribution, questions can be raised concerning the meaningfulness of data on percentages of free versus plasma-protein-bound drug as measured in patients. The studies of tissue accumulation of phenothiazines are also relevant to this point. It is also reported that brain tissue itself can carry out many of the metabolic reactions of phenothiazines, which in a sense further increases the complexity of the problem facing the clinician attempting to interpret blood level data. Another aspect of the problem is highlighted in the paper dealing with the metabolism of imipramine by the liver and the effects of the interactions of other drugs on this metabolism. From a clinical point of view, this is a phenomenon often overlooked at our peril since a large percentage of patients in any clinical popu-

lation may also be taking, from time to time, other drugs. To the extent that these drugs alter the metabolism of phenothiazines and antidepressants, they can present problems in interpretation of clinical-pharmacological data. In a study of blood levels of butaperazine, the investigators were able to predict the steady-state drug level from the decay curve after a single dose. This experiment is closely related to the data presented by others indicating the usefulness of pharmacokinetic calculations for prediction of ultimate steady-state blood levels of tricyclic antidepressants. Problems in interpreting single-dose kinetic studies are caused by the multiple phases of disappearance and by the difficulty in determining the half-life given a multiphase disappearance curve. In a review of the attempts that have been made in recent years to correlate plasma levels of tricyclic antidepressants with clinical response, it was pointed out that there is still considerable variability in the results of different studies in this area. Of particular importance in the view of some investigators is the issue of binding to plasma proteins, since it is felt that the physiologically active drug resides in the unbound portion. Thus small changes in the percentage bound would make large changes in the absolute amount of drug which is unbound, since more than 90% of the drug can be bound to plasma protein.

(5) During the sessions dealing with clinical effects there was an interesting debate concerning the issue of target symptoms and whether or not specific drugs could correlate with specific target symptoms in schizophrenia. Some felt that nothing significantly useful had come of this research, except for the overall statement that certain drugs were better in hypoactive, whereas others were better in hyperactive schizophrenics. In contrast, there was a report from a related approach to specificity, namely, a study in which a number of significant correlations between animal behavioral paradigms and clinical efficacy were found. It was acknowledged that no one-to-one correlations exist between clinical efficacy and animal behavioral effects, but that in fact one might increase the odds of picking the right drug by attending to such data. One thing of particular interest in this study is that the symptomatology best correlated with the largest number of animal behavioral tests was that of "change in affect." This is of interest in relation to the question of overlap between the central core pathology of schizophrenia and that of the affective disorders.

Naturally, in a field as rich and varied as this, there is never enough time to fully develop every area within a single volume. One area that we all would have liked more time to discuss is the issue of the animal or human (drug) models of schizophrenia and what these various models may tell us about the mechanism of action of the phenothiazine drugs. Of particular importance is the question concerning the relevance of the chronic amphetamine psychosis model as opposed to the LSD hallucination model. There is also the more recent and intriguing 6-hydroxydopamine model of schizophrenia presented by Stein and Wise. The possible relationship between schizophrenia and affective illness in terms of symptomatology, drug effects, or neurobiological substrates is also of increasing importance in light of recent data on genetic overlap. This problem becomes all the more compelling given the convergence of data from both these major groups of psychoses on the central neurotransmitter amines.

Finally, there is the question that was implicit in many of the presentations during this symposium: Just what is it the phenothiazine drugs *do* in schizophrenia? Should they be considered curative or only palliative drugs? Is there a prevailing consensus among clinicians in this field on this question? It is, of course, an enormously important question both practically and theoretically. Are these drugs really reversing the schizophrenia syndrome, or are they merely blunting or diminishing some of the symptoms? I do not ask this as a rhetorical question, but rather because I really do not, myself, have the answer.

Finally, a few overall observations. It seems that we are at a threshold where a large amount of animal and basic biochemical data has been collected but that as yet we lack the critical understanding to provide unifying hypotheses to which these data can be linked and through which these data can be more fully understood and interpreted. In this regard, I suggest that it is time to direct more attention toward the development of techniques for the direct study of the effects of these drugs on various biochemical systems in the central nervous system of *man,* particularly because we are dealing with systems which are known to have wide species variation. I think it will be important to pay attention to the problems of differentiating state-dependent from state-independent variables in human studies. Further, I would remind us all that schizophrenia is, of course, known to involve some genetically determined predisposition, or vulnerability, at least in the majority of cases. What then are the biological correlates of this predisposition to schizophrenia? Are we, perhaps, misleading ourselves by studying people only once they are schizophrenic, that is, once they already have the various symptoms making up this complex syndrome. Perhaps we should develop experimental models that would allow us to test, in schizophrenia-prone individuals, the possibility that there are abnormal neurochemical responses to environmental stress.

One gets the overall impression that the wealth of data in the various fields exemplified in this symposium is in need of synthesis. It is apparent that the tendency for cross-fertilization expressed in individual careers is increasing, although much more remains to be accomplished in this direction.

SUBJECT INDEX

SUBJECT INDEX

A

Acanthosis nigricans, nicotinic acid and, 295-299

Aceperone, spectra of, 77-95

Acetophazine, albumin binding, 175-188

Acetophenazine in schizophrenia, 667-672

Acetylcholine
  chlorpromazine interaction, 16-22, 26, 27, 28, 769-776
  drug effect on, in brain, 707-714, 727
  in temperature regulation, 719-728
  turnover, *in vivo*, 769-776

Acid phosphatase, chlorpromazine and, 229-242

ACTH, drug effect on, 739-747

Adenyl cyclase activity, 731-766

Agranulocytosis, fluphenazine and, 307

Akathisia
  evolutionary origin, 255-267
  fluphenazine and, 301-309
  sex differences, 249-253

Albumin, drug binding to, 165, 175-188

Alcohol withdrawal, 685-690

Aldrin, chlorpromazine metabolism, 197, 198

Alimemazine, structure-activity, 6-9

Amino acid oxidase, activation, 547-559

Aminoglutethimide, 739-747

Amitryptiline
  monoamine in blood, effect on, 379-388
  norepinephrine, effect on, 479

steroidogenesis inhibition, 739-747

structure, 10

cAMP, drug effect on, 731-766

Amphetamine, blocking of effect, 474

Antibodies, development of, 363-376

Antiemetic effect, 475

Apomorphine, dopamine metabolism and, 475

Arginine, chlorpromazine and, 237

Artifacts in chlorpromazine oxidation, 315-322

Aryl hydrocarbon hydroxylase, 717

ATP
  chlorpromazine and membrane stability, 239
  oxygen uptake in brain, 609-615

ATPase $(Na^+ + K^+)$ inhibition, 633-639

Atropine, effect on monoamines, 379-388

Autoradiography, chlorpromazine, 413-423

Azobenzene, effect on chlorpromazine, 198

B

Behavior
  avoidance, rat, 473, 597, 617-630
  chlorpromazine derivatives and, 617-630
  imipramine effect in children, 425-430
  open field, rat, 597
  thiothixene in children, 519-533

Benperidol, spectra of, 77-95

Benzquinamide in schizophrenia, 667-672